Impacts of Information Technology on Patient Care and Empowerment

Roger W. McHaney
Kansas State University, USA

Iris Reychev
Ariel University, Israel

Joseph Azuri
Maccabi Healthcare Services, Israel

Mark E. McHaney
U.S. Air Force, USA

Rami Moshonov
Assuta Medical Centers, Israel

A volume in the Advances in Medical Technologies and Clinical Practice (AMTCP) Book Series

IGI Global
DISSEMINATOR OF KNOWLEDGE

Published in the United States of America by
IGI Global
Medical Information Science Reference (an imprint of IGI Global)
701 E. Chocolate Avenue
Hershey PA, USA 17033
Tel: 717-533-8845
Fax: 717-533-8661
E-mail: cust@igi-global.com
Web site: http://www.igi-global.com

Library of Congress Cataloging-in-Publication Data

Names: McHaney, Roger, editor. | Reychav, Iris, 1969- editor. | Azuri, Joseph, 1972- editor. | McHaney, Mark E., editor. | Moshonov, Rami, editor.
Title: Impacts of information technology on patient care and empowerment / Roger W. McHaney, Iris Reychav, Joseph Azuri, Mark E. McHaney, and Rami Moshonov, editors.
Description: Hershey, PA : Medical Information Science Reference (an imprint of IGI Global), [2020] | Includes bibliographical references.
Identifiers: LCCN 2019015419| ISBN 9781799800477 (hardcover) | ISBN 9781799800484 (ebook)
Subjects: | MESH: Medical Informatics--trends | Patient Care Management | Patient Participation | Telemedicine
Classification: LCC R855.3 | NLM W 26.5 | DDC 610.285--dc23 LC record available at https://lccn.loc.gov/2019015419

This book is published in the IGI Global book series Advances in Medical Technologies and Clinical Practice (AMTCP) (ISSN: 2327-9354; eISSN: 2327-9370)

British Cataloguing in Publication Data
A Cataloguing in Publication record for this book is available from the British Library.

All work contributed to this book is new, previously-unpublished material. The views expressed in this book are those of the authors, but not necessarily of the publisher.

For electronic access to this publication, please contact: eresources@igi-global.com.

Advances in Medical Technologies and Clinical Practice (AMTCP) Book Series

Srikanta Patnaik
SOA University, India
Priti Das
S.C.B. Medical College, India

ISSN:2327-9354
EISSN:2327-9370

Mission

Medical technological innovation continues to provide avenues of research for faster and safer diagnosis and treatments for patients. Practitioners must stay up to date with these latest advancements to provide the best care for nursing and clinical practices.

The **Advances in Medical Technologies and Clinical Practice (AMTCP) Book Series** brings together the most recent research on the latest technology used in areas of nursing informatics, clinical technology, biomedicine, diagnostic technologies, and more. Researchers, students, and practitioners in this field will benefit from this fundamental coverage on the use of technology in clinical practices.

Coverage

- Neural Engineering
- Nursing Informatics
- Clinical Nutrition
- Diagnostic Technologies
- Medical Imaging
- Biomechanics
- Biomedical Applications
- E-Health
- Clinical High-Performance Computing
- Patient-Centered Care

IGI Global is currently accepting manuscripts for publication within this series. To submit a proposal for a volume in this series, please contact our Acquisition Editors at Acquisitions@igi-global.com or visit: http://www.igi-global.com/publish/.

The Advances in Medical Technologies and Clinical Practice (AMTCP) Book Series (ISSN 2327-9354) is published by IGI Global, 701 E. Chocolate Avenue, Hershey, PA 17033-1240, USA, www.igi-global.com. This series is composed of titles available for purchase individually; each title is edited to be contextually exclusive from any other title within the series. For pricing and ordering information please visit http://www.igi-global.com/book-series/advances-medical-technologies-clinical-practice/73682. Postmaster: Send all address changes to above address.

Titles in this Series

For a list of additional titles in this series, please visit:
https://www.igi-global.com/book-series/advances-medical-technologies-clinical-practice/73682

Early Detection of Neurological Disorders Using Machine Learning Systems
Sudip Paul (North-Eastern Hill University Shillong, India) Pallab Bhattacharya (National Institute of Pharmaceutical Education and Research (NIPER) Ahmedabad, India) and Arindam Bit (National Institute of Technology Raipur, India)
Medical Information Science Reference • copyright 2019 • 376pp • H/C (ISBN: 9781522585671) • US $265.00 (our price)

Incivility Among Nursing Professionals in Clinical and Academic Environments Emerging Research and Opportunities
Cheryl Green (Southern Connecticut State University, USA)
Medical Information Science Reference • copyright 2019 • 181pp • H/C (ISBN: 9781522573418) • US $195.00 (our price)

Computational Methods and Algorithms for Medicine and Optimized Clinical Practice
Kwok Tai Chui (City University of Hong Kong, Hong Kong) and Miltiadis D. Lytras (Effat University, Saudi Arabia)
Medical Information Science Reference • copyright 2019 • 290pp • H/C (ISBN: 9781522582441) • US $245.00 (our price)

Advanced Classification Techniques for Healthcare Analysis
Chinmay Chakraborty (Birla Institute of Technology Mesra, India)
Medical Information Science Reference • copyright 2019 • 424pp • H/C (ISBN: 9781522577966) • US $285.00 (our price)

Tele-Audiology and the Optimization of Hearing Healthcare Delivery
Elaine Saunders (Blamey Saunders Hears, Australia)
Medical Information Science Reference • copyright 2019 • 274pp • H/C (ISBN: 9781522581918) • US $225.00 (our price)

Design and Implementation of Healthcare Biometric Systems
Dakshina Ranjan Kisku (National Institute of Technology Durgapur, India) Phalguni Gupta (National Institute of Technical Teachers Training and Research, India) and Jamuna Kanta Sing (Jadavpur University, India)
Medical Information Science Reference • copyright 2019 • 300pp • H/C (ISBN: 9781522575252) • US $265.00 (our price)

IGI Global
DISSEMINATOR OF KNOWLEDGE

701 East Chocolate Avenue, Hershey, PA 17033, USA
Tel: 717-533-8845 x100 • Fax: 717-533-8661
E-Mail: cust@igi-global.com • www.igi-global.com

Table of Contents

Detailed Table of Contents

With the spread of telecommunications infrastructure, telemedicine has attracted attention from both healthcare and IT industries. Telemedicine has shown a potential to improve health maintenance, enhancement, as well as healthcare cost reduction. Many governments are boosting telemedicine applications through regulations. The purpose of this chapter is to review the major telemedicine technologies—telemedicine, wearable devices, and emerging innovative health equipment—and current issues of the impact on the patient care in the healthcare industry, the business opportunities, and threats from telemedicine.

The exponential development of Information Technologies revolutionized healthcare. A significant aspect of this revolution is the access to health information in the Internet. The Internet World Stats estimates that 56.8% of the world population used the Internet in March 2019, an increase of 1,066% from 2000. According to The Pew Research Center survey of 2012 81% of Americans used the internet and 72% of them searched for health information. Even though there is a lack in more recent data on the percentage of online health information seekers, it is clear that this trend is on the rise. This chapter focuses on the characteristics of the search for online health information by patients and providers, investigates features related to the quality of health web sites, and discusses the impact of these searches on healthcare.

EHRs, IRIS registry, and MIPS. Recognizing patterns would aid in predicting preventative measures for an increased holistic and personalized patient care. Although big data proves to have endless beneficial applications, it can bring into question the ownership of this information. Additionally, big data poses a risk for security breaches, and thus, precautionary measures will also be discussed. Ultimately, the emergence of big data creates an exhilarating frontier for healthcare with its unlimited possibilities.

This chapter explores gamification and its potential to address leading health and healthcare issues, to promote healthy behaviors and empower patients to take charge of their own health. It discusses some of the key advantages of gamification over past iterations of technology-based behavioral health interventions, including personal informatics and serious games. The advantages discussed in this chapter include: 1) a greater emphasis on the promotion of intrinsic motivation through quality, intentional game design; 2) broader accessibility to patients through mobile technology and advancing sensor systems; and 3) broader applicability to tackle a variety of health challenges. This chapter is useful for those hoping to gain a deeper understanding of the promise that drives the excitement in gamification as a method for addressing the health challenges of the modern world, as well as the work that is still required to fulfill that promise.

No-shows are patients who miss scheduled Specialist Outpatient Clinic (SOC) appointments. No-shows can impact patients' access to care and appointment lead time. This chapter describes a data-driven strategy of improving access to specialist care through first developing a stratified predictive scoring model to identify patients at risk of no-shows; second, studying the impact of a dynamic overbooking strategy that incorporates the use of the no-show prediction model using discrete event simulation (DES) on lead time. Seventeen variables related to new SOC appointments for subsidized patients in 2016 were analyzed. Multiple logistic regression (MLR) found eight variables independently associated with no-shows with area under receiver operation curve (AUC) 70%. The model was tested and validated. DES model simulated the appointment overbooking strategy as applied to the top highest volume specialties and concluded that lead time of Specialty 1 and 2 can be shortened by 27.5 days (49% improvement) and 21.3 (33%) respectively.

The current study analyzes the information collected and the lessons learned during the first six months of the CONNECARE project in Israel, in order to assess the use of the mobile technology by patients, their motivations and obstacles; as well as their satisfaction. As of the middle of February 2019, 59 patients were recruited and 18 discharged from the project and completed the feedback questionnaires. Based on preliminary data presented in this chapter, as measured against the McGaughey et al. Research Framework, it can be concluded that the usage of the CONNECARE mobile platform can be rated as moderate. The analysis together with insights from the literature, suggest that usage of the CONNECARE app could be improved by introducing additional features that would increase patients' motivation to use the system as well as its full integration into usual healthcare processes.

The World Health Organization lauds mobile health (mHealth) technology as a means of creating stronger healthcare systems and improving health-related outcomes. This chapter reports on an action research study examining the development of a mHealth technology hypertension app to help people living in India's urban slums and rural villages take better care of their health. The collaboration involved a multidisciplinary team of U.S.-based academic researchers, and India-based healthcare and technology professionals. This study suggests that traditional Western-based project management approaches alone are insufficient when developing technology for social good. Specifically, the study finds that team, process, and technology adaptability are key to successfully developing healthcare technology to serve at-risk populations in resource-constrained areas. Implications of these findings to systems development research are discussed.

Encouraging patients to play a more active role in their health care is crucial for healthcare planning and for the design of services. This chapter shifts the scholarly focus from practitioners' decision making to that of laypersons' trying to make sense of the lab results available on their EPRs. The authors developed a methodology to capture the relationship between information formats (graph, numeric, or verbal), laypersons' assessment of the conditions' gravity, and their preferred course of action. Focusing on the effect of "not knowing" on laypersons' preferred courses of action, our findings show that formats that left respondents less able to understand the results—namely, the numeric and verbal formats—produced a lower sense of urgency, and correspondingly, less inclination to actively seek professional help. The chapter takes a step toward deriving practical recommendations as to how personal clinical information should be communicated, to improve laypersons' interpretation of the information's significance.

Advances in information technology, be it by way of social media or use of the electronic medical information systems, has changed the way we deal with patient confidential information. The hitherto clear professional relationship with the patient has been blurred using social media, just like the unprecedented rate at which electronic health information is used to access and share patient's confidential information among healthcare professionals. However, given the special professional relationship of confidence which traditionally bonds the healthcare practitioner with the patient, use of these technologies by the healthcare professionals portends the risk of breach of that duty of confidentiality. Although the patient's right to demand confidentiality of his information is not absolute, an unlawful breach could result in a crime, actionable tort, or become a subject of disciplinary action. This chapter undertakes a general review of the benefits and dangers of embracing these new information technologies and their impact on the confidentiality of sensitive health data.

Preface

INTRODUCTION

Modern technologies impact the way health care providers and patients interact in dramatic ways. The Internet and World Wide Web provide varying levels of accessible information that enable patient self-diagnosis---whether correct or incorrect. Social media permits patients to discuss their providers, health care facilities, and their experiences in a variety of positive and negative ways. Mobile devices, wearable technologies, gamification, and the Internet of Things (IOT) offer unprecedented mechanisms for patients to monitor their own vital signs, habits, and actions; and pass these to their health care providers. Big data offer insights and better understanding of both micro and macro level health concerns but create situations where confidential data could be at risk. Simulation techniques allow health and IT researchers to glimpse the future through evaluating different scenarios with varying probabilities of occurrence. Educational materials are widely available and communication links to expert and non-expert advisors have emerged. Changes occurring at the personal technology level alter the way patients view their health care experiences. New technologies empower and frustrate; and, educate and confuse the modern patient. The gap between what is possible and what has been done is a subject of great importance that this book addresses from several perspectives: academic researcher; healthcare professional; practitioner; and patient. Overall, this book explores new approaches to empowerment in ways that can help reduce mistakes and problems; and improve overall health care in various venues such as patient care, data security, information accessibility, communication, and adaptation of new technologies.

BACKGROUND

Health care today has been irrevocably altered by patient access to information technology. Not only to do patients seek out health-related information using Internet-based sources, they also expect to have access to technology that facilitates all aspects of their health care experiences. These expectations range from information availability prior to interaction with their health care providers, extends into their waiting room experiences, informs their physician interactions, and impacts their treatment options. It advises their choices on both procedural and decision-making matters; and affects their follow-up care. Gamification, Internet of Things, Mobile Computing, Big Data, Social Media and other technologies form the core of their expectations whether they realize it or not. More than ever, patients are empowered to shape their own health care experiences and this trend shows no signs of slowing down or reversing.

However, a healthcare utopia is far from realization. Disaffected healthcare recipients find themselves on the wrong side of the digital divide. To them, new technologies are confusing and add to the stress of their healthcare situations. They may lack the skills to use healthcare portals or be unable to afford, acquire or use new technologies taken for granted by many people. They may view data collection suspiciously and believe their healthcare information may be used for purposes counter to their best interests.

This book compiles a snapshot of current patient experience-centered practical and research viewpoints and offers ideas for the future of this field from a broad, international perspective. Health-related information technologies have created new venues for patients and their families to interact with health care providers, actively manage their care, and subsequently experience better outcomes. These new technologies offer different ways for physicians to partner with their patients for improved quality of care in transformative ways. This book examines existing challenges as well as potential opportunities for improving patient care, empowerment, personalization, and outcomes through emerging health information technology.

It is important to recognize that while new technologies may facilitate empowerment, they are not solely responsible for patient experiences. Rather, empowerment is a phenomenon that this book's authors suggest come from within a patient. It is up to healthcare providers to find ways to use the best new technology to create an environment where empowerment and sound healthcare choices can emerge. From here, better health outcomes can result, and new forms of interaction can develop. But, ultimately, this requires patient buy-in and active participation.

Patients come from all walks of life and nations. They may be: professionals; scientists; physically challenged individuals fighting for their lives; economically disadvantaged and suspicious people from troubled neighborhoods; illegal immigrants; school children; warriors; women expecting their first child; HIV-positive young men; elderly with dementia; or, women feeling uncertain about having to discuss their most personal issues with someone they do not know. Ultimately, patients want to find ways to feel good about their healthcare options and understand what provides the best path to resolve their current issues. They want to remain in control of their lives as much as possible and maintain their lifestyles. Our authors and physician editors suggest this relates to patient empowerment: giving the patient power to utilize reliable information and come away with more knowledge and understanding which they take to meetings with their healthcare providers. Finding confidence and a self-advocating voice ensures patients become part of the decision-making process: they become their own best supporter---not needing to rely solely on doctors. They can participate in choices that provide the best way forward for their situation---holistically. Confidence in one's knowledge and capability to engage in medical decision-making enhances an individual's self-efficacy. This means the patient believes in her or his abilities, and in more specific terms, in his or her capability to successfully and knowledgably take on healthcare challenges in ways that result in successful outcomes (Bandura, 2002).

Patient empowerment can be difficult to describe regarding technology because it does not come from the technology specifically. Instead, it results from a complex relationship between healthcare providers, patients, and those providing tools and techniques to facilitate interaction and information exchange.

TOPICS

This book, *Impacts of Information Technology on Patient Care and Empowerment,* is organized into four sections based on content, author role, and chapter goals; and intends to help international researchers, practitioners, healthcare providers and patients holistically view recent developments in technology noting both successes and remaining challenges. Contributors include an international mix of academics, practitioners, and industry specialists.

We start the book with an overview section offering background information and a state-of-the art literature review in various broad areas where technology and patient empowerment intersect. Section two dives into cutting edge technology examples that suggest directions for healthcare and patient experiences. Section three offers specific case studies and research projects furthering the field; and finally, the last section lists challenges brought about by the intersection of technology, healthcare and society. The editors believe the chapters provided by our authors, with a variety of practical and academic expertise, offer excellent reference material and provide sound advice for healthcare practice as well as a starting point for future research.

Section 1: Technology Overview

The first section, *Technology Overview*, provides background information with an intention to inform practitioners and update researchers. This section comprises four chapters with overviews in complementary areas. Each provides a conceptual view related to current technologies in healthcare, with an emphasis on patient experience and empowerment.

Chapter 1 describes telemedicine concepts with its potential to improve health maintenance, enhance health outcomes and reduce costs. Healthcare regulations are covered briefly, together with concerns that the speed of technology development, particularly in wearable devices, innovative health equipment, and related data transmission/collection have outpaced regulatory capabilities. In general, telemedicine offers a paradigm shift: healthcare's move from acute care to preventive care and health management. As the chapter suggests, patients today receive medical care at a hospital or a clinic. However, the primary venue could shift to our homes or offices due to the advent of technologies including mHealth, video conferencing, wearable devices, and other telemedicine innovations.

Chapter 2 looks at the explosive rise of healthcare technologies related to web-based information. Individuals seeking health information online have created new dynamics affecting the authority of health practitioners in unexpected ways. The widely varying quality of health web sites, incorrect information and bad advice have major impacts as patients search for health information online. On one hand, access to health information can contribute to patient empowerment. However, it also negatively impacts people that access questionable sources. For some, information-seeking can reach levels beyond the occasional, with excessive and repeated searches triggering health-anxiety. The tendency to conduct obsessive online health information searches coupled with health anxiety is called cyberchondria. People may find information confusing, have difficulties in navigating from site to site, and feel stressed not finding answers for their questions. So, web-based information offers interesting research opportunities going forward.

Chapter 3 explores mobile health initiatives which give patients more medical information and can empower them to proactively manage medical treatments and interact with healthcare providers. This chapter also considers challenges such as information overload and lack of digital literacy which have created a digital healthcare divide. A wide array of mobile health options has emerged, and the authors review researchers' definitions used to characterize mobile health and its nexus to patient empowerment. The chapter makes it clear that mobile health applications have the potential to improve care service quality, but challenges remain. Policymakers have begun to address these, and their attention appears to be shifting from productivity to positive patients' experiences based on personal preferences. As such, the World Health Organization (WHO) has developed a definition for quality of care as "the extent to which health care services provided to individuals and patient populations improve desired health outcomes. In order to achieve this, health care must be safe, effective, timely, efficient, equitable and people-centered". This definition provides researchers and practitioners with a direction, that combined with new technologies, encourages patient empowerment.

The first section of this book concludes with *Chapter 4*: a review of mHealth tools available for mental health care. The chapter offers an assessment of current studies, publications trends, and research gaps in the existing literature; and includes technologies such as mobile devices, smartphones, and mobile apps. The findings from this extensive literature search suggest text messaging and SMS have been used for mental health intervention as a cost-effective method. Other more sophisticated approaches also are described but cautions regarding technology literacy and access are provided.

Section 2: Cutting-Edge Technologies in Patient Care

Section 2 of this book moves into cutting edge technologies used in healthcare and offers specific examples of current use by practitioners and researchers. Among topics covered are Big Data, Gamification, Simulation, and Deep Learning. These topics comprise Chapters 5 through 8.

Big data refers to the vast amount of data collected from an array of technologies proliferating in healthcare-related areas. The sources include medical devices, wearables, social media, web sites, communications devices, and more. In recent years, healthcare providers, insurers, governments, and researchers have begun exploration into the latent value of these data stores. However, our authors caution that big data encompasses more than just collection and quantity. Analysis requires techniques that pull together data from wide ranging sources that vary in complexity, diversity, and relativity in ways that reveal patterns, trends, and associations. The large volume of data accessible to healthcare providers can aid patients in the decision-making processes throughout the duration of their treatment plans. Large data repositories have emerged and enable clinicians to utilize structured, semi-structured, and unstructured data to better diagnose or treat a patient. Structured data is information easily stored or formatted by a machine, whereas unstructured data is not organized in a specific way (e.g. text, notes, and more). Not only does this provide clinicians with the opportunity to make more informed decisions, it also allows providers the chance to detect a disease early on. Awareness of health issues at earlier stages increases the likelihood of diseases being more manageable and treatable. In turn, this generally results reduced healthcare expenditures.

Another approach to healthcare infused with technology utilizes gamification. Gamification takes on challenges of poor patient adherence to physician recommended regimens and medical non-adherence which pose significant hurdles in optimizing care, improving health outcomes and reducing overall health management costs. The idea uses game design elements in real-world contexts to reward patients each time they take medication (or adhere to other treatment elements) in order to motivate them to continue the desired behavior. Gamification depends upon psychological factors built into game design elements to drive positive behavior changes. It is a dynamic and mechanical way to help non-adherence and increase patient compliance. Further, these technologies can be used to monitor patient behavior and provide tracking data.

Another cutting-edge technology, simulation, helps healthcare researchers and practitioners better understand how various strategies and operational tactics impact utilization of health resources. The simulation chapter in this book looks at patient no-show management strategies. In this case, no-shows are patients who miss scheduled, specialist outpatient clinic appointments. No-shows impact more than just that patient's health. The ripple effect limits access to care for others and increases everyone's appointment lead times. Using a data-driven strategy improves overall access to specialist care and ultimately reduces costs for clinics and its patients.

The last chapter in the section exploring emerging technologies takes us into deep learning. Deep learning technology can solve complex medical problems that require more than a simple set of rubrics to arrive at choices. For example, deep learning can address the need for more medical professionals in healthcare fields. It fits naturally with telemedicine applications where artificial intelligence and other approaches assist diverting patients requiring routine care away from seeking specialist medical professionals and instead to those specializing in basic care. In general, integrating deep learning technologies into telemedicine services will increase the number of patients that these services assist.

Section 3: Cases With Empowerment Through IT

The third section of the book looks at several specific cases to provide examples of patient empowerment facilitated with technology. Several chapters report successes and others, failures. Chapter 9 starts this section by looking at ways that patient-centered empowerment is enhanced through evidence-based engagement in stressful medical situations. The goal of this study was to ensure accessibility and understandability of information in a gynecology clinic specializing in sensitive medical conditions such as HPV. The approach used mobile technology in the waiting room and demonstrated that promoting specialized information in the clinic with high quality, relevant, physician-vetted resources led to better engagement inside the clinic. Empowerment resulted from more confident patients.

Chapter 10 focuses on patients with multiple sclerosis (MS) and provides a literature review of relevant studies on digital health information and information usability. It also presents key findings from a mixed methods study that explored how people with MS access and use health digital information when trying to manage their condition. The chapter provides useful findings and identifies how technology can facilitate shared decisions. It also points out gaps in related research and suggests future study. The approach used in this chapter could be extended to nearly any sub-specialty area of medical care.

Chapter 11 provides insights from the design and development of a mobile-based intelligent pain management system (IPMS) app used for cancer patient pain in a rural hospital in China. Using an app permitted real-time pain recording and timely intervention by healthcare providers. The study also described the app's development lifecycle and emphasized that healthcare professionals' input was crucial throughout the process. The idea that smartphones and mobile apps have been introduced to pain management, together with the option for real time consultation with the healthcare professionals and medication reminders, enables proactive pain management.

In Chapter 12, we visit a healthcare facility that focuses on an underserved community. The development and release of a new healthcare portal at Einstein Medical Center Philadelphia (EMCP) are reported. Its implementation offered promise to enhance patient empowerment but resulted in challenges related to managing trust. These challenges were examined in the contexts of poor social determinants of health (SDOH), unique social factors, and other issues facing unique inner-city populations which included dealing cultural diversity, perceived lack of respect, and poor health literacy.

Chapter 13 discusses the challenges faced by the Children's Hospital of Philadelphia (CHOP). This pediatric medical institution attempted to develop a partnership with a local school district to provide access to pediatric care through a telemedicine unit embedded in the nurses' offices of various schools within the district. Perceptions in the target community lead to reservations about sharing sensitive personal health information. Fears derived from immigration status and from perceptions that collected data could be used for purposes other than their children's healthcare. The benefits of the program would have empowered community members and included fewer missed school days for students and reduced burdens on parents having to take time off work. In the desired model, nurses would use a telemedicine unit with a computer monitor and camera for video conferencing with a physician and smart medical tools which relay information back to the physician in real time. The unit would allow the physician to complete basic screening procedures. An encrypted HIPAA-secure connection added protection for student's health information. Parent distrust in the school district, in CHOP, and in the government led to underutilization of a potentially beneficial system.

Chapter 14 continues with the theme of healthcare professional interaction leveraging the concept of doctor-patient social networking using the Diagnostic Modality Interface Portal (DMIP). This study suggests that effective communication and coordination among medical doctors, specialists and other caregivers can have a lasting impact on patients. Using a new digital health technology paradigm based on social networking can improve care coordination. It also enables data integration across diagnostic modalities to simplify the process of accessing information and reporting medical interpretations and treatment recommendations. The combination of data and social networking helps care providers improve patient outcomes by facilitating initial risk stratification, reducing admissions and readmissions, and making patient care more effective. The current state of the art involves a variety of systems that doctors need to access to order diagnostic tests for patients, track status, review and interpret results, clarify treatment options and suggestions, and communicate with the patient. DMIP integrates these different sources to facilitate care by presenting healthcare providers with a unified view of patient medical events, diagnostic data and images. Thus, the patient and his or her caregivers can communicate through social networking interaction for questions and answers, and general information sharing about a patient's specific history and treatment.

Section 4: Underserved Populations

The final section of our book looks at underserved populations. This refers to people who lack modern infrastructure or fear collected data might be misused. The chapters in this section provide insight into efforts to improve the way health care is delivered to at-risk populations. First, Chapter 15 focuses on the issues and opportunities that exist using mobile technologies with older patients. The chapter reports on lessons learned during the first 6 months of the CONNECARE project in Israel. This process assessed the use of mobile technology by older patients, their motivations and obstacles; as well as their satisfaction. The project suggests that citizen empowerment with digital tools for user feedback and person-centered care empowers people to look after their health, enhance prevention and engage in feedback and interaction with their healthcare providers. The project also suggests how the system could be improved by introducing additional features to increase patients' motivation to use the system as well as its full integration into usual healthcare processes. This study concludes that the movement toward digitalization of healthcare must include considerations that meet the growing needs of an expanding elderly population with an increasing chronic disease burden.

Chapter 16 provides an overview of how mHealth collaboration results in social good. This chapter draws on WHO's suggestions that mobile technology has the potential to create stronger healthcare systems and ultimately improve patient health. This chapter reports the development of a hypertension app that helps people living in India's urban slums and rural villages improve their health practices; and suggests traditional Western-based project management approaches are insufficient when developing technology for social good in emerging countries. Instead, team, process and technology adaptability are keys to successful implementation of healthcare technology to serve at-risk populations in resource-constrained areas.

Chapter 17 shifts the focus to laypersons attempting to make sense of their lab results. The authors provide a methodology to capture the relationship between information formats (graph, numeric or verbal), a potential patient's assessment of their condition gravity, and their preferred course of action. The study shows that not understanding medical information had an effect opposite of empowerment. Essentially, report formats that were less understandable, reduced patient inclination to seek professional help. This chapter suggests that making medical information more understandable to the non-expert is very important in encouraging patients to take ownership of their healthcare.

The final chapter of this section and of the book reviews very important issues relating to confidentiality rights. The benefits and dangers of embracing the new information technologies, and its impact on the confidentiality of sensitive health data has not always been protected consistently by laws. Laws vary by region, country and culture. Laws are not able to keep up with the revolution in the information technology sector. The growing gap has resulted in unresolved gray areas. Advances in information technology, both in formal medical records systems and informal social media or mobile computing, have changed the way society deals with patient confidential information. Formerly clear professional relationships between patient and caregiver have blurred. Further, electronic health information is used to access and share patient's confidential information among healthcare professionals sometimes without patient knowledge or consent. Much work needs to be done in this area as the author suggests.

DOCTORS' PERSPECTIVES

This book is unique because it pulls together the collective knowledge of medical professionals, academics from health and information systems fields, and practitioners in medical-related areas. While perspectives vary, the overarching goal of all groups is to ensure better healthcare outcomes through enhanced patient experiences and empowerment. Technology can play a part in making this happen. The next section of our Preface provides the viewpoint of our team of physician editors.

Empowerment

Empowerment has two sources: (1) to be given power by someone or something; and, (2) to realize one's own potential and therefore to empower oneself. In the world of fantasy, superheroes often rely on the former definition and individuals embrace the idea of being rescued. This also coincided with societal viewpoints and expectations for and amongst physicians, sometimes casting them as heroes that performed miracles and saved the day (Chambers, 1999, pp. 27–28; Clark, 1990, pp. 520–521; MacNulty & Kennedy, 2008). Many experts point out the danger of accepting the mantle of physician-hero and just like the comic book archetypes, these physicians discover this role leads to dire consequences (Drummond, 2015; Privitera, Rosenstein, Plessow, & LoCastro, 2014). Instead, the best superhero perhaps is the one that enables others to step up and realize their own potential (Loewen, 2007). This is our latter source of empowerment where an individual will gain the confidence to take control of their healthcare possibilities leveraging physician interactions, technology, information, self-confidence and best practices to positively impact their own outcomes. These individuals firmly believe that empowerment is not something from outside but something that happens internally, so the patients became the heroes inside the medical encounter while receiving sound advice and communication with their healthcare providers and other experts.

A recent example from Dr. Mark McHaney, a family practice physician in the U.S. Air Force Medical Service illustrates. He recently had a patient interaction that demonstrated how appropriately leveraging information technology and a sense of internal modern medicine can help empower an individual. In this case, a 36-year-old woman was empaneled into a small, remote rural clinic as part of military practice. She had a strange lump in her chest that the local doctor had reassured her was a benign cyst and nothing to worry about. Due to her location, that was the only healthcare she had available to her.

Regardless of what she was told, she still felt something wrong. She took it upon herself to continue to push toward diagnosis of the condition by seeking more information and reaching out to experts. She was able to contact her prior women's health physician and held a telemedicine encounter – done like a face to face appointment, but through cellphones using FaceTime. During that encounter, they felt that she needed to get further imaging, and the women's health physician was able to put the order into the local radiology unit remotely. When they did the imaging, and subsequent analysis, they found stage IV breast cancer that had moved to the spine.

From there, the patient saw oncology virtually, and they worked on getting her medications that would suppress the condition. Four years have elapsed, and she is alive and well. Technology options provided her with the ability to become her own hero. She was empowered to push ahead even when a member of her local healthcare team was reluctant, and other nearby options did not exist. She believes she owes her life to her empowerment. She felt that she could continue to push and advocate for herself using remote medicine despite local issues.

This is an example of how technology empowered the patient – it gave her options that previously did not exist and enabled her to truly participate in her care through non-conventional options. True empowerment comes from the ability to advocate for oneself and have people listen. Technology allows people to reach out, listen and see, no matter the distance.

The other physicians on our editorial team, Dr. Joseph Azuri, Department of Family Medicine, Maccabi Health Services and Dr. Rami Moshonov, Head of Gynecology, Assuta Medical Center provide a short definition of patient empowerment from their perspective as being: *to incorporate or collaborate with the patient in order to enhance our health providers and healthcare systems and enable these to provide better quality medicine and healthcare outcomes*. Our physicians offer observations and advice on ways to help move patients toward self-advocacy and empowerment.

Patient Information Searches

Healthcare providers must recognize that 'the informational search train has already left the station', especially considering adolescents and young adults. Patients are more knowledgeable and sometimes it seems they already know what the physician has to say next. Young people are better trained to extract data and make more intelligent web searches. This allows them, as patients, to ask more intelligent questions and avoid medical pitfalls by making a better treatment selection or identifying treatment side effects. Elderly patients or those with computer phobias will probably never move into this space and will depend more on their medical providers to assist them in developing confidence and finding ways to make technology-based systems more user-friendly to enable better empowerment.

Dr. Moshonov suggests that giving information lowers anxiety and fear in a patient. They can ask questions more freely and are more likely to comply with treatment recommendations. They will respond to requests better and understand why certain actions are important to their outcomes. This approach enables a better context with the patient. They better understand what will happen during the procedures/treatment and this helps ensure the patient will do what is needed to be successful. This is especially true when visual information is provided. The best occasion to start this process is when the patient makes the appointment. This can be done using a smartphone or other technology. The information provided can include how to prepare; what to expect; and where to get reliable information on the Web. That way, when the patient arrives to the appointment, she is ready to communicate and understand the treatment better with less anxiety.

This also means patient knowledge can be enhanced to a higher level because the background information is complete. More can come from the same visit. Again, knowledge will decrease anxiety and the 'state of shock' will be passed. The visit can be used more constructively for this reason. And the patient will be more compliant with treatment recommendations. The uncertainty is removed.

Anxiety can result from: not knowing why they need the appointment in a correct way; from getting wrong information from the web or even the physician referring them to the procedure (for example sometimes a low change in a screening test might be misinterpreted by the referring physician making the patient very worried).

Dr. Azuri provided comments on web-based information: often patients get incorrect information from the Web. However, sometimes they do come to a physician knowing exactly what they want. Or at least they think they know what they want. They may know what medication they need. They expect the doctor to recommend things they have found on the Internet. A good goal in this era is to guide patients in finding good, reliable information. Family physicians have the privilege of seeing patients with a wide range of conditions. Therefore, it makes sense to instruct a patient on how to examine sites to determine if their source is accurate or reliable. The wide range of conditions makes it difficult to assess all sites. Many times, a patient comes with their research on conditions that a physician will not yet have had time to review because it is a first encounter. This might frighten some physicians, but that is the reality of the current era of patients.

The goal then becomes to guide the patient to accurate information; to the important information that can be relied upon. Physicians must teach the patient to become good at gathering information from reliable sites in the right way. Likewise, it is important to realize that patients can be correct. This is particularly true when dealing with family practice medicine where such a wide range of situations can be encountered.

Dr. Moshonov suggests that in specialty medicine areas, interaction with the patient is much narrower so guiding them to specific, reliable information becomes easier than perhaps for someone in family medicine. In this case, it becomes possible for the doctor to push out information prior to the visit: preferably this is accurate, visual information for the patient. When they come to the visit they will already be informed and ready to talk. They will be more compliant and ready to understand with specific questions. It is best for them to receive the right information from the clinic, so they will not need to look for information. If they do feel they need to search, it is best to give them links to sites on the Internet where information is accurate and relevant to their condition. Physicians could provide those links and make it easier to push the information to patients. That way, they will come to the visit understanding why they need the procedure and what will be done. They can ask better questions. And know why future treatments and visits will be required.

So, in general the family doctor deals with broader issues that might involve more Internet searches in a wide range of areas which means guiding the patient in conducting educated searches. The specialist, on the other hand, can guide the patient proactively to more specific information. Both approaches are needed depending on the situation. Both approaches provide less anxiety; and a more compliant patient who is more likely to adhere to the treatment plan and more willing to work with the doctor closely.

Big Data

According to the doctors on our editorial team, big data still is more of a research tool for making better decisions based on real information. Healthcare industries are moving into an evidence-based medical era that helps with patient treatment. Currently, it is not a diagnostic tool in real time but may be some day. Big data is not a replacement for doctors at the current time (although the future for big data usage could look very different). Patient/doctor relations are still crucial when considering the human side of treatment and the use of big data. Overall, it will help healthcare providers understand what has happened in the past and inform decisions in the future. Maybe someday, big data will be used real time during doctor-patient interaction. But more work is needed first.

Changes to Patient Care Through Empowerment

The future holds great promise regarding patient empowerment. This conclusion came about during a brainstorming session with the doctors on our editorial team. They suggested this best practice: when making an appointment, accurate information should be pushed instantly out to the patient on a smartphone to reduce anxiety and confirm reasons for treatment. A one-minute video clip on what to expect would help a great deal. Additionally, good links to accurate information would help direct the patient's urge to search the web. This would help them formulate good treatment questions and make better use of time later during an appointment. Reliably graded websites for accurate content would help greatly. Patients will search but enabling them to understand how to judge 'good' information would greatly enhance their process. This would reduce anxiety and help them become better informed. This is particularly true when a time lag exists between appointments.

The main point is to push the correct information to the patient in real time. The use of technology becomes a continuous element. The doctor needs to be sure there is a continual information influx to remind and reinforce the message to the patient. Each time they visit, a physician should say, "Okay now it is important to do the next thing. If you don't then this could happen. Look at these sites and places for the next information." Empowerment through education is a continuous thing!

CONCLUSION AND CALL TO ACTION

Patient empowerment is desirable. Modern healthcare operates in a dramatically different environment now with the advent of personal technologies, ubiquitous access to information and widespread communication capabilities. The era of society viewing the physician as a superhero has been supplanted with a viewpoint where the physician mentors the new superhero, the patient herself.

Empowerment can encourage enhanced health outcomes and can leverage technology to promote the best available medical treatment in line with patients' preferences and values. A communicative relationship between physicians and patients is an important component in high quality care service that meets patients' needs. Big data, mobile technologies, deep learning, gamification, social media, medical websites, video conferencing, and other technologies facilitate access to customized and expert-vetted information based on care path and needs of a patient receiving specific medical treatment. A once unidirectional flow of information from health professional to patient has been supplanted by an information-rich ecosystem. This book contributes to seminal studies in empowerment and helps operationalize this concept in healthcare-related environments. First, empowerment is a motivational construct, and individuals need to have control to cope with changes in their life. Second, empowerment is an enabling process- highlighting personal efficacy and the internal development of confidence that health goals can be achieved. Finally, empowerment has psychological constructs and provides patients with an energetic and participative role in their healthcare solution. Patient empowerment both enables and transforms people's ability to meet their own preferences and to mobilize resources for gaining control over their healthcare to better comply and adhere to medical treatment. Patient empowerment is a capacity-building process, in which patients play an active role in decision-making and their health management processes. It focuses on enhancing care-provider and patient relationships.

In short, empowerment represents the process by which patients gain control over their care path and feel that they can adequately cope with events and situations. Feelings of empowerment lead a patient to better accomplish the required tasks. This book explores the implications of empowerment in a rapidly changing, technology and data rich healthcare environment.

Roger McHaney
Kansas State University, USA

Iris Reychav
Ariel University, Israel

Joseph Azuri
Maccabi Healthcare Services, Israel

Mark McHaney
U.S. Air Force, USA

Rami Moshonov
Assuta Medical Centers, Israel

REFERENCES

Bandura, A. (2002). Social foundations of thought and action. In D. F. Marks (Ed.), *The health psychology reader* (pp. 94–106). London, UK: Sage. doi:10.4135/9781446221129.n6

Chambers, C. (1999). Superheroes don't take sick leave. *Health Dialogue*, (11). Retrieved from https://www.asms.org.nz/wp-content/uploads/2015/11/Presenteeism_A5-Final-for-Print_164753.pdf

Clark, R. E. (1990). Who, hobbies, and heroes. *The Annals of Thoracic Surgery*, *49*(4), 515–521. doi:10.1016/0003-4975(90)90293-F PMID:2322042

Drummond, D. (2015). Physician burnout: Its origin, symptoms, and five main causes. *Family Practice Management*, *22*(5), 42–47. PMID:26554564

Loewen, A. (2007). Ma's story: Finding superhero power. *Canadian Family Physician Medecin de Famille Canadien*, *53*(8), 1344.

MacNulty, A., & Kennedy, D. (2008). Beyond the models: investing in physician-hospital relationships: communication, physician involvement in decision making, and physician leadership development are as critical to strong hospital-physician partnerships as the organizational models for these relationships. *Healthcare Financial Management*, *62*(12), 72–78. PMID:19069325

Privitera, M. R., Rosenstein, A. H., Plessow, F., & LoCastro, T. (2014). Physician burnout and occupational stress: An inconvenient truth with unintended consequences. *Journal of Hospital Administration*, *4*(1), 27–35. doi:10.5430/jha.v4n1p27

Acknowledgment

The editors of this book wish to acknowledge the help and efforts of the following key organizations and individuals:

Dr. Bella Azaria, Chief Medical Director at Assuta Medical Centers, for providing ideas, inspiration, and other general support. She enabled and supported the HPV project described in this book.

Dr. Batami Sadan, ILAMI Representative and Chair, for supporting this project. She provided exposure during our early stages in ways that permitted us to find contributors, authors, reviewers and other key individuals. It was particularly important for us to have the support of Israel health community. For more information about IMIA see: https://imia-medinfo.org/wp/the-israeli-association-for-medical-informatics/

The Association of Information Systems and its SIG-Health that provided distribution lists for health, HCI, ILAIS. See https://aisnet.org/ and http://www.aissighealth.com for more information.

We also could not have completed the project without the help and support of the following reviewers and supporters: Abba Elgujja, Alon Hagsall, Amit Rechavi, Andreas Hedrén, Aviv Shachak, Christopher Gantz, Dafana Raban, Darina Slattery, David Gefen, Dezhi Wu, Eghosa Edogun, Gali Naveh, Gia Park, Gina Green, Gloria Iyawa, Guillaume Faddoul, Güney Gürsel, Ilana Lavy, Izabella Lejbkowicz, Jeremy Kagan, Joseph Buckman, Lin Zhu, Megan Lindstrom, Michael J. May, Mor Peleg, Nasser Shahrasbi, Shelby Garner, Shirly Bar-Lev, Taiki Nishihara, Tai-Yin Chi, Terry Saint Marie, Viviana Bastidas, Y. Ken Wang, and Zonayed Mahid. Thank you so much.

Section 1
Technology Overview

Chapter 1
Improving Patient Care With Telemedicine Technology

Edward T. Chen
University of Massachusetts – Lowell, USA

ABSTRACT

With the spread of telecommunications infrastructure, telemedicine has attracted attention from both healthcare and IT industries. Telemedicine has shown a potential to improve health maintenance, enhancement, as well as healthcare cost reduction. Many governments are boosting telemedicine applications through regulations. The purpose of this chapter is to review the major telemedicine technologies—telemedicine, wearable devices, and emerging innovative health equipment—and current issues of the impact on the patient care in the healthcare industry, the business opportunities, and threats from telemedicine.

INTRODUCTION

With the spread of telecommunications infrastructure, digital health has attracted the attention of the healthcare and IT industries. According to the U.S. Food and Drug Administration (FDA), digital health includes various technologies such as mobile health, telemedicine, wearable devices, and personalized medicine. The use of digital health technologies would provide us with innovative ways to treat our diseases, monitor our health, and give us greater access to healthcare information. Patients are expected to receive innovative medical treatment and preventive medical care, and track health and wellness related activities (Kimball, 2018). Healthcare providers could increase the quality of services, reduce costs, improve access to healthcare information, and make medicine more personalized for patients through the progress of digital health. Digital health has the potential to break conventional healthcare: Therefore, a variety of companies are entering this space including primary healthcare related organizations such as pharmaceutical companies, medical equipment manufacturers, hospitals, etc., and electronics device manufacturers, communication companies, and IT companies. According to Thilo Kaltenbach (2016), the digital health market was 79 billion USD in 2015, but it is expected to grow to 206 billion USD in 2020 with an annual growth rate of 21%.

DOI: 10.4018/978-1-7998-0047-7.ch001

This chapter reviews a component of digital health: telemedicine technologies - telemedicine, wearable devices, and emerging innovative health equipment, and discusses related impact on patient care, business opportunities, and threats.

TELEMEDICINE

Telemedicine is changing the lives of patients by making healthcare more accessible than ever before. The Internet is completely changing the way people look at managing their health. As technology advances, individuals can integrate telemedicine more seamlessly. For example, the Apple Watch has the capability to track heart rates and feed it to smart phones. This information can be sent to primary care physicians to give them real time data on how their patient's body is performing. Patients with chronic illnesses like diabetes and heart disease now can be monitored more closely with the help of wearable health devices and interactive patient portals.

Scheduling and completing appointments is now easier than ever before. Patients can log on and send an email rather than call and speak with someone directly. They can schedule an appointment from an automated calendar rather than do so with a medical secretary. Patients can complete a follow up health survey with questions related to their in-office visit a few weeks after the fact rather than return to the office for a follow up visit. Conversely, a physician can answer a handful of emails much faster than they can see the same number of patients since each would need to come in, check in, confirm their information, make their payment, get their vitals taken, speak with the physician, debrief with an assistant, pay for their visit, and schedule the next one. A virtual visit is as easy as answering a few questions or reading a message. The process is much easier than in-person visits. This encourages patients to check in with their doctors more frequently. Therefore, patients should be able to sustain a better level of health (Rupp, 2017; Sanyal, 2018).

How Telemedicine Works

The first positive effects of telemedicine were seen in the late 1800s when appointments began to be completed via telephone. Hugo Gernsback predicted that in the future, doctors would utilize not only the telephone but also TV and radio to treat and reach patients. Flash forward to Pennsylvania in the 1940's when radiology images were sent via telephone wire over 24 miles. It was not until the 1950's that telemedicine was used to send out neurological exams at the University of Nebraska. Also, in the 1950's in Nebraska, closed circuit TVs began being used by psychiatric practitioners to complete patient consultations. Because video conferencing with physicians is just now hitting the mainstream, these doctors were ahead of their time. Telemedicine remained largely stagnant until the age of the Internet. Since the inception of Web 2.0 and legislation in the Affordable Care Act of 2010, telemedicine options are now nearly endless (Rupp, 2017).

Alexa, Amazon's voice assistant, will probably soon be able to refill prescriptions at the pharmacy down the street. Telemedicine allows health care professionals to use telecommunications to meet with, evaluate, diagnose, and treat patients remotely through technology. Telemedicine may be utilized on many different applications like smartphones, video conferencing, mobile applications, and high definition televisions to conduct virtual appointments. This technology was originally created to address medical professional shortages, and to reach patients that live far from traditional medical facilities.

Today's patient wants to spend less time in a waiting room and get immediate care for minor but urgent conditions. Telemedicine can fill in the gap between supply and demand, opening a whole new market for physicians and healthcare organizations alike.

Benefits of Telemedicine

Telemedicine aims to: solve care accessibility issues (time spent getting to and from the doctors, time off from work, and traveling long distances for some patients, etc.), reduce healthcare cost, and improve health for patients in vulnerable and underserved populations. Telemedicine has been a game changer for many patients across the U.S. and the world. Some may think of personal health as something that only affects themselves, but this is not true. Rising healthcare costs are of concern on a wider scale. High risk and high cost patients raise premiums for everyone. It is in society's best interest to increase the health of others that may not traditionally be able to do so with the healthcare infrastructure of the past.

Telemedicine services are designed to be very easy to use. People can lose hours of their day to go to a physical doctor's appointment with delays in traffic, long routes or inclement weather. With telemedicine, patients can be diagnosed from their beds. Usually a person can create an online profile on a patient portal or call a toll-free phone number to speak with a healthcare specialist. The patient will then request a visit by submitting basic information on their condition as well as on their general health. The physician will then accept, deny or schedule it for the future. Correspondence is typically completed via messaging and email, which oftentimes is built right into the patient portal. This will cut down on calls to the office, and it is more secure than sending confidential messages through a third-party email provider. Keeping communication within the patient application helps to avoid security breaches. A visit that can take upwards of 30 minutes can now be reduced to an online interaction that takes a few minutes.

University of California Davis conducted a study on the time saving effects of telemedicine. The study looked at data from over 19,000 consultations from 11,281 patients. "Telemedicine visits resulted in a total travel distance savings of 5,345,602 miles, a total travel time savings of 4,708,891 minutes or 8.96 years, and a total direct travel cost savings of $2,882,056" (Dullet et al., 2017). There is new use of telemedicine in public school settings. Assessment devices include otoscopes that are connected to video devices. The school nurse can place the otoscope in the child's ear, and the physician, physician assistant (PA) or nurse practitioner (NP) at a telemedicine connected remote site can see the inner ear through the telehealth connection (Mousseau, Lapointe, & Gravel, 2018).

Many regions of the United States are clinically underserved, meaning there are not enough physicians in that area to adequately treat the entire population. To address this, the Health Resources and Service Administration promotes the use of telemedicine programs in areas of physician shortages. One of the resources offered through the Federal Office of Rural Health Policy is the Rural Community Health Information Hub. The RHIhub is a resource that supports those interested in putting together a telemedicine healthcare model for their area. It has guides and models that can assist in creating and implementing telemedicine programs in underserved areas (Health Resources and Service Administration, 2019). Setting up a virtual patient gateway is much easier than setting up a physical brick and mortar practice that is staffed with physical people.

Virtual practices allow practitioners to reach patients from any proximity. Patients that may have had to drive hours or days to receive medical care now check in with their doctor with a click of a button. Medical conditions that may have previously been ignored by the patient due to difficulty of obtaining care can now be addressed with relative ease. All the patient needs to be seen is a smartphone, computer, or other smart device with an Internet connection. This has especially hopeful implications for patients with chronic illnesses that need frequent monitoring. For example, diabetic patients are now able to track and monitor their blood sugar levels using wearable medical devices and secure patient portals. A patient that was difficult to monitor from afar would be able to upload their blood sugar data within the span of a few minutes or seconds depending on the technology and their proficiency level.

General medicine is not the only area that benefits. Specialties and psychological care also can benefit from technological advances associated with telemedicine. Patients who live in rural areas now have access to mental health care. Usage is on the rise and expected to grow in the years to come. Research suggests that the usage levels vary significantly across states. Katherine Igoe (2017) wrote, "The number of telemedicine visits increased from 2,365 in 2004 to 87,120 in 2014. An average of 5 out of 100 rural beneficiaries with a mental health condition had a telemedicine visit, and the number was even higher—12 out of 100—for patients with serious mental illnesses" (Igoe, 2017, p.1).

Psychological care clinicians are in an excellent position to utilize virtual visits. Some patients fear going to a psychiatrist or psychologist because they do not want to be stigmatized or judged. Being able to visit with a qualified clinician from their home's comfort could minimize this worry. Through a different lens, virtual visits may be ideal for those who are afraid to or unable to leave their house. For some, chatting with a clinician online or on the phone may make a huge difference in their life. It is unlikely for psychological care to take off the same way general medicine care has until the government starts reimbursing better for behavioral healthcare.

Psychological care access is just one example of an increase in access to specialty care. The U.S. Department of Veterans Affairs has one of the nation's largest telemedicine programs, which reaches about 700,000 VA patients virtually per year (Lapowsky, 2017). In May 2018, The Department of Veterans Affairs announced an expansion of their services, which would allow doctors to treat patients across state lines. This change is the result of a new federal rule, titled "Authority of Health Care Providers to Practice Telehealth," which permits VA clinicians to administer care to patients via telemedicine regardless of what state the patient or clinician was located. Also, in this announcement was the unveiling of the VA's new service, VA Video Connect, which allows patients and clinicians to interface via live video (Office of Public and Intergovernmental Affairs, 2018).

This is a big step toward patient empowerment. Veterans are notoriously underserved and are more vulnerable than others to certain psychiatric afflictions, which may result in substance use disorders or homelessness. *The Military Times* reports that between 2015 and 2016, suicide rates for young U.S. Veterans jumped 10 percent (Shane, III., 2018). There is a clear need for an intervention among this demographic. What has been done in the past is clearly not working (The Military Times, 2019).

Issues And Limitations Of Telemedicine

Telemedicine is nearly a complete solution for problems associated with routine check-ups and visits, but it is not a total solution to replace physically visiting the doctor for all ailments. Telemedicine cannot replace emergency rooms or hospitals. As the technology stands now, a patient cannot get a telemedicine surgery, or many life-saving medical interventions. There is no replacement at this time for emergency care. However, telemedicine technology is becoming increasingly more common in emergency departments. "Rather than replace the physical ICU outright, the tele-ICU, as it is called, provides a "second set of eyes" for nurses or physicians who must treat several patients at once amid alarms and other distractions that may make them miss a medication dose, sudden change in blood pressure or other important signal" (Eastwood, 2012).

Telemedicine in the emergency department could mean extra support for nurses and doctors when staffing is low. This could result in better patient outcomes and more efficient patient care. A second set of eyes can make all the difference for clinicians that work in high volume hospitals. For instance, this could help address the severe Registered Nurse shortage currently impacting Massachusetts. Had the Nurse Staffing act passed, virtual nurses could have possibly bridged the gap for community hospitals or nursing facilities that could not afford new nurse staffing minimums.

One issue with telemedicine is that it all hinges on the reliability of the patient. It only works if they accurately report their symptoms and honestly report metrics like weight, blood pressure, pulse, etc. This technology also assumes that patients have ready access to smartphones, wearables, computers, and the Internet. Individuals in rural areas may not always have access to the Internet. Also, every patient is not in the financial position to own a device that can complete a telemedicine visit.

Another issue is even if the patient is in possession of this type of device, they may not be fully proficient in using it. Navigating patient portals is an easy task for some users, but for other it is difficult to just turn their devices on. This may lessen as technology becomes more ubiquitous. Currently, many people did not grow up with technology and are not fluent in its usage. Often, older patients are impacted by the digital divide, which presents a problem because this demographic needs the most care. This can be partially addressed by making sure that patient portals and access points for virtual visits are easy to navigate for a patient at any level of technology proficiency. Organizations should be sure to evaluate their websites through the eyes of a technology novice. This can help to bring that barrier down. The more the patients use it, the more proficient they will become. The user problem should go away with time as patients become "native" technology users.

Another problem to consider is the safety of patient data. Personal information sells for a premium on the dark web, and organizations need to make sure they have the correct information systems infrastructure in place before they launch a telemedicine initiative. This would be a barrier for smaller organizations that may not have limited resources.

WEARABLE DEVICES

Wearable devices can aid and assist in monitoring and recording healthcare measurements. This phenomenon "achieved mainstream popularity with the Bluetooth headset in 2002. Between 2006 and 2013, iconic wearable technology devices Nike+, Fitbit and Google Glass were released. In 2014, dubbed 'The Year of Wearable Technology' by several media outlets, activity trackers grew in popularity and the Apple Watch was introduced. Other wearable technology devices, such as those that track seizures or sunlight exposure, continued expanding the industry" (Grace College, 2019).

An abundance of choices exists, largely because many organizations have expanded their capabilities to involve healthcare. For example, in 2009, a Company called Glacier Computers introduced the W200 Wearable Computer. This device was able to appeal to emergency response services. It was water-resistant and weighed approximately 10 ounces. One year later, Philips Lifeline was introduced, and this technology was worn around the user's neck. This device had the ability to call emergency personnel should a senior fall or need of assistance and could not reach a phone. Smart watches were developed a few years later, which changed the way users looked at healthcare within the context of wearable devices. Today, wearables can call emergency services; to track heart rate, activity, seizure monitoring; and, much more.

How Wearable Devices Work

At a high level, a wearable device has the ability track an individual's movements along with certain body measurements. The wearable accomplishes this through the device's hardware technology in conjunction with an algorithm specifically designed for that device's main functions. For example, numerous fitness trackers use gyroscopes to determine the orientation of an object, a compass to determine the cardinal direction, an altimeter sensor for measuring altitude including an aneroid barometer designed to register changes in atmospheric pressure, and an accelerometer sensor for detecting and measuring vibrations.

After the data has passed through the micro-electronics and is processed through the algorithms, the data is presented to the end-user in a user-friendly layout. An example of a positively reviewed user interface is Apple Health app for both iPhone and Apple Watch. Collected health data is broken into four key components: Sleep, Nutrition, Mindfulness, and Activity. These are correlated in ways that lead to a satisfying experience for the end-user (Walker, Hickey, & Freedson, 2016).

Benefits of Wearable Devices

Wearable technology can reduce problems and resolve issues associated healthcare delivery as this technology becomes more prevalent within people's daily lives. One of the benefits of new wearable technology is that healthcare providers can better monitor the older-adult demographic. The U.S. Census Bureau estimates that the population over 65 years old will double from 2012 to 2050, to approximately 83.7 million (Lewis & Neider, 2017). The growth of this demographic is driven by the baby boomer generation that has seen the emergence of wearable technology and has the potential to remain tech-savvy through their later years if shown the benefits of wearable devices in regard to healthcare. One of the major issues with adults over the age of 65 where wearable technology could make a significant impact relates to medication regimens including drug specific requirements. As noted by the American Society of Consultant Pharmacists, adults over the age of 65 are responsible for approximately 40% of all medication consumption (Lewis & Neider, 2017).

In addition to identifying a need with a medication regimen, wearable technology also can assist the older demographic, with common concerns such as activity tracking, sleep monitoring, cognitive processes, and health metrics. An example of these benefits is to use activity tracking and goal setting through a wearable device to help alleviate symptoms associated with ailments such as Parkinson's or arthritis. With arthritis, movement has been known to help keep ligaments and tendons flexible, which has been shown to help improve the range and motion of the body. It is important as close to 50% of adults 65 years of age or older suffer from some form of arthritis (Lewis & Neider, 2017).

Another benefit of new wearable technology is that healthcare can now transition from a disease treatment mindset to a prevention mindset by proactively monitoring patient data. Healthcare organizations continue to invest in remote monitoring apps and virtual care programs. CCS Insight indicates that 411 million smart wearable devices will be sold in 2020. Hence, the wearable device market has the potential to reach a large portion of the population (Lamkin, 2016). Many wearable devices in the market will contain sensors that allow monitoring of healthcare ailments such as diabetes, sleep disorders, high blood pressure, obesity, cardiovascular disease, epilepsy, anxiety disorders, and asthma.

The use of collected information will assist patients and healthcare providers in two different fashions. At the user level, wearable technology can use biosensors to identify physical or mental attributes that could be affecting an individual's health state and notify the user if imbalances exist. For example, Lief

Therapeutics designed a wearable health technology that senses and measures an individual's breathing and heart rate so that the individual can better train their mental and physical responses to stress, thereby reducing anxiety. By using Lief throughout the day an individual can positively improve their ability to monitor and control their emotions, thoughts in-the-moment, and behaviors which in turn could reduce the negative effects of anxiety. This could lead to a reduction in several physiological conditions such as heart disease, stroke, and insomnia (Kimball, 2018).

At the healthcare level, the use and interpretation of continuously measured physiological data provides a broader range of data for medical professionals to analyze. In this past, this was often limited to a small sample set collected during a single doctor's visit. Through access to a broad range of data, healthcare professionals can more accurately diagnose their patients and supply them with better preventative care methods. With use of big data, the healthcare industry would have the potential to make major advances in overall health benefits. If a healthcare provider was able to monitor biosensors in real time and identify warning signs of illness or disease, the potential to increase the average life expectancy of their patients exists. That would directly influence insurance and healthcare costs in a positive manner. With additional preventative data, the early stage preventative treatments would be significantly lower than the treatment costs for a disease recognized at a later stage.

Issues and Limitations of Wearable Devices

Currently, companies are developing products for specialization and industrial uses. For example, Biostrap is a technological company that has developed a wearable wristband. This wristband has many healthcare capabilities including: sleep and activity monitoring, heart and respiratory rates assessment, and oxygen saturation monitoring (Biostrap, 2019). They have partnered with Wavelet Health to conduct industry analysis and develop cloud-based computing that provides a private network for users to share data with healthcare professionals and trainers. Wavelet Health's website states that "[r]aw and processed, time-series sensor data is accessible at any time via our web application. Data can also be easily extracted and uploaded into other data management systems" (Wavelet Health, 2019). This represents the direction that healthcare is headed. The changes are both beneficial and potentially damaging considering security and privacy of patients' healthcare records.

Wearable devices have gained popularity, especially within the U.S. In a 2016 article in Forbes, Paul Lamkin suggests the market for wearable technology will double by the year of 2022. He cites that there is "critical mass adoption" taking place across the U.S. and it is becoming a staple in the American society. Lamkin (2017) also reports that a report from Forrester predicts the market for wearable technology will grow from a $4.8 billion business to $9 billion during the year of 2022 alone (Lamkin, 2017).

Privacy and confidentiality must be considered when implementing wearable technology for healthcare purposes. In 2015, there was a national security breach in health systems where 112 million patient records went missing, were stolen, or improperly disclosed (Blau, 2017). This is a major issue with this technology when used for healthcare. Since healthcare providers are developing wearable devices and establishing networks, privacy issues fall under the purview of Health Insurance Portability and Accountability Act of 1996 (HIPAA) and its privacy laws. HIPAA is United States legislation that provides data privacy and security provisions for safeguarding medical information. Jack Malloy, Vice President of Henry Ford Health System, says "any device that connects to our network has to have some authentication code… If a hacker got that, there's a potential to get into our network and insert malware" (Blau, 2017).

Wearable devices have great potential in healthcare for monitoring and evaluating a person's health and vitals. It is important to note that the data acquired by the device may be skewed or altered based upon how it sits on a patient's wrist or how it is worn. Today most wearable devices are smartwatches or fitness watches that monitor heart rate, number and type of steps taken (e.g. flights of stairs or cardio actions). They are connected to other devices, typically a mobile phone.

Users must be conscientious of the privacy of their data and its accuracy. Walker et al. (2016) discuss the use of these devices with cancer survivors and state that, "if survivors use devices that dramatically underestimate activity and energy expenditure, they may overcompensate by over exercising and risk exhaustion or injury. Over estimation of total energy expenditure could also lead survivors to reduce activity levels and adherence to activity prescriptions" (Walker, Hickey, & Freedson, 2016). The idea that wearable devices are completely accurate or may be subject to inaccuracies may lead to real health issues and the implications could lead to discomfort, injuries or reinjury for the patient.

USE CASES OF EMERGING DIGITAL HEALTH TECHNOLOGY

In addition to telemedicine and wearable devices, there are many emerging digital health technologies available to improve patient care. Several use cases of digital health using the framework of "Prevention/Early Diagnosis," "Intervention," and "Monitoring" follow. This framework is useful to clarify digital health in three segments of patient care and has an impact on pharmaceutical companies.

Use Case: Prevention/Early Diagnosis

IDx-DR: Software Program Powered by Artificial Intelligence to Detect Diabetic Retinopathy

Diabetic retinopathy (DR) primarily causes working-age population's visual loss and blindness. Approximately 24,000 people per year lose their vision in the U.S. alone. To diagnose DR early, it is important for patients to have regular eye examinations, so they can have treatment for DR as soon as possible (Fong, Aiello, Gardner, King, Blankenship, Cavallerano, Ferris, & Klein, 2003; The Centers for Disease Control and Prevention, 2017). However, less than 50% of patients with diabetes regularly visit an eye doctor to have eye examinations in accordance with the recommended schedule and this results in delayed diagnosis, blindness and visual loss (Bragge, Gruen, Chau, Forbes, & Taylor, 2011; The Centers for Disease Control and Prevention, 2011). IDx Technologies, Inc. developed IDx-DR which is a software program powered by artificial intelligence (AI) to detect DR from images of retina without the need for a clinician.

IDx-DR has two core algorithms: 1) Image Quality AI-based Algorithm and 2) Diagnostic Algorithm. The Image Quality AI-based Algorithm works as multiple independent detectors for retinal area validation (Mehta & Rahimy, 2018). The algorithm contributes to detecting sufficient image quality for the Diagnostic Algorithm to identify more than mild DR. Once the digital images of patient's retinas are submitted to a cloud server running IDx-DR, it analyzes the images and provides results in less than a minute.

In the pivotal clinical study of IDx-DR involving 900 patients with diabetes, IDx-DR was 87.4% successful in identifying more than mild DR. and 89.5% successful in identifying patients who did not have more than mild DR as well (Abràmoff, Lavin, Birch, Shah, & Folk, 2018). Based on these results, the FDA approved IDx-DR as the first medical device to use AI to detect more than mild DR in adults with diabetes in April 2018 (FDA News Release, 2018). IDx-DR does not require an eye doctor. Patients can be diagnosed with DR even in primary care offices. If DR is detected by IDx-DR, it will recommend a referral visit for the patient to see an eye doctor for further diagnosis and possible treatment, promptly. IDx-DR is expected to contribute to early diagnosis and reduce the development of blindness or visual loss in patients with diabetes.

Use Case: Intervention

EVO (AKL-T01): Potential Prescription Digital Medicine for the Treatment of Pediatric Attention Deficit/ Hyperactivity Disorder (ADHD)

An American start-up company, Akili Interactive Labs, Inc., has been developing a therapeutic video game called EVO (AKL-T01) designed to cure cognitive conditions including attention deficit hyperactivity disorder (ADHD) and Alzheimer's disease. In this game, a user navigates an alien avatar down a course by inclining a mobile device such as an iPad or smartphone back and forth and responds to targets by tapping the screen. Dr. Adam Gazzaley, a neuroscientist at the University of California San Francisco, and colleagues discovered that people can improve concentration power by playing challenging video games (Anguera, Boccanfuso, Rintoul, Al-Hashimi, Faraji, Janowich, Kong, Larraburo, Rolle, Johnston, & Gazzaley, 2013). Dr. Gazzaley and his team trained elderly people aged 60 to 85 with the game Neuro Racer. In the multitasking version of the game, players are required to quickly press the key or controller if they notice that a green sign appears on roadside, while simulating driving a winding road. For comparison, another group was given the single task version of the game that eliminates a winding street and only requests reaction to the green sign.

The group who received the multitasking version training evenly for a total of 12 hours doubled their efficiency of switching concentration compared to their staring levels. This means they achieved great improvement. Later their efficiency was comparable to those in their twenties who were not trained in Neuro Racer. The test group remained in an improved condition after six months. Also, this multitasking group showed unexpected brain improvement. Their ability to concentrate and their short-term memory also improved. Training was not aimed at improving these functions, but these effects appeared. In contrast, people who trained in the single task version improved their ability to detect signatures, but the efficacy did not affect their short-term memory or concentration levels.

Similar technologies have been used in for the treatment of ADHD. The video game, Evolution Championship Series (*Evo AKL-T01*) stimulates the target cognitive nervous systems in the prefrontal cortex, which is the front part of the brain known to be deficient in ADHD. In the proof of concept study, EVO improved the Attention Performance Index in pediatric patients with ADHD (Davis, Bower, & Kollins, 2018). Since EVO contributes to treatment of ADHD directly, it would be classified as digital therapeutics and this technology surely competes with pharmaceutical products. This could have a big impact on pharmaceutical companies.

Use Case: Monitoring

Recently, various types of wearable devices have been launched to monitor patients' vital signs. Apple Watch is one of them. Apple Watch is a waterproofed smart watch with a heart rate sensor. Its sensor detects heart rate (HR) and heart rhythm using green LED lights flashing hundreds of times per second. A light-sensitive photodiode senses the amount of blood flowing through the blood vessel of the wrist

(Apple Inc., 2017). Subsequently, when the sensor collects signals from four locations on the wrist and combines these with software algorithms, Apple Watch detects heart rhythms distinguishable from other noises. According to research assessing the accuracy of seven commercially available wrist-worn devices in estimating heart rate (HR), Apple Watch achieved the lowest overall error in HR (Shcherbina et al., 2017).

In 2017, Apple launched the Apple Heart Study app to collect data on irregular heart rhythms and notify users who may be experiencing atrial fibrillation (AFib). AFib causes about 130,000 deaths and 750,000 hospitalizations in the U.S. every year, but AFib often goes undiagnosed because many people do not feel any symptoms (Apple Inc., 2017). If Apple Watch detects AFib using the sensor and app, it contributes to early diagnosis and treatment which could significantly result in healthcare cost reduction. In 2018, Apple announced that the FDA-approved two new technologies for Apple Watch. One is a technology to monitor heart activities called an electrocardiogram, and the other is the technology to detect and notify the user of an irregular heart rhythm. Moreover, Apple has been granted a patent for a wearable blood pressure monitor in 2018 (Sullivan et al., 2018). This means that Apple clearly tries to make Apple Watch a wearable healthcare device and Apple is diving into the healthcare industry. Apple's movement and its products could have an impact on other healthcare competitors in the near future.

GOVERNMENT REGULATIONS RELATED TO TELEMEDICINE

Since telemedicine has the potential to contribute to health maintenance, enhancement, and healthcare cost reduction, the government is boosting digital health, which includes telemedicine through regulations. The Center for Devices and Radiological Health (CDRH) of the U.S. Food and Drug Administration launched the Digital Health Innovation Action Plan in 2017 (U.S. Food and Drug Administration, 2017). The purpose of this plan is to find ways to ensure that all Americans, including patients, consumers and other medical clients have access to high quality, safe, and effective digital health products. The FDA has the following vision to promote digital health innovation while continuing to protect and promote public health:

- Issuing guidance to provide clarity on medical software provisions of the 21st Century Cures legislation;
- Launching an innovative pilot precertification program to work with customers to develop a new approach to digital health technology oversight,
- Building FDA's bench strength and expertise in CDRH's digital health unit.

Then, FDA launched a guide "Software as a Medical Device (SaMD): Clinical Evaluation - Guidance for Industry and Food and Drug Administration Staff" in December 2017. The guide utilizes SaMD clinical evaluation principles and recommendations issued by the International Medical Device Regulators Forum (IMDRF). U.S. regulators intend to use this guide as a basis for developing more specific SaMD clinical evaluation guidance in the future. In addition, the guide suggests that SaMD developers monitor safety, effectiveness and performance on a continuous basis via their products' in-depth levels of connectivity. These regulation supports will help the development of digital health and the future healthcare revolution (Eisenhart, 2019).

IMPLICATIONS AND FUTURE DIRECTION OF TELEMEDICINE

Telemedicine is already having positive impacts on improving access to healthcare for the current population. Telemedicine is much cheaper than office visits; logging on to check a patient health survey or reply to a patient question via email is much quicker than physically checking in and meeting with multiple patients. This has resulted in a reduction in healthcare costs, which has convinced the government that this is something worth supporting. Legislation has been passed to make it easier for doctors licensed in one state to treat patients virtually in other states. It has also made it easier for physicians to share information and quickly diagnose patients. According to the Public Health Institute, all 50 states and Washington, D.C. provide reimbursement for some form of live video in Medicaid fee-for-service (Public Health Institute, 2018).

In the next six years the global telemedicine market is expected to reach $93.45 billion (MarketWatch, 2018). The possibilities for this technology's success are unprecedented. In the future, virtual hospitals or the use of voice recognition devices such as Alexa or app like Siri to will be used to diagnose patients' symptoms. A person who is not feeling well and is unsure whether to go to an urgent care will be able to say " Hey, Alexa" and describe the condition. From there Alexa, or a different artificial intelligence robot, will be able to research the severity of the symptoms and from there diagnose or have the person get to a physical physician right away. The AI robot can make the appointment or run through a prescription at a local pharmacy. Eventually, artificial intelligence will be extended to the examining room. The idea centers around the machine "listening", understanding and notating the conversation between the patient and the doctor, which will decrease time spent in the hospital. Doctors nowadays spend an extraordinarily large amount of time writing down notes between and during patient visits.

A new concept in the works, virtual hospitals, has been gaining increasing attention. According to Forrester Research, 55 percent of healthcare organizations are making a new investment or increasing funds in virtual care technologies, which they view as crucial to patient acquisition and retention (Boulton, 2018). The virtual hospital has no beds. Doctors and nurses will see their patients through a computer screen that will display patient data and list problems it thinks doctors should monitor. Keeping patients out of the physical hospital can assist in reducing hospitalizations for patients who have chronic diseases. When their bodies are fragile and susceptible to germs in the hospital, these people can avoid the consequences of exposure by staying in their home.

Millennials are especially open to telemedicine, 74 percent said they would prefer to see a doctor virtually (Pennic, 2015). In another study, 40 percent reported that telemedicine is an extremely or very important option to have in their health care coverage. To attract and retain millennials, it is critical that companies partner with a health plan that offers telemedicine. Millennials are not the only relevant age group. In the next 30 years, the number of people aged 60 and older is expected to increase from 605 million to 2 billion. One of the main beneficiaries of telemedicine will be this group of population. Companies like Comarch, American Well, and Global Med are building doctor video chat programs targeted at the elderly (Sanyal, 2018). With access to routine care, mental health visits, diagnose-related inquiries, and reduced costs, telemedicine will outpace outpatient care.

Wearable devices, while convenient and helpful, may provide another avenue for hackers to get control of data or privacy within the cloud between patient and practitioner. The privacy infringement and security of private, confidential patient data is very important and could slow the implementation of wearable devices within the healthcare industry. What is important here is that the information is very sensitive and important and must be protected by the healthcare network and healthcare providers such as hospitals and physicians. While telemedicine and wearables are convenient and may prevent many serious issues within the patient's life, the privacy and security of their health records are very important as well. Both areas are essential for future research and improvement.

CONCLUSION

Telemedicine can help reduce health care costs by decreasing the number of people who attend avoidable office visits, readmissions, and by providing easier access to routine care. Cost-benefit analysis is a great tool to determine how well the return offsets funding needed for research and development. Cost-benefit analysis of telemedicine shows the benefits in the long term will provide economic viability. There is a huge barrier to entry with telemedicine, requiring an investment in IS infrastructure and employee training. Organizations would need to pay special attention to the systems that are storing the files.

With many evolving and developing technologies, there are benefits and limitations that may project or impair the growth of the technology. Wearable devices have many benefits that could revolutionize the healthcare industry and make it more of a cohesive and integrated system. The convenience of wearable technology can benefit not only the patient but the practitioner as well by limiting administrative and medical costs as well as providing real time data on the patient for the practitioner to analyze without a waiting period. The practitioner can limit required visits for patients as they will be able to closely monitor the patient's health status by utilizing the data generated by these devices. That convenience comes at a cost. The privacy and security of the patient's information may be a problem with the technology moving forward. It is important that healthcare companies and technology companies work closely to develop a secure network in which to house and share patient data from the device to the practitioner. The transfer of information is at risk of being interrupted or stolen by hackers. Wearable devices and technology have real potential to be successful recreationally, for fitness, and in healthcare. The healthcare industry, being one of the biggest industries in many countries, is accelerating the speed of technology evolution day by day. Digital health could be a main driver of the healthcare revolution. Medical care could be transferred from acute care to preventive care and health management. Today, patients receive medical care at a hospital or a clinic. However, medical venues could become our homes or offices due to the advent of digital health technologies such as wearable devices, and telemedicine. Not only pharmaceutical products but also digital therapeutics could become an option in medical treatment. Patients and practitioners will seek the most appropriate medicine from a wider array of options. IT companies have begun to move into healthcare to act as suppliers for traditional players including hospitals, payers, pharmaceutical companies. However, IT companies are not stopping here. Some have begun to provide patients with medical care.

The healthcare revolution could become a threat to many pharmaceutical companies because the pharmaceutical market could shrink due to preventive medical care and early diagnosis driven by digital health. Digital therapeutics could compete with pharmaceutical products. However, the healthcare revolution could also provide opportunities for pharmaceutical companies. To make good use of these opportunities, pharmaceutical companies should innovate with digital health technology through partnerships with IT companies and become total solution providers in the healthcare industry.

REFERENCES

Abràmoff, M. D., Lavin, P. T., Birch, M., Shah, N., & Folk, J. C. (2018). Pivotal trial of an autonomous AI-based diagnostic system for detection of diabetic retinopathy in primary care offices. *npj Digital Medicine*, *1*(39), 1-8.

Anguera, J. A., Boccanfuso, J., Rintoul, J. L., Al-Hashimi, O., Faraji, F., Janowich, J., ... Gazzaley, A. (2013). Video game training enhances cognitive control in older adults. *Nature*, *501*(7465), 97–101. doi:10.1038/nature12486 PMID:24005416

Apple Inc. (2017). Apple Heart Study launches to identify irregular heart rhythms. Retrieved from https://www.apple.com/newsroom/2017/11/apple-heart-study-launches-to-identify-irregular-heart-rhythms/

Biostrap. (2019). Hack your health: Biostrap helps you measurably improve your sleep, recovery, and performance. Retrieved from https://biostrap.com/

Blau, M. (2017). Health wearables raise new privacy concerns. *The Boston Globe*. Retrieved from https://www.bostonglobe.com/business/2017/08/09/health-wearables-raise-new-privacy-concerns/0W2X9iNuLttoa7dUTFTzLJ/story.html

Boulton, C. (2018). Virtual healthcare gets real, as telehealth turns to AI. *CIO*. Retrieved from https://www.cio.com/article/3321736/health-care-industry/virtual-healthcare-gets-real-as-telehealth-turns-to-ai.html

Bragge, P., Gruen, R. L., Chau, M., Forbes, A., & Taylor, H. R. (2011). Screening for presence or absence of diabetic retinopathy: A meta-analysis. *Archives of Ophthalmology*, *129*(4), 435–444. doi:10.1001/archophthalmol.2010.319 PMID:21149748

Davis, N. O., Bower, J., & Kollins, S. H. (2018). Proof-of-concept study of an at-home, engaging, digital intervention for pediatric ADHD. *PLoS One*, *13*(1). doi:10.1371/journal.pone.0189749 PMID:29324745

Dullet, N. W., Geraghty, E. M., Kaufman, T., Kissee, J. L., King, J., Dharmar, M., ... Marcin, J. P. (2017). Impact of a university-based outpatient telemedicine program on time savings, travel costs, and environmental pollutants. *Value in Health*, *20*(4), 542–546. doi:10.1016/j.jval.2017.01.014 PMID:28407995

Eastwood, B. (2012). 10 ways telemedicine is changing healthcare IT. *CIO*. Retrieved from https://www.cio.com/article/2390576/healthcare/10-ways-telemedicine-is-changing-healthcare-it.html

Eisenhart, S. (2019). Final guidance from US FDA on clinical evaluation of software as a medical device (SaMD). *Emergo*. Retrieved from https://www.emergobyul.com/blog/2017/12/final-guidance-us-fda-clinical-evaluation-software-medical-device-samd

FDA News Release. (2018). FDA permits marketing of artificial intelligence-based device to detect certain diabetes-related eye problems. Retrieved from https://www.fda.gov/NewsEvents/Newsroom/PressAnnouncements/ucm604357.htm

Fong, D. S., Aiello, L., Gardner, T. W., King, G. L., Blankenship, G., Cavallerano, J. D., ... Klein, R. (2003). Diabetic retinopathy. *Diabetes Care*, *26*(1), 226–229. doi:10.2337/diacare.26.1.226 PMID:12502685

Grace College. (2019). Rapid Growth: The past, present and future of wearable technology. Retrieved from https://online.grace.edu/news/business/the-past-present-future-of-wearable-technology/

Health Resources & Services Administration. (2019). Telehealth programs. Retrieved from https://www.hrsa.gov/rural-health/telehealth/index.html

Igoe, K. (2017). Mental health on the line: use of telemedicine for mental health in rural areas on the rise but uneven. Retrieved from https://hms.harvard.edu/news/mental-health-line

Kaltenbach, T. (2016). Digital and disrupted: All change for healthcare. *Roland Berger Publication: Think Act*. Retrieved from https://www.rolandberger.com/de/Publications/Digital-and-disrupted-All-change-for-healthcare.html

Kimball, T. G. (2018). How wearable technology changes our approach to healthcare. *MAP Health Management*. Retrieved from https://thisismap.com//insights/map-blog/how-wearable-technology-changes-our-approach-healthcare

Lamkin, P. (2016). Wearable tech market to be worth $34 billion by 2020. *Forbes*. Retrieved from https://www.forbes.com/sites/paullamkin/2016/02/17/wearable-tech-market-to-be-worth-34-billion-by-2020/#67333e973cb5

Lamkin, P. (2017). Smartwatch sales to double in next 5 years. *Forbes*. Retrieved from https://www.forbes.com/sites/paullamkin/2017/11/29/smartwatch-sales-to-double-in-next-5-years/#2a7c2b8d35ed

Lapowsky, I. (2017). The VA's new app tries to reach vets wherever they live. *Wired*. Retrieved from https://www.wired.com/story/va-video-telemedicine-app/

Lewis, J. E., & Neider, M. B. (2017). Designing wearable technology for an aging population. *Ergonomics in Design*, *25*(3), 4–10. doi:10.1177/1064804616645488

MarketWatch. (2018). The global telemedicine market is accounted for $21.56 billion in 2017 and is expected to reach $93.45 billion by 2026 growing at a CAGR of 17.7% during the forecast period. *PRNewswire*. Retrieved from https://www.marketwatch.com/press-release/the-global-telemedicine-market-is-accounted-for-2156-billion-in-2017-and-is-expected-to-reach-9345-billion-by-2026-growing-at-a-cagr-of-177-during-the-forecast-period-2018-08-30

McGinnis, J. M., Russo, P. M., & Knickman, J. R. (2002). The case for more active policy attention to health promotion. *Health Affairs*, *21*(2), 78–93. doi:10.1377/hlthaff.21.2.78 PMID:11900188

Mehta, N., & Rahimy, E. (2018). Artificial intelligence for automated detection of diabetic retinopathy. Retina Roundup. Retrieved from https://retinaroundup.com/2018/06/08/artificial-intelligence-for-automated-detection-of-diabetic-retinopathy/

Mousseau, S., Lapointe, A., & Gravel, J. (2018). Diagnosing acute otitis media using a smartphone otoscope; a randomized controlled trial. *The American Journal of Emergency Medicine*, *36*(10), 1796–1801. doi:10.1016/j.ajem.2018.01.093 PMID:29544905

Munie, K., & Thakur, S. (2017). Digital affect ability: Therapeutic lens on value. *Accenture Strategy*. Retrieved from https://www.accenture.com/t20170321T020154__w__/ie-en/_acnmedia/PDF-47/Accenture-Strategy-Digital-Affectability-PoV.pdf

Office of Public and Intergovernmental Affairs. (2018). VA expands telehealth by allowing health care providers to treat patients across state lines. Retrieved from https://www.va.gov/opa/pressrel/pressrelease.cfm?id=4054

Pennic, F. (2015). 66% of Americans would use mobile health apps to manage their health. *HIT Consultant.* Retrieved from https://hitconsultant.net/2015/02/24/66-of-americans-would-use-mobile-health-apps/#.XGxlKeRKiUk

Public Health Institute. (2018). State telehealth laws and reimbursement program policies. Retrieved from http://www.phi.org/resources/?resource=state-telehealth-laws-and-medicaid-program-policies

Rupp, S. (2017). A quick look at the history of telemedicine. Retrieved from https://www.nuemd.com/news/2017/01/04/quick-look-history-telemedicine

Sanyal, S. (2018). 5 surprising ways in which telemedicine is revolutionizing healthcare. *Forbes.* Retrieved from https://www.forbes.com/sites/shourjyasanyal/2018/10/31/5-surprising-ways-in-which-telemedicine-is-revolutionizing-healthcare/#68a924e156be

Schroeder, S. A. (2007). We can do better - Improving the health of the American people. *The New England Journal of Medicine, 357*(12), 1221–1228. doi:10.1056/NEJMsa073350 PMID:17881753

Shane, L., III. (2018). VA: Suicide rate for younger veterans increased by more than 10 percent. *Military Times.* Retrieved from https://www.militarytimes.com/news/pentagon-congress/2018/09/26/suicide-rate-spikes-among-younger-veterans/

Shcherbina, A., Mattsson, M. C., Waggott, D., Salisbury, H., Christle, J. W., Hastie, T., ... Ashley, E. A. (2017). Accuracy in wrist-worn, sensor-based measurements of heart rate and energy expenditure in a diverse cohort. *Journal of Personalized Medicine, 7*(2), 1–12. doi:10.3390/jpm7020003 PMID:28538708

Sullivan, T. J., Karaki, H. S., Kimoto, R. C., Koch, R. H., Harrison-Noonan, T. J., & Montgomery, R. K. (2018). Cuff designs and methods. *United States Patent application publication.* Retrieved from http://pdfaiw.uspto.gov/.aiw?docid=20180153418

The Centers for Disease Control and Prevention. (2011). *National diabetes fact sheet, 2011.* Retrieved from https://www.cdc.gov/diabetes/pubs/pdf/ndfs_2011.pdf

The Centers for Disease Control and Prevention. (2017). *Diabetes Report Card 2017.* U.S. Department of Health and Human Services. Retrieved from https://www.cdc.gov/diabetes/pdfs/library/diabetesreportcard2017-508.pdf

The Military Time. (2019). Commandos to counselors: A response to the special operations forces mental health crisis. Retrieved from https://www.militarytimes.com/opinion/commentary/2019/02/14/commandos-to-counselors-a-response-to-the-special-operations-forces-mental-health-crisis/

U.S. Food and Drug Administration. (2017). Digital health innovation action plan. Retrieved from https://www.fda.gov/downloads/medicaldevices/digitalhealth/ucm568735.pdf

Walker, R., Hickey, A., & Freedson, P. (2016). Advantages and Limitations of Wearable Activity Trackers: Considerations for Patients and Clinicians. *Clinical Journal of Oncology Nursing*, *20*(6), 606–610. doi:10.1188/16.CJON.606-610 PMID:27857250

Wavelet Health. (2019). Technology: A fundamentally different approach. Retrieved from https://wavelethealth.com/technology/#data

ADDITIONAL READING

Aas, E. (2017). Prepare providers for telemedicine: 3 critical training areas. Retrieved June 2, 2019 from *Managed Healthcare Executive*: http://managedhealthcareexecutive.modernmedicine.com/managed-healthcare-executive/news/prepare-providers-telemedicine-3-critical-training-areas

Addady, M. (2016). A new study of telemedicine services finds bad diagnoses. Retrieved June 5, 2019 from *Fortune*: http://fortune.com/2016/05/16/telemedicine-services/

Akiyama, M., & Byung-Kwang, Y. (2016). A Systematic review of the economic evaluation of telemedicine in Japan. *Journal of Preventive Medicine and Public Health*, *49*(4), 183–196. doi:10.3961/jpmph.16.043 PMID:27499161

Bhardwaj, R., Nambiar, A., & Dutta, D. (2017). A study of machine learning in healthcare. Proceedings of *2017 IEEE 41st Annual Computer Software and Applications Conference*, Torino, Italy: IEEE Computer Society, 236-241. 10.1109/COMPSAC.2017.164

Chang, J., Savage, S. J., & Waldman, D. M. (2017). Estimating willingness to pay for online health services with discrete-choice experiments. *Applied Health Economics and Health Policy*, *15*(4), 491–500. doi:10.100740258-017-0316-z PMID:28290107

Chen, J. (2017). Playing to our human strengths to prepare medical students for the future. *Korean Journal of Medical Education*, *29*(3), 193–197. doi:10.3946/kjme.2017.65 PMID:28870022

Cilliers, L. (2014). Using the cloud to provide telemedicine services in a developing country. *South African Journal of Information Management*, *16*(1), 1–7. doi:10.4102ajim.v16i1.611

Daugherty Douglas, M., Xu, J., Heggs, A., Wrenn, G., Mack, D., & Rust, G. (2016). Assessing telemedicine utilization by using Medicaid claims data. *Psychiatric Services (Washington, D.C.)*, *68*(2), 173–178. doi:10.1176/appi.ps.201500518 PMID:27691381

De Cnudde, S., Martens, D., & Provost, F. (2018). An exploratory study towards applying and demystifying deep learning classification on behavioral big data. *University of Antwerp Working Paper*, 1-32.

Dinesen, B., Nonnecke, B., Lindeman, D., Toft, E., Kidholm, K., Jethwani, K., ... Nesbitt, T. (2016). Personalized telehealth in the future: A global research agenda. *Journal of Medical Internet Research*, *18*(3), 1–31. doi:10.2196/jmir.5257 PMID:26932229

Gheorghe, M. (2014). Mobile cloud computing for telemedicine solutions. *Informações Econômicas*, *18*(4), 50–61. doi:10.12948/issn14531305/18.4.2014.05

Hoyt, R., Snider, D., Thompson, C., & Mantravadi, S. (2016). IBM Watson Analytics: Automating visualization, descriptive, and predictive statistics. *JMIR Public Health and Surveillance*, *2*(2), 1–27. doi:10.2196/publichealth.5810 PMID:27729304

Jo, S. M., & Chung, K. Y. (2015). Design of access control system for telemedicine secure XML documents. *Multimedia Tools and Applications*, *74*(4), 2257–2271. doi:10.100711042-014-1938-x

Khanna, S., Sattar, A., & Hansen, D. (2013). Artificial intelligence in health – the three big challenges. *The Australasian Medical Journal*, *6*(5), 315–317. doi:10.4066/AMJ.2013.1758 PMID:23745154

Lafolla, T. (2017). *History of Telemedicine Infographic*. Retrieved June 5, 2019 from *eVisit*: http://blog.evisit.com/history-telemedicine-infographic

Marshall, D. A., Burgos-Liz, L., Pasupathy, K. S., Padula, W. V., IJzerman, M. J., Wong, P. K., ... Osgood, N. D. (2016). Transforming healthcare delivery: Integrating dynamic simulation modelling and big data in health economics and outcomes research. *PharmacoEconomics*, *34*(2), 115–126. doi:10.100740273-015-0330-7 PMID:26497003

Maxmen, A. (2018). *Deep learning sharpens views of cells and genes*. Retrieved June 4, 2019 from *Scientific American*: https://www.scientificamerican.com/article/deep-learning-sharpens-views-of-cells-and-genes/

Michaud, T. L., Zhou, J., McCarthy, M. A., Siahpush, M., & Su, D. (2018). Costs of home-based telemedicine programs: A systematic review. *International Journal of Technology Assessment in Health Care*, *34*(4), 410–418. doi:10.1017/S0266462318000454 PMID:30058505

Panlaqui, O., Broadfield, E., Champion, R., Edington, J., & Kennedy, S. (2017). Outcomes of telemedicine intervention in a regional intensive care unit: A before and after study. *Australian Society of Anaesthetists*, *45*(5), 605–610. PMID:28911290

Pegah, N. B., Mahdavi, M., Shahram, E. B., & Arasteh, S. (2018). Security analysis of a key based color image watermarking vs. a non-key based technique in telemedicine applications. *Multimedia Tools and Applications*, *77*(24), 31713–31735. doi:10.100711042-018-6218-8

Pham, T., Tran, T., Phung, D., & Venkatesh, S. (2017). Predicting healthcare trajectories from medical records: A deep learning approach. *Journal of Biomedical Informatics*, *69*, 218–229. doi:10.1016/j.jbi.2017.04.001 PMID:28410981

Razzak, M., Naz, S., & Zaib, A. (2017). *Deep learning for medical image processing: overview, challenges and future*. Retrieved June 5, 2019 from arXiv: https://arxiv.org/ftp/arxiv/papers/1704/1704.06825.pdf

Saigi-Rubió, F., Jiménez-Zarco, A., & Torrent-Sellens, J. (2016). Determinants of the intention to use telemedicine: Evidence from primary physicians. *International Journal of Technology Assessment in Health Care*, *32*(2), 29–36. doi:10.1017/S0266462316000015 PMID:27472158

Sims, J. M. (2018). Communities of practice: Telemedicine and online medical communities. *Technological Forecasting and Social Change*, *126*(C), 53–63. doi:10.1016/j.techfore.2016.08.030

Srivastava, S., Soman, S., & Rai, A., Srivastava, & Praveen. (2017). Deep learning for health informatics: recent trends and future directions. *Proceedings of 2017 International Conference on Advances in Computing, Communications and Informatics (ICACCI)*, Udupi, India. DOI: 10.1109/ICACCI.2017.8126082

KEY TERMS AND DEFINITIONS

Accessibility: The availability of good health services within reasonable reach of those who need them and of opening hours, appointment systems and other aspects of service organization and delivery that allow people to obtain the services when they need them.

Affordability: A measure of people's ability to pay for services without financial hardship. It considers not only the price of the health services but also indirect and opportunity costs such as the costs of transportation to and from facilities and of taking time away from work.

Affordable Care Act (ACA): The comprehensive health care reform law enacted in the U.S. in March 2010, sometimes known as ACA, PPACA, or "Obamacare". The law has 3 primary goals: make affordable health insurance available to more people; expand the Medicaid program to cover all adults with income below 138% of the federal poverty level; and, support innovative medical care delivery methods designed to lower the costs of health care generally.

Artificial Intelligence: The theory and development of computer systems able to perform tasks normally requiring human intelligence, such as visual perception, speech recognition, decision-making, and translation between languages.

Digital Health: The convergence of digital technologies with health, healthcare, living, and society to enhance the efficiency of healthcare delivery and make medicines more personalized and precise.

Digital Therapeutics: A health discipline and treatment option that utilizes a digital and often online health technologies to treat a medical or psychological condition.

Health Insurance Portability and Accountability Act (HIPAA): A U.S. federal law enacted in 1996 that protects continuity of health coverage when a person changes or loses a job, that limits health-plan exclusions for preexisting medical conditions, that requires that patient medical information be kept private and secure, that standardizes electronic transactions involving health information, and that permits tax deduction of health insurance premiums by the self-employed.

Information Accessibility: The right of a patient to seek, receive and impart information and ideas concerning health issues. This access to information, however, should not impair the right to have personal health data treated with confidentiality.

Privacy: Medical privacy or health privacy is the practice of maintaining the security and confidentiality of patient records. It involves both the conversational discretion of health care providers and the security of medical records.

Smartwatch: A smartwatch is a wearable computer in the form of a wristwatch. Modern smartwatches provide a local touchscreen interface for daily use, while an associated smartphone app provides for management and telemetry such as long-term biomonitoring.

Telemedicine: Telemedicine is the use of telecommunication and information technology to provide clinical health care from a distance. It has been used to overcome distance barriers and to improve access to medical services that would often not be consistently available in distant rural communities.

Wearable Devices: A wearable device is a technology that is worn on the human body. Wearable devices are also known as wearable gadgets, wearable technology or simply wearables.

Chapter 2
Web-Based Information for Patients and Providers

Izabella Lejbkowicz
Independent Researcher, Israel

ABSTRACT

The exponential development of Information Technologies revolutionized healthcare. A significant aspect of this revolution is the access to health information in the Internet. The Internet World Stats estimates that 56.8% of the world population used the Internet in March 2019, an increase of 1,066% from 2000. According to The Pew Research Center survey of 2012 81% of Americans used the internet and 72% of them searched for health information. Even though there is a lack in more recent data on the percentage of online health information seekers, it is clear that this trend is on the rise. This chapter focuses on the characteristics of the search for online health information by patients and providers, investigates features related to the quality of health web sites, and discusses the impact of these searches on healthcare.

OVERVIEW

The following chapter provides a review of the current literature on online healthcare information and its nexus to empowerment. More than ever, patients have new mechanisms to become informed about their conditions and treatment options. Providers bear a responsibility to understand and support emerging needs that may be driven by both underlying human psychology and by limited access to healthcare. The reader is presented herein to an interesting compilation of how the world wide web, social media, health informatics, AI, automated search tools and other technologies both promote and inhibit patient empowerment from a conceptual standpoint. The chapter concludes with a call to action echoed by many physicians: How can we ensure patients have available, reliable, high-quality health information that contributes to their empowerment?

DOI: 10.4018/978-1-7998-0047-7.ch002

Characteristics of Patients' Online Search of Health Information

The number of Internet users worldwide has been estimated as 4.4 billion in March 2019, representing 56.8% of the world population- an increase of 1,114% since year 2000 (Miniwatts Marketing Group, 2019). The main factors considered as contributors to this increase were the reduced computers prices, the increased usage of smartphones, and the broad access to the Internet in public places.

Alongside the increase in Internet usage, the percentage of population seeking online for health information also has enlarged. The US nationwide 2012 Pew Research survey reported that 72% of Internet users in America searched for health information (Fox & Duggan, 2013). This high percentage emphasizes the importance of characterizing the online search of health information and understanding its effects on healthcare.

Regarding the topics of most interest among online health information seekers, the 2012 Pew Survey reported that 52% of them were looking for information about specific diseases or medical problems, 43% were looking for information related to a specific treatment or medical procedure, 27% searched for weight loss/control and 25% searched for information on medical insurance (Fox & Duggan, 2013).

Several other studies investigated the topics of interest on online searches for health information in specific population groups. Ayakhot and Carolan-Olah (2016) reviewed the literature for quantitative studies of pregnant women searching for pregnancy related online information that were published from 2004 to 2014. In the 7 studies included in their investigation, the most searched topics were: stages of childbirth and fetal development, pregnancy complications, antenatal care and nutrition during pregnancy. Those most likely to search for information were women in their first pregnancy and/or in early pregnancy stages. Regarding demographics, women with higher education, those employed, and those within the age group of 25-34 were most likely to search for information. Frequency of searches varied from once a month to 10 or more a month. This variation may be due to the time gap since the first studies and the last studies investigated, implying in the changes occurred in the frequency of Internet usage.

In another systematic review of health-related Internet use by children and adolescents, researchers analyzed 19 studies selected from major databases across different countries. The results indicate that time spent online on health issues changes with age. Overall, 82.8% of youth in the age range of 11 to 18 years reported 1 to 4 hours/day online (Park & Kwon, 2018). Also, a high frequency of health-related Internet use was reported in all studies. Sixty-four percent of teens aged 10 to 26 in the UK stated they use the Internet every day, and 26% used it at least once or twice a week. In the US, 97% of the participants reported using the Internet at least once a month, with 87% of them reporting usage once a week. Results of most of the studies show that a high percentage of youth use the Internet for health-related purposes and the use is more frequent in teens over 15. The main topics of searches were everyday health-related issues (such as sport injuries, flu, asthma) chronic diseases, physical well-being, sexual health, mental health, social problems, and culturally and religiously sensitive topics. Some evidence suggests that teens avoid searching online for issues that make them feel uneasy. For emotional difficulties they generally opt for help and related information from peers online. Youth with chronic diseases search online information for symptoms and treatments related to their condition. Supportive communities for a specific health condition are well accepted, as well as health-related online activities, including messaging and connecting with others, networking, and receiving information. Notably over 60% preferred an online support group to in-person meetings. A Swedish study of hospitalized diabetic children also indicated interest in using the Internet for support networking and for interpersonal contacts with their nondiabetic peers. (Nordwall, Ekberg, & Bertero, 2013) These results point to the Internet as an important tool in adolescence and early adulthood support.

In yet another study of health information seeking online, Biernatzki et al. (2018) performed a meta-analysis of 25 published studies of the information needs of diabetes mellitus patients. The main topics sought by the patients were 'treatment-process', 'course of disease', 'abnormalities of glucose metabolism', 'diabetes through the life cycle', 'pathophysiology of diabetes', 'research', 'coping', 'support', and 'prevention'. 'Treatment process' searches included questions on 'medication', 'diabetes self-management' and 'nutrition'. The 'course of disease' was the second highest topic reported, particularly searches on the 'consequences of diabetes', including consequences concerning physical health, lifestyle and social life. Four studies reported searches related to 'coping' and 'support', while two reported searches on 'prevention' (Biernatzki et al., 2018). Since this investigation was based on multiple studies, associations between demographics and search topics could not be inferred.

These studies indicate topics that are especially meaningful to patients and therefore are most frequently searched online. Patients no longer wait for information from healthcare providers but instead actively seek the information they need. Health providers therefore should address these topics with their patients and provide them with related reliable sources of information. Appropriate empowerment can only happen when the information is reliable, valid, applicable, correct and relevant to the patient interests.

Patients' Strategies for Searching for Online Health Information

The strategy employed for searching online information may affect the quality of the information retrieved. The 2012 Pew Internet survey reports that 77% of the health information seekers attested to beginning their searches using a general search engine such as Google, Bing, or Yahoo. An additional 13% said they begin their searches at a site that specializes in health information, like WebMD, which are expected to connect the user to links of high quality of health content. Just 2% say they would go to a general site like Wikipedia. Search on social media was reported by 1% of the survey participants. As far as we know, there are no reports of changes in these numbers over time, but additional studies are in need.

The same study suggests using a search engine is associated with being younger. Eighty two percent of online health seekers aged 18 to 29 years old said they used Google, Bing, Yahoo, or another search engine, while only 73% of those age 50 and older reported the use of search engines. These results suggest an association between age and the usage of search engines. Interestingly, the first Pew Internet survey conducted in the year 2000 presented similar results regarding searching habits of the middle-agers.

An additional source of health-related information is social media. With the emergence of Web 2.0, interactive Internet based activities, such as social media, became available. Patients, their proxies and the general public approach social media to seek information, to share experiences, to assist others and to feel supported. (Zhao & Zhang, 2017). While in traditional web sites content is distributed from one source (the site authors) to many receivers (the Internet users), in social media there are many sources and many receivers. Users create their own profile and communicate within online social networks by connecting to other users profiles. Examples of popular social media websites are Facebook, YouTube, Twitter, LinkedIn and Instagram (Wikipedia, 2019). In 2017, 71% of Internet users reported social network usage and this figure is expected to grow. North America ranks first among regions where social media is highly popular, with a social media penetration rate of 66%. In 2016, more than 81% of the United States population had a social media profile (Statista, 2019).

Zhao and Zhang (2017) characterized health-related social media activities in a review of studies published from 2011 to 2016 on health information search on social media. Their results indicated that growing numbers of health information searchers are present on social media, but still less than on the WWW. In most of the studies reviewed, searches focused mainly on specific diseases, and their causes and treatments, similarly to web site searches. Participants of different studies expressed the added benefit of the social support they find in social media, again emphasizing the role of the Internet as a support tool. Others emphasized the significance of exchanging information with people facing similar challenges (Zhao & Zhang, 2017). More research is required in this evolving field.

Quality of Online Health Information

An impediment to empowerment based on knowledge acquisition relates to the quality of information (Akerkar & Bichile, 2004). This is particularly true in healthcare. More than ever, the leading status of the Internet as a source of health-related information stresses the importance of assuring that the information available is trustworthy.

However, assessing the quality of the information presents several challenges. First, the criteria to be analyzed to evaluate the information should be determined. Second, the appropriate methodology to analyze these criteria, taking into consideration both objective and subjective criteria, should be chosen. While reliability of objective criteria can be measured by intra and inter agreement rates, subjective criteria should be tested by determining the agreement among multiple experts. Finally, the assessment of information quality is a manual process, hence it is time expensive. Besides quality considerations, the information must be of value for the patient and fulfill his information needs. In many cases, information's value has to be determined by an expert in the area (Suarez-Almazor, Kendall, & Dorgan, 2001; Visser, Bleijenbergh, Benschop, Riel, & Bloem, 2016).

The development of the WWW in the 1990's and the emergence of broadly available health information were followed by the development of methods to assess the quality of online health information. For example, in 1996 the HON Foundation, a Switzerland non-governmental organization, launched HONcode as an initiative to encourage quality health information on the web. The code evaluates site quality based on eight principles: authority, complementarity, confidentiality, attribution, justifiability, transparency, financial disclosure, and advertising. Web authors can apply for the code seal to the HON Foundation and, if approved, can place it on their homepage (Boyer, Selby, & Appel, 1998).

Studies on the presence and use of the HONcode seal have indicated subject-dependent differences that vary greatly. For instance, Wozney et al. (2018) found that 24% of selected websites on child and adolescent mental health used the seal. Pass et al. (2018) on the other hand, found no use of the seal for selected sites with information on sclerotherapy for venous malformations. Salem et al. (2018) found HONcode coverage on 27% of the most frequented sites for viewing information on bladder cancer. In general, due to the vast number of sites covering health topics, any study includes a very small proportion of the sites available. Therefore, different studies on the same subject may reveal discrepancies on the percentage of HONcode coverage.

The use of HONcode is in general, limited. This may be attributed to several factors. First, due to the voluntary nature of the application for the HONcode seal and potential costs involved in adherence to code requirements, web authors must be highly committed to the quality of information to apply for certification. Second, HONcode identification of trustworthy health websites and follow up of certified sites is limited by the expensive time-consuming procedure of the manual process evaluation by the Foundation staff.

Presently, there are a few tools available to maximize the impact of the HONcode seal. The first tool, the HONcode toolbar extension, allows identification of HONcode certified web sites while browsing, as well as in the search results of the major search-engines, like Google and Bing. The second tool is KConnect. The KConnect search engine was developed under the European Union's Horizon 2020 research and innovation program. KConnect searches within an Internet environment of curated sites with quality information. The third tool is Health Trust Indicator which is a free browser extension that functions as a health search engine. It selects web sites according to quality of content, instead of popularity (Health On the Net Foundation, 2017; Kwag, González-Lorenzo, Banzi, Bonovas, & Moja, 2016).

Several authors have studied the impact of HONcodes on web searches. For example, Corfield et al. (2018) applied the Google search engine embedded with the HONcode toolbar and accessed 1350 Web sites using the keywords "bladder cancer", "ileal conduit" and "orthotopic neobladder" in English, Italian and Spanish. The first 150 results of each search were identified and screened. They found that less than 20% of English, Italian and Spanish "bladder cancer" and urinary diversion ("ileal conduit" and "orthotopic neobladder") websites were HON-accredited. HON-accredited web sites featured preferentially in the first 50 search results for bladder cancer (P=0.0001) and ileal conduit (P=0.03) web sites. Comparing 2016 results to 2009, percentage of HON-accreditation has shown a non-statistically significant decrease of 13% while overall number of search results has increased by 44%. This indicates a proliferation of non-vetted health care information (Corfield et al., 2018).

An additional instrument to assess the quality of written information on treatments in both printed and online forms, DISCERN, was funded by the National Health Service (United Kingdom) in 1999. The first step in the development of DISCERN was the choice by an expert team of the criteria to evaluate health information. In a second step, a national sample of health information providers and self-help group members used these criteria to evaluate a range of consumer health information about treatment choices. The final tool consisted of 3 sections (reliability, quality and overall rating) in a total of 16 questions scored from 1-No, through 5-Yes. (Charnock, Shepperd, Needham, & Gann, 1999). DISCERN was the first standardized quality score of consumer health information that could be used both by health professionals and patients to appraise written information on treatment choices.

A short version, called *Brief DISCERN*, was later developed and validated for sites without treatment related information. It has six items graded on a five-point scale for a maximum score of 30; two of those items involved reliability, while the other four evaluated website content (Tangri & Chande, 2011). A Brief DISCERN score of 16 or more out of 30 indicates good quality (Khazaal et al., 2009).

Recognizing the need to automate the evaluation of online health information, Allam et al. (2017) addressed two key issues essential to construct automated DISCERN classifiers: (1) generation of a robust DISCERN training corpus useful for training classification algorithms, and (2) assessment of the usefulness of the current DISCERN scoring schema as a metric for evaluating the performance of these algorithms (Allam et al., 2017). Studies of automated evaluations were not found when searching PubMed with the term DISCERN.

An additional early system for evaluation of health information sites was established by the Journal of the American Medical Association in 1997. The JAMA benchmark criteria assessed the presence or absence of four elements: authorship, clear attribution with specific references, whether information is up to date (i.e., how recent it was published), and if authors have reported disclosures of conflicts of interest (Silberg, Lundberg, & Musacchio, 1997).

Breckons et al. (2008) investigated questionnaire-based evaluation tools for health web site quality. The authors observed the presence of hundreds of such tools in the literature. They found similarity and high inter-agreement rates among the questionnaires criteria. The majority of questionnaires however, were available online for a limited time window (Breckons et al., 2008).

Besides quality, readability is essential for the comprehension of available information. The NIH recommends reading levels consistent with grade 7 to 8 as appropriate to health web sites for adult consumers. The Flesch reading-ease test (FLESCH, 1948) and the Flesch–Kincaid Grade Level Formula are two standard tests to assess readability in English. In the first, higher scores indicate text that is easier to read; lower numbers mark passages that are more difficult to read. Scores go from 100 to 0. 100-90 is 5th grade level, 50-30 college and under 30 college graduates. The second test presents a score parallel to U.S. school grade levels, making it easier to compare the readability level of texts. If the score result is greater than 10, it can also indicate the number of years of education required to understand the text (Kincaid, Fishburne, Rogers, & Chissom, 1975). Readability tests are available in a few other languages such as READ-IT (Italian), Spaulding, modified Fry graph, and Crawford formula (Spanish), and Lix Readability Formula (Swedish).

Several studies have attempted to employ multiple evaluation systems together to assess website quality. For example, Roughead et al. (2016) assessed the quality of websites with recommendations on pre-operation fasting using the JAMA Benchmark criteria, the DISCERN score, and the HONcode certification. Readability was scored using the Flesch Reading Ease score and Flesch–Kincaid Grade Level. Eighty-seven websites were included in the analysis. More than half these sites (55%) provided at least 1 recommendation that contradicted established guidelines, with websites from health care institutions being most likely to make inaccurate recommendations. Only 17% of websites encouraged preoperative hydration, in spite of its proven benefits. Quality and readability were poor and the HONcode certification was present in 10% of the sites only. Even though Anesthesia Society websites and scientific articles had higher DISCERN scores, readability was lower than websites from health care institutions. These results indicate incongruences between guidelines and online fasting recommendations are frequent and may confuse patients on how to proceed before a surgery, reducing their sense of empowerment and increasing confusion instead.

A study of asthma websites evaluated the quality of the information through the BRIEF DISCERN instrument and by ascertaining the presence of the HONcode seal (Banasiak & Meadows-Oliver, 2017). Readability was assessed by employing Flesch-Kincaid grade level and Flesch reading ease tools using Microsoft Office Word 2013 software. The study included 22 English sites (15 unsponsored and 7 sponsored) found in the first page of searches for the word "asthma" with the most used search engines such as Google and Bing, so to mimic a regular patient search. Sixty-eight percent of the sites scored BRIEF DISCERN scores of 16 and higher. The Flesch-Kincaid grade level scores ranged from 2.9 to 15.4, with an average reading grade score of 9.49 (SD =2.7). Only four of the 22 sites (18%) had reading grade levels below the eighth-grade reading level, as recommended by the NIH. The Flesch reading ease scores ranged from 17 to 82.7, with an average reading ease score of 53.57, while 50-30 is the reading ease score for college educated readers (SD =15.03). Only five sites (22.7%) were HONcode certified. The study indicated higher BRIEF DISCERN scores for unsponsored sites as well as for HONcode certified sites. The results provided evidence of good quality information on sites with BRIEF DISCERN score over 16 and the HONcode seal. However, the study was limited by the number of websites investigated. Regarding readability, reading scores demonstrated the information was not at the comprehension level recommended for health consumers (Banasiak & Meadows-Oliver, 2017).

Overall, research suggests that reliable health-related information remains limited and out of reach for many patients. Methods developed over the past years to assure online health information reliability are not currently widespread. No reliable system for rating information and passing that to patients is available to provide enhanced empowerment through increased knowledge (Grando, Rozenblum, & Bates, 2015).

Patients' Reasons for Online Information Searches and Effects on Patient-Provider Relationship

Personal involvement in health increasingly is expected both by patients and by the healthcare system. The advent of health information that is accessible on the Internet is considered as the main trigger for patient demand to take part on medical decision-making regarding his own health.

The increase in the number of patients with chronic diseases together with the high costs associated with the care of these diseases, has induced healthcare management organizations to promote health self-management. Besides the potential of decreasing costs, several studies have demonstrated the benefits of patient engagement and empowerment, including: better adherence to treatment, satisfaction with care, satisfaction with decision-making and improved outcomes (van Dijk, Groenewegen, Rademakers, de Jong, & Brabers, 2017).

However, most physicians were not prepared for this information revolution. From an environment where the physician held the knowledge, hence the power to decide, the informed patient began to demand participation in the decision-making process.

Patients have experienced a variety of reactions to the availability of information online. For example, some well-informed patients omitted the information they found online (Rosis & Barsanti, 2016). In fact, some patients were afraid that their physician would consider that searching for information online meant they lacked confidence in him. As a result, patients were exposed to health information with questionable reliability without discussing the information with their physician.

Health Providers point to lack of time during medical encounters as one of the main reasons they cannot discuss online information assessed by the patients nor indicate reliable online sources of information (Tan & Goonawardene, 2017). However, since well informed, empowered patients can discuss their fears and stress their opinions, enhancing their relationship with their health provider, the availability of reliable information for patients should be considered of interest both for patients and the medical system.

Tan and Goonawardene (2017) reviewed 18 studies that investigated the effects of patient search of online health information on the patient provider relationship. They concluded that most patients gather information to be prepared prior to the medical encounter, even though only some of them will report their findings to the physician. Table 1 summarizes the patient-related and physician-related barriers to patient-provider communication reviewed in the literature (Rosis & Barsanti, 2016; Tan & Goonawardene, 2017).

Sayakhot and Carolan-Olah (2016) concluded in their review of pregnancy-related online information that few women discuss the information collected with their attending providers. This creates a potential for misinformation and needless anxiety about pregnancy.

While the access to health information is believed to contribute to patient empowerment, it has been described to have a negative impact on some people. Information seeking can reach levels beyond the occasional, with excessive and repeated searches that cause increasing levels of health-anxiety. The tendency to conduct obsessive online searches of health information coupled with health anxiety has been coined cyberchondria (Starcevic & Berle, 2013). It is not clear if existing anxiety causes excessive

Table 1. Barriers to discussing retrieved online information with providers

Barriers
Patient-related Barriers: Embarrassment Fear it may interfere with the flow of the consultation Feeling it turns them into problematic patients Feeling strange to ask questions to the doctor
Physician-related Barriers: Feeling disapproved by the Physician Feeling discouraged by the Physician Fear that it may insult the Physician Fear that the Physician may feel challenged Fear that the Physician may feel criticized Feeling that physician dismiss the discussion to assert his authority
Other Barriers: Lack of time during the consultation Forgetfulness

searching or, if the access to health-information leads some patients to high levels of health anxiety and they turn back to the Internet feeling that more information will make them feel secure. In both cases, the number of searches increases with time while they attempt to alleviate their distress. But instead, these behaviors have the opposite effect (Starcevic, 2017).

Even though the name cyberchondria derives from hypochondria, it is not generally accepted as a digital version of the later. Intensive online searches for health information is probably part of a hypochondriac personality. However, the main characteristic of cyberchondria is the excessive amount of time devoted to online information seeking, preventing the affected person from engaging in other normal activities.

In addition to personality traits pre-disposed to high health anxiety, several issues related to online information may trigger anxiety. People may find information confusing, can have difficulties in navigating from site to site, and can feel stressed for not finding the answers for their questions. Research on cyberchondria is still limited. Only one assessment tool was developed so far, the Cyberchondria Severity Scale which takes into consideration dimensions such as compulsion and distress (McElroy & Shevlin, 2014). Additional studies on how to help mediate health anxiety and overcome excessive health information seeking are needed.

Other research suggests people seek online health information due to an increasing difficulty to access healthcare services. Recent research demonstrates that people in Britain are turning to Google instead of seeing a health provider to diagnose medical problems (Tkachenko et al., 2017). Google UK reports that 21.8% of people in 2015 choose to self-diagnose online via search engines, rather than consulting their family, friends or even a professional GP. The main reason for self-diagnosing online, according to the analysis of 61 million Google searches and a survey of 1013 adults, is the difficulty in getting access to medical professionals. The British Medical Association estimates that 20% of the population may be self-diagnosing online today. They believe this phenomenon does not put the public at risk, since they can count with reliable sites from the NHS Direct. The Australian Patients Association expresses an opposite opinion, attesting concerns about self-diagnosis. Inferring from doubtable reliability information without discussing it with a health provider can lead to wrong conclusions and even harming consequences (Tkachenko et al., 2017).

The 2012 Pew Internet Survey reports that 59% of those looking for health information online (35% of all-American adults) stated that they have searched for a medical condition affecting themselves or someone else. The survey investigated participants' steps following their online diagnosis and asked if the search result led them to consider consulting a health professional. Forty-six percent said the condition needed medical attention, 38% said they could care for the condition at home, and 11% answered both ways or none. Regarding confirmation of their diagnosis by a healthcare professional, 41% answered yes, an additional 18% said a healthcare professional either did not agree or offered a different opinion about the condition. 2% said a healthcare professional partially confirmed their diagnosis while 35% said they did not visit a clinician. One percent said their conversation with the health professional was inconclusive and the professional was unable to diagnose them (Fox & Duggan, 2013). It should be taken into consideration that the Pew Internet survey was performed a few years ago. However, Internet access and health information searching has increased over these years, while healthcare services have not become easier to access under limited budgets and growing chronic diseases populations. It is expected that the trend reported in the US survey has continued.

In short, the exact reasons behind online self-diagnosis remain to be discovered through research and further study. Researchers suspect it could relate to causes such as cyberchondria or because health care access is limited. But other causes may also exist. Without proper oversight, high-levels of health-related anxiety could lead patients to diagnose themselves online, fearing to go to a physician and to be diagnosed with a serious disease. This appears to have the opposite effect of patient empowerment.

Usage of Patient Data Accumulated During Online Searches

Besides possible positive and negative aspects of online self-diagnosis for the single individual, the collective accumulation of patient symptomology in search engines may become valuable. For example, reported data can be explored with the use of AI techniques to preview a medical condition. Tkachenko et al. (2017) made use of the Experian geodemographic Mosaic dataset to extract variables possibly associated with the risk of Type 2 diabetes and compared their temporal relationships with the search keywords used to describe early symptoms of the disease on Google. Their results indicate that Google Trends has the capability of providing early detection of diabetes 2 by monitoring the presence of combinations of keywords (Tkachenko et al., 2017).

Likewise, online self-diagnosis may improve if we better understand patient differences. For example, patients differ in their attitude regarding involvement in their health-management (van Dijk et al., 2017). Several factors may be associated with patients' positions toward issues such as: patient-provider relationships, health-status, age and health literacy. In a study on Multiple Sclerosis, patients reported differences in patterns of information searching according to their degree of disability. Patients stated that they increased online searches when disease worsens. Higher disability was associated with interest on peers' information about coping strategies with the disease and with interest to communicate with health providers through the Internet. Study participants who reported not searching for information were divided into two groups. In the first group, patients used the Internet but did not search for health-related topics. They stated that the information would stress them. In the second group, some of the patients reported not having an Internet equipped computer to perform the searches. Other patients reported lack of computer literacy (Lejbkowicz, Paperna, Stein, Dishon, & Miller, 2010).

Patients lacking health literacy will probably have more search difficulties in their quest for information about their conditions, and as they attempt to understand medical terms in ways that empower them to feel secure in medical decision participation. van Dijk et al. (2017) studied the association between self-reported participation in medical decisions and health literacy. In the study, health literacy was evaluated with a validated questionnaire. The study results suggest that critical health literacy, i.e. literacy that goes beyond basic text comprehension, is an important factor in medical decision-making involvement. Given the association between health-literacy and improved health outcomes, further research on strategies to increase health literacy should be advanced (Lejbkowicz, Caspi, & Miller, 2012).

Online Information for Healthcare Providers

Medical care has always demanded continuous education for its professionals. New challenges faced by providers are the inspiration for research, leading to new findings and hopefully to solutions to medical problems. While in the past, providers had to keep updated so they could exercise optimal care, recently an additional perspective has been added as patients have access to more information than ever before. Thus, besides the significance of information for the advancement of healthcare practice, it can enhance the patient-provider-relationship and empower both providers and patients

With the advent of the Internet, the publication of information for health providers turned gradually digital. Online information has the potential of being available everywhere, being easy to update, easy to search and generally of free access. Most peer-review medical journals, medical news journals, physicians' manuals and textbooks are currently published online, sometimes coupled to hard copy editions. In addition, healthcare organizations, hospitals, medical schools and medical organizations have web sites oriented to healthcare professionals. Continuing medical education courses are also offered online. A novel technology based on secured data storage and transmission, Blockchain, has the potential to enable improved tracking of course creators, content and participants. Institutions adopting blockchain technology will be able to provide certification and credentialing of health care professionals with no intermediaries. This new technology may be the key to advance online medical education (Funk, Riddell, Ankel, & Cabrera, 2018). Likewise, it may provide advances in patient record management.

A critical time for the provider to obtain reliable and updated information takes place during initial and subsequent encounters with the patient. Hence, information is needed at the point of care. However, to make use of the most updated information, and the ever-expanding medical literature accessible online, providers need tools to accelerate their searches without compromising the quality and the reliability of the information retrieved. Commercial tools have been developed to offer information summaries specifically designed to deliver pre-digested, rapidly accessible, comprehensive, and periodically updated information. These tools are becoming increasingly common and study data suggests that the implementation of such tools may contribute to improved patients outcomes (Isaac, Zheng, & Jha, 2012).

Kwag et. al (2016) investigated commercial tools offering information summaries by searching on Medline, Google, librarian association websites, and conference proceedings from August 2012 to December 2014. Web-based, regularly updated, point-of-care information summaries defined as evidence-based, were retrieved. Data on the general characteristics and content presentation of the products was extracted. Extent of disease coverage, editorial quality, and evidence-based methodology were assessed. From 26 tools screened, a quarter were developed after 2012. Twenty-three products were analyzed in the study for content presentation and quantitative dimensions. It is interesting to note that most summaries were developed by major publishers in the United States and the United Kingdom, but none originated in low-income countries where needs may be the greatest. The main target audience of the tools were physicians. Nurses and physiotherapists were target of a few tools, with an increased proportion over the years. The tools "Best Practice", "Dynamed", and "UptoDate" achieved the highest scores for all dimensions evaluated, while most of the other tools presented low scores. In fact, only a moderate positive correlation between editorial quality and evidence-based methodology was found (r=.41, P=.0496). However, all dimensions improved from a previous evaluation performed on 2008: editorial quality (P=.01), evidence-based methodology (P=.015), and the volume of diseases and medical conditions included in the summaries went up significantly (P<.001). The authors concluded that publishers of medical and scientific literature understand the importance of point of care summaries. They devoted resources to their development and maintenance, and consequently both the number and the quality of these products have increased. Nevertheless, the study indicated differences in quality among the available tools. It is important to assess these regularly since their quality may change over time (Kwag et al., 2016). Tools were developed in high-income countries and are available mostly in these countries, while health care providers in low-income countries would probably take advantage of free access to such tools. Nevertheless, it is not clear if the tools would align with the information needs of the countries' providers. First, because users may lack Internet connection, and second, since health conditions supported in the summaries may differ from those most common in the local population (Hudspeth & Morse, 2017). Hence, point-of-care tools consistent with a broad range of countries' needs should be developed. Further research into the development of such tools within less-equipped, low-income countries is needed, as is the further investigation of the results of their implementation.

Even through tools with predigested summaries can facilitate physicians' searches at the point of care, the possibilities offered are limited when compared to the amount of information available. Additional tools are yet in need.

DISCUSSION: CALL TO ACTION

This chapter characterizes online searches for health information in view of the benefits and drawbacks for the patient-provider relationship and for patients' outcomes.

Most patients want to be well informed. However, studies indicate that the average reliability and quality of online health information is poor and not all patients discuss the information they gather with their providers. Therefore, they may be misguided by the information collected.

Information Technology (IT) and Artificial Intelligence (AI) based systems able to increase the reliability, quality, and readability of online health information should be considered priority projects in healthcare. They are needed to empower patients and to diminish the current risks of non-reliable information online.

In addition, the moment seems technologically and psychologically mature to enable the integration of AI into Electronic Health Records (EHR). This development has the potential to retrieve patient specific information and become a major engine to drive change. Personalized information which is derived from the patient's record could pave the way to maximize point of care resources. Such patient-provider interaction would contribute to patient engagement and empowerment.

CONCLUSION: KEY MESSAGES

The percentage of health information searchers using the Internet has increased over the years transforming the Internet into a significant source of health information. The importance of online health information is recognized by healthcare organizations and by providers, however studies have demonstrated that quality and reliability of sites have yet to improve.

The current methods used to evaluate reliability and quality of online health information are based on manual evaluation. Even though a few automatic methodologies were developed, they cannot technically be applied in extended numbers of websites.

Much of the information available has therefore not been evaluated by health experts and that is a reason for the poor quality. Advanced methodologies appropriated to the evaluation of the ever-increasing number of health-related web sites are desperately needed.

Patients may feel embarrassed or discouraged to share information they gathered on the web with a provider. Hence, they may be exposed to poor information without the benefit of a provider's advice about it. Providers should discuss the validity of information gathered by their patients and refer them to reliable sites.

Health information available online can pave the way to patient empowerment and engagement for his or her own healthcare. Research demonstrated that engaged patients have better outcomes.

Even though the number of Internet users around the World has rapidly increased, a digital gap exists among populations regarding their usage of health information. This gap may be due to limited access to the Internet, to lack of health literacy or to lack of online resources appropriate to the specific population.

Online clinical information is a significant asset to health providers. Information is important at all stages of healthcare but is still most needed at the point of care. Additional efforts should be made to increase the accessibility and the usability of point of care information for health providers.

Empowerment is a two-way street. Information can empower patients to be more engaged in their treatment and care; and it can empower healthcare providers to make better, more holistic decisions with patient collaboration and buy-in.

REFERENCES

Akerkar, S. M., & Bichile, L. S. (2004). Health information on the internet: Patient empowerment or patient deceit? *Indian Journal of Medical Sciences*, *58*(8), 321–326. PMID:15345885

Allam, A., Schulz, P. J., & Krauthammer, M. (2017). Toward automated assessment of health Web page quality using the DISCERN instrument. *Journal of the American Medical Informatics Association*, *24*(3), 481–487. doi:10.1093/jamia/ocw140 PMID:27707819

Banasiak, N. C., & Meadows-Oliver, M. (2017). Evaluating asthma websites using the Brief DISCERN instrument. *Journal of Asthma and Allergy*, *10*, 191–196. doi:10.2147/JAA.S133536 PMID:28670135

Biernatzki, L., Kuske, S., Genz, J., Ritschel, M., Stephan, A., Bächle, C., ... Icks, A. (2018). Information needs in people with diabetes mellitus: A systematic review. *Systematic Reviews*, *7*(1), 1–21. doi:10.118613643-018-0690-0 PMID:29444711

Boyer, C., Selby, M., & Appel, R. D. (1998). The Health On the Net Code of Conduct for medical and health web sites. *Studies in Health Technology and Informatics*, *52*(Pt 2), 1163–1166. PMID:10384641

Breckons, M., Jones, R., Morris, J., & Richardson, J. (2008). What do evaluation instruments tell us about the quality of complementary medicine information on the internet? *Journal of Medical Internet Research*, *10*(1), e3. doi:10.2196/jmir.961 PMID:18244894

Charnock, D., Shepperd, S., Needham, G., & Gann, R. (1999). DISCERN: An instrument for judging the quality of written consumer health information on treatment choices. *Journal of Epidemiology and Community Health*, *53*(2), 105–111. doi:10.1136/jech.53.2.105 PMID:10396471

Corfield, J. M., Abouassaly, R., & Lawrentschuk, N. (2018). Health information quality on the internet for bladder cancer and urinary diversion: A multi-lingual analysis. *Minerva Urologica e Nefrologica = The Italian. Journal d'Urologie et de Nephrologie*, *70*(2), 137–143. doi:10.23736/S0393-2249.17.02952-6 PMID:28707843

De Rosis, S., & Barsanti, S. (2016). Patient satisfaction, e-health and the evolution of the patient – general practitioner relationship : Evidence from an Italian survey. *Health Policy (Amsterdam)*, *120*(11), 1279–1292. doi:10.1016/j.healthpol.2016.09.012 PMID:27836231

Flesch, R. (1948). A new readability yardstick. *The Journal of Applied Psychology*, *32*(3), 221–233. doi:10.1037/h0057532 PMID:18867058

Fox, S., & Duggan, M. (2013). Health Online 2013. *Pew Internet and American Life Project*, 1–55.

Funk, E., Riddell, J., Ankel, F., & Cabrera, D. (2018). Blockchain Technology: A Data Framework to Improve Validity, Trust, and Accountability of Information Exchange in Health Professions Education. *Academic Medicine : Journal of the Association of American Medical Colleges*, *93*(12), 1791–1794. doi:10.1097/ACM.0000000000002326 PMID:29901658

Grando, M. A., Rozenblum, R., & Bates, D. W. (2015). Information technology for patient empowerment in healthcare. Berlin, Germany: H. Walter de Gruyter GmbH & K. G. Co. doi:10.1515/9781614514343

Health On the Net Foundation. (2017). HONcode Toolbar. Retrieved from https://www.hon.ch/HONcode/Patients/Visitor/visitor.html

Hudspeth, J., & Morse, M. (2017). Health Information and Global Health Inequity: Point-of-Care Knowledge Systems as a Foundation for Progress. *Journal of General Internal Medicine*, *32*(5), 572–575. doi:10.100711606-016-3909-6 PMID:27798781

Isaac, T., Zheng, J., & Jha, A. (2012). Use of UpToDate and outcomes in US hospitals. *Journal of Hospital Medicine*, *7*(2), 85–90. doi:10.1002/jhm.944 PMID:22095750

Khazaal, Y., Chatton, A., Cochand, S., Coquard, O., Fernandez, S., Khan, R., ... Zullino, D. (2009). Brief DISCERN, six questions for the evaluation of evidence-based content of health-related websites. *Patient Education and Counseling*, *77*(1), 33–37. doi:10.1016/j.pec.2009.02.016 PMID:19372023

Kincaid, J. P., Fishburne, R. P., Rogers, R. L., & Chissom, B. S. (1975). *Derivation of New Readability Formulas (Automated Readability Index, Fog Count and Flesch Reading Ease Formula) for Navy Enlisted Personnel*. Memphis, TN. doi:10.21236/ADA006655

Kwag, K. H., González-Lorenzo, M., Banzi, R., Bonovas, S., & Moja, L. (2016). Providing Doctors With High-Quality Information: An Updated Evaluation of Web-Based Point-of-Care Information Summaries. *Journal of Medical Internet Research, 18*(1), e15. doi:10.2196/jmir.5234 PMID:26786976

Lejbkowicz, I., Caspi, O., & Miller, A. (2012). Participatory medicine and patient empowerment towards personalized healthcare in multiple sclerosis. *Expert Review of Neurotherapeutics, 12*(3), 343–352. doi:10.1586/ern.11.161 PMID:22364333

Lejbkowicz, I., Paperna, T., Stein, N., Dishon, S., & Miller, A. (2010). Internet Usage by Patients with Multiple Sclerosis: Implications to Participatory Medicine and Personalized Healthcare. *Multiple Sclerosis International, 2010*, 1–7. doi:10.1155/2010/640749 PMID:22096625

McElroy, E., & Shevlin, M. (2014). The development and initial validation of the cyberchondria severity scale (CSS). *Journal of Anxiety Disorders, 28*(2), 259–265. doi:10.1016/j.janxdis.2013.12.007 PMID:24508033

Miniwatts Marketing Group. (2019). Statistics about the Internet. Retrieved from https://www.internetworldstats.com/stats.htm

Nordfeldt, S., Ängarne-Lindberg, T., Nordwall, M., Ekberg, J., & Berterö, C. (2013). As Facts and Chats Go Online, What Is Important for Adolescents with Type 1 Diabetes ?, *PLoS ONE 8*(6). doi:10.1371/journal.pone.0067659

Park, E., & Kwon, M. (2018). Health-related internet use by children and adolescents: Systematic review. *Journal of Medical Internet Research, 20*(4), 1–30. doi:10.2196/jmir.7731 PMID:29615385

Pass, J. H., Patel, A. H., Stuart, S., Barnacle, A. M., & Patel, P. A. (2018). Quality and readability of online patient information regarding sclerotherapy for venous malformations. *Pediatric Radiology, 48*(5), 708–714. doi:10.100700247-018-4074-3 PMID:29396791

Roughead, T., Sewell, D., Ryerson, C. J., Fisher, J. H., & Flexman, A. M. (2016). Internet-based resources frequently provide inaccurate and out-of-date recommendations on preoperative fasting: A systematic review. *Anesthesia and Analgesia, 123*(6), 1463–1468. doi:10.1213/ANE.0000000000001590 PMID:27644057

Salem, J., Paffenholz, P., Bolenz, C., von Brandenstein, M., Cebulla, A., Haferkamp, A., … Heidenreich, A. (2018). Websites on Bladder Cancer: An Appropriate Source of Patient Information? *Journal of Cancer Education: The Official Journal of the American Association for Cancer Education*. doi:10.100713187-017-1316-2

Sayakhot, P., & Carolan-Olah, M. (2016). Internet use by pregnant women seeking pregnancy-related information: A systematic review. *BMC Pregnancy and Childbirth, 16*(1), 65. doi:10.118612884-016-0856-5 PMID:27021727

Silberg, W. M., Lundberg, G. D., & Musacchio, R. A. (1997, April). Assessing, controlling, and assuring the quality of medical information on the Internet: Caveant lector et viewor--Let the reader and viewer beware. *JAMA*. USA.

Starcevic, V. (2017). Cyberchondria: Challenges of Problematic Online Searches for Health-Related Information. *Psychotherapy and Psychosomatics*, *86*(3), 129–133. doi:10.1159/000465525 PMID:28490037

Starcevic, V., & Berle, D. (2013). Cyberchondria: Towards a better understanding of excessive health-related Internet use. *Expert Review of Neurotherapeutics*, *13*(2), 205–213. doi:10.1586/ern.12.162 PMID:23368807

Statista. (2019). Number of social media users worldwide. Retrieved from https://www.statista.com/statistics/278414/number-of-worldwide-social-network-users/

Suarez-Almazor, M. E., Kendall, C. J., & Dorgan, M. (2001). Surfing the Net--information on the World Wide Web for persons with arthritis: Patient empowerment or patient deceit? *The Journal of Rheumatology*, *28*(1), 185–191. PMID:11196523

Tan, S. S. L., & Goonawardene, N. (2017). Internet health information seeking and the patient-physician relationship: A systematic review. *Journal of Medical Internet Research*, *19*(1), e9. doi:10.2196/jmir.5729 PMID:28104579

Tangri, V., & Chande, N. (2011). Quality of Internet-based information on gastrointestinal diseases. *Canadian Journal of Gastroenterology*, *25*(2), 93–96. doi:10.1155/2011/345076 PMID:21321681

Tkachenko, N., Gupta, N., Chotvijit, S., Gilks, C., Jarvis, S., Crosby, H., ... Guo, W. (2017). Google Trends can improve surveillance of Type 2 diabetes. *Scientific Reports*, *7*(1), 1–10. doi:10.103841598-017-05091-9 PMID:28694479

van Dijk, L., Groenewegen, P. P., Rademakers, J. J., de Jong, J. D., & Brabers, A. E. M. (2017). What role does health literacy play in patients' involvement in medical decision-making? *PLoS One*, *12*(3). doi:10.1371/journal.pone.0173316 PMID:28257472

Visser, L. M., Bleijenbergh, I. L., Benschop, Y. W. M., Van Riel, A. C., & Bloem, B. R. (2016). Do online communities change power processes in healthcare? Using case studies to examine the use of online health communities by patients with Parkinson's disease. doi:10.1136/bmjopen-2016-012110

Wikipedia. (2019). Web 2.0. Retrieved from https://en.wikipedia.org/wiki/Web_2.0

Wozney, L., Radomski, A. D., & Newton, A. S. (2018). The Gobbledygook in Online Parent-Focused Information about Child and Adolescent Mental Health. *Health Communication*, *33*(6), 710–715. doi:10.1080/10410236.2017.1306475 PMID:28402141

Zhao, Y., & Zhang, J. (2017). Consumer health information seeking in social media: A literature review. *Health Information and Libraries Journal*, *34*(4), 268–283. doi:10.1111/hir.12192 PMID:29045011

Chapter 3
Empowering Patients Through Digital Technologies:
The Case of Mobile Health Applications

Cristina Trocin
https://orcid.org/0000-0002-0710-8351
Ca' Foscari University of Venice, Italy

Enrica Croda
Ca' Foscari University of Venice, Italy

ABSTRACT

Mobile health initiatives aim to give patients more medical information and to empower them over their medical treatments. However, information overload and lack of digital literacy may hinder patient empowerment. This chapter investigates opportunities and challenges of patient empowerment and mobile health. The authors analyze the different definitions used in the literature to characterize patient empowerment and mobile health, discussing implications for all the care actors involved. Although the adoption rate of mobile technologies is at its infant stage and challenges still outweigh the benefits of patient empowerment, mobile health apps can foster the progress towards patient-centered care.

INTRODUCTION

The introduction and worldwide adoption of new information technologies are changing healthcare around the globe. A powerful combination of factors is driving this change. These include rapid advances in mobile technologies and applications, cloud-based computing and the exponential growth in coverage of mobile cellular networks (Dadgar & Joshi, 2018; Fox & Connolly, 2018; WHO, 2011).

In recent years, especially since the advent of smartphones, a vast number of apps have been developed to address different aspects of disease management or prevention including screening, symptoms tracking, stress management, medical support, habit building and providing a routine to give patients more power and control over their healthcare path (Varshney, 2014). There were more than 325,000

DOI: 10.4018/978-1-7998-0047-7.ch003

mobile health applications available in major apps stores and over 3.5 billion downloads in 2017 alone, reflecting a growth rate of 16% compared to the previous year (Research2Guidance, 2018). Researchers have attempted to understand the increasing use of mobile health applications and the way patients' role is changing by analyzing the adoption, the use and the consequences of mobile apps in the healthcare context, reviewing scientific literature, collecting empirical evidence of specific apps or conducting randomized controlled trials (Cerezo et al., 2016; Eskildsen et al., 2017; Klecun, 2016).

The pervasiveness of mobile apps in the healthcare industry suggests that their use has enriched doctor-patient communications and improved the delivery of care services (Boonstra & Broekhuis, 2010). The focus of care providers is shifting from productivity to quality of care and to positive experience for patients. This can be reached through timely health advice (Perera et al., 2011), promotion of compliance and adherence to medical treatments (Free et al., 2013), staying connected with health care provider(s), personal health management (Chatterjee et al., 2018; Dadgar & Joshi, 2018), self-care (Storni, 2014), and remote consultation (Manda & Herstad, 2015). Consequently, mobile health is composed of advanced technological tools with several benefits such as portable access to continuous streams of information, interactive functionality of the apps, monitoring patients remotely, and sending electronic alerts for disease control (Klasnja & Pratt, 2012).

Although the proliferation of mobile devices is continuously increasing because of reduced costs and diminished waiting times (Reychav et al., 2018), this phenomenon has not reached maturity yet. Some patients have had a positive experience using mobile apps to manage chronic diseases, while others have had a negative feedback because they became more dependent on care professionals, thus losing some of the advantages of patient empowerment. For instance, Ghosh and colleagues (2014) demonstrated how digital integration enhanced patients' psychological empowerment to manage a chronic disease.

Patients may benefit from using mobile apps as they acquire higher awareness of their care path or they are being facilitated in accomplishing routine tasks (Prgomet et al., 2009; Noteboom & Al-Ramahi, 2018; Marcolino et al., 2018). In contrast, others face several challenges with mobile apps because of the potential information overload due to cognitive constraints (Iyengar & Lepper, 2000) and the lack of expertise or digital literacy (van den Broek & Sergeeva, 2018; Fox & Connolly, 2018). Additionally, a recent study demonstrated that patient empowerment is an elusive ideal and on the contrary patients become more dependent on care professionals (van den Broek & Sergeeva, 2018).

The terms *patient empowerment* and *mobile health* have been used for several years, during which patients and medical staff have interpreted their meanings in different and sometimes contrasting ways. The absence of consensus over the definitions has led to misunderstandings among healthcare practitioners, researchers, policy makers and stakeholders alike. To make progress, it is crucial to take stock of existing knowledge.

This chapter investigates opportunities and challenges of patient empowerment and mobile health and discusses implications for care actors. After presenting the research methods, the authors review definitions of patient empowerment and mobile health. For each of these dimensions of "mobile health revolution", they examine the main benefits and challenges experienced by care actors. Finally, they conclude with the discussion of the implications of mobile health technologies for different stakeholders and directions for future research.

METHODS

The authors conducted a literature review in Information Systems (IS) and Management journals using as keywords: mobile health, mHealth, m-health, empowerment, psychological empowerment, patient empowerment, health apps, care apps, healthcare apps (Webster & Watson, 2002). The search included 8 leading IS journals: Management Information Systems Quarterly (MISQ), Information Systems Research (ISR), Journal of the Association for Information Systems (JAIS), Journal of Management Information Systems (JMIS), Information Systems Journal (ISJ), Journal of Information Technology (JIT), European Journal of Information Systems (EJIS), and Journal of Strategic Information Systems (JSIS). The Management journals included are the following: Organization Science (Org. Sci), Management Science (MS), Strategic Management Journal (Strat. Mgmt. J), Organization Studies (Org. Stud), Administrative Science Quarterly (ASQ), Journal of Management Studies (JMS), and Journal of Management (JM).

Besides Management and IS, mobile health and empowerment are covered also in other disciplines such as healthcare. Therefore, the authors included healthcare journals that focused explicitly on the use of mobile technology. To have an up to date source of information, they considered conference papers as well. The search was also conducted with the main online academic data basis EBSCOhost Business, Searching Interface, Web of Science, Scopus, ACM Digital Library.

After having selected the papers according to this strategy, the authors identified the definitions of patient empowerment and mobile health and proceeded to analyze the main benefits and challenges faced patients while using mobile health technology.

DISCUSSION

Psychological Empowerment in Patients

The spread of digital health technology brings about a fundamental change in patient information flow. Traditionally, there used to be a unidirectional flow of information from health professional to patient. The mobile health apps are now turning this communication into a dialogue, which may involve information flowing back from patient to health professional or may manifest as communication between patients themselves. Mobile health also allows patients to obtain information about their conditions that was previously accessible only by health professionals. These changes have the potential to empower patients.

Definitions and Factors of Patient Empowerment[1]

The concept of empowerment is not new and has been used and investigated in different contexts and domains (Maynard et al., 2012). The interest in this topic has continued to increase in management and organizational fields because the practice of empowerment is considered a principal component of organizational effectiveness (Conger & Kanungo, 1988). This section analyzes the concept of empowerment through its historical evolution (Table 2).

Three seminal studies introduced the concept of empowerment and how to operationalize it (Conger & Kanungo, 1988; Spreitzer, 1995; Thomas & Velthouse, 1990). Conger and Kanungo (1988) considered empowerment as a *motivational construct* because when individuals perceive themselves to have control and cope with social life events, they believe they adequately can confront with other people. They consider empowerment as an *enabling process* rather than a delegating one because it increases the motivation of subordinates to accomplish several tasks while highlighting personal efficacy.

Thomas and Velthouse (1990) further developed this concept. They proposed a cognitive model of empowerment and operationalized it in terms of *intrinsic task motivation*. They referred to those experiences that individuals gather and value as positive for accomplishing specific tasks. They added three more notions more notions: *impact, choice* and *meaning*.

Spreitzer (1995) built on these previous studies and coined the term *psychological empowerment* with the related cognitive dimensions, arguing that psychological empowerment is a *multifaceted motivational* construct composed of four cognitions that provide an energetic role to the employee.

The concept of empowerment implies three underlying assumptions. First, psychological empowerment may take different forms in different people because the population can be differentiated in multiple ways based on age, job position, education and different characteristics of the target population (Zimmerman, 1995). Second, psychological empowerment might take different forms in different contexts across different life domains, which might require different skills, knowledge, competences in order to have an active role inside a particular organization. Third, psychological empowerment is a variable construct that might change over time because an individual initially might experience the feeling of empowerment and later disempowerment or vice versa. Moreover, they might become empowered over time. Zimmerman argues that a universal measure of empowerment for all cases is not a realistic option and not appropriate (Zimmerman, 1995).

Starting from the core definitions and operationalization of the concept of psychological empowerment, multiple research projects have further developed and contextualized it according to specific case study, or field or situation. Initially, it has been studied in organizational and management domains with a focus on the ways to increase the motivation of employees to better perform their tasks and achieve better results. Later on, the term psychological empowerment spread among different settings such as education, innovation, healthcare, strategy, and crowdsourcing. Table 1 provides a summary of the most recognized definitions of patient empowerment in the healthcare industry (Bulsara et al., 2006; Deng et al., 2016; Maynard et al., 2012).

Based on the analysis of the definitions, the authors identified four crucial factors that better describe the concept of patient empowerment (see Table 2). It has been defined as an enabling and transformative process of promoting and enhancing people's ability to meet own preferences and to mobilize resources for gaining control over their healthcare to better comply and adhere to the medical treatment (McAllister et al., 2012). Some researchers have listed patients' abilities required to possess or to develop empowerment (Permwonguswa et al., 2017). Others conceived it as a process, which involves patients, medical staff, and family members (Anderson & Funnell, 2010; Castro et al., 2016; Khuntia et al., 2017; Zimmerman, 1995); or, it has been considered an outcome to be achieved for increasing healthcare quality (Wentzer & Bygholm, 2013).

The process of patient empowerment can be analyzed from the caregivers-patient's perspective and from the patients' viewpoint alone (Aujoulat et al., 2007). If we take into account the caregiver-patient interaction, it is considered a communicative process through a collaborative and fair relationship, where values and decisions are shared (Galanakis et al., 2016; Singh et al., 2011). Instead, if the definition is considered only from the patients' points of view, the process of empowerment is considered a process of change from a passive towards an active role (Table 2). Additionally, patient empowerment has been

Table 1. Definitions of patient empowerment

References	Definitions
Holmström & Röing (2010)	*"Patient empowerment may place greater demands on the caregivers. It requires of caregivers to first develop educational skills in empowering people to make informed choices about their own health. Patient empowerment requires that caregivers learn self-management education and the teaching of problem-solving skills to patients as a complement to traditional patient education, in order to increase patients' understanding of their situations, and consequently, enhance lasting change in the patients' lives. Patient empowerment can be said to have an important function for people with disabilities. It can help them reject the passive 'sick role' status relegated on them by past medical and health professions."*
Castro, Van Regenmortel, Vanhaecht, Sermeus, & Van Hecke (2016)	*"a process that enables patients to exert more influence over their individual health by increasing their capabilities to gain more control over issues that they themselves define as important."*
Deng, Khuntia & Ghosh (2013)	*"The concept of psychological empowerment has been viewed from both relational and motivational perspectives. Empowerment means delegating authority to, or sharing resources with subordinates. This view treats empowerment as psychologically enabling, and enhancing an individual's internal efficacy."*
Chiauzzi, DasMahapatra, Cochin, Bunce, Khoury, & Dave (2016)	*"Key factors in patient empowerment are positive patient– provider interactions and knowledge and personal control—were identified. Levels of these empowerment factors varied across disease type."*
Segal, Silverman, & Temkin (1993)	*"a process of 'gaining control over one's life situation influencing the organizational and societal structure in which one lives".*
Aujoulat, d'Hoore, & Deccache (2007)	*"Empowerment may be defined as a complex experience of personal change. It is guided by the principle of self- determination and may be facilitated by health-care providers if they adopt a patient-centered approach of care which acknowledges the patients' experience, priorities and fears."*
McAllister, Dunn, Payne, Davies, & Todd (2012)	*"Combining this broader definition of rational decision-making with a patient empowerment approach would require clinicians to be more open minded and explicit about what outcomes patients might want, what norms and constraints the patient feels are important, the values and uncertainties the patient considers apply to themselves and the world."*
Khuntia, Yim, Tanniru, & Lim (2017)	*Patient empowerment is nothing but a capacity-building process. Empowered patients believe that they can play an active role in the management of their own health and make decisions related to it. As a result, they experience greater control over their health management process.*
Funnell & Anderson (2004)	*Empowerment is a patient-centered, collaborative approach tailored to match the fundamental realities of diabetes care. Patient empowerment is defined as helping patients discover and develop the inherent capacity to be responsible for one's own life"*
Funnell, Anderson, Arnold, Barr, Donnelly, M., Johnson, ... White (1991)	*"We have defined the process of empowerment as the discovery and development of one's inherent capacity to be responsible for one's own life. People are empowered when they have sufficient knowledge to make rational decisions, sufficient control and resources to implement their decisions, and sufficient experience to evaluate the effectiveness of their decisions. Empowerment is more than an intervention or strategy to help people make behavior changes to adhere to a treatment plan. Fundamentally, patient empowerment is an outcome. Patients are empowered when they have knowledge, skills, attitudes, and self-awareness necessary to influence their own behavior and that of others in order to improve the quality of their lives"*
Anderson & Funnell (2010)	*"Patient empowerment is a process designed to facilitate self-directed behavior change. The empowerment approach involves facilitating and supporting patients to reflect on their experience of living with diabetes. Self-reflection occurring in a relationship characterized by psychological safety, warmth, collaboration, and respect is essential for laying the foundation for self-directed positive change in behavior, emotions, and/ or attitudes"*
Zimmerman (1995)	*"Empowerment is a process by which people, organizations, and communities gain mastery over issues of concern to them' and 'PE (Psychological Empowerment) is a feeling of control, a critical awareness of one's environment, and an active engagement in it."*
Small, Bower, Chew-Graham, Whalley, & Protheroe (2013)	*"An enabling process or outcome arising from communication with the health care professional and a mutual sharing of resources over information relating to illness, which enhances the patient's feelings of control, self-efficacy, coping abilities and ability to achieve change over their condition. empowerment is a psychological state that occurs as a result of effective communication in health care, and which acts as a determinant of consequent participation and self-management."*

continues on following page

Table 1. Continued

References	Definitions
Wentzer & Bygholm (2013)	*"A collaborative approach in which health professionals help patients acquire the knowledge necessary to make informed decisions and whose outcome is a patient who is responsible for the management of his/ her illness."*

Source: Authors' elaboration

Table 2. Key factors of patient empowerment

Key factors	Definitions	References
Motivation	*"Empowerment means delegating authority to, or sharing resources with subordinates. This view treats empowerment as psychologically enabling, and enhancing an individual's internal efficacy."* *"When individuals perceive themselves to have control and cope with social life events, they believe they adequately can confront with other people."* *"Psychological empowerment is a multifaceted motivational construct composed of four cognitions that provide an energetic role to the employee."*	(Kwon et al., 2017; Deng et al., 2013; Klasnja & Pratt, 2012; Alpay et al., 2011; Spreitzer, 1995; Thomas & Velthouse, 1990; Konger & Kanungo, 1988)
Self-efficacy	Empowered patients are defined as those individuals that are aware of their health conditions and have the capacity to make decisions about their health, and to take control over their life in order to reach their goals related to health conditions. The concept of self-efficacy is the most used and studied measure related to the concept of empowerment. This means to make more rational decisions, to decrease their dependence on health services and achieve the desired outcome.	(Reychav et al., 2019; Galanakis et al., 2016; McAllister et al., 2012)
Ownership	*"The ownership domain assesses the extent to which a person feels responsible for his or her own health. [...]consumers with high ownership scores were more likely to look up their health symptoms online before going to the doctor, compared to those with low ownership scores."*	(Lynch et al., 2016)
Navigation	*"The navigation domain measures how skilled a person is at using the health care system. [.....], those with high navigation scores were more than twice as likely to arrive at a health care visit with a prepared list of questions for the doctor as those with low navigation scores."*	(Lynch et al., 2016)

Source: Authors' elaboration

defined as a capacity-building process, in which patients play an active role in decision making and their health management process (Khuntia et al., 2017). For instance, Khuntia believes it goes beyond care management and focuses on enhancing care-provider and patient relationships.

Patient empowerment[2] has been conceived also as an outcome related to medical treatments, which can be reached through self-management (Funnell et al., 1991), self-efficacy (Galanakis et al., 2016), self-determination (see Table 4, Appendix 1; Aujoulat et al., 2007), self-esteem (Rogers et al., 1997), or active participation in decision making (Small et al., 2013). Self-efficacy is one of the most used concepts in the definitions (see Table 4, Appendix 1). It is considered at the individual level referring to personal levels of performance in disease and treatment behaviors.

Some definitions focus on common goals such as: patients who are empowered are healthier; will take more rational decisions; will contribute to more cost-effective healthcare resources; and, will receive higher care quality services (Holmström & Röing, 2010; McAllister et al., 2012). Others refer to patients' quality of life during medical treatments or in the follow up phase. This includes capabilities to cope with negative feelings, and personal satisfaction. Other authors focus on capabilities and actions to be taken to empower patients through education, patient-centered care, or active participation in design phase (Holmström & Röing, 2010).

Benefits and Challenges of Patient Empowerment

Psychological empowerment is a complex process that has been investigated at micro (patients, medical staff), meso (healthcare organizations or entities) and macro levels (healthcare industry) (Castro et al., 2016). Previous empirical studies investigated the benefits and challenges of those patients who feel empowered.

Prior studies investigated the consequences of patient empowerment with relation to a specific target population, which includes mental health (Rogers et al., 1997), long term conditions in primary care (Small et al., 2013), HIV patients (Johnson et al., 2012; Webb et al., 2001; Wilson et al., 2018), patients with chronic diseases (Maunsell et al., 2014; Galanakis et al., 2016), and patients with cancer (Bulsara & Styles, 2013).

The main benefits experienced by empowered patients consist of emotional empowerment, autonomy, self-efficacy and feeling connected.

- **Emotional Empowerment:** The process of giving power to patients over their medical treatment means to give more decisional, cognitive, emotional control, and hope to improve personal quality of life (Doll & Deng, 2010; Huang & Ran, 2014; Wilson et al., 2018). This enables patients not only to better understand their care path but also to take actions and to have an impact on their own path (Anders & Cassidy, 2014; Aujoulat et al., 2007; Loukanova et al., 2007).
- **Autonomy:** Complete and updated medical information allows patients to acknowledge the areas of their life more affected by their illness (see Table 4, Appendix 1). Then they can autonomously determine the best and most suitable decisions and tasks to have meaningful outcomes in their life (Aujoulat et al., 2007). The medical treatment changes patients' habits and routines, which consequently might decrease self-confidence and the ability to make decisions in an autonomous way. Mobile technologies facilitate patients' routines and medical treatments, for managing medical prescriptions or for other administrative purposes and to give the opportunity to patients to complete tasks and procedures in an autonomous way (Holmström & Röing, 2010).
- **Self-Efficacy:** Empowered patients are defined as those individuals that are aware of their health conditions and have the capacity to make decisions about their health, and to take control over their life in order to reach their goals related to health conditions (see Table 4, Appendix 1). This means to make more rational decisions, to decrease their dependence on health services and achieve the desired outcome (McAllister et al., 2012). The concept of self-efficacy is the most used and studied measure related to the concept of empowerment (Reychav et al., 2019).
- **Feeling Connected:** During the medical treatment, patients might face hard times and might be in need of support not only from family members but also from external actors. This refers to medical staff while monitoring patients' health with the help of mobile technologies but also refers to other patients with the same pathology. One antecedent of feeling empowered is to feel connected with the rest of the society, including family, friends, colleagues and other people in their same condition (Bravo et al., 2015).

The approach of patient empowerment is not entirely shared and supported by practitioners mostly because it imposes additional elements on their time and efforts since it challenges physicians' autonomy.

- **Time and Effort:** Medical information is created and managed by care professionals, who can benefit from shared data if they implement it. Therefore, they are required to change the results of medical visits on the platform and send it to mobile apps. This requires a higher involvement and effort, considering the time required to create digital versions of medical data and then transmit it further (Sandlund et al., 2016; Miller et al., 2016). Higher investments are needed in terms of time and effort to learn the platforms and explain the information to patients. This might be frustrating and time consuming, especially in the initial stage of implementation. In fact, one of the key barriers to mobile technologies adoption is the creation of accounts, and legal authorization of data sharing (Dadgar & Joshi, 2018)
- **Physicians' Authority is Challenged:** Not only does the decreased information asymmetry between patients and physicians yields more opportunities for empowerment, it also challenges the role of physician authority and expertise. Indeed, more information increases patients' awareness regarding medical treatments, but, at the same time, patients have the opportunity to question physicians' knowledge and suggestions. This happens especially in those situations, when patients are not able to contextualize medical information and might be willing to choose a past treatment for a new disease based on positive outcomes or vice versa.

Implications for Care Givers and Care Receivers

The patient empowerment approach involves shared decision making, which can increase existing knowledge, provide more accurate risk perceptions, make the decisions in line with patients' preferences, reduce internal decisional conflict for patients, and diminish passive or undecided patients. It also creates the opportunity to address the problem of over-diagnosis and overtreatment. When patients know that they have several options available for the best treatment such as a screening test or diagnostic procedure, they are more willing to engage with the clinicians in the decision making process (Liberati et al., 2015).

The creation of an ecosystem offering digital healthcare services focused on the collaboration and participation of healthcare professionals leveraging on their expertise, on the co-creation of ideas and on the co-design, service directly involving the end-users. The contribution of the patients represents the keystone to create useful and usable services for everyday healthcare activities and at the same time ends up with enriching the construction of the healthcare digital ecosystem.

The innovativeness of mobile applications lays in the integration of different needs of all involved categories/stakeholders in an open space for dialogue, listening, co-creating and negotiating proposals for common, innovative solutions. The key concept of the mobile application is to offer a tailored service for digital health that directly and predominantly involves the patient (patient-centered-healthcare-ecosystem). It offers the possibility to access a dematerialized medical prescription, to manage personal medical information, monitor the process of personal continuous healthcare, be aware of the healthcare process, understand how the healthcare system works (transparency), and be responsible for the personal medical data management (patient empowerment and awareness).

Generation, storage and processing of data is the lifeblood of digital disruption and represents an opportunity for many industries including healthcare, which by definition is a knowledge-intensive and information-intensive industry. Information and Communication Technologies (ICT) shape both the execution of company activities and the organization of information flows and services. More specifically, ICT allows the exploitation of different advantages such as intra and inter-organizational distribution of limited resources with a patient-centered perspective, monitoring the company's performance, facilitating the interactions between the many actors involved, and optimizing internal processes to offer a more efficient service of higher quality. Significant challenges remain, and many new approaches and ideas are needed to ensure potential benefits materialize within healthcare organizations. In the meanwhile, investment in this area continues (Atasoy et al., 2017).

Mobile Health

Mobile applications in the healthcare sector share common goals. For example, they have the potential to increase the quality of the care services through shared medical information (Reychav et al., 2018), to increase healthcare efficiency and efficacy while increasing patients' satisfaction (Varshney, 2014), to facilitate the care service delivery, to offer patients tailored services, and to provide more convenient access to needed health information (Rai et al., 2013).

The development of mobile care apps follows a multidimensional and multidisciplinary approach that takes into consideration technical aspects as well as their effects on the final users. The goal is twofold: fostering an active engagement of the final users in the process and empowering the users while satisfying real needs as a cornerstone of the process of innovation.

There is a tendency to create a medical app in response to a specific need, fostering the concept of tailored care service and creating a user-driven innovation to represent value and impactful delivery of care services. So far, mobile device projects have been implemented on a pilot basis with a collaborative and participatory approach of healthcare professionals leveraging their expertise, on the co-creation of ideas and on the co-design of service directly involving the end-users (Marcolino et al., 2018; Yaraghi et al., 2014).

The pervasiveness of mobile health apps has been encouraged by policy makers, who have emphasized the fact that the patients' voice can gain control over factors that might affect their health and lives through the use of mobile technologies (Castro et al., 2016; WHO, 2011; WHO, 2016).

Definitions and Key Characteristics of Mobile Health

Over the last two decades this term has been used in many fields from health sciences to computers and human behavior, information systems, and information management. However, to date, no standardized definition of mHealth has been established. The authors selected nineteen different definitions reported in Table 3.

Some scholars have embraced a technical view. For example, Zhao and colleagues (2018) defined mobile health services as tools for "providing health services and information through the use of mobile communication technology, such as smart phones, 3G/4G mobile networks and satellite communications". Studies adopting this view, have highlighted mobile technologies' technical functions such as networking capabilities, convenient access to medical information, cloud-based computing systems, medical sensors, and satellite communications (Liu et al., 2018; Meng et al., 2018; Wu et al., 2007; Yen et al., 2011).

Other scholars have conceptualized mobile health apps based on non-technical perspectives by focusing on their consequences and on the interactions and information exchange among different groups. Specifically these scholars have studied health promotion, prevention, chronic disease care enhancement,

Table 3. Definitions of mobile health

References	Definitions
Liu, Guo, & Ju (2018)	*"mHealth is defined as one type of healthcare service that can provide mobile device users with ubiquitous and pervasive access to medical advice and information. It changes the spectrum of healthcare services from crisis intervention to health promotion, prevention, and self-management."*
World Health Organization (2011)	*"The Global Observatory for eHealth (GOe) defined mHealth or mobile health as medical and public health practice supported by mobile devices, such as mobile phones, patient monitoring devices, personal digital assistants (PDAs), and other wireless devices."*
Reychav, Parush, McHaney, Hazan, & Moshonov (2018)	*"m-Healthcare solutions are used in the remote monitoring of patients, delivering care, reducing costs, saving time, and increasing accessibility and geographical coverage of services"*
Meng, Guo, Lai, & Zhao (2018)	*"mHealth service can be defined as the use of mobile information and communication technologies (ICTs) endowed with the capability of managing and delivering health information timely, between end-users and health professionals to improve patient safety and the quality of healthcare"*
Fox & Connolly (2018)	*"the utilization of mobile technologies to realize health objectives,ealth encompasses a variety of mobile applications, wearable devices, and health record systems. Mobile health can provide additional benefits including removing geographic barriers to health information, facilitating access to customized information, and removing the stigmatization often associated with other medical devices"*
Kwon, Dewan, Oh, & Kim (2017)	*"mobile apps enable users to upload their records immediately after an event occurs, thereby alleviating concerns associated with inaccuracies that potentially emanate from remembering the activities that people engage in over the long-term"*
Reychav, Beeri, Balapour, Raban, Sabherwal, & Azuri (2019)	*"Mobile computing offers fairly cheap and accessible outlets with wide-spread functionalities that are adopted in business and healthcare. In healthcare, especially in the most recent years, mobile devices are used extensively to improve patient life quality and health. Mobile healthcare or m-Healthcare solutions are used in the remote monitoring of patients, delivering care, reducing costs, saving time, and increasing accessibility and geographical coverage of services"*
Kwon, Lee, & Lee (2014)	*"Through mobile personal health record (mPHR) applications, users can access their health information easily. They enable patients to get their health information whenever and wherever they are. Patients are able to record and update their health conditions such as weight, blood pressure, and blood glucose level, and keep track of such information for themselves. This information can be shared with physicians, helping them check the patient's current conditions, give instructions that patients are supposed to follow, and provide more precise and customized care services."*
Wu, Li, & Fu (2011)	*"The use of mobile healthcare is closely related to the patients' health and life. Mobile healthcare is an emerging technology for personal use which is often used voluntarily. It involves both technological and organizational aspects on the level of individual."*
Nouri, Niakan, Kalhori, Ghazisaeedi, Marchand, & Yasini (2018)	*"Mobile health can be defined as the use of wireless communication devices to support public health and clinical practice or soft wares that are incorporated into smartphones to improve health outcome, health research, and health care services."*
Lim, Xue, Yen, Chang, Chan, Tai, & Choolani (2011)	*"health applications facilitate the public's self-management of their own health by offering a rich library of health information which educate users on disease prevention, promote fitness and offer tips on wellness."*
Rai, Chen, Pye, & Baird (2013)	*"Mobile health is defined as the use of mobile communication technology to aid health services delivery. mHealth could increase their control over their health care, provide more convenient access to needed health information, and ultimately improve their health care costs and quality."*
Wu, Wang, & Lin (2007)	*"Mobile IT/IS applications in health care can be recognized as both emerging and enabling technologies that have been applied in several countries for emergency care or general health care."*
Sun, Wang, Guo, & Peng (2013)	*"Mobile health services (MHS) can be defined as a variety of healthcare services, including health consulting, hospital registering, and location-based services delivered through mobile communications and network technologies."*
Li, Wu, Gao, & Shi (2016)	*"Healthcare wearable devices includes both, fitness and medical wearable devices. There are two main kinds of healthcare wearable devices in the market, fitness and medical wearable devices. Users can monitor their health conditions such as sleep, calories burned, heart rate, and distance traveled in real time."*

continues on following page

Table 3. Continued

References	Definitions
Hoque & Sorwar (2017)	*"mHealth is considered to be an easy, low cost, and affordable solution to improve access to healthcare services especially for those with shortage healthcare resources. "*
Pung, Fletcher, & Gunn (2018)	*"Mobile apps are emerging as tools with the potential to revolutionize the treatment of mental health conditions such as depression. Apps are advanced technological tools with multiple capabilities and have been postulated to revolutionize mental health treatment in myriad ways, such as by allowing for the affordable and accessible delivery of interventions, providing real-time diagnostic and monitoring support, enhancing therapeutic relationships, augmenting engagement with treatments, and even acting as "virtual coaches"."*
Zhao, Ni, & Zhou (2018)	*"Mobile health services (MHS) have been defined as providing health services and information through the use of mobile communication technology, such as smart phones, 3G/4G mobile networks and satellite communications. Mobile health could track health condition of people, evaluate the trend of its evolution and provide timely treatment. Mobile health services can save the time and cost of diagnosis. It plays a positive role in improving the quality and the efficiency of medical resources. "*
Eng & Lee (2013)	*"Mobile health, referred to as mHealth, is defined as mobile computing, medical sensor and communication technologies that can enhance chronic disease care beyond the traditional out-patient physician-patient encounter. This includes applications that run on mobile phones, sensors that track vital signs, health activities and cloud-based computing systems."*

Source: Authors' elaboration

saved time and cost of diagnosis, enhanced therapeutic relationships, improved access to healthcare services and low cost affordable solutions (Eng et al., 2013; Hoque & Sorwar, 2017; Pung et al., 2018). Some of them have also investigated information and timely interventions, and effective communication between the care providers and receivers (Rai et al., 2013).

Certain characteristics of mobile health apps are common to all the definitions reported in the Table 3. For example, most researchers argue that mobile health apps have the potential to facilitate the delivery of care services, to improve the quality of the care, to share timely medical information, to meet patients' needs with pervasive access to medical information and to improve patient-physician' interactions. Moreover, scholars have highlighted that shared medical information facilitates remote monitoring of patients, delivering care, reducing costs, saving time, and increasing accessibility and geographical coverage of services (Reychav et al., 2019).

The uptake of mobile apps is rapidly increasing thanks to their core characteristics, which are the following:

- Mobility provides an access to medical information without physical and temporal constraints (Prgomet et al., 2009).
- Ubiquity, a consequence of mobility, provides a direct access to multiple information anytime and anywhere (Middleton et al., 2014).
- Connectivity allows the exchange of medical information among multiple actors not only in the healthcare system but also with the personal network of the patient like family, friends, other patients with similar diseases regardless time and location (Dadgar & Joshi, 2018).
- Transparency and accuracy are achieved via information storage, analysis and consultation (Dadgar & Joshi, 2018). Some information may be retrieved from previous medical visits or laboratory results thus avoiding the duplication tests (Adjerid et al., 2018).

- Coping with perpetual tasks increases patients' autonomy because once the medical treatment has been selected, mobile technologies allow patients to better adhere to the medical treatment (Dadgar & Joshi, 2018).

Benefits and Challenges of Mobile Health

Recent studies have demonstrated that mobile health applications have the potential to improve the quality of the care services through shared medical information (Reychav et al., 2018), to increase healthcare efficiency and efficacy while increasing patients' satisfaction (Varshney, 2014), to facilitate care service delivery, to offer patients tailored services and to provide more convenient access to needed health information (Rai et al., 2013; Klasnia & Pratt, 2012). Therefore, the authors analyze benefits and challenges that care actors experience using mobile health applications to accomplish daily tasks. The main benefits range from enhanced care quality, to the removal of geographic barriers, to the facilitation of access to customized information, to the remote monitoring of patients.

- **Enhancing Care Quality:** Policy makers are shifting their attention about care performance from productivity to positive patients' experience based on their preferences. The World Health Organization[3] defines the quality of care as "the extent to which health care services provided to individuals and patient populations improve desired health outcomes. In order to achieve this, health care must be safe, effective, timely, efficient, equitable and people centered." The return of desired health outcomes refers to the best available medical treatment in line with patients' preferences and values. The underlying assumption is that the care service that meets patients' needs and health conditions enhances the care quality. According to this approach, the focus of care organizations shifts from care professional controlled care to professional managed care, creating the concept of patient-centered care service (Varshney, 2014; Peleg et al., 2017).
- **Removing Geographic Barriers to Health Information or Geographical Coverage of Services:** Mobile health apps facilitate patient-care professional interactions which can take place from different locations (Varshney, 2014). Temporal and locational constraints can be removed as the diagnosis sent by the primary care physician to the patient can be consulted in different moments by the patient and by other physicians. This is particularly useful for routine activities (i.e. chronic disease, medical prescriptions), emergency cases and during holidays in different locations. In fact, a patient suffering from chronic disease during the holidays can get the prescribed medicine in any pharmacy around the vacation location. Moreover, in emergency cases, patients can remotely access their medical history thanks to Health Information Exchange platforms or Electronic Health Records (Peleg et al., 2017; Peleg et al., 2018). Therefore, mobile health applications have the potential to remove the time and location constraints under the condition that digital platforms and mobile technologies are implemented in all care organizations and have interoperable systems, which requires economic, time and effort investments (Trocin et al., 2018).
- **Facilitating Access to Customized Information:** Mobile health apps are considered extensions of digital care services for providing timely patient-tailored care. The access to a complete medical information may make the difference for the diagnosis of a disease, the management of chronic disease and for handling an emergency case. For example, Health Information Exchanges facilitate the sharing of medical information and their access by multiple care actors such as general and specialized physicians, nurses, and administrative staff for different purposes, based on their

account characteristics (Peleg et al., 2018). Moreover, mobile technologies further facilitate access to information which can be updated and customized based on care path and the reaction of the patient to the specific medical treatment (Reychav et al., 2018).

- **Facilitating Decision Making:** One of the major goals of mHealth is to facilitate decision making (Nouri et al., 2018). Access to recent medical information can improve the quality of decisions and decrease duplicated tests, which leads to efficiency improvements (Ayabakan et al., 2017). Mobile systems can reduce task completion time significantly. Healthcare professionals consider multiple sources of information before making a diagnosis. These include symptoms, medical history, lab results and tests (Peleg et al., 2017). This information is shared with the patient and the decision-making process moves forward in collaboration with the patient. Multiple care actors are involved in the decision-making process, thus mobile technologies facilitate processing and updating pertinent medical information. This is particularly useful for patients simultaneously affected by multimorbidity, which can be facilitated by mobile health technology (Peleg et al., 2018).
- **Remote Monitoring of Patients:** Mobile health applications provide opportunities to deliver care services beyond the physicians' offices and hospital setting thus reshaping the boundaries of care organizations and care services (Singh et al., 2011). For instance, in the past, patients were released from a hospital during working days and the medicine prescribed during traditional working hours. Nowadays, patients can be released and buy the necessary medicine without temporal constraints. In case of necessity, physicians can prescribe additional medicine through the mobile app and patients can get them from pharmacies. For chronic diseases, patients can self-monitor their health status with the mobile apps and their physicians can check them through the apps (Reychav et al., 2018).

Example of apps that have been used for the remote monitoring of patients are personal weight management apps. Kwon and colleagues (2017) studied the efficacy of such an app. They followed a Markov modeling approach to capture the intrinsic motivation, or state of self-regulation, of individuals engaged in losing weight. They demonstrated that use of the mobile app is more effective than the PC to influence the behavior of the patients. An intensive use of the mobile application increases the probability of losing weight but after a threshold of 80% of the time engaged in this activity.

Beyond the aforementioned benefits, mobile health applications also raise challenges that might inhibit their adoption. The major challenges arise from privacy concerns, digital divide and digital health literacy.

- **Privacy Concerns:** The act of sharing medical information among multiple care actors on digital platforms and mobile apps requires legal authorization from patients, which involves a sequence of steps and might be considered a barrier to adopt mobile technologies. Account creation, collection of medical information from previous visits and later update requires higher involvement and effort from all care actors (Sandlund et al., 2016). Moreover, legislation on the ownership of medical data and on the extent to which it can be shared is not clearly defined. The boundaries of dealing with medical information on digital platforms and on mobile technologies are blurred, thus patients might not feel protected enough and might not want to use these tools. Health data privacy concerns are considered barriers to mHealth adoption (Fox & Connolly, 2018, McKinsey, 2013). For example, reminders on patients' mobile devices help patients to do regularly specific tasks and improve medical adherence. They have the potential to increase motivation and the probability of being effective during the care path (Klasnja and Pratt, 2012). In case someone can see the recipients' phone, patients need a privacy-preserving also in the reminder option of mobile apps. Otherwise, they will not use them and the potential for increased medical adherence will not be realized (Jean et al., 2018; Wu et al., 2007).

- **Digital Divide:** The pervasiveness of mobile health apps facilitates access to medical information but also leads to a digital divide (Fox and Connolly, 2018; Kenny and Connolly, 2017). The digital divide is stronger along the age dimension. Older patients are those who could benefit from mobile technologies for chronic diseases such as diabetes, which increase with age. However, research shows that, rather than using apps to manage chronic health conditions, they prefer to use apps for fitness and dieting. They are concerned about privacy and lack trust and do not want to disclose personal data. Recently, some scholars found that older patients tend to avoid mobile health apps (Fox & Connolly, 2018; Srivastava et al., 2015).

The digital divide arises when some needs are ignored or not satisfied. As a consequence, some patients remain excluded from the potential advantages of mobile health (Kenny & Connolly, 2017).

- **Digital and Health Literacy:** Platforms and mobile apps collect and generate an increasing amount of medical information. On one side, this enriches patients' medical history and allows a more accurate diagnosis (Bravo et al., 2015). On the other side, this might create confusion for patients, who might lack digital skills and health literacy. Patients might not possess knowledge and medical expertise to contextualize received information and make sense of it (van den Broek & Sergeeva, 2018). Moreover, some patients may not have the skills needed to use digital platforms or mobile apps, no matter how intuitive they are (Alpay et al., 2011).

If the goal of policy makers is to increase mhealth adoption rates, digital and health literacy are big challenges.

Implications for Care Givers and Care Receivers

Mobile health apps facilitate the sharing of information for decision making and the responsibilities of selected medical treatments. For some care paths, patients' preferences are less taken into consideration because there is one treatment that is clearly superior. For instance, appendicitis requires an immediate surgery, and meningitis requires specific antibiotics (Reychav et al., 2018). However, most of the medical decisions entail different combinations of possible therapeutic choices. This leads to higher involvement of the patient thus adding value to the treatment because it is more consistent with their preferences and values (Sandlund et al., 2016; Miller et al., 2016). In determining the care path, multiple actors such as clinicians, patients and/or their family and other clinical staff are all engaged.

There are several implications for care givers and receivers because such mobile technologies require higher involvement (Miller et al., 2016). The act of sharing information starts with the clinician, who explains the disease and treatment options available, highlighting benefits and risks. In the same way, patients share their beliefs and values with the medical staff and with the help of the clinician, they better understand their preferences for a specific treatment. In this process, not only the information is shared but also the responsibilities linked to the selected care path while empowering the engaged actors.

Beyond the aims of improving the reach of healthcare, the decision-making process and management of chronic diseases, the increasing use of mobile applications is witnessing a shift in care service delivery that ranges from care professionals-controlled to care professionals-managed (Varshney, 2014). Contrary to common wisdom, the use of mobile applications is not limited only to the consultation of personal medical information but also includes a plethora of other care services such as disease prevention, mobile decision making, emergency intervention, monitoring the care path, healthcare data access, and mobile telemedicine just to mention the main services (Viswanathan et al., 2017).

CONCLUSION AND FUTURE WORK

This chapter has reviewed the definitions of patient empowerment and mobile health, discussing their main benefits and challenges. In this sense, it can provide common ground on which the academic community and stakeholders can build.

There is still little understanding about how mobile health apps empower patients and about the characteristics of those patients who are empowered. Since the concept of empowerment varies across settings, context and times, longitudinal studies should be conducted to assess the extent of the level of empowerment in different time frames and to understand the key characteristics that affect feelings of empowerment. In particular, little is known about the technological features that influence this feeling. Research should also be conducted on the association between mobile apps and Electronic Healthcare Records (EHR) or Health Information Exchange (HIE) platforms since apps' performance depends on the quality of the information provided. Actual and granular information from the mobile apps logins or patient behavior within the apps should be collected in related questionnaire data or semi-structured interviews.

Mobile health applications are not expected to reduce all care costs, but they provide several benefits that facilitate care service delivery from multiple perspectives. They have the ability to extend the reach of the care services, improve decision making, help prevent and manage chronic diseases and ensure faster emergency care (WHO, 2016; Varshney, 2014, Dadgar, & Joshi, 2018). Care organizations have made significant investments to develop and deploy mobile applications and in the process, have become closer to the users' needs. In this context, the apps have played the role of mediators between the information made available on web sites and the information users are demanding (Baird et al., 2018; Fox & Connolly, 2018).

This chapter has implications for healthcare providers, policy makers and technology developers. Mobile technologies can support healthcare providers to better serve their patients by providing home care assistance and personnel training to reduce the need for hospitalization. Hospitals and post-acute care providers can enhance patients' capabilities for off-site monitoring and self-management. Regulations have yet to fully address the new challenges introduced by mHealth. Policy makers deal with fragmented and complex regulatory environments. The authors believe that guarantying privacy and security in mHealth should have top priority. Another important issue is the communication among multiple care actors. Technology developers have led the way in mHealth innovation, specifically targeting individuals with health and wellness apps. However, the ultimate value of the apps themselves depends on interoperability and the connection with existing Electronic Health Records. It is therefore crucial that developers focus on these issues (Deloitte, 2017).

To conclude, mobile health could radically change the way healthcare is viewed, managed and delivered. This chapter has focused on two dimensions of the phenomenon that are fundamentally linked: the use of patient empowerment and mHealth technology. The success of the "mobile health revolution" will depend on the extent to which the use of mHealth products and services lead to better health outcomes at lower costs for the population. To this end, a coordinated collective effort by all stakeholders on promoting digital health education and engagement and protecting data privacy and security of patients' information is becoming more and more urgent (WHO, 2016).

ACKNOWLEDGMENT

The authors are grateful to Giovanni Vaia for encouraging them to work on the topic and for helpful comments. They also thank the anonymous reviewers for constructive feedback.

REFERENCES

Adjerid, I., Adler-Milstein, J., & Angst, C. (2018). Reducing Medicare spending through electronic health information exchange: The role of incentives and exchange maturity. *Information Systems Research, 29*(2), 341–361. doi:10.1287/isre.2017.0745

Alpay, L., Van Der Boog, P., & Dumaij, A. (2011). An empowerment-based approach to developing innovative e-health tools for self-management. *Health Informatics Journal, 17*(4), 247–255. doi:10.1177/1460458211420089 PMID:22193825

Anders, C., & Cassidy, A. (2014). Effective organizational change in healthcare: Exploring the contribution of empowered users and workers. *International Journal of Healthcare Management, 7*(2), 132–151. doi:10.1179/2047971913Y.0000000061

Anderson, R. M., & Funnell, M. M. (2010). Patient empowerment: Myths and misconceptions. *Patient Education and Counseling, 79*(3), 277–282. doi:10.1016/j.pec.2009.07.025 PMID:19682830

Atasoy, H., Greenwood, B. N., & McCullough, J. S. (2018). The digitization of patient care: A review of the effects of electronic health records on health care quality and utilization. *Annual Review of Public Health, 40*(1), 487–500. doi:10.1146/annurev-publhealth-040218-044206 PMID:30566385

Aujoulat, I., D'hoore, W., & Deccache, A. (2007). Patient empowerment in theory and practice: Polysemy or cacophony? *Patient Education and Counseling, 66*(1), 13–20. doi:10.1016/j.pec.2006.09.008 PMID:17084059

Ayabakan, S., Bardhan, I. R., & Zheng, Z. (2017). A data envelopment analysis approach to estimate it-enabled production capability. *Management Information Systems Quarterly, 41*(1), 189–205. doi:10.25300/MISQ/2017/41.1.09

Boonstra, A., & Broekhuis, M. (2010). Barriers to the acceptance of electronic medical records by physicians from systematic review to taxonomy and interventions. *BMC Health Services Research, 10*(1), 231. doi:10.1186/1472-6963-10-231 PMID:20691097

Bravo, P., Edwards, A., Barr, P. J., Scholl, I., Elwyn, G., & Mcallister, M. (2015). Conceptualising patient empowerment: A mixed methods study. *BMC Health Services Research*, *15*(1), 525. doi:10.118612913-015-0907-z PMID:26126998

Bulsara, C., Styles, I., Ward, A. M., & Bulsara, M. (2006). The Psychometrics of Developing the Patient Empowerment Scale. *Journal of Psychosocial Oncology*, *24*(2), 1–16. doi:10.1300/J077v24n02_01 PMID:17046803

Castro, E. M., Van Regenmortel, T., Vanhaecht, K., Sermeus, W., & Van Hecke, A. (2016). Patient empowerment, patient participation and patient-centeredness in hospital care: A concept analysis based on a literature review. *Patient Education and Counseling*, *99*(12), 1923–1939. doi:10.1016/j.pec.2016.07.026 PMID:27450481

Cerezo, P. G., Juvé-Udina, M.-E., & Delgado-Hito, P. (2016). Concepts and measures of patient empowerment: A comprehensive review. *Revista da Escola de Enfermagem da U S P.*, *50*(4), 667–674. doi:10.1590/S0080-623420160000500018 PMID:27680054

Chatterjee, S., Byun, J., Dutta, K., Pedersen, R. U., Pottathil, A., & Xie, H. (2018). Designing an Internet-of-Things (IoT) and sensor-based in-home monitoring system for assisting diabetes patients: Iterative learning from two case studies. *European Journal of Information Systems*, *27*(6), 670–685. doi:10.1080/0960085X.2018.1485619

Conger, J. A., & Kanungo, R. N. (1988). The empowerment process: Integrating theory and practice. *Academy of Management Review*, *13*(3), 471–482. doi:10.5465/amr.1988.4306983

Dadgar, M., & Joshi, K. D. (2018). The role of Information and Communication Technology in self-management of chronic diseases: An Empirical Investigation through Value Sensitive Design. *Journal of the Association for Information Systems*, *19*(2), 86–112. doi:10.17705/jais1.00485

Deng, X., Joshi, K. D., & Galliers, R. D. (2016). The Duality of Empowerment and Marginalization in Microtask Crowdsourcing: Giving Voice to the Less Powerful Through Value Sensitive Design. *Management Information Systems Quarterly*, *40*(2), 279–302. doi:10.25300/MISQ/2016/40.2.01

Deng, X., Khuntia, J., & Ghosh, K. (2013). Psychological Empowerment of Patients with Chronic Diseases: The Role of Digital Integration. *Thirty Fourth International Conference on Information Systems* (pp. 1–20).

Doll, W., & Deng, X. (2010). A technology empowerment model for engineering work. *ACM SIGMIS Database: the DATABASE for Advances in Information Systems*, *41*(4), 52–74. doi:10.1145/1899639.1899643

Eng, D., Lee, J. M., Eng, D. S., & Lee, J. M. (2013). The promise and peril of mobile health applications for diabetes and endocrinology. *Pediatric Diabetes*, *14*(4), 231–238. doi:10.1111/pedi.12034 PMID:23627878

Eskildsen, N. B., Joergensen, C. R., Thomsen, T. G., Ross, L., Dietz, S. M., Groenvold, M., & Johnsen, A. T. (2017). Patient empowerment: A systematic review of questionnaires measuring empowerment in cancer patients. *Acta Oncologica*, *56*(2), 156–165. doi:10.1080/0284186X.2016.1267402 PMID:28077053

Fox, G., & Connolly, R. (2018). Mobile health technology adoption across generations: Narrowing the digital divide. *Information Systems Journal*, *28*(6), 995–1019. doi:10.1111/isj.12179

Free, C., Phillips, G., Galli, L., Watson, L., Felix, L., Edwards, P., ... Haines, A. (2013). The Effectiveness of Mobile-Health Technology-Based Health Behaviour Change or Disease Management Interventions for Health Care Consumers: A Systematic Review. *PLoS Medicine*, *10*(1). doi:10.1371/journal.pmed.1001362 PMID:23349621

Funnell, M. M., Anderson, R. M., Arnold, M. S., Barr, P. A., Donnelly, M., Johnson, P. D., ... White, N. H. (1991). Empowerment: An idea whose time has come in diabetes education. *The Diabetes Educator*, *17*(1), 37–41. doi:10.1177/014572179101700108 PMID:1986902

Galanakis, M., Tsoli, M., & Darviri, S. (2016). The Effects of Patient Empowerment Scale in Chronic Dis-eases. *Psychology (Irvine, Calif.)*, *7*(11), 1369–1390. doi:10.4236/psych.2016.711138

Ghosh, K., Khuntia, J., Chawla, S., & Deng, X. (2014). Media Reinforcement for Psychological Empowerment in Chronic Disease Management. CAIS, 34, 22.

Greenspun, H., & Coughlin, S. (2012). mHealth in an mWorld: How mobile technology is transforming health care. Deloitte Center for Health Solutions, 1-21.

Holmström, I., & Röing, M. (2010). The relation between patient-centeredness and patient empowerment: A discussion on concepts. *Patient Education and Counseling*, *79*(2), 167–172. doi:10.1016/j.pec.2009.08.008 PMID:19748203

Hoque, R., & Sorwar, G. (2017). Understanding factors influencing the adoption of mHealth by the elderly: An extension of the UTAUT model. *International Journal of Medical Informatics*, *101*, 75–84. doi:10.1016/j.ijmedinf.2017.02.002 PMID:28347450

Huang, K.-Y., & Ran, W. (2014). Not Just for Support: Companionship Activities in Healthcare Virtual Support Communities. *Communications of the Association for Information Systems*, *34*(29).

Iyengar, S., & Lepper, M. (2000). When Choice is Demotivating: Can One Desire Too Much of a Good Thing? *Journal of Personality and Social Psychology*, *79*(6), 995–1006. doi:10.1037/0022-3514.79.6.995 PMID:11138768

Jean, B., Koffi, B., Yazdanmehr, A., & Mahapatra, R. (2018). Mobile Health Mobile Health Privacy Concerns-A Systematic Review. *Twenty-fourth Americas Conference on Information Systems.*

Johnson, M. O., Rose, C. D., Dilworth, S. E., & Neilands, T. B. (2012). Advances in the conceptualization and measurement of Health Care Empowerment: Development and validation of the Health Care Empowerment inventory. *PLoS One*, *7*(9). doi:10.1371/journal.pone.0045692 PMID:23029184

Kenny, G., & Connolly, R. (2017). Towards an Inclusive World : Exploring M-Health Adoption Across Generations. *Twenty-fifth European Conference on Information Systems (ECIS)*, Guimarães, Portugal, (pp. 1129-1144).

Khuntia, J., Yim, D., Tanniru, M., & Lim, S. (2017). Patient empowerment and engagement with a health infomediary. *Health Policy and Technology*, *6*(1), 40–50. doi:10.1016/j.hlpt.2016.11.003

Klasnja, P., & Pratt, W. (2012). Healthcare in the pocket: Mapping the space of mobile-phone health interventions. *Journal of Biomedical Informatics*, *45*(1), 184–198. doi:10.1016/j.jbi.2011.08.017 PMID:21925288

Klecun, E. (2016). Transforming healthcare: Policy discourses of IT and patient-centred care. *European Journal of Information Systems*, *25*(1), 64–76. doi:10.1057/ejis.2014.40

Kwon, H. E., Dewan, S., Oh, W., & Kim, T. (2017). Efficacy of a Health App for Obesity and Overweight Management: A Hidden Markov Model. *International Conference on Information Systems*, 1-17.

Liberati, E. G., Gorli, M., Moja, L., Galuppo, L., Ripamonti, S., & Scaratti, G. (2015). Exploring the practice of patient centered care: The role of ethnography and reflexivity. *Social Science & Medicine*, *133*, 45–52. doi:10.1016/j.socscimed.2015.03.050 PMID:25841094

Liu, F., Guo, X., & Ju, X. (2018). Routine Use of Mobile Health Services: Promotion or Prevention. *International Conference on Information Systems* (pp. 1–10).

Loukanova, S., Molnar, R., & Bridges, J. F. P. (2007). Promoting patient empowerment in the healthcare system: Highlighting the need for patient-centered drug policy. *Expert Review of Pharmacoeconomics & Outcomes Research*, *7*(3), 281–289. doi:10.1586/14737167.7.3.281 PMID:20528314

Manda, T. D., & Herstad, J. (2015). Enacting technology: Accounting for the interplay between mHealth solutions and existing paper-based data reporting practices. *Information Technology & People*, *28*(3), 442–465. doi:10.1108/ITP-02-2014-0045

Marcolino, M. S., Oliveira, J. A. Q., D'Agostino, M., Ribeiro, A. L., Alkmim, M. B. M., & Novillo-Ortiz, D. (2018). The impact of mHealth interventions: Systematic review of systematic reviews. *JMIR mHealth and uHealth*, *6*(1), e23. doi:10.2196/mhealth.8873 PMID:29343463

Maunsell, E., Lauzier, S., Brunet, J., Pelletier, S., Osborne, R. H., & Campbell, H. S. (2014). Health-related empowerment in cancer: Validity of scales from the Health Education Impact Questionnaire. *Cancer*, *120*(20), 3228–3236. doi:10.1002/cncr.28847 PMID:24988944

Maynard, M. T., Gilson, L. L., & Mathieu, J. E. (2012). Empowerment-Fad or Fab? A Multilevel Review of the Past Two Decades of Research. *Journal of Management*, *38*(4), 1231–1281. doi:10.1177/0149206312438773

McAllister, M., Dunn, G., Payne, K., Davies, L., & Todd, C. (2012). Patient empowerment: The need to consider it as a measurable patient-reported outcome for chronic conditions. *BMC Health Services Research*, *12*(1), 157. doi:10.1186/1472-6963-12-157 PMID:22694747

McKinsey. (2013). mHealth: A new vision for healthcare. McKinsey & Company, 1-20.

Meng, F., Zhang, X., Guo, X., Lai, K. H., & Zhao, X. (2019). How Do Patients with Chronic Diseases Make Usage Decisions regarding Mobile Health Monitoring Service? *Journal of Healthcare Engineering*, 2019. PMID:30931088

Middleton, C., Scheepers, R., & Tuunainen, V. K. (2014). When mobile is the norm: Researching mobile information systems and mobility as post-adoption phenomena. *European Journal of Information Systems*, *23*(5), 503–512. doi:10.1057/ejis.2014.21

Miller, A. D., Pollack, A. H., & Pratt, W. (2016). Bursting the information bubble: Identifying opportunities for pediatric patient-centered technology. *American Medical Informatics Association Annual Symposium Proceedings, 2016*, 894. PMID:28269886

Noteboom, C., & Al-Ramahi, M. (2018). What are the Gaps in Mobile Patient Portal? Mining Users Feedback Using Topic Modeling. *Proceedings of the 51st Hawaii International Conference on System Sciences*, 1-16. 10.24251/HICSS.2018.072

Nouri, R., Niakan, R., Kalhori, S., Ghazisaeedi, M., Marchand, G., & Yasini, M. (2018). Criteria for assessing the quality of mHealth apps: A systematic review. *Journal of the American Medical Informatics Association*, *25*(8), 1089–1098. doi:10.1093/jamia/ocy050 PMID:29788283

Peleg, M., Michalowski, W., Wilk, S., Parimbelli, E., Bonaccio, S., O'Sullivan, D., ... Carrier, M. (2018). Ideating Mobile Health Behavioral Support for Compliance to Therapy for Patients with Chronic Disease: A Case Study of Atrial Fibrillation Management. *Journal of Medical Systems*, *42*(11), 234. doi:10.100710916-018-1077-4 PMID:30317403

Peleg, M., Shahar, Y., Quaglini, S., Fux, A., García-Sáez, G., Goldstein, A., ... Parimbelli, E. (2017). MobiGuide: A personalized and patient-centric decision-support system and its evaluation in the atrial fibrillation and gestational diabetes domains. *User Modeling and User-Adapted Interaction*, *27*(2), 159–213. doi:10.100711257-017-9190-5

Perera, G., Holbrook, A., Thabane, L., Foster, G., & Willison, D. J. (2011). Views on health information sharing and privacy from primary care practices using electronic medical records. *International Journal of Medical Informatics*, *80*(2), 94–101. doi:10.1016/j.ijmedinf.2010.11.005 PMID:21167771

Permwonguswa, S., Khuntia, J., Yim, D., & Gregg, D. (2017). Empowerment and knowledge sharing in health infomediary: empirical evidence from reconstructive surgery patients. In *Twenty-third Americas Conference on Information Systems*, Boston, MA.

Prgomet, M., Georgiou, A., & Westbrook, J. I. (2009). The impact of mobile handheld technology on hospital physicians' work practices and patient care: A systematic review. *Journal of the American Medical Informatics Association*, *16*(6), 792–801. doi:10.1197/jamia.M3215 PMID:19717793

Pung, A., Fletcher, S. L., & Gunn, J. M. (2018). Mobile app use by primary care patients to manage their depressive symptoms: Qualitative study. *Journal of Medical Internet Research*, *20*(9). doi:10.2196/10035 PMID:30262449

Rai, A., Chen, L., Pye, J., & Baird, A. (2013). Understanding determinants of consumer mobile health usage intentions, assimilation, and channel preferences. *Journal of Medical Internet Research*, *15*(8), e149. doi:10.2196/jmir.2635 PMID:23912839

Research2Guidance. (2018). mHealth Economics 2017/2018 – Connectivity in Digital Health. *Research2Guidance*, 1-17.

Reychav, I., Beeri, R., Balapour, A., Raban, D. R., Sabherwal, R., & Azuri, J. (2019). How reliable are self-assessments using mobile technology in healthcare? The effects of technology identity and self-efficacy. *Computers in Human Behavior*, *91*, 52–61. doi:10.1016/j.chb.2018.09.024

Reychav, I., Parush, A., McHaney, R., Hazan, M., & Moshonov, R. (2018). The use of mobile technology in waiting rooms to leverage women's empowerment: A conceptual context. *Health Informatics Journal, 24*(3), 277–292. doi:10.1177/1460458216671561 PMID:27738260

Rogers, S., Chamberlin, J., Ellison, M. L., & Crean, T. (1997). A consumer-constructed scale to measure empowerment among users of mental health services. *Psychiatric Services (Washington, D.C.), 48*(8), 1042–1047. doi:10.1176/ps.48.8.1042 PMID:9255837

Sandlund, M., Lindgren, H., Pohl, P., Melander-Wikman, A., Bergvall Kåreborn, B., & Lundin Olsson, L. (2016). Towards a mobile exercise application to prevent falls: A participatory design process. *International Journal of Child Health and Human Development, 9*(3), 389–398.

Singh, R., Mathiassen, L., Stachura, M. E., & Astapova, E. V. (2011). Capabilities in Home Health : IT-Enabled Transformation of Post-Acute Care. *Journal of the Association for Information Dynamic, 12*(2), 163–188. doi:10.17705/1jais.00257

Small, N., Bower, P., Chew-Graham, C. A., Whalley, D., & Protheroe, J. (2013). Patient empowerment in long-term conditions: Development and preliminary testing of a new measure. *BMC Health Services Research, 13*(1), 263. doi:10.1186/1472-6963-13-263 PMID:23835131

Spreitzer, G. M. (1995). Psychological Empowerment in the Workplace: Dimensions, Measurement, and Validation. *Academy of Management Journal, 38*(5), 1442–1465.

Srivastava, S. C., Shainesh, G., Barrett, M., Davidson, E., Prabhu, J., & Vargo, S. L. (2015). Bridging the Service Divide Through Digitally Enabled Service Innovations: Evidence from Indian Healthcare Service Providers. *Management Information Systems Quarterly, 39*(1), 245–267. doi:10.25300/MISQ/2015/39.1.11

Storni, C. (2014). Diabetes self-care in-the-wild: Design challenges for personal health record systems and self-monitoring technologies. *Information Technology & People, 27*(4), 397–420. doi:10.1108/ITP-02-2013-0032

Thomas, K. W., & Velthouse, B. A. (1990). Cognitive elements of empowerment: An "interpretive" model of intrinsic task motivation. *Academy of Management Review, 15*(4), 666–681.

Trocin, C., Arkhipova, D., Lee, G., Vaia, G., & Saccavini, C. (2018). The Effect of Network Centrality of Medical Specialists on Their Performance: Evidence from an Italian Health Information Exchange Platform. *International Conference on Information Systems Proceedings*, San Francisco, CA.

van den Broek, E., & Sergeeva, A. (2018). Empowering Patients Through Data: Promise versus Practice. Academy of Management Global Proceedings, 97.

Varshney, U. (2014). Mobile health: Four emerging themes of research. *Decision Support Systems, 66*, 20–35. doi:10.1016/j.dss.2014.06.001

Viswanathan, V., Hollebeek, L. D., Malthouse, E. C., Maslowska, E., Jung Kim, S., & Xie, W. (2017). The dynamics of consumer engagement with mobile technologies. *Service Science, 9*(1), 36–49. doi:10.1287erv.2016.0161

Webb, D. G., Horne, R., & Pinching, A. J. (2001). Treatment-related empowerment: Preliminary evaluation of a new measure in patients with advanced HIV disease. *International Journal of STD & AIDS*, *12*(2), 103–107. doi:10.1258/0956462011916875 PMID:11236098

Webster, J., & Watson, R. (2002). Analyzing the Past to Prepare for the Future: Writing a Literature Review. *MIS Quarterly, 26*(2), 13-23.

Wentzer, H. S., & Bygholm, A. (2013). Narratives of empowerment and compliance: Studies of communication in online patient support groups. *International Journal of Medical Informatics*, *82*(12), e386–e394. doi:10.1016/j.ijmedinf.2013.01.008 PMID:23523082

Wiljer, D., Urowitz, S., Apatu, E., DeLenardo, C., Eysenbach, G., Harth, T., ... Leonard, K. (2008). Patient accessible electronic health records: Exploring recommendations for successful implementation strategies. *Journal of Medical Internet Research*, *10*(4), e34. doi:10.2196/jmir.1061 PMID:18974036

Wilson, T. E., Kay, E. S., Turan, B., Johnson, M. O., Kempf, M. C., Turan, J. M., ... Goparaju, L. (2018). Healthcare empowerment and HIV viral control: Mediating roles of adherence and retention in care. *American Journal of Preventive Medicine*, *54*(6), 756–764. doi:10.1016/j.amepre.2018.02.012 PMID:29656911

Kay, M., Santos, J., & Takane, M. (2011). mHealth: New horizons for health through mobile technologies. *World Health Organization, 64*(7), 66-71.

World Health Organization. (2016). Global diffusion of eHealth: making universal health coverage achievable: report of the third global survey on eHealth (No. 9789241511780). World Health Organization.

Wu, J.-H., Wang, S.-C., & Lin, L.-M. (2007). Mobile computing acceptance factors in the healthcare industry: A structural equation model. *International Journal of Medical Informatics*, *76*(1), 66–77. doi:10.1016/j.ijmedinf.2006.06.006 PMID:16901749

Yaraghi, N., Du, A. Y., Sharman, R., Gopal, R. D., & Ramesh, R. (2014). Health information exchange as a multisided platform: Adoption, usage, and practice involvement in service co-production. *Information Systems Research*, *26*(1), 1–18. doi:10.1287/isre.2014.0547

Yen, C. C., Chang, L., Tai, B. C., Chan, H. C., Choolani, M., Lim, S., ... Xue, L. (2011). A study on Singaporean women's acceptance of using mobile phones to seek health information. *International Journal of Medical Informatics*, *80*(12), e189–e202. doi:10.1016/j.ijmedinf.2011.08.007 PMID:21956003

Zhao, Y., Ni, Q., & Zhou, R. (2018). What factors influence the mobile health service adoption? A meta-analysis and the moderating role of age. *International Journal of Information Management*, *43*, 342–350. doi:10.1016/j.ijinfomgt.2017.08.006

Zimmerman, M. A. (1995). Psychological empowerment: Issues and illustrations. *American Journal of Community Psychology*, *23*(5), 581–599. doi:10.1007/BF02506983 PMID:8851341

KEY TERMS AND DEFINITIONS

Digital Health: Digital health refers to the act of providing care services through the use of digital platforms such as Electronic Healthcare Records (EHR), Health Information Exchanges (HIE) and mobile devices to allow patients to self-manage their care path.

Digital Literacy: Digital literacy refers to the knowledge and capabilities of all care actors with a specific focus on patients to use digital tools, platforms and devices for self-managing their care path.

Emotional Empowerment: "The process of giving power to patients over their medical treatment means to give more decisional, cognitive, emotional control, and hope to improve personal quality of life" (i.e. Doll & Deng, 2010; Huang & Ran, 2014; Wilson et al., 2018).

Empowerment: "Empowerment is a process by which people, organizations, and communities gain mastery over issues of concern to them" (i.e. Zimmerman, 1995).

Health Literacy: Health literacy refers to the knowledge and capabilities of patients to accomplish specific tasks to improve personal health status according to the indications of the personal physician.

Mobile Application: The key concept of the mobile application is to offer a tailored service for digital health that directly and predominantly involves the patient (patient-centered-healthcare-ecosystem).

Mobile Health: "Mobile health is defined as medical and public health practice supported by mobile devices, such as mobile phones, patient monitoring devices, personal digital assistants (PDAs), and other wireless devices" (i.e. WHO, 2016).

Patient Empowerment: "Patient empowerment is a process designed to facilitate self-directed behavior change. The empowerment approach involves facilitating and supporting patients to reflect on their experience of living with diabetes."

Psychological Empowerment: "Psychological Empowerment is a feeling of control, a critical awareness of one's environment, and an active engagement in it" (i.e. Spreitzer, 1995).

ENDNOTES

1 It is important to notice that the concept of patient empowerment is similar, but it is not interchangeable with the concept of patient engagement. Empowerment represents the process by which patients gain control over their care path and feel that they can adequately cope with events and situations. The feel of empowerment leads the patient to better accomplish the required tasks. Engagement is the act of health providers and patients working together to contribute to improved health conditions. This includes better education, better motivation, creating a better healthcare experience, and driving better and shared decision-making (Peleg et al., 2018).

2 For examples of successful implementation of these concepts and key factors of patient empowerment seeKlasnja and Pratt (2012); Wiljer et al (2008); Reychav et al (2019).

3 The definition can be retrieved from the following link:https://www.who.int/maternal_child_adolescent/topics/quality-of-care/definition/en/

APPENDIX

Table 4. Self-determination, autonomy and self-efficacy definitions

Terminology	Definition	References
Self-determination	*A patients' sense of having choice in initiating and regulating tasks and processes*	(Aujoulat et al., 2007; Doll & Deng, 2010)
Autonomy	*The degree of choice patients have in using mobile technology for their healthcare conditions*	(Aujoulat et al., 2007; Holmström & Röing, 2010; Dadgar & Joshi, 2018)
Self-efficacy	*A patients' belief in his/her ability to use the mobile health technology for own healthcare path*	(McAllister et al., 2012; Small et al., 2013; Galanakis et al., 2016; Reychav et al., 2019)

Source: Authors' elaboration

Chapter 4
mHealth as Tools for Development in Mental Health

Gloria Ejehiohen Iyawa
Namibia University of Science and Technology, Namibia

Julie Langan-Martin
University of Glasgow, UK

Stephen Sevalie
University of Sierra Leone, Sierra Leone

Wanano Masikara
https://orcid.org/0000-0002-4328-0570
Nanosoft Designs, Botswana

ABSTRACT

This chapter provides an assessment of studies on mobile health (mHealth) tools for development in addressing diseases relating to mental health, informs the current publications trends, identifies research gaps in the existing literature, and suggests a future research agenda that can help address these gaps. We, therefore, assessed empirical studies using a Systematic Mapping Study approach. We searched five academic databases as well as Google Search Engine and Google Scholar. Based on the inclusion and exclusion criteria, 54 full-text papers were included in this chapter. The findings suggest a growing trend in the use of various mHealth tools for mental health, such as mobile apps and text messaging. The findings also suggest that the responsibility of health monitoring and management can be shared between the medical practitioner and the patient in mental healthcare. Research gaps were identified and areas for future research are proposed.

DOI: 10.4018/978-1-7998-0047-7.ch004

INTRODUCTION AND BACKGROUND

Mental Health

The World Health Organization (WHO) (2014) defines mental health as a "state of well-being in which every individual realizes his or her own potential, can cope with the normal stresses of life, can work productively and fruitfully, and is able to make a contribution to her or his community." However, several conditions can greatly impact on the mental health of a person, including mental illnesses such as depression (Hellman, 2018), post-traumatic stress disorder (PTSD) (Bisson et al., 2015), schizophrenia (Rasool et al., 2018) and psychosis (Chan, 2017). Mental health is a serious health issue; however, countries have paid little attention to the burden of mental health (Tomlinson & Lund, 2012). Russell and Patrick (2018) emphasize the importance of addressing mental health issues as these cause a financial strain on health systems.

One of the United Nations' Sustainable Development Goals (SDGs) is to ensure that populations of the world live a healthy life as stated in the SDG 3, to maintain "good health and well-being" (United Nations Development Programme, 2016). To achieve these goals, countries have taken innovative approaches. Some efforts include the use of technologies in diagnosing, managing and aiding the treatment of diseases (Hoffmann & Svenaeus, 2018). Iyawa, Herselman and Botha (2017a) propose Digital Health Innovation Ecosystems as a practical approach for meeting these goals. Digital Health Innovation Ecosystems emphasize the use of digital health technologies in the delivery of healthcare services where both patients and key healthcare stakeholders interact in a digital platform with evidence of the "principles of innovation" (Iyawa et al., 2016a; 2017d, p. 433).

Iyawa et al. (2016a, p.249) define Digital Health Innovation Ecosystems as a "a network of digital health communities consisting of interconnected, interrelated and interdependent digital health species, including healthcare stakeholders, healthcare institutions and digital healthcare devices situated in a digital health environment, who adopt the best-demonstrated practices that have been proven to be successful, and implementation of those practices through the use of information and communication technologies to monitor and improve the wellbeing and health of patients, to empower patients in the management of their health and that of their families." This definition suggests that all healthcare stakeholders are involved in the healthcare process which includes both medical practitioners and patients. Involving patients in healthcare delivery processes have shown to improve health outcomes (Vahdat et al., 2014). While Herselman et al. (2016) advocate for a Digital Health Innovation Ecosystem for South Africa, Iyawa et al. (2017b) validate the components of a Digital Health Innovation Ecosystem in Namibia and present a framework for implementing such an ecosystem in the Namibian context (Iyawa, 2017c). Other studies on Digital Health Innovation Ecosystems highlight the benefits of implementing such an ecosystem. Some of the benefits include the sharing of information between healthcare stakeholders such as patients and doctors and improved healthcare services (Iyawa et al., 2017b; Iyawa et al., 2019).

Digital Health Innovation Ecosystems are important in ensuring that patients are involved in the healthcare process through digital health technologies with innovative approaches. Iyawa et al. (2016b) present the components of a digital health innovation ecosystem which includes digital health, innovation and digital ecosystems as shown in Figure 1. An example of digital health technologies is the use of mobile technologies for healthcare purposes (mHealth) as shown in Figure 1 (Iyawa et al., 2016b). The

Figure 1. Components of a digital health innovation ecosystem (Iyawa et al., 2016b)

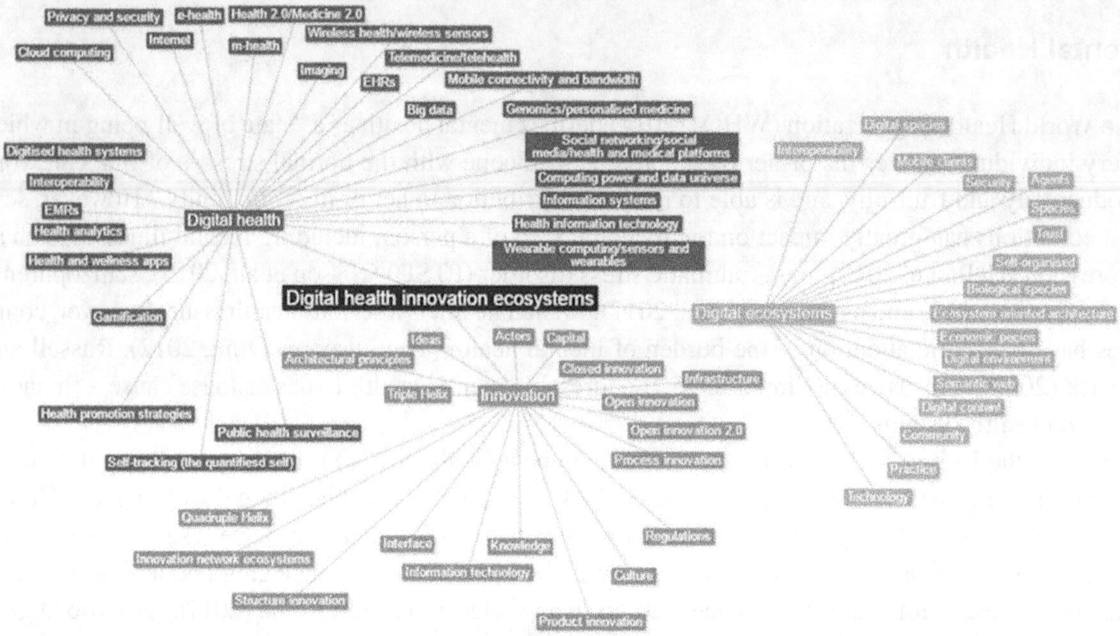

focus of this chapter is on applying a component of Digital Health Innovation Ecosystems, mHealth, for mental healthcare and explore how different healthcare stakeholders such as patients and medical practitioners make use of mHealth as tools for development in mental health.

mHealth

mHealth is an element of digital health and Digital Health Innovation Ecosystems, which leverages mobile technologies in the provision of healthcare services (Botha & Booi, 2016; Vesel et al., 2015). While other definitions of mHealth suggest that mobile technologies and devices are included in the provision of healthcare services (WHO's Global Observatory for eHealth (GOe), Istephanian, Jovanov and Zhang (2004) explain that mHealth is not just about the application of mobile devices for health care but the application of sensor technologies as well. Sensors in mobile devices have provided a new dimension in improving the health and well-being of patients. Application of mobile technologies in improving the health of patients include the use of mobile phones for educating pregnant and postpartum women (Su et al., 2016; Alam et al., 2017; Iyawa & Hamunyela, 2019), the use of mobile phones for health promotion (Kaplan and Stone, 2013) and apps that aid identification of diseases (Jutel & Lupton, 2015). mHealth encompasses a wide range of mobile technologies including low-end tablets (O'Donovan et al., 2018), mobile phones (Zimic et al., 2009) especially in developing countries where the majority of the population may not have access to sophisticated mobile technologies. For the purpose of this study, mHealth is defined as the use of any mobile device including mobile phones, smartphones, mobile or phone-based sensors for providing and receiving healthcare services such as healthcare monitoring, diagnosis, management and prediction of diseases. One of the reasons why mobile technologies have been adopted for healthcare is the rapid expansion of mobile phone access worldwide, including in low-income countries (Davey & Davey, 2014). With this growing potential, mobile technologies have been adopted in the healthcare sector for health care purposes.

mHealth and Mental Health

mHealth has been used to monitor and support mental health and mental illnesses. For example, managing mental disorders such as depression (Carswell et al., 2018), psychosis (Stamate et al., 2017), and schizophrenia (Ben-Zeev et al., 2016). Recently, there has been an increase in the use of mobile technologies in providing care to patients. From healthcare service delivery (DeSouza et al., 2015) to diagnosis and monitoring of diseases (Alepsis & Lambrinidis, 2013), mobile technologies have been incorporated in healthcare. One reason for the adoption of this technology is the accessibility of mobile technologies by a considerable proportion of the population, especially in rural and medically underserved communities (Sylvester, 2016; Afolayan et al. 2015). Campbell et al. (2015) also found that mobile phone usage among people with mental health issues was high and also recommended the use of text messaging as a technique to support patients with mental health problems. Despite reviews summarizing and evaluating these technologies in mental healthcare (Sedrati et al., 2016; Chandrashekar, 2018), there is still no study focusing on the current trends in publications of mHealth tools for mental health. This mapping study is useful in identifying research gaps in the literature regarding the use of mobile technologies in mental health and developing a future research agenda. This chapter provides an assessment of studies of mHealth tools for mental health conditions, assesses the current publications trends, researches gaps in the existing literature and identifies future research agenda that can help address the gaps identified.

RESEARCH QUESTIONS

For the main objectives to be achieved, the following research questions were posed:

- What are the publication trends in mental health mHealth research over the last decade?
    - This question aimed to investigate how many papers have been published on the application of mHealth tools for mental health purposes within the last ten years.
- In what ways are mHealth tools being used to address mental health issues?
    - This question aimed to investigate the different mental illnesses in which mHealth tools have been applied and how these technologies are being applied.
- What are the different types of mHealth technologies and applications that have been employed in mental health interventions?
    - This question aimed to investigate various mobile technologies and tools that are being used for mental health interventions.
- In what settings have mobile technologies been used in mental healthcare interventions?
    - This question aimed to identify the different settings in which mHealth has been applied in mental health.
- What are the main publication outlets for publishing research on mHealth for mental health?
    - This question aimed to identify the main publication outlets for publishing research on mHealth for mental health

A systematic mapping study approach was used to achieve the main aim of this chapter. Hence, this chapter contributes to the literature on mHealth for mental health by mapping out current trends of published research on the subject.

This chapter is structured as follows: the research methodology is presented in the next section. Then, results and discussion of the findings are presented. Finally, this chapter concludes with recommendations and future work.

RESEARCH METHODOLOGY

The systematic mapping study review method was applied to assess mHealth studies in mental health. Other review methods have been used to assess empirical studies in mental health. Examples include, systematic literature reviews of mHealth for mental health services (Aldridge & McChesney, 2018; Karasouli & Adams, 2014), scoping review of the mental health of immigrants (Guruge & Butt, 2015; Goldner et al., 2015) and critical review of mental health policies (Wong et al., 2014). A systematic mapping study aims to "map out and categorize existing literature on a particular topic, identifying gaps in research literature from which to commission further reviews and/or primary research" (Grant & Booth, 2009, p. 97). Systematic mapping reviews have been conducted in different fields including wearable technologies (Iyawa, Velusamy, & Palanisamy, 2019) and software engineering (Petersen et al., 2008). The concept of systematic mapping reviews is to explain the trends of particular research (Grant and Booth, 2009) and is in line with the objective of this chapter. As such, the systematic mapping review was the appropriate methodology to apply in this context.

This systematic mapping review adopted guidelines for conducting systematic mapping studies as outlined by Petersen et al. (2008). This will be detailed in the subsequent sections.

SEARCH FOR RELEVANT PAPERS

Data Sources

We searched five academic databases, namely, IEEE Xplore, ScienceDirect, PyschINFO, Scopus and ACM. We also searched Google Scholar and Google Search engine. A total of 3887 papers were retrieved. After the removal of duplicate records, 3252 papers were identified. We conducted the search in three phases, title, abstract and full-text. We first searched for relevant titles and removed papers with an irrelevant title. In this process, 1822 papers were excluded. 1430 papers remained. These abstracts were read for relevance. In this process, 803 papers were removed. 627 full-text articles were analysed and based on inclusion and exclusion criteria, 54 relevant papers were included in this study. We conducted the search from February 2019 to April 2019.

Inclusion and Exclusion Criteria

- We included papers on mHealth specifically focusing on mental health
- We included articles published between 2009 and 2019
- We included journal articles and conference papers

Our exclusion criteria are listed as follows:

- We excluded papers not written in English
- We excluded papers with mental health focus outside the context of mHealth
- We excluded papers which are not explicitly focused on the mental health of patients
- We excluded Masters and PhD theses

RESULTS

RQ 1: What are the Publication Trends in Mental Health mHealth Research over the Last Decade?

The findings show, in general, an increase in publications in mHealth for mental health research over the past decade. For example, in the first 5 years (2010-2015 inclusive), we retrieved 18 papers relevant to our study and in the second 4 years (2016-2019 inclusive), we retrieved 36 papers relevant to our study. For 2019, we retrieved data published till April 2019. The publication trends of mHealth studies on mental health are illustrated in Figure 2.

RQ2: In What Ways are mHealth Being Used to Address Mental Health Issues?

The literature suggests that mHealth tools and technologies including mobile phones, smartphones, and mobile apps have been used to provide a variety of mental health services. The subsequent sections of this chapter explain the different ways mHealth is being applied to address mental health issues.

Determining the Mental State of a Patient

Mankodiya et al. (2013) assessed the feasibility of assessing emotions and the mental state of patients through the use of a smartphone camera to determine the presence of mental illnesses as early as possible. Chow et al. (2019) piloted the use of mobile apps to support the mental health of patients with

Figure 2. Publication trends in the last decade

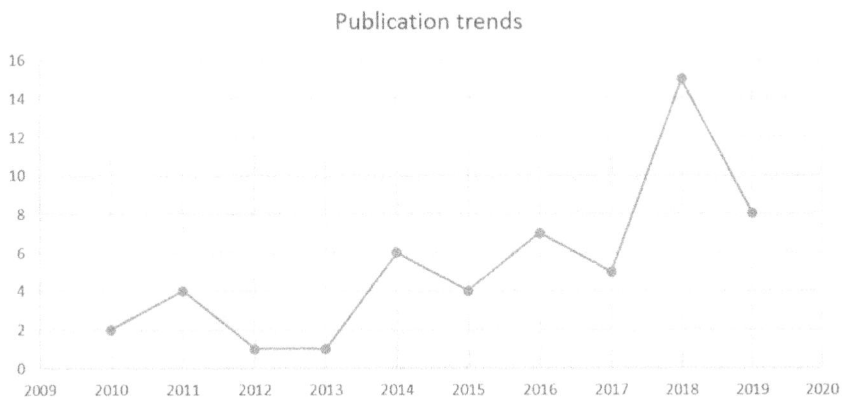

breast cancer. Epp et al. (2011) developed a mobile app to support nursing trainees in understanding the processes of assessing the mental state of a patient. An evaluation of the app revealed that it improved nursing students' learning.

Treatment of Patients With Dementia

Laird et al. (2018) evaluated the use of a mobile app to support patients living with dementia and the study found that it improved the mental health of these patients.

Early Prediction, Prevention, and Treatment of Depression

mHealth tools such as mobile apps have been used for treating depression (Osma & Plasma, 2014). Mobile apps have also been used to facilitate healthy living in patients with depression and diabetes (Hartzler et al., 2016) as well as support postnatal mothers suffering from depression (Sawyer et al., 2018). Apart from mobile apps, other techniques such as short message service (SMS) and text messaging have been used for the early prevention of depression and violence in young people (Chu et al., 2018; Ranney et al., 2018). A study by Lipschitz et al. (2019) shows that mobile apps can be easily adopted for the treatment of depression. Burns et al. (2011) developed a mobile app based on machine learning algorithms to predict the mood of patients, as such, predict depression in patients.

Suicide Prevention and Monitoring

Indigenous mobile apps have been designed and developed for specific communities in Australia, such as the Aboriginals for suicide prevention (Larsen et al., 2015). Nuij et al. (2018) investigated the possibility of using mobile phones to monitor patients that are at risk of suicide.

Treatment of Bipolar Disorder

Torri et al. (2015) explored the requirements of a mobile app to support the treatment of bipolar disorder. Sensor-based mHealth approaches have been used to monitor diseases such as bipolar disorder and depression (Seppala et al., 2019). Menon et al. (2018) evaluated the use of text messaging to ensure patients with bipolar I disorder take their medication. Prociow and Crowe (2010) utilized a mobile app to facilitate self-monitoring of patients with bipolar disorder.

Detection, Prediction, and Management of Psychosis

Smartphones (Stamate et al., 2017) and smartphone apps (Niendam et al., 2018) have been used to detect psychosis and report mental health symptoms of young patients with psychosis. Niendam et al. (2018) evaluated the use of smartphone apps to report health symptoms of young patients with psychosis. Välimäki et al. (2012) evaluated the Mobile.Net short message service (SMS) as an intervention to improve treatment for people with schizophrenia. The impact of the intervention is that it allowed customized messages to facilitate medication adherence and follow-up.

Maintaining Mindfulness

Maintaining mindfulness is one of the goals of researchers working on technology to support mental disorder. For example, Sanchez et al. (2015) developed a mobile app to help older people maintain mindfulness, while Wolf et al. (2016) investigated user actions on their phones to determine mindfulness in depressed patients. Garcia et al. (2017) also developed an app to train people on mindfulness and improve their mental health. Lee and Jung (2018) evaluated the effectiveness of a mindfulness-based app ("DeStressify") to support university students with mental health challenges.

Monitoring and Management of Patients with Schizophrenia

Ben-Zeev et al. (2016) found that mobile phones can be used by clinicians to engage patients in the management of schizophrenia in distant locations. Wang et al. (2016) evaluated crosscheck, a mobile app for the early detection of schizophrenia.

Monitoring Patients with Parkinson's Disease

Cancela et al. (2016) proposed the development of a mobile app to support different specialists in monitoring patients with Parkinson's disease.

Monitoring of Anxiety

Lipschitz et al. (2019) indicate that patients are willing to use mobile apps for monitoring of anxiety. mHealth tools have also supported patients suffering from anxiety. For example, Firth et al. (2017) presented the use of smartphones to alleviate anxiety. Some mobile apps have been developed to support patients with anxiety, for instance, Stoll et al. (2017) and Almadovar et al. (2018) used a mobile app to manage anxiety in young people. Harrison et al. (2011) assessed the efficacy of mobile apps to improve anxiety and low mood, which contains an SMS reminder. Using a mobile app, Teng et al. (2018) enforced an attention training mechanism to improve anxiety symptoms among people between the ages of 20 and 35 years old.

Borderline Personality Disorder and Self-Injury

Lederer et al. (2014) developed a prototype for developing a mobile app for borderline personality disorder and self-injury. Stallard et al. (2018) evaluated BlueIce, a mobile app to encourage activities that boost young people's mood and as such discourage them from engaging in self-harm behaviours.

Cognitive Behavourial Therapy Sessions

A mobile app was developed to facilitate cognitive behavioral therapy sessions between patients and their therapists (Michelle, Jarzabek, & Wadhwa, 2014).

Rehabilitation

Rizia et al. (2014) developed a mobile peering app, iPeer, to aid in the rehabilitation of veterans to facilitate mental help.

Improving the Quality of Care in Child Mental Health Treatment

mHealth tools have also been applied to the care of children with mental health problems. An example is the use of tablet technology to provide trauma–focused cognitive-behavioral therapy for children (Davidson et al., 2019).

General Mental Health

Mobile apps have been used generally to support and monitor patients with mental illnesses (Tuli et al., 2016). Such apps include recording of disabilities caused as a result of mental health issues (Hebert et al., 2016). Washington et al. (2015) further suggest a method for conducting mHealth trials with mobile apps. Studies have evaluated how patients with mental health issues use mobile apps (Torous et al., 2018; Atallah et al., 2018) and it was identified that the use of mobile apps for mental health is low when patients are out of the hospital. The benefits and challenges of using mobile apps for mental health have also been discussed (Brian & Ben-Zeev, 2014; Jain et al., 2015). Feasibility studies on the use of mHealth apps for mental health in countries such as Finland and Palestine have been conducted (Simila et al., 2018; Ben-Zeev et al., 2017). A mobile app was community co-designed to assist the youth in addressing their mental health issues (Waterman et al., 2018). Other areas of study include the development of a mobile app to monitor side effects of psychotropic medications (Rojnic et al., 2018) and the use of a mobile app to aid the collection of research data for mental health research. Mobile phones have also been used to aid the treatment of patients with serious mental illness to support their full recovery (Noel et al., 2019), to reduce stress (Mak et al., 2019) and for mood reporting (Morris et al., 2010).

RQ 3: What are the Different Types of mHealth Technologies and Applications That Have Been Employed in Mental Healthcare Intervention?

To answer this research question, we grouped the technology types we identified in the literature. However, some articles we identified in the search did not state explicitly the type of technology used (Torri et al., 2015; Cancela et al., 2015). The mobile technologies which have been used to support mental health include mobile apps, smartphones, text messaging/SMS, mobile phones, sensors and mobile phone-based sensors. mHealth technologies and applications for mental health intervention are presented in Figure 3.

RQ 4: In What Settings Have Mobile Technologies Been Applied in Mental Healthcare Intervention?

Several articles did not indicate the settings where the studies were conducted. However, some studies mentioned the United States (n=11), Australia (n=3), or the United Kingdom, Canada and Finland (n=2 for each). Other countries such as Taiwan, Singapore, Sierra Leone, New Zealand, Saudi Arabia,

Figure 3. mHealth tools and technologies used for mental health intervention

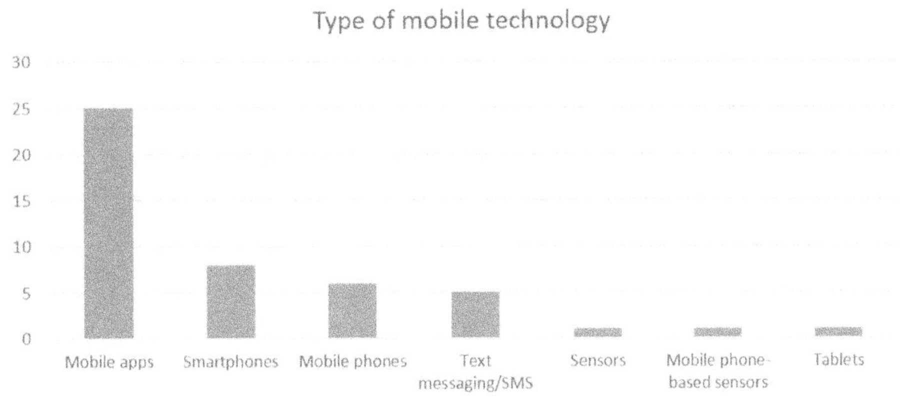

India, Croatia, China, Serbia, Palestine, and Netherlands were the settings for single studies exploring mHealth for mental health. The number of countries in which mHealth for mental health intervention have been discussed is illustrated in Figure 4.

RQ 5: What are the Main Publication Outlets for Publishing Research on mHealth for Mental Health?

The majority of studies on mHealth for mental health have been published in journals (n=36), while other studies have been presented at conferences which are depicted in Table 1.

DISCUSSION

This chapter assessed literature on the use of mHealth tools for mental health conditions, to inform the current publications trends, research gaps in the existing literature and identify future research agenda that can help address the research gaps identified. This chapter, thus, contributes to the literature on mHealth for mental health by mapping out the current trends of published research on the subject.

Figure 4. Countries in which mHealth for mental health have been discussed

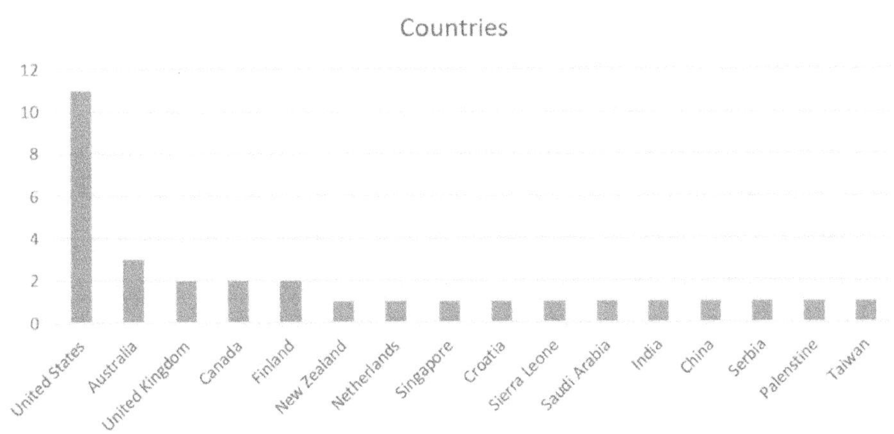

Table 1. List of publishing outlets

Outlet Type	Journal/Conference name	# Publications
Journals	JMIR Mental Health (7)	36
	Journal of Psychiatric Research (2)	
	Journal of Affective Disorders (1)	
	JMIR Research Protocols (3)	
	Computer Methods and Programs in Biomedicine (1)	
	Asian Journal of Psychiatry (3)	
	Geriatric Nursing (1)	
	Schizophrenia Research (1)	
	JMIR mHealth and uHealth (2)	
	International Journal of Medical Informatics (1)	
	Journal of Medical Internet Research (2)	
	Mental Health & Prevention (1)	
	Hong Kong Medical Journal (1)	
	Internet Interventions (1)	
	BMC Family Practice (1)	
	Personal and Ubiquitous Computing (2)	
	Clinical Psychological Science (1)	
	Journal of Mental Health (1)	
	Cognitive and Behavioral Practice (1)	
	Behavior Therapy (1)	
	BMC Public Health (1)	
	Procedia Computer Science (1)	
Conferences	IEEE 10th International Conference on Ubiquitous Intelligence & Computing and 2013 IEEE 10th International Conference on Autonomic & Trusted Computing (1)	18
	IEEE-EMBS International Conference on Biomedical and Health Informatics (1)	
	IEEE Global Humanitarian Technology Conference - South Asia Satellite (1)	
	IEEE International Conference on Collaborative Computing: Networking, Applications and Worksharing (1)	
	IEEE 3nd International Conference on Serious Games and Applications for Health (1)	
	Hawaii International Conference on System Sciences (1)	
	Annual international conference of the IEEE engineering in Medicine and biology society (1)	
	International conference on pervasive computing technologies for healthcare (1)	
	IET International Conference on Technologies for Active and Assisted Living (1)	
	International Workshop on Service Science for e-Health (1)	
	Annual International Conference of the IEEE Engineering in Medicine and Biology Society (2)	
	IEEE Global Humanitarian Technology Conference (1)	
	IEEE International Conference on Machine Learning and Applications (1)	
	ACM CHI Conference on Human Factors in Computing Systems (1)	
	ACM International Joint Conference on Pervasive and Ubiquitous Computing: Adjunct (1)	

continues on following page

Table 1. Continued

Outlet Type	Journal/Conference name	# Publications
	European Conference on Technology Enhanced Learning (1)	
	IEEE Annual International Conference of the IEEE Engineering in Medicine and Biology (1)	

This chapter found that research on mHealth for mental health has evolved over the last decade. The findings suggest there is a progressive growth in the mobile mental health research domain (Torous et al., 2018; Ranney et al., 2018; Chu et al., 2018; Niendam et al., 2018; Atallah et al., 2018). The findings on the publication trends in the last decade suggest a slight decline in 2012 and 2013. This could be as a result of our inclusion and exclusion criteria; as such, the authors could not find relevant papers for that period. This shows that research on mHealth for mental health is emerging. The findings also show that mHealth has been used to monitor and manage different mental health disorders such as depression (Osma & Plasma, 2014), schizophrenia (Ben-Zeev et al., 2016), anxiety disorder (Firth et al., 2017), psychosis (Niendam et al., 2018) and bipolar disorder (Torri et al., 2015).

Mobile technologies have also been used for prediction of mental disorders as well as tracking compliance to medications as well as to identify the side effects of certain medications (Menon et al., 2018; Burns et al., 2011). However, there was a lack of studies on the use of mHealth for a variety of mental disorders, such as eating disorders, obsessive-compulsive disorder, post-traumatic stress disorder and seasonal affective disorder. These areas of mental health disorders represent some of the mental health disorders where mHealth research is lacking. However, mHealth may be of potential value in monitoring and treatment of these mental disorders. Furthermore, there was a lack of research on using mHealth as a strategy for addressing the mental health and well-being of patients in displaced communities, victims of sexual and gender-based violence, especially in low-resource settings.

Various mHealth technologies and tools have been used to support mental health. Examples include text messaging/SMS (Harrison et al., 2011). This represents the easiest way of providing mental health service. Text messaging/SMS is often used to inform and remind patients of appointments or to improve drug adherence (Menon et al., 2018). mHealth can thus be used to facilitate medication adherence among patients, thereby improving the efficiency of mental health care. Mobile applications have also been heavily used for mental health care as evidenced by the findings. Mobile apps, thus, show great potential for development in mental health care. Mobile apps facilitate a wide range of activities such as tracking and early detection of mental illnesses. The difference between mobile apps and other forms of mHealth tools and technologies is that mobile apps are often programmed, to perform specific functions, using algorithms and models, such as machine learning and deep learning. The importance of such algorithms is that they are useful for diagnosis, prediction and prescriptive analysis, offering more capabilities for mHealth in mental health. However, such technologies can mostly be used in urban areas, where people have access to smartphones. Hence, more research should focus on improving the capability of basic mobile phones to perform specific functions to support mental health care.

Mobile phone-based sensors show great potential for mental health. However, the literature suggests that they are seldom used probably because it is a new and emerging area. Researchers can make use of mobile phone-based sensors to optimize mental health care as these sensors can be used to collect relevant data which can be helpful in the early diagnosis and detection of mental health problems (Wang et al., 2016).

Studies on mHealth for mental health has been conducted in various contexts, although the contexts were not mentioned in the majority of the studies. Countries, where mHealth for mental health have been discussed included the United States, United Kingdom, Singapore, Australia, Netherlands, New Zealand, Canada, Finland, Croatia, Sierra Leone, Saudi Arabia, China, India, Taiwan, Serbia, and Palestine. Nine of these countries represent high-income countries. Low-income countries should endeavor to carry out and publish research on mHealth tools for mental health care, as mobile phone penetration is high in these countries (James, 2010), and there is a great need for mental health support as the majority of developing countries often lack mental health resources such as skilled staff, health information systems and ability to capture data for research and mental health service improvement (Bruckner et al., 2011).

The findings of the study show that more papers on mHealth for mental health have been published in journals than conferences, which is similar to other fields where publications rates in journals are much higher than publications in conferences (Iyawa et al., 2019).

The application of mHealth for mental health shows that patients can be empowered to manage their health. This provides a different perspective on how the responsibility of healthcare can be shared between the healthcare practitioner and the patient. mHealth tools can significantly improve the healthcare process as patients are given the opportunity to take part in the diagnosis and monitoring of their health and provide early diagnosis and monitoring of mental health related diseases.

CONCLUSION

In conclusion, this chapter assessed the publication trends of studies exploring mHealth for mental health. The chapter also highlighted the years of active publications, countries in which active research on mHealth for mental health was conducted in the last ten years, areas of research on mHealth tools for addressing mental health disorders, specific mHealth tools and technologies, and publication outlets for disseminating the findings on the subject. This chapter, therefore, suggests that mHealth tools and technologies have indeed, been used for development in mental health as these tools have facilitated treatment and management of mental health conditions.

This study was, however, limited in some ways. First, our findings were based on a search from 2009 to 2019; as such, this might have put a constraint on the publications included in this study. We might have excluded relevant papers as we used only five academic databases. We might have excluded some essential findings from Masters and PhD theses as our inclusion and exclusion criteria did not permit these studies. The keywords we used might have also put a constraint on the papers retrieved.

The authors, therefore, based on the gaps and challenges identified in the current research, recommend mHealth research in other areas of mental health such as obsessive-compulsive disorder, post-traumatic stress disorder and seasonal affective disorder.

The findings from the literature search suggest that text messaging and SMS have been used for mental health intervention. Although mobile apps seemed to be more popular, text messaging and SMS could be a cost-effective approach and relevant in rural areas where the majority of the population do not have access to smartphones.

The findings of this chapter indicate that there is less research in the application of mHealth tools and technologies for mental health intervention in developing countries, and as such, researchers should focus on conducting research in these countries, owing to the huge potential benefits in reducing treatment gap in low-resource settings.

REFERENCES

Afolayan, T., Aiterebhe, E. F., & Mejabi, V. (2015). Mobile phone usage in rural communities in Kwara state, Nigeria. *Inform Technolt*, *12*(2), 1–15.

Alam, M., D'Este, C., Banwell, C., & Lokuge, K. (2017). The impact of mobile phone based messages on maternal and child healthcare behaviour: A retrospective cross-sectional survey in Bangladesh. *BMC Health Services Research*, *17*(1), 434. doi:10.118612913-017-2361-6 PMID:28645278

Alepis, E., & Lambrinidis, C. (2013). M-health: Supporting automated diagnosis and electonic health records. *SpringerPlus*, *2*(1), 103. doi:10.1186/2193-1801-2-103 PMID:23556144

Almodovar, A. S., Surve, S., Axon, D. R., Cooper, D., & Nahata, M. C. (2018). Self-directed engagement with a mobile app (Sinasprite) and its effects on confidence in coping skills, depression, and anxiety: Retrospective longitudinal study. *JMIR mHealth and uHealth*, *6*(3), e64. doi:10.2196/mhealth.9612 PMID:29549066

Atallah, N., Khalifa, M., El Metwally, A., & Househ, M. (2018). The prevalence and usage of mobile health applications among mental health patients in Saudi Arabia. *Computer Methods and Programs in Biomedicine*, *156*, 163–168. doi:10.1016/j.cmpb.2017.12.002 PMID:29428068

Ben-Zeev, D., Fathy, C., Jonathan, G., Abuharb, B., Brian, R. M., Kesbeh, L., & Abdelkader, S. (2017). mHealth for mental health in the Middle East: Need, technology use, and readiness among Palestinians in the West Bank. *Asian Journal of Psychiatry*, *27*, 1–4. doi:10.1016/j.ajp.2017.02.010 PMID:28558877

Ben-Zeev, D., Scherer, E. A., Gottlieb, J. D., Rotondi, A. J., Brunette, M. F., Achtyes, E. D., & Mohr, D. C. (2016). mHealth for schizophrenia: Patient engagement with a mobile phone intervention following hospital discharge. *JMIR Mental Health*, *3*(3), 1–9. doi:10.2196/mental.6348 PMID:27465803

Bisson, J., Cosgrove, S., Lewis, C., & Roberts, N. P. (2015). Post-traumatic stress disorder. *Clinical Review*, *351*, 1–7. PMID:26611143

Brian, R. M., & Ben-Zeev, D. (2014). Mobile health (mHealth) for mental health in Asia: Objectives, strategies, and limitations. *Asian Journal of Psychiatry*, *10*, 96–100. doi:10.1016/j.ajp.2014.04.006 PMID:25042960

Bruckner, T. A., Scheffler, R. M., Shen, G., Yoon, J., Chisholm, D., Morris, J., & Saxena, S. (2011). The mental health workforce gap in low-and middle-income countries: A needs-based approach. *Bulletin of the World Health Organization*, *89*(3), 184–194. doi:10.2471/BLT.10.082784 PMID:21379414

Burns, M. N., Begale, M., Duffecy, J., Gergle, D., Karr, C. J., Giangrande, E., & Mohr, D. C. (2011). Harnessing context sensing to develop a mobile intervention for depression. *Journal of Medical Internet Research*, *13*(3), e55. doi:10.2196/jmir.1838 PMID:21840837

Campbell, B., Caine, K., Connelly, K., Doub, T., & Bragg, A. (2015). Cell phone ownership and use among mental health outpatients in the USA. *Personal and Ubiquitous Computing*, *19*(2), 367–378. doi:10.100700779-014-0822-z

Cancela, J., Mascato, S. V., Gatsios, D., Rigas, G., Marcante, A., Gentile, G., & Konitsiotis, S. (2016). Monitoring of motor and non-motor symptoms of Parkinson's disease through a mHealth platform. Paper presented at the *38th Annual International Conference of the IEEE Engineering in Medicine and Biology Society*, Orlando, FL. 10.1109/EMBC.2016.7590789

Carswell, K., Harper-Shehadeh, M., Watts, S., van't Hof, E., Ramia, J. A., Heim, E., ... van Ommeren, M. (2018). Step-by-Step: A new WHO digital mental health intervention for depression. *mHealth*, *4*, 1–7. doi:10.21037/mhealth.2018.08.01 PMID:30225240

Chan, V. (2017). Schizophrenia and psychosis: Diagnosis, current research trends, and model treatment approaches with implications for transitional age youth. *Child and Adolescent Psychiatric Clinics*, *26*(2), 341–366. doi:10.1016/j.chc.2016.12.014 PMID:28314460

Chandrashekar, P. (2018). Do mental health mobile apps work: Evidence and recommendations for designing high-efficacy mental health mobile apps. *mHealth*, *4*, 1–4. doi:10.21037/mhealth.2018.03.02 PMID:29682510

Chow, P. I., Showalter, S. L., Gerber, M. S., Kennedy, E., Brenin, D. R., Schroen, A. T., ... Cohn, W. F. (2019). Use of Mental Health Apps by Breast Cancer Patients and Their Caregivers in the United States: Protocol for a Pilot Pre-Post Study. *JMIR Research Protocols*, *8*(1). doi:10.2196/11452

Chu, J. T. W., Whittaker, R., Jiang, Y., Wadham, A., Stasiak, K., Shepherd, M., & Bullen, C. (2018). Evaluation of MyTeen–a SMS-based mobile intervention for parents of adolescents: A randomised controlled trial protocol. *BMC Public Health*, *18*(1), 1–8. doi:10.118612889-018-6132-z PMID:30367613

Davey, S., & Davey, A. (2014). Mobile-health technology: Can it Strengthen and improve public health systems of other developing countries as per Indian strategies? A systematic review of the literature. *International Journal of Medicine and Public Health*, *4*(1), 40–45. doi:10.4103/2230-8598.127121

Davidson, T. M., Bunnell, B. E., Saunders, B. E., Hanson, R. F., Danielson, C. K., Cook, D., ... Walker, J. H. (2019). Pilot Evaluation of a Tablet-Based Application to Improve Quality of Care in Child Mental Health Treatment. *Behavior Therapy*, *50*(2), 367–379. doi:10.1016/j.beth.2018.07.005 PMID:30824252

Dennis, T. A., & O'Toole, L. J. (2014). Mental health on the go: Effects of a gamified attention-bias modification mobile application in trait-anxious adults. *Clinical Psychological Science*, *2*(5), 576–590. doi:10.1177/2167702614522228 PMID:26029490

DeSouza, S. I., Rashmi, M. R., Vasanthi, A. P., Joseph, S. M., & Rodrigues, R. (2014). Mobile phones: The next step towards healthcare delivery in rural India? *PLoS One*, *9*(8). doi:10.1371/journal.pone.0104895 PMID:25133610

Epp, C. D., Horne, J., Scolieri, B. B., Kane, I., & Bowser, A. S. (2018, September). PsychOut! a Mobile App to Support Mental Status Assessment Training. In *European Conference on Technology Enhanced Learning* (pp. 216-230). Cham, Switzerland: Springer.

Gaggioli, A., Pioggia, G., Tartarisco, G., Baldus, G., Corda, D., Cipresso, P., & Riva, G. (2013). A mobile data collection platform for mental health research. *Personal and Ubiquitous Computing*, *17*(2), 241–251. doi:10.100700779-011-0465-2

García, I. P., Sánchez, C. M., Espílez, Á. S., García-Magariño, I., Guillén, G. A., & García-Campayo, J. (2017). Development and initial evaluation of a mobile application to help with mindfulness training and practice. *International Journal of Medical Informatics*, *105*, 59–67. doi:10.1016/j.ijmedinf.2017.05.018 PMID:28750912

Goldner, E. M., Jeffries, V., Bilsker, D., Jenkins, E., Menear, M., & Petermann, L. (2011). Knowledge translation in mental health: A scoping review. *Healthcare Policy*, *7*(2), 83. PMID:23115572

Grant, M. J., & Booth, A. (2009). A typology of reviews: An analysis of 14 review types and associated methodologies. *Health Information and Libraries Journal*, *26*(2), 91–108. doi:10.1111/j.1471-1842.2009.00848.x PMID:19490148

Guruge, S., & Butt, H. (2015). A scoping review of mental health issues and concerns among immigrant and refugee youth in Canada: Looking back, moving forward. *Canadian Journal of Public Health*, *106*(2), e72–e78. doi:10.17269/CJPH.106.4588 PMID:25955675

Harrison, V., Proudfoot, J., Wee, P. P., Parker, G., Pavlovic, D. H., & Manicavasagar, V. (2011). Mobile mental health: Review of the emerging field and proof of concept study. *Journal of Mental Health (Abingdon, England)*, *20*(6), 509–524. doi:10.3109/09638237.2011.608746 PMID:21988230

Hartzler, A. L., Venkatakrishnan, A., Mohan, S., Silva, M., Lozano, P., Ralston, J. D., & Pirolli, P. (2016). Acceptability of a team-based mobile health (mHealth) application for lifestyle self-management in individuals with chronic illnesses. Paper presented at the *38th Annual International Conference of the IEEE Engineering in Medicine and Biology Society (EMBC)*, Orlando, FL. 10.1109/EMBC.2016.7591428

Hebert, E., Ferguson, W., McCullough, S., Chan, M., Drobakha, A., Ritter, S., & Mehta, K. (2016). mBody health: Digitizing disabilities in Sierra Leone. Paper presented at the *IEEE Global Humanitarian Technology Conference (GHTC)*, Seattle, WA. 10.1109/GHTC.2016.7857357

Hellman, M. (2018). Social causes of depression, anxiety and stress. *Nordisk Alkohol- & Narkotikatidskrift*, *35*(3), 149–151. doi:10.1177/1455072518773613

Herselman, M., Botha, A., Toivanen, H., Myllyoja, J., Fogwill, T., & Alberts, R. A digital health innovation ecosystem for South Africa. Paper presented at 2016 IST Africa Conference, Durban, South Africa.

Hofmann, B., & Svenaeus, F. (2018). How medical technologies shape the experience of illness. *Life Sciences, Society and Policy*, *14*(1), 3. doi:10.118640504-018-0069-y PMID:29397458

Iyawa, G. E. (2017c). *A Namibian digital health innovation ecosystem framework.* (PhD thesis, University of South Africa).

Iyawa, G. E., Botha, A., & Herselman, E. (2016b). Identifying and defining the terms related to a Digital Health Innovation Ecosystem. In M. Herselman, & A. Botha (Eds.), *Strategies, Approaches and Experiences: Towards Building a South African Digital Health Innovation Ecosystem* (pp. 30–54). Pretoria, South Africa: CSIR.

Iyawa, G. E., & Hamunyela, S. (2019). mHealth apps and services for maternal healthcare in developing countries. Paper presented at *2019 IST Africa Conference*, Nairobi, Kenya.

Iyawa, G. E., Herselman, M., & Botha, A. (2016a). Digital health innovation ecosystems: From systematic literature to conceptual framework. *Procedia Computer Science*, *100*, 244–252. doi:10.1016/j.procs.2016.09.149

Iyawa, G. E., Herselman, M., & Botha, A. (2017a). A scoping review of digital health innovation ecosystem. Paper presented at *2017 IST Africa Conference*, Windhoek, Namibia. 10.23919/ISTAFRICA.2017.8102325

Iyawa, G. E., Herselman, M., & Botha, A. (2017b). Identifying essential components of a digital health innovation ecosystem for the Namibian context: Findings from a Delphi study. *The Electronic Journal on Information Systems in Developing Countries*, *82*(1), 1–40. doi:10.1002/j.1681-4835.2017.tb00601.x

Iyawa, G. E., Herselman, M., & Botha, A. (2017d). Potential stakeholders and perceived benefits of a Digital Health Innovation Ecosystem for the Namibian context. *Procedia Computer Science*, *121*, 431–438. doi:10.1016/j.procs.2017.11.058

Iyawa, G. E., Herselman, M., & Botha, A. (2019). Digital Health Innovation Ecosystem: Identifying key participants, benefits, challenges and guidelines for the Namibian context. *International Journal of Reliable and Quality E-Healthcare*, *8*(2), 1–14. doi:10.4018/IJRQEH.2019040101

Iyawa, G. E., Velusamy, V., & Palinasamy, S. (2019). Wearable technologies for glucose monitoring: A systematic mapping study of publication trends. In: The IoT and the Next Revolution Automating the World.

Jain, N., Singh, H., Koolwal, G. D., Kumar, S., & Gupta, A. (2015). Opportunities and barriers in service delivery through mobile phones (mHealth) for Severe Mental Illnesses in Rajasthan, India: A multi-site study. *Asian Journal of Psychiatry*, *14*, 31–35. doi:10.1016/j.ajp.2015.01.008 PMID:25701069

James, J. (2010). Penetration and growth rates of mobile phones in developing countries: An analytical classification. *Social Indicators Research*, *99*(1), 135–145. doi:10.100711205-009-9572-0 PMID:20835391

Jutel, A., & Lupton, D. (2015). Digitizing diagnosis: A review of mobile applications in the diagnostic process. *Diagnosis*, *2*(2), 89–96. doi:10.1515/dx-2014-0068 PMID:29540025

Kaplan, R. M., & Stone, A. A. (2013). Bringing the laboratory and clinic to the community: Mobile technologies for health promotion and disease prevention. *Annual Review of Psychology*, *64*(1), 471–498. doi:10.1146/annurev-psych-113011-143736 PMID:22994919

Karasouli, E., & Adams, A. (2014). Assessing the Evidence for e-Resources for Mental Health Self-Management: A Systematic Literature Review. *JMIR Mental Health*, *1*(1), e3. doi:10.2196/mental.3708 PMID:26543903

Laird, E. A., Ryan, A., McCauley, C., Bond, R. B., Mulvenna, M. D., Curran, K. J., & Gibson, A. (2018). Using Mobile Technology to Provide Personalized Reminiscence for People Living with Dementia and Their Carers: Appraisal of Outcomes from a Quasi-Experimental Study. *JMIR Mental Health*, *5*(3), e57. doi:10.2196/mental.9684 PMID:30206053

Larsen, M. E., Cummins, N., Boonstra, T. W., O'Dea, B., Tighe, J., Nicholas, J., . . . Christensen, H. (2015). The use of technology in suicide prevention. Paper presented at the *37th annual international conference of the IEEE engineering in Medicine and Biology Society (EMBC)*, Milano, Italy. 10.1109/EMBC.2015.7320081

Lederer, N., Grechenig, T., & Baranyi, R. (2014). unCUT: bridging the gap from paper diary cards towards mobile electronic monitoring solutions in borderline and self-injury. Paper presented at the *IEEE 3nd International Conference on Serious Games and Applications for Health (SeGAH)*, Rio de Janeiro, Brazil. 10.1109/SeGAH.2014.7067092

Lee, R. A., & Jung, M. E. (2018). Evaluation of an mHealth App (DeStressify) on University Students' Mental Health: Pilot Trial. *JMIR Mental Health*, *5*(1), e2. doi:10.2196/mental.8324 PMID:29362209

Lipschitz, J., Miller, C. J., Hogan, T. P., Burdick, K. E., Lippin-Foster, R., Simon, S. R., & Burgess, J. (2019). Adoption of Mobile Apps for Depression and Anxiety: Cross-Sectional Survey Study on Patient Interest and Barriers to Engagement. *JMIR Mental Health*, *6*(1), e11334. doi:10.2196/11334 PMID:30681968

Mak, W. W. S., Wong, C. C. Y., Chan, A. T. Y., & Lau, J. T. F. (2019). Mobile self-compassion programme for promotion of public mental health: A randomised controlled trial. *Hong Kong Medical Journal*, *25*(1Supplement 2). PMID:30674702

Mankodiya, K., Sharma, V., Martins, R., Pande, I., Jain, S., Ryan, N., & Gandhi, R. (2013, December). Understanding User's Emotional Engagement to the Contents on a Smartphone Display: Psychiatric Prospective. Paper presented at *2013 IEEE 10th International Conference on Ubiquitous Intelligence and Computing and 2013 IEEE 10th International Conference on Autonomic and Trusted Computing*, Sorrento Pennisula, Italy. 10.1109/UIC-ATC.2013.98

Menon, V., Selvakumar, N., Kattimani, S., & Andrade, C. (2018). Therapeutic effects of mobile-based text message reminders for medication adherence in bipolar I disorder: Are they maintained after intervention cessation? *Journal of Psychiatric Research*, *104*, 163–168. doi:10.1016/j.jpsychires.2018.07.013 PMID:30081390

Michelle, T. Q. Y., Jarzabek, S., & Wadhwa, B. (2014, September). CBT Assistant: mHealth App for Psychotherapy. Paper presented at *IEEE Global Humanitarian Technology Conference-South Asia Satellite*, Trivandrum, India.

Morris, M. E., Kathawala, Q., Leen, T. K., Gorenstein, E. E., Guilak, F., DeLeeuw, W., & Labhard, M. (2010). Mobile therapy: Case study evaluations of a cell phone application for emotional self-awareness. *Journal of Medical Internet Research*, *12*(2), e10. doi:10.2196/jmir.1371 PMID:20439251

Niendam, T. A., Tully, L. M., Iosif, A. M., Kumar, D., Nye, K. E., Denton, J. C., & Pierce, K. M. (2018). Enhancing early psychosis treatment using smartphone technology: A longitudinal feasibility and validity study. *Journal of Psychiatric Research*, *96*, 239–246. doi:10.1016/j.jpsychires.2017.10.017 PMID:29126059

Noel, V. A., Acquilano, S. C., Carpenter-Song, E., & Drake, R. E. (2019). Use of mobile and computer devices to support recovery in people with serious mental illness: Survey study. *JMIR Mental Health, 6*(2), 1–5. doi:10.2196/12255 PMID:30785401

Nuij, C., van Ballegooijen, W., Ruwaard, J., De Beurs, D., Mokkenstorm, J., van Duijn, E., ... Kerkhof, A. (2018). Smartphone-based safety planning and self-monitoring for suicidal patients: Rationale and study protocol of the CASPAR (Continuous Assessment for Suicide Prevention and Research) study. *Internet Interventions, 13*, 16–23. doi:10.1016/j.invent.2018.04.005 PMID:30206514

Osma, J., Plaza, I., Crespo, E., Medrano, C., & Serrano, R. (2014). Proposal of use of smartphones to evaluate and diagnose depression and anxiety symptoms during pregnancy and after birth. Paper presented at *IEEE-EMBS International Conference on Biomedical and Health Informatics*, Valencia, Spain. 10.1109/BHI.2014.6864423

Petersen, K., Feldt, R., Mujtaba, S., & Mattsson, M. (2008). Systematic mapping studies in software engineering. *EASE, 8*, 68–77.

Prociow, P. A., & Crowe, J. A. (2010). Development of mobile psychiatry for bipolar disorder patients. In *2010 Annual International Conference of the IEEE Engineering in Medicine and Biology* (pp. 5484-5487). IEEE. 10.1109/IEMBS.2010.5626759

Ranney, M. L., Thorsen, M., Patena, J. V., Cunningham, R. M., Boyer, E. W., Walton, M. A., . . . Morrow, K. (2015). "You Need to Get Them Where They Feel it": Conflicting Perspectives on How to Maximize the Structure of Text-Message Psychological Interventions for Adolescents. Paper presented at *2015 48th Hawaii International Conference on System Sciences*, Kauai, Hawaii.

Rasool, S., ZeeshanZafar, M., Ali, Z., & Erum, A. (2018). Schizophrenia: An overview. *Clinical Practice (Therapy), 15*(5), 847–851.

Reid, S. C., Kauer, S. D., Hearps, S. J., Crooke, A. H., Khor, A. S., Sanci, L. A., & Patton, G. C. (2011). A mobile phone application for the assessment and management of youth mental health problems in primary care: A randomised controlled trial. *BMC Family Practice, 12*(1), 131–145. doi:10.1186/1471-2296-12-131 PMID:22123031

Rizia, R., Johnson, N., Patwary, A. K., Ahsan, G. M. T., Ahamed, S. I., Franco, Z., & Flower, M. (2014). Mobile peer-mentoring: An approach to make veterans seek mental health-care support a normality. Paper presented at *10th IEEE International Conference on Collaborative Computing: Networking, Applications and Worksharing*, Miami, Florida.

Rojnic, K. M., Andlauer, O., Burmeister, K., Dvoracek, B., Lencer, R., Koelkebeck, K., & Aukst, M. B. (2018). Effective assessment of psychotropic medication side effects using PsyLOG mobile application. *Schizophrenia Research, 192*, 211–212. doi:10.1016/j.schres.2017.04.038 PMID:28457773

Russell, E., & Patrick, K. (2018). Mental health needs our attention. *CMAJ: Canadian Medical Association Journal, 190*(2), E34. doi:10.1503/cmaj.171469 PMID:29335259

Sánchez, A., Plaza, I., Medrano, C. T., & Garcia-Campayo, J. (2015). Proposal of a mobile application for mindfulness practice in elder people. Paper presented at the *IET International Conference on Technologies for Active and Assisted Living*, London, UK. 10.1049/ic.2015.0143

Sawyer, A. C., Kaim, A. L., Reece, C. E., McDonald, D., Le, H. N., Clark, J., ... Sawyer, M. G. (2019). Evaluating the Effectiveness of an App-Based Nurse-Moderated Program for New Mothers with Depression and Parenting Problems (eMums Plus): Protocol for a Pragmatic Randomized Controlled Trial. *JMIR Research Protocols*, *8*(1). doi:10.2196/11549 PMID:30664487

Sedrati, H., Nejjari, C., Chaqsare, S., & Ghazal, H. (2016). Mental and physical mobile health apps. *Procedia Computer Science*, *100*, 900–906. doi:10.1016/j.procs.2016.09.241

Seppala, J., De Vita, I., Jamsa, T., Miettunen, J., Isohanni, M., Rubinstein, K., … Bulgheroni, M. (2019). Mobile Phone and Wearable Sensor-Based mHealth Approaches for Psychiatric Disorders and Symptoms: Systematic Review. *JMIR Mental Health, 6*(2), 1-14.

Similä, H., Immonen, M., Toska-Tervola, J., Enwald, H., Keränen, N., Kangas, M., & Korpelainen, R. (2018). Feasibility of mobile mental wellness training for older adults. *Geriatric Nursing*, *39*(5), 499–505. doi:10.1016/j.gerinurse.2018.02.001 PMID:29530292

Stallard, P., Porter, J., & Grist, R. (2018). A smartphone app (BlueIce) for young people who self-harm: Open phase 1 pre-post trial. *JMIR mHealth and uHealth*, *6*(1), e32. doi:10.2196/mhealth.8917 PMID:29382632

Stamate, D., Katrinecz, A., Alghamdi, W., Stahl, D., Delespaul, P., van Os, J., & Guloksuz, S. (2017). Predicting Psychosis Using the Experience Sampling Method with Mobile Apps. Paper presented at the *IEEE International Conference on Machine Learning and Applications*, Cancun, Mexico. 10.1109/ICMLA.2017.00-84

Stoll, R. D., Pina, A. A., Gary, K., & Amresh, A. (2017). Usability of a smartphone application to support the prevention and early intervention of anxiety in youth. *Cognitive and Behavioral Practice*, *24*(4), 393–404. doi:10.1016/j.cbpra.2016.11.002 PMID:29056845

Su, Y., Yuan, C., Zhou, Z., Heitner, J., & Campbell, B. (2016). Impact of an SMS advice programme on maternal and newborn health in rural China: Study protocol for a quasi-randomised controlled trial. *BMJ Open*, *6*(8). doi:10.1136/bmjopen-2015-011016 PMID:27515750

Sylvester, G. (2016). *Use of mobile phones by the rural poor: gender perspectives from selected Asian countries*. Ottawa, Canada: IDRC.

Teng, M. H., Hou, Y. M., Chang, S. H., & Cheng, H. J. (2019). Home-delivered attention bias modification training via smartphone to improve attention control in sub-clinical generalized anxiety disorder: A randomized, controlled multi-session experiment. *Journal of Affective Disorders*, *246*, 444–451. doi:10.1016/j.jad.2018.12.118 PMID:30599367

Tomlinson, M., & Lund, C. (2012). Why does mental health not get the attention it deserves? An application of the Shiffman and Smith framework. *PLoS Medicine*, *9*(2). doi:10.1371/journal.pmed.1001178 PMID:22389632

Torous, J., Wisniewski, H., Liu, G., & Keshavan, M. (2018). Mental Health Mobile Phone App Usage, Concerns, and Benefits Among Psychiatric Outpatients: Comparative Survey Study. *JMIR Mental Health*, *5*(4), 1–11. doi:10.2196/11715 PMID:30446484

Torri, E., Mayora, O., Cobo, J., & Palao, D. (2015). Requirements identification for the development of a design involving adaptive ICTs for supporting bipolar disorder treatment in different healthcare contexts. Paper presented at the *Proceedings of the 9th International Conference on Pervasive Computing Technologies for Healthcare*, Istanbul, Turkey. 10.4108/icst.pervasivehealth.2015.259238

Tuli, A., Singh, P., Sood, M., Deb, K. S., Jain, S., Jain, A., & Verma, R. (2016). Harmony: close knitted mhealth assistance for patients, caregivers and doctors for managing SMIs. Paper presented at the *ACM International Joint Conference on Pervasive and Ubiquitous Computing: Adjunct*, Heidelberg, Germany. 10.1145/2968219.2968301

United Nations Development Programme. (2014). Good health and well-being. Available at https://www.undp.org/content/undp/en/home/sustainable-development-goals/goal-3-good-health-and-well-being.html

Vahdat, S., Hamzehgardeshi, L., Hessam, S., & Hamzehgardeshi, Z. (2014). Patient involvement in health care decision making: A review. *Iranian Red Crescent Medical Journal, 16*(1). doi:10.5812/ircmj.12454 PMID:24719703

Välimäki, M., Hätönen, H., & Adams, C. E. (2012). Mobile. net: mobile telephone text messages to encourage adherence to medication and to follow up with people with psychosis: methods and protocol for a multicenter randomized controlled two-armed trial. *JMIR Research Protocols, 1*(2), e8. doi:10.2196/resprot.2136 PMID:23611874

Wang, R., Aung, M. S., Abdullah, S., Brian, R., Campbell, A. T., Choudhury, T., & Tseng, V. W. (2016). CrossCheck: toward passive sensing and detection of mental health changes in people with schizophrenia. Paper presented at the *ACM International Joint Conference on Pervasive and Ubiquitous Computing*, Heidelberg, Germany.

Washington, P., Kumar, M., Tibrewal, A., & Sabharwal, A. (2015). ScaleMed: A methodology for iterative mHealth clinical trials. Paper presented at the *17th International Conference on E-health Networking, Application and Services*, Boston, MA. doi:10.1145/2971648.2971740

Waterman, L., Szatala, S., Motta, B. D., Son, C. H., & To, J. (2018). Mellow: A mobile application to help youth in crisis. Extended Abstracts presented at the *2018 CHI Conference on Human Factors in Computing Systems,* Quebec, Canada.

Wolf, M., Kraft, S., Tschauner, K., Bauer, S., Becker, T., & Puschner, B. (2016). User activity in a mobile phone intervention to assist mindfulness exercises in people with depressive symptoms. *Mental Health & Prevention, 4*(2), 57–62. doi:10.1016/j.mhp.2016.02.003

Wong, D. F. K., Zhuang, X. Y., Pan, J. Y., & He, X. S. (2014). A critical review of mental health and mental health-related policies in China: More actions required. *International Journal of Social Welfare, 23*(2), 195–204. doi:10.1111/ijsw.12052

World Health Organisation. (2014). Mental health: A state of well-being. Available at https://www.who.int/features/factfiles/mental_health/en/

Zimic, M., Coronel, J., Gilman, R. H., Luna, C. G., Curioso, W. H., & Moore, D. A. (2009). Can the power of mobile phones be used to improve tuberculosis diagnosis in developing countries? *Transactions of the Royal Society of Tropical Medicine and Hygiene*, *103*(6), 638–640. doi:10.1016/j.trstmh.2008.10.015 PMID:19036392

ADDITIONAL READING

American Psychiatric Association (APA). (1980). *Diagnostic and statistical manual of mental disorders* (3rd ed.). Washington, DC: APA.

Arciniegas, D. B. (2015). Psychosis. *Continuum: Lifelong Learning in Neurology*, *21*(3), 715–736. PMID:26039850

Chandrashekar, P. (2018). Do mental health mobile apps work: Evidence and recommendations for designing high-efficacy mental health mobile apps. *mHealth*, *4*(3). PMID:29682510

Lui, J. H., Marcus, D. K., & Barry, C. T. (2017). Evidence-based apps? A review of mental health mobile applications in a psychotherapy context. *Professional Psychology, Research and Practice*, *48*(3), 199–210. doi:10.1037/pro0000122

Torous, J., Wisniewski, H., Liu, G., & Keshavan, M. (2018). Mental health mobile phone app usage, concerns, and benefits among psychiatric outpatients: Comparative survey study. *JMIR Mental Health*, *5*(4), e11715. doi:10.2196/11715 PMID:30446484

KEY TERMS AND DEFINITIONS

Digital Health: Digital health is an "improvement in the way healthcare provision is conceived and delivered by healthcare providers through the use of information and communication technologies to monitor and improve the wellbeing and health of patients and to empower patients in the management of their health and that of their families" (Iyawa et al., 2016a, p.246).

Digital Health Innovation Ecosystems: Digital health is a "network of digital health communities consisting of interconnected, interrelated and interdependent digital health species, including healthcare stakeholders, healthcare institutions and digital healthcare devices situated in a digital health environment, who adopt the best-demonstrated practices that have been proven to be successful, and implementation of those practices through the use of information and communication technologies to monitor and improve the wellbeing and health of patients, to empower patients in the management of their health and that of their families" (Iyawa et al., 2016a, p.249).

Mental Disorder: A mental disorder is a "syndrome characterized by clinically significant disturbance in an individual's cognition, emotion regulation, or behavior that reflects a dysfunction in the psychological, biological, or developmental processes underlying mental functioning" (American Psychiatric Association, 2013, p. 20).

Mental Health: Mental health is "the state of well-being in which every individual realizes his or her own potential, can cope with the normal stresses of life, can work productively and fruitfully, and is able to make a contribution to her or his community" (WHO, 2014).

Mobile Apps: Mobile apps refer to a software program designed to run on mobile devices.

Mobile Health (mHealth): mHealth is the use of any mobile device including mobile phones, smartphones, mobile or phone-based sensors for providing and receiving healthcare services such as healthcare monitoring, diagnosis, management and prediction of diseases.

Mobile Technologies: Mobile technologies refer to portable hand-held devices used for communication purposes.

Psychosis: Psychosis is the "presence of delusions, hallucinations without insight, or both" (Arciniegas, 2015, p. 717).

Systematic Mapping Study: A systematic literature review aims to "map out and categorize existing literature on a particular topic, identifying gaps in research literature from which to commission further reviews and/or primary research" (Grant and Booth, 2009, p. 97).

Text Messaging: Text messaging refers to the use of mobile devices to compose messages which can be sent to another party through a telecommunication channel.

Section 2
Cutting-Edge Technologies in Patient Care

Chapter 5
Big Data:
Its Implications on Healthcare and Future Steps

Shannon Wai Yi Yee
University of California – Davis, USA

Carolina Gutierrez
University of California – Los Angeles, USA

Caroline Narae Park
University of California – Davis, USA

Danny Lee
University of California – Berkeley, USA

Scott Lee
University of California – Berkeley, USA

ABSTRACT

In the last three decades, big data has been applied to diverse fields, such as the government, international development, and education. It is only now that the US healthcare system has begun to explore its under-utilized data. Big data is not only referencing the quantity, but also the complexity, diversity, and relativity of the information. This information may be analyzed to reveal patterns, trends, and associations that may be applicable to the healthcare field. This information can be gathered through sources, such as EHRs, IRIS registry, and MIPS. Recognizing patterns would aid in predicting preventative measures for an increased holistic and personalized patient care. Although big data proves to have endless beneficial applications, it can bring into question the ownership of this information. Additionally, big data poses a risk for security breaches, and thus, precautionary measures will also be discussed. Ultimately, the emergence of big data creates an exhilarating frontier for healthcare with its unlimited possibilities.

DOI: 10.4018/978-1-7998-0047-7.ch005

INTRODUCTION

Big data, in consideration of the healthcare field, are massively large sets of health data sets with varied potentiality for in-depth analysis. The information gathered from these analyses present trends that healthcare professionals, patients, and pharmaceutical companies can utilize to improve patient care, mortality rates, and costs. Gathering data is done with a flow of information from one sector to another.

Since Census Day, April 1st, 2010, the U.S. population has grown by 6.31% or 19,485,799 to the current 2019 population (U.S. Census Bureau, 2019). To put things into perspective, the U.S. is expected to increase in population by one person every 19 seconds when considering birth, death, immigration, and emigration rates (U.S. Census Bureau, 2019). From this increasingly large population, 85.9% of persons had one or more health care visits, whereas only 14.1% had no health care visits in 2016 (U.S. Department of Health and Services Services, 2018). Furthermore, the percentage is predicted to be higher in the future as morbidity rates in all ages and certain risk factors, such as heart disease, obesity, and diabetes have shown an upward trend in recent years (U.S. Department of Health and Services Services, 2018). With the sheer volume of patients being seen nationally, the need for a more organized method of maintaining health information moves beyond the capability of paper records. Thus, practices turn to digitized solutions: smart phones, tablets, and web-based devices. From a study conducted by the U.S. Department of Health and Human Services in 2001, 18.2% of the practices surveyed had some form of Electronic Health Records System (EHRS) implemented (Hsiao & Hing, 2012). By 2013 this had risen drastically to 78.4%, varying in percentage depending on different states (Hsiao & Hing, 2015). One attribution of this upward trend was the demand for patient information consolidation between different practices to better gauge an individual's overall health, and for comparison of benchmarks between practices. This meant a large untapped database of patient information, stored in a centralized location, was becoming available. The stored data includes medical visits of all time periods, past and concurrent illnesses and diseases, and types of insurance plans held by patients (Raghupathi & Raghupathi, 2014). Individually or together, these categories can be used to analyze patterns, help improve cost and efficiency of practices, and provide overall better patient care. For example, Kaiser Permanente's complete implementation of their EHRS, HealthConnect, has not only made it easier to share pertinent medical information across all the Kaiser Permanente regions, but has also significantly decreased cost and improved health. McKinsey reported one example: Kaiser Permanente saved an estimated $1 billion by reducing repetitive lab tests and thus the number of office visits while simultaneously improving the end results of cardiovascular disease (Lebied, 2018).

DATA COLLECTION SYSTEMS

In this section, different types of data collection are discussed beginning with a broad view provided by an EHRS that moves toward a specialty view provided by the IRIS Registry. The advantages and disadvantages of each big data collection process are discussed in detail.

EHRS vs EMRS

Electronic Health Records Systems (EHRS) and Electronic Medical Records Systems (EMRS) are easily confused. EMRS comprise a clinical data repository, clinical decision support, controlled medical vocabulary, order entry, computerized provider order entry, pharmacy, and clinical documentation applications (Garets & Davis, 2006). EMRS, on the other hand, are intraorganizational systems used by healthcare professionals to document, monitor, and manage care of their patients. Ultimately, the data from EMRS are legal records of patient experiences at the care delivery organization (CDO) and are owned by the CDO. EHRS, are interorganizational systems and contain a subset of information from various CDOs that patients have utilized. For EHRS, the data generally is owned by the patient, which allows for greater access and the ability to supplement the information. EMRS are sources of data for EHRS, while EHRS allow sharing of medical information between patient, CDO, and stakeholders (Garets & Davis, 2006).

Electronic Health Records System (EHRS)

EHRS are systematized collections of all patients' medical histories, diagnoses, medications, treatment plans, immunization dates, allergies, radiology images, and laboratory and test results (HealthIT.gov, 2019). EHRS are synonymous with the basic system of paper records but has leveraged advantages through adaption to smart devices. Depending on the type of EHRS adopted, providers can curate their own statistics looking at their patient population to find the most effective strategies to implement their practice. Focusing on one EHRS, DrChrono, practices can filter patient visits through any time period, find commonly performed procedures and testing, and query overall monetary earnings. This type of database can inform providers on whether a patient is at risk for a particular disease, help document the progression of an illness, or identify patients who would or would not benefit from surgery. Additionally, the accuracy and speed of intercommunication between different practices produces a more complete patient record than its physical counterpart. As a result, clinicians provide patients with a comprehensive consideration of their health, rather than just their own diagnoses. Despite the benefits offered by the EHRS, there are still barriers that prevent its adoption.

A challenge to EHRS adoption is selection of appropriate software that best fits the practice. Among notable software companies are: Epic, which focuses on middle to large sized practice; Allscripts, which caters to small to middle sized practices; and Practice Fusion, which offers features like billing and scheduling. Thus, the selection process is a daunting task for practices to identify which system caters to the needs of their clinicians and patients, in addition to having basic requirements such as Health Insurance Portability and Accountability Act (HIPAA) compliance, ICD-10, and CPT codes. Additionally, the direct and indirect costs in implementing EHRS serve as major barriers to its adoption. According to a survey conducted by National Center for Health Statistics, the largest barriers for non-adoptees include: the upfront cost of purchasing an EHRS (73%), loss of productivity (59%), annual maintenance cost (46%), and adequacy of training (40%) (U.S. Department of Health and Services Services, 2018). Based on the survey, most challenges focus on short term costs and inefficiency. For example, upfront costs can be extremely detrimental and may be as high as $33,000 with an annual cost of $4,000 (Green, 2019). This can be a relatively large setback for beginning and small practices that cannot afford the price immediately, as compared to more established and profitable practices. On the other hand, inefficiency is a deterrent for larger practices. The time it takes to train employees to learn new software can take time, cut down on productivity, and result in adverse mistakes.

Despite drawbacks of EHRS, there has been a push for adoption through the Health Information Technology for Economic and Clinical Health (HITECH) Act of 2009 (Birkhead, Klompas, & Shah, 2015). HITECH provides $30 billion in incentives for the adoption of EHRS by both hospitals and practices (Birkhead et al., 2015). In the ten years following HITECH, 84% of hospitals and 87% of individual practices have adopted some basic and certified form of EHRS (Jamoom & Yang, 2016). EHRS provide valuable information in terms of patient care by minimizing error, increasing efficiency, and improving care coordination, while providing an extensive source of data for research. The large masses of data collected from EHRS can be separated into structured and unstructured categories. The structured category is limited to billing and administrative purposes, in which well-defined codes are used for medical concepts (International Statistical Classification of Diseases and Related Health Problems (ICD)) and procedures encountered during the visit (Current Procedural Terminology (CPT)) (Shickel, Tighe, Bihorac, & Rashidi, 2017). On the other hand, unstructured data include clinical notes that are primarily used for detailed documentation of admission notes, discharge summaries, and transfer orders (Shickel et al., 2017). Unstructured data include heterogeneous formatting, abundant typing and spelling errors, violation of natural language grammar, rich domain-specific abbreviations, acronyms, and idiosyncrasies (P.-Y. Wu et al., 2016). The distinction between data types also relates to degree of extractability: structured data is easily filtered and sorted through established codes in the U.S.; whereas unstructured data requires intensive manual organization and engineering (P.-Y. Wu et al., 2016). Regardless, the recent availability of patient data through EHRS provides increasing diversity for population studies and trends.

An example is the adoption of genomics data in EMRS for precision medicine. The Electronic Medical Records and Genomics (eMERGE) Network consortium helps identify causal genomic variants for EMR-based phenotypes and helps integrate identified genotype-phenotype associations into the EMR system. Unfortunately, the consortium faces challenges. Among these are the millions of changing variants between individuals. Because of this, in the inclusion of false positives and exclusion of false negatives can impact studies (P.-Y. Wu et al., 2016). Furthermore, EMRS are associated only with local clinics and hospitals and that limits access and results in data not representative of the entire population (P.-Y. Wu et al., 2016). Thus, additional improvements and adjustments are needed to make EMRS more feasible.

Fortunately, other methods used to organize medical data are being investigated through specific database applications. Among these are the Merit-Based Incentive Payment System (MIPS) used by USA's Medicare and Medicaid programs, and the IRIS Registry.

Merit-Based Incentive Payment System (MIPS)

MIPS, employed by USA's Medicare and Medicaid, allows eligible clinicians and their practices to maintain current and updated patient information. MIPS provides preset, organized clinical data categories which include (Department of Health and Human Services USA, 2019):

- **Quality**: Categorizes the quality of care a clinician delivers to their patients. This section requires clinicians to report six measures the practice best performs. This requires active coding of measures with individual claims and final submission through the Quality Payment Program (QPP).

- **Improvement Activities**: Assesses activities that clinicians have undertaken to: improve care processes; enhance patient engagement in care; and, increase access to care. Clinicians choose from a list of nine subcategories covering over 100 activities and are encouraged to select the ones that are most applicable to their practice.
- **Promoting Interoperability**: Focuses on patient engagement and electronic exchange of health information using certified electronic health record technology (CEHRT) with other coordinating clinicians and patients.
- **Cost**: Gauges total cost of care based on Medicare Claims submitted by clinicians during the year or hospital stay.

Achieving maximum points in each category yields a total MIPS score of 100. The scoring determines penalties and rewards based on a sliding scale to determine the practice's total Medicare/Medi-Cal payments. MIPS incorporates data collection and compiles current information through real-time reporting and yields consistent outputs in response to rewards and penalties. The data produced from MIPS enable clinicians to gauge and adjust accordingly to the quality of care provided as well as allow intrapersonal and interpersonal communication between the clinician, other healthcare professionals, and their patients (Department of Health and Human Services USA, 2019). MIPS does have a downside. As it becomes a requirement for practices accepting patients with USA federal government insurance, the possibility of inaccurate and false data input by clinicians is possible and this can impact correlations. However, with such large sample sizes, the effect of these outliers generally is minimal.

IRIS Registry

The Intelligent Research in Sight (IRIS) Registry is an electronic health record-based registry focusing on eye diseases and conditions. The IRIS Registry utilizes both the EHR system and MIPS to create a comprehensive and extensive database for ophthalmologists and other eligible providers. The integration of a practice's EHR system with the IRIS registry allows ophthalmologists and eligible providers to streamline their patient visits and input data into the registry through any device. With this information, providers can track and evaluate their performances, implement effective care strategies, identify trends in their patient demographics, and compare their results with benchmarks generated by other clinicians (American Academy of Ophthalmology, 2019). With the aid of a data registry such as IRIS, participating providers can continue to provide effective patient care.

In addition to improvements at the practice level, this type of data collection can be essential for future research in ophthalmology. Collected information allows for generalizability since it is input in real-time from practices throughout the U.S. As of 2017, the IRIS Registry grants researchers large and variable sample sizes through its records of 148 million patient visits with 37.3 million unique patients. This makes it one of the largest single-specialty clinical data registries in the world (Parke, Rich, Sommer, & Lum, 2017). The success of the IRIS Registry is attributed to several general factors (Department of Health and Human Services USA, 2019):

1. No initial cost for physician participation.
2. Ease of integrating a practice's EHR system with the registry
3. No manual entry of patient data.
4. Confidential benchmarking of a practice's process of care and outcome of care.

5. Use of data registry for scientific research and discoveries.
6. Potential use for patient reported outcomes.
7. Coordination with MIPS for substantial Medicare reimbursements (Groves, Kayyali, Knott, & Kuiken, 2013).

These factors emphasize simplicity, convenience, and long-term potentiality. As individual providers have their own practices to operate, data recording for each patient becomes an infeasible task. The IRIS registry encourages active participation by its users by providing a easy user interface and bonuses from coordination with MIPS. Thus, other specialty-oriented data registries can follow suit of the IRIS Registry by applying similar strategies. Like MIPS, IRIS data may become contaminated due to user error through incorrect or false data input. Since it is a highly specialized system, this means the false data can lead to misleading correlations with rare eye conditions and can further impact research studies. Regardless, the sample sizes are large and generally able to account for these deviations.

PROCESSING BIG DATA

Big Data involves storing data at high volumes. However, the value of such data is dependent upon how it is managed. Relevant, organized data that lends itself to easy analysis requires data processing. Data processing optimizes the management of healthcare data and enhances its potential for analysis. However, traditional data processing methods are unable to manage such high volumes of at high velocities and variety (Oracle, 2019).

Since big data compiles information from multiple sources, it needs to be processed and formatted uniformly (Oracle, 2019). To integrate such data, methods such as extract, transform, and load (ETL) are performed to create a data warehouse---storage repository of data collected and integrated from many sources (SAS, 2019a). Any clinical data warehouse sourcing its data from databases utilizes ETL processing in some manner (Denney, Long, Armistead, Anderson, & Conway, 2016). Through ETL processing, data is extracted from its source, transformed into a single format, and loaded into a single location, usually using a common data model for its structure (Ong, Kahn, et al., 2017). Data can be analyzed simultaneously using streaming analytics techniques (e.g. analyzing a moving stream of data in near real time).

According to SAS Institute Inc. (2019b), key components of ETL processing include, data migration, data flows, control flows, parallel processing, and recoverability. Data migration is the movement of data from one storage device to another. In contrast, data flows are the movement of data from one place to another. Control flows maintain the order of processing steps. With parallel processing, volumes of data can be managed by executing operations simultaneously. With *Big Data*, data loss is a big concern. In addition to parallel processing, data can be split into parts, run in parallel, and be tagged for failure points. Failure points allow the ETL process to return to the last successful processing event should an error occur.

Different tools are needed to adapt to new data sources. As a result, different integration tools are employed, such as "deduping", or deleting duplicate data, during the transformation stage (Morgan, 2018). Like ETL, another approach called extract, load, and transform (ELT) has been used to speed up data processing, as extracted data is transformed after it has been loaded. This permits leveraging the processing power of the data store (Morgan, 2018).

Big data presents certain challenges during integration using ETL processing, especially when there is separation between the data source and ETL processor. One of the biggest challenges is terminology mapping (Ong, Pradhananga, Holve, & Kahn, 2017). The wide variety of tool and structures used to process the data prevents uniformity. In addition, with multiple data sources, data syncing can be difficult with different synchronization schedules. According to FlyData Inc. (2019), the management of such data requires a big data structure that is easy to navigate, especially during extraction. Accessing the data during extraction requires making sense of it. Quality data is organized and consistent, which does not easily occur when many different electronic health systems are utilized (Benson, 2014).

BIG DATA ANALYTICS IN HEALTHCARE

The increasing ease of collecting and processing data has resulted in a corresponding increase in health data analytics. Additionally, increasing implementation of electronic health records in the US has facilitated its access. Big data analytics of medical records can predict and assess issues earlier, and this can help get patients more involved in their health care (Lebied, 2018). With machine learning, the work of healthcare professionals, such as radiologists, is facilitated and stronger evidence-based decisions are made. Big data analytics of medical records unfold many possibilities, ranging from personalized medicine to health promotion. Analytics have the potential to improve the quality of life overall. For example, China has examined the economic and clinical burden of chronic diseases, and established the China Kidney Disease Network through a data-sharing initiative (Zhang, Wang, Li, Zhao, & Zhan, 2018). Because of such data, healthcare models have shifted focus from treatment to prevention. In another example, data scientists have identified 724 risk factors for patients likely to abuse opioids using insurance and pharmacy data (Lebied, 2018).

However, there are many challenges when analyzing medical records. The structure and organization of EHRs do not necessarily lend themselves to analytics, especially with the wealth of information stored. Furthermore, EHRs are not user-intuitive or friendly. Family physicians spend more time updating their EHRs than interacting with patients (Young, Burge, Kumar, Wilson, & Ortiz, 2018). According to Archer Software (2019), EHRs are not usually designed to integrate or manage data. To analyze medical records, data needs to be extracted into a data warehouse. A data warehouse consolidates data and contains important features including common linkable identifiers, security, and metadata, which can be sent to be prepared, cleaned, normalized, and processed. Semantic data integration technology can add context and allow deeper integration. Distributed processing can be implemented to simplify the amount of data (Raghupathi & Raghupathi, 2014). Analytics of records can involve routine analytics scaled up for larger amounts of data. Various analyses between clinical features and outcomes can be modeled with regression analysis, classification, and associate rule learning (J. Wu, Hou, & Jin, 2017). Statistical regression estimates the relationship between independent and dependent variables. Classification builds statistical models that assign a new observation to a class, using techniques such as decision trees. Association rule learning discovers frequent associations. Temporal relationships should be considered using techniques such as temporal association rule mining. Open source platforms, such as Hadoop have been used in healthcare, to aggregate, organize and analyze data (J. Wu et al., 2017). There are many approaches to analysis, depending on the context, including predictive or descriptive analytics (Khennou, Khamlichi, & Chaoui, 2018). Additionally, the data must be modeled and visualized in a user-friendly way, such as in the form of a medical dashboard.

Data mining looks for data patterns and relationships with individual data in a dataset, which comes with the risk of uncovering identifying patient information. With the Health Insurance Portability and Accountability Act (HIPAA) in the USA, patient information can be used if identification details are removed. Common practices include de-identification, which is removing key characteristics from a patient's record before it is released (Motiwalla & Li, 2013). However, non-sensitive characteristics can be used to uncover a patient's identity. One challenge with removing identifiers becomes the lack of a common identifier across data systems. Data-masking, where values are altered to hide sensitive data but still maintain its integrity, is an effective way to protect privacy, as results mirror those based on original data (Motiwalla & Li, 2013). Other methods include noise-based perturbation, data swapping, cell suppression, k-anonymity, and microaggregation. Another approach to protecting data is encryption. In contrast to data masking, which prevents intrusion when data is stored, encryption prevents interpretation when the data is shared (Motiwalla & Li, 2013). Much of privacy research focuses on policy rather than the design or tools, so there is a need for more research on the application of privacy preserving data mining (Motiwalla & Li, 2013). For instance, identity-based anonymization either encrypts or removes identifiers from data so subjects are anonymous (Abouelmehdi, Beni-Hessane, & Khaloufi, 2018). The trade-off between data quality and privacy also must be considered when deciding which analytic tools to use.

USES OF BIG DATA

With the various modalities of acquiring big data comes numerous potential uses. The correct applications of big data can lend themselves to a revolution in healthcare and enhance the culture of medicine. Though many healthcare providers have been resistant to the increasing use of big data, more and more hospitals and physicians are understanding its benefits, in both an individual and holistic sense. In this section, the array of possible ways to utilize big data are discussed.

Clinical Decision Making

The large volume of data accessible to providers aid patients in the decision-making process throughout the duration of a patient's disease or sickness. With access to data repositories such as EMRS and EHRS, clinicians can utilize structured, semi-structured, and unstructured data to better diagnose or treat a patient. Consequently, being able to view medical records, MRI and CT scans, in addition to information from blogs or social media can give physicians a more holistic and comprehensive understanding of possible next steps without running the risk of repeating efforts made by other contributing doctors. Additionally, analyzing patients' social and medical characteristics can influence physician behavior by altering treatment plans that are most financially and medically appropriate for the patient (Raghupathi & Raghupathi, 2014).

Not only does this provide clinicians with the opportunity to make more informed decisions, it also allows providers the opportunity to detect a disease early on. By detecting it at an earlier stage, the likelihood of the disease being in a more manageable and treatable form is greater. In turn, this can lead to reduced healthcare expenditures. According to McKinsey and Company, analyzing big data effectively can create greater than $300 billion in value, annually (Manyika et al., 2011).

Research and Development

Big data also can be utilized to discover overall trends to make informed predictions. This can be applied to numerous aspects of healthcare, including analysis of cost-effectiveness of a drug or device, or identifying and targeting certain demographics or populations for specific treatment protocols (Raghupathi & Raghupathi, 2014). By analyzing the safety or number of adverse events of a drug or product, developers are able to streamline the process of putting a new product out on the market (B. Chen & Butte, 2016). Big data also can be utilized to accelerate the process of new drug discovery. Former President Obama's Cancer Moonshot program made use of big data with the hopes of making progress in the cure to cancer in half the time (Lebied, 2019). Medical researchers were then able to analyze which treatment programs had the highest success rate and how certain cancer proteins interact with different types of treatment. Thus, the task of analyzing these trends became easier to do with a greater population to study. Desipramine, an antidepressant, was unexpectedly found to contribute to the treatment of certain types of lung cancer (Lebied, 2019).

Population Health and Surveillance

Another use that will benefit healthcare on a more global scale is the use of advanced analytics to better track and survey disease progressions in different populations and geographic locations (Raghupathi & Raghupathi, 2014). By tracking disease outbreaks, epidemiologists and other public health officials can better track the spread of different diseases. With this knowledge, quicker response times and more targeted solutions can contribute to treating the disease and preventing it in the future. Furthermore, the large amounts of data can help policymakers better triage the diseases and gain a better idea of what diseases to allocate more funds to.

Not only does the use of these massive amounts of data help understand and reduce disease spread, it can also shine light on the population which is at a higher risk of medical complications. In appropriately monitoring these groups, additional measures can be taken to better educate the patient and prevent negative consequences, such as some causes of morbidity and mortality.

Detecting Fraud

With the help of various data registries, such as MIPS, EHRS, and EMRS, information on billing claims and types of appointments coded can easily give insight into possible types of fraud. Analyzing and categorizing large quantities of codes using big data gives insurance companies the opportunity to better understand whether or not providers are intentionally overcoding visits (HealthIT.gov, 2019).

All in all, the potential uses of big data do not stop here. As the field of medicine and healthcare is growing and evolving, so is the future of big data. In gaining access to such a vast repository of information, when used correctly, big data can help streamline many processes, such as developing a patient's care protocol, identifying and tracking a disease, and preventing and catching fraud. Moreover, the pros of utilizing big data can help physicians and allow better communication for a more unified standard of care.

Prediction Capabilities

Evidence driven decisions are the foundation for patient care (Chen, Elenee-Argentinis, & Weber, 2016). However, there are issues with data collection and organization done by a human as opposed to machine. A human may not sift through all the evidence available and may harbor a bias towards conflicting information. As a result, a human is much less holistic in evidence discrimination compared to a computer. One such cognitive computing tool is Watson by IBM.

Watson is a cognitive computing technology that integrates and analyzes big datasets, including medical literature, patents, genomics, and chemical and pharmacological data (Y. Chen, Argentinis, & Weber, 2016). According to Y. Chen et al. (2016), IBM aggregates data into a single repository called the Watson Corpus which in turn normalizes, cleans, and formats the information into a dataset that can be used for analysis. What makes Watson a cognitive versus an automated system is its ability to learn. In the case of the drug Valium, Watson not only recognizes its chemical structure, but also more than 100 synonyms for it, like its related compounds, generic or brand names (Y. Chen et al., 2016). Furthermore, its cognitive system can leverage known vocabulary to deduce the meaning of new terms based on the contextual clues.

An example application of Watson is in the exploration of cancer kinases. Watson was taught to recognize protein kinases that phosphorylated P53 based on previously published evidence. It was then allowed to read and discriminate all articles discussing the known kinases. Watson was able to identify 9 potential kinases that phosphorylated p53, 7 of 9 that were discovered and validated through published experiments during the following decade. The findings suggest that the usage of cognitive computing technology and its ability to learn, understand, and organize large datasets can accelerate newfound discoveries especially in the healthcare field (Y. Chen et al., 2016).

Google Trends

An additional organizational form of Big Data comes from Google Trends. Google Trends is a freely accessible online portal which provides insight into population behavior and health related phenomena. Additionally, there is flexibility with Google Trends as it allows individuals to specify their searches geographically and temporally (Nuti et al., 2014). Thus, the ability to consolidate massive amounts of information and readily streamline it to the user holds potentiality for larger scale projects, especially in the prediction of infectious diseases. One such study is influenza prevalence and incidence rates conducted solely through Google Trends. In 2009, Google Flu Trends (GFT) was able to anticipate flu illness rates just by analyzing Google searches (Viceconti, Hunter, & Hose, 2015).

However, it was not always accurate (Walsh, 2014). The lack of review of its applications, methodologies, and reproducibility of results serve as a limitation in the usage of Google Trends in research as discussed by Nuti et al. (2014). Nevertheless, Google Trends is useful in identifying causations and surveying; it is a pivotal tool which encourages researchers to ask questions and guides them to discover meaningful insights about the population and its health.

Preventative Measures

Big data can be used for preventative medicine. Specifically, it can aid in predicting disease or a sudden increase in diagnosis of a disease. Understanding a person's genetics, environment, and lifestyle can help configure the best approach in preventing and treating diseases. Possessing the understanding of big data as well as its pros can improve the quality of healthcare worldwide.

Due to the nature of large data sets, the healthcare industry will be highly dependent on machine learning and artificial intelligence (AI). According to Skymind (2019), AI currently is used worldwide due to its ability to imitate intelligent human behavior, which has proven a crucial asset to society. Machine learning is known as a subset system of AI that automatically learns programs from data (Domingos, 2012). This has become increasingly popular in the field of computer science leading to developments in various algorithms. As these systems become finely tuned, they will be able to sustain the large influx of big data and accurately organize data, similarly to how the human brain processes data. The goal is to use these systems to quickly rule out the list of differentials and decide on a diagnosis. Recently, Google developed a machine learning program algorithm that helps identify cancerous tumors on mammograms (Corbett, 2017). Algorithms are continuously created as they are crucial to machine learning. In order to have a successful algorithm, a vast resource of data where patterns can be detected is required. From the data, algorithms can create artificial maps which create accessible information (Andreu-Perez, Poon, Merrifield, Wong, & Yang, 2015). Consequently, great strides have been made in the healthcare field with such technological advances.

CONSEQUENCES OF BIG DATA

Although big data holds vast amount promise to improve healthcare by improving patient care, it still is only in the beginning stages of doing so. One of the main reasons that healthcare professionals are turning to big data relates to the nearly limitless information it offers. But with the promise, arise multiple problems, such as an overwhelming amount of data, the lag of real-time data, and increasing IT costs (Frost & Sullivan, 2011). As of now, big data contains a vast amount of potentially useful information that is not well organized nor easily accessible. Consequently, professionals feel overwhelmed by the velocity, volume and variety of data available. There is a constant influx of data coming from a variety of sources, such as research and insurance companies (Frost & Sullivan, 2011). Additionally, even more information can come from medical equipment like MRIs and CT scans. These medical tools provide numerous visual images that could be very useful to professionals, but they are not available in a streamlined manner to provide beneficial information. Along with the volume and velocity of big data, the variety of data also presents a problem in terms of accessibility (Raghupathi & Raghupathi, 2014). Because the data can be collected from various sources as well as in different formats, such as structured and unstructured records, the inability to easily interact with and manipulate the data presents an issue. Consequently, healthcare professionals need to discover a way to filter big data an organized, accessible, and easy-to-use format (Raghupathi & Raghupathi, 2014). Moreover, big data needs to be constantly cleansed of old and unusable information. This will decrease the overwhelming volume of data that healthcare professionals have to sort through. Consequently, the data will then need to be in a format that is user-friendly. Big data is found on multiple platforms that are always compatible. By having a single database or user-friendly program, big data can be accessed much more quickly and prove to be even more beneficial (Frost & Sullivan, 2011).

Another issue that healthcare professionals are facing with using big data is the lag of real-time data. Big data often is unorganized and unfiltered, which in turn causes real time data to be inevitably inaccessible. The real-time data may be lost because it needs to be organized properly and the volume of data causes the organization to proceed slowly. Therefore, real-time data needs to be accessible instantly for healthcare professionals to truly take advantage of the latent information.

Resolving these issues will inevitably be costly and this could affect all practices from small and private clinics to large and public ones. The healthcare system needs to include IT costs into daily expenses. As big data becomes more organized and accessible, it will exist on platforms such as a cloud-based computer programs or online database systems. Furthermore, professionals need to invest in different data storage methods. New expenditures could, in turn, detrimentally affect the patient by increasing the cost of healthcare as providers must compensate for a greater list of costs.

Additionally, the question of security and privacy also come into question. Professional healthcare providers need to collaborate with IT companies to ensure their data is secured and had received proper maintenance. Although healthcare professionals need to overcome many obstacles to successfully acquire and use big data to improve patient care, they are moving in the right direction.

SECURITY ISSUES

The use of big data in healthcare has exploded with data sets, stored in various electronic health systems and documents. The question of compatibility and security practices arises with the various modalities in which big data is stored. HIPAA, the longstanding standard dictating patient privacy, has been called into question whether it is up-to-date with today's technology. Furthermore, the sharing and analysis of big data on a mass scale raises questions about patient privacy, data security, liability, and policy. In 2004, Iceland's supreme court decided that including a dead man's health information in a proposed genetic database would violate the privacy of the man's descendants (Abbott, 2004).

In general, the sheer size of big data inherently increases the possibility and severity of security breaches. The risk continues to increase as big data often is organized and processed via distributed computing (Parms, 2017). Overall, privacy challenges can be broken down into four main categories: infrastructure security, data privacy, and data management (Parms, 2017).

- **Infrastructure Security**: Because big data is accessed via a distributed computing framework, the opportunities for a security breach automatically increase. A distributed computing framework consists of different network computers coordinating their actions to achieve a common goal, which is in this case to organize and analyze health information. Strict authentication procedures and Mandatory Access Control (MAC), which limit the tasks of each computer can help resolve this issue, in addition to using encryption techniques (Parms, 2017).
- **Data Privacy**: Organizations that own data are held legally responsible for ensuring the security measures used to protect patient privacy comply with all standards. Because many government agencies, outside companies, and business partners use the data for analytical and research purposes, it is even more crucial to ensure patient privacy. Again, the standard form of encryption

plus new, emerging forms of encryption such as homomorphic encryption allows working computers to utilize encrypted data (Parms, 2017). As a result, this ensures the protection of patient information.

- **Data Management**: Big data often consists of petabytes of data due to acquiring information from multiple sources. To effectively and efficiently manage this massive amount of information, auto-tiering has become increasingly used. Auto-tiering automatically categorizes data into different levels, or tiers, of storage devices based on pre-established policies (Parms, 2017). However, this presents an issue as critical patient information can be automatically moved to a lower tier, which has a lower level of security. But, performing routine audits can help identify any potential privacy breaches and prevent it in the future. Technology is available to protect patient information. The problem arises due to the lack of an all-encompassing framework that can protect all aspects of big data use (Parms, 2017).

Concerns about insurance coverage based on pre-existing conditions and discrimination based on factors such as HIV status have long caused patient hesitation to disclose information (Abbot, 2004). Anonymizing identifying information according to HIPPA standards has already been implemented for analysis purposes. With big data, however, data points and small details analyzed together may risk patient identification (Parms, 2017). Even though all identifiers are stripped from the data, the relationships between the data can still reveal a person (Epic.org, 2019). For example, some patients would stand out in a data set if sexual orientation and social media information were looked at together. The anonymization of information, especially genomics, poses a future challenge to the expansion of big data analysis.

Additionally, private consumer data, such as information collected from smart devices, have been primarily used by companies to analyze trends. However, data from public sources such as Medicare have the potential to transform the healthcare industry. Incorporating multiple data sources should be encouraged to not only enhance a company's assets, but also to improve the quality of data analyzed. Companies holding consumer data are not subject to the same degree of HIPAA compliance as healthcare providers. Private data collected by companies may seem more valuable but publicly accessible data has wider applications. The intersection between publicly accessible data and consumer data is an avenue to be further explored in the future, as companies seek to expand their market reach.

Currently in the USA, there have been initiatives to address the needs of each state through health information exchanges (Epic.org, 2019). However, with differing approaches and policies for each state to protect patients, national data sharing becomes complex. Laws in conjunction with HIPAA, must be interpreted state by state. As such, the sharing of big data nationwide remains unpredictable. The General Data Protection Regulation implemented by the European Union (EU) in 2016 is an example of a regulation which governs how personal information is processed. It sets common standards for everyone in the EU (Epic.org, 2019). A national framework like GDPR will facilitate future big data analysis and collaboration.

While there are valid privacy concerns with the increased amount of data collected and analyzed, there is a need to streamline data sharing to ensure consumer and patient data is both protected and accessible to qualified stakeholders. Increased transparency of how the data is collected and shared would allow patients to make informed choices and knowingly consent to such practices. Thus, a uniform set of regulations and procedures would make collecting such data more efficient, promoting collaboration between researchers and those in the industry, all while requiring less data collection by different stakeholders. Furthermore, with increased data flow and collection, the risks of data breaches increase and the question of liability remains. HIPAA does not apply to consumer health information therefore a set of required security policies would decrease liability. However, this also might discourage collaboration. Both increased protections for patients and companies is necessary for big data analysis to thrive. The tradeoffs between privacy and convenience must not be compromised. With the potential of big data comes the potential of improving its infrastructure and the policies surrounding it.

CONCLUSION

Now that the advantages and disadvantages to the uses of big data are known, it is important to consider both sides as the field of medicine advances. In combining conventional, structured data with big data, the opportunity to provide patients with the best quality of care presents itself. In learning more about the varying implications of big data on multiple facets of the healthcare system, big data will continue to propel the future of medicine in the right direction. However, privacy breaches and idealistic, but not practical, obstacles stand in the way of its further integration. Nevertheless, one must first clearly understand what big data is in order to truly appreciate and utilize it appropriately in the future.

REFERENCES

Abbott, A. (2004). Icelandic database shelved as court judges' privacy in peril. London, UK: Nature Publishing Group. doi:10.1038/429118b

Abouelmehdi, K., Beni-Hessane, A., & Khaloufi, H. (2018). Big healthcare data: Preserving security and privacy. *Journal of Big Data*, *5*(1), 1. doi:10.118640537-017-0110-7

American Academy of Ophthalmology. (2019). About the IRIS@ registry. Retrieved from https://www.aao.org/iris-registry/about

Andreu-Perez, J., Poon, C. C. Y., Merrifield, R. D., Wong, S. T. C., & Yang, G.-Z. (2015). Big data for health. *IEEE Journal of Biomedical and Health Informatics*, *19*(4), 1193–1208. doi:10.1109/JBHI.2015.2450362 PMID:26173222

Archer. (2019). The importance of healthcare data analytics in an EMR. Retrieved from https://www.archer-soft.com/en/blog/importance-healthcare-data-analytics-emr

Benson, B. (2014). ETL challenges within healthcare business intelligence. Retrieved from https://www.hitechanswers.net/etl-challenges-within-healthcare-business

Birkhead, G. S., Klompas, M., & Shah, N. R. (2015). Uses of electronic health records for public health surveillance to advance public health. *Annual Review of Public Health*, *36*(1), 345–359. doi:10.1146/annurev-publhealth-031914-122747 PMID:25581157

Chen, B., & Butte, A. J. (2016). Leveraging big data to transform target selection and drug discovery. *Clinical Pharmacology and Therapeutics*, *99*(3), 285–297. doi:10.1002/cpt.318 PMID:26659699

Chen, Y., Argentinis, J. D. E., & Weber, G. (2016). IBM Watson: How cognitive computing can be applied to big data challenges in life sciences research. *Clinical Therapeutics*, *38*(4), 688–701. doi:10.1016/j.clinthera.2015.12.001 PMID:27130797

Corbett, E. (2017). The real-world benefits of machine learning in healthcare. Retrieved from https://www.healthcatalyst.com/clinical-applications-of-machine-learning-in-healthcare

Denney, M. J., Long, D. M., Armistead, M. G., Anderson, J. L., & Conway, B. N. (2016). Validating the extract, transform, load process used to populate a large clinical research database. *International Journal of Medical Informatics*, *94*, 271–274. doi:10.1016/j.ijmedinf.2016.07.009 PMID:27506144

Department of Health and Human Services USA. (2019). Merit-based Incentive Payment System (MIPS) overview. Retrieved from https://qpp.cms.gov/mips/overview

Domingos, P. M. (2012). A few useful things to know about machine learning. *Communications of the ACM*, *55*(10), 78–87. doi:10.1145/2347736.2347755

Epic.org. (2019). Big data and the future of privacy. Retrieved from https://epic.org/privacy/big-data/

FlyData. (2019). The 6 challenges of big data integration. Retrieved from https://www.flydata.com/the-6-challenges-of-big-data-integration/

Frost & Sullivan. (2011). *Drowning in big data? Reducing information technology complexities and costs for healthcare organizations*. Mountain View, CA. Retrieved from https://www.emc.com/collateral/analyst-reports/frost-sullivan-reducing-information-technology-complexities-ar.pdf

Garets, D., & Davis, M. (2006). Electronic medical records vs. electronic health records: Yes, there is a difference. Retrieved from https://www.google.com/url?sa=t&rct=j&q=&esrc=s&source=web&cd=2&ved=2ahUKEwjHka6xjsjiAhVNnKwKHai7DhsQFjABegQIARAC&url=https%3A%2F%2Fwww.aao.org%2Fasset.axd%3Fid%3D8e9b1f20-0ed6-4d2b-92f8-e28fbaf378ec%26t%3D634962799822530000&usg=AOvVaw2IZUASCFHwbgR_kQ7BLvfo

Green, J. (2019). How much EHR costs and how to set your budget. Retrieved from https://www.ehrinpractice.com/ehr-cost-and-budget-guide.html

Groves, P., Kayyali, B., Knott, D., & Kuiken, V. S. (2013). *The "big data" revolution in healthcare. Accelerating value and innovation*. Retrieved from http://www.pharmatalents.es/assets/files/Big_Data_Revolution.pdf

Health, I. T. gov. (2019). What is an electronic health record (EHR)? Retrieved from https://www.healthit.gov/faq/what-electronic-health-record-ehr

Hsiao, C.-J., & Hing, E. (2012). Use and characteristics of electronic health record systems among office-based physician practices: United States, 2001-2012. *National Center for Health Statistics Data Brief*, *111*(December), 1–8. Retrieved from https://www.cdc.gov/nchs/data/databriefs/DB111.pdf

Hsiao, C.-J., & Hing, E. (2015). *Use and characteristics of electronic health record systems among office-based physician practices: United States, 2001--2013. NCHS data brief, no 143. Hyattsville, MD: National Center for Health Statistics. 2014*. Hyattsville, MD: National Center for Health Statistics. Available at Http://Www.Cdc.Gov/Nchs/Data/Databriefs/Db143.Htm

Jamoom, E., & Yang, N. (2016). *Table of electronic health record adoption and use State Variation in Electronic Sharing of Information in Physician Offices: United States, 2015*. Atlanta, GA. Retrieved from https://www.cdc.gov/nchs/products/databriefs/db261.htm

Khennou, F., Khamlichi, Y. I., & Chaoui, N. E. H. (2018). Improving the Use of Big Data Analytics within Electronic Health Records: A Case Study based OpenEHR. *Procedia Computer Science*, *127*, 60–68. doi:10.1016/j.procs.2018.01.098

Lebied, M. (2018). 12 examples of big data analytics in healthcare that can save people. Retrieved from https://www.datapine.com/blog/big-data-examples-in-healthcare/

Lebied, M. (2019). Examples of big data in healthcare that can save people.

Manyika, J., Chui, M., Brown, B., Bughin, J., Dobbs, R., Roxburgh, C., & Byers, A. H. (2011). *Big data: The next frontier for innovation, competition, and productivity*. Seoul Korea. Retrieved from https://www.mckinsey.com/~/media/McKinsey/Business Functions/McKinsey Digital/Our Insights/Big data The next frontier for innovation/MGI_big_data_full_report.ashx

Morgan, L. (2018). What is ETL: Extract, transform, load. Retrieved from https://www.datamation.com/big-data/what-is-etl-extract-transform-load.html

Motiwalla, L., & Li, X.-B. (2013). Developing privacy solutions for sharing and analyzing healthcare data. *International Journal of Business Information Systems*, *13*(2), 199–216. doi:10.1504/IJBIS.2013.054335 PMID:24285983

Nuti, S. V., Wayda, B., Ranasinghe, I., Wang, S., Dreyer, R. P., Chen, S. I., & Murugiah, K. (2014). The use of google trends in health care research: A systematic review. *PLoS One*, *9*(10). doi:10.1371/journal.pone.0109583 PMID:25337815

Ong, T., Kahn, M. G., Kwan, B. M., Yamashita, T., Brandt, E., Hosokawa, P., ... Schilling, L. M. (2017). Dynamic-ETL: A hybrid approach for health data extraction, transformation and loading. *BMC Medical Informatics and Decision Making*, *17*(1), 134. doi:10.118612911-017-0532-3 PMID:28903729

Ong, T., Pradhananga, R., Holve, E., & Kahn, M. G. (2017). A framework for classification of electronic health data extraction-transformation-loading challenges in data network participation. *EGEMs: The Journal for Electronic Health Data and Methods*, *5*(1), 10. doi:10.5334/egems.222 PMID:29930958

Oracle. (2019). What is big data? Retrieved from https://www.oracle.com/big-data/guide/what-is-big-data.html

Parke, D. W. II, Rich, W. L. III, Sommer, A., & Lum, F. (2017). The American Academy of Ophthalmology's IRIS®Registry (Intelligent Research in Sight Clinical Data): A look back and a look to the future. *Ophthalmology*, *124*(11), 1572–1574. doi:10.1016/j.ophtha.2017.08.035 PMID:29055362

Parms, J. (2017). More info, more problems: Privacy and security issues in the age of big data. Retrieved from https://www.business.com/articles/privacy-and-security-issues-in-the-age-of-big-data/

Raghupathi, W., & Raghupathi, V. (2014). Big data analytics in healthcare: Promise and potential. *Health Information Science and Systems*, *2*(1), 3. doi:10.1186/2047-2501-2-3 PMID:25825667

SAS. (2019a). Data warehouse: What it is and why it matters. Retrieved from https://www.sas.com/en_us/insights/data-management/data-warehouse.html

SAS. (2019b). ETL: What it is and why it matters. Retrieved from https://www.sas.com/en_us/insights/data-management/what-is-etl.html

Shickel, B., Tighe, P. J., Bihorac, A., & Rashidi, P. (2017). Deep EHR: A survey of recent advances in deep learning techniques for electronic health record (EHR) analysis. *IEEE Journal of Biomedical and Health Informatics*, *22*(5), 1589–1604. doi:10.1109/JBHI.2017.2767063 PMID:29989977

Skymind. (2019). Artificial intelligence (AI) vs. machine learning vs. deep learning. Retrieved from https://skymind.ai/wiki/ai-vs-machine-learning-vs-deep-learning

U.S. Census Bureau. (2019). *Census Bureau projects U.S. and world populations on New Year's Day*. Retrieved from https://www.census.gov/newsroom/press-releases/2019/new-years-population.html

U.S. Department of Health and Services. (2018). *Health, United States, 2017 with special feature on mortality*. Hyattsville, MD. Retrieved from https://www.cdc.gov/nchs/data/hus/hus17.pdf

Viceconti, M., Hunter, P., & Hose, R. (2015). Big data, big knowledge: Big data for personalized healthcare. *IEEE Journal of Biomedical and Health Informatics*, *19*(4), 1209–1215. doi:10.1109/JBHI.2015.2406883 PMID:26218867

Walsh, B. (2014, March). Google flu trends failure shows drawbacks of big data. *Time.Com*. Retrieved from http://time.com/23782/google-flu-trends-big-data-problems/

Wu, J., Hou, S., & Jin, M. (2017). Social Support and User Roles in a Chinese Online Health Community: A LDA Based Text Mining Study. In *International Conference on Smart Health* (pp. 169–176). Retrieved from 10.1007/978-3-319-67964-8_16

Wu, P.-Y., Cheng, C.-W., Kaddi, C. D., Venugopalan, J., Hoffman, R., & Wang, M. D. (2016). --Omic and electronic health record big data analytics for precision medicine. *IEEE Transactions on Biomedical Engineering*, *64*(2), 263–273. PMID:27740470

Young, R., Burge, S., Kumar, K., Wilson, J., & Ortiz, D. (2018). A time-motion study of primary care physicians' work in the electronic health record era. *Family Medicine*, *50*(2), 91–99. doi:10.22454/FamMed.2018.184803 PMID:29432623

Zhang, L., Wang, H., Li, Q., Zhao, M.-H., & Zhan, Q.-M. (2018). Big data and medical research in China. *BMJ (Clinical Research Ed.)*, *360*, j5910. doi:10.1136/bmj.j5910 PMID:29437562

KEY TERMS AND DEFINITIONS

Computerized Tomography (CT) Scans: Combines a series of x-ray images taken from different angles around a patient's body and uses computer processing to create cross-sectional images (slices) of the bones, blood vessels and soft tissues inside the body.

Human Immunodeficiency Virus (HIV): A virus that weakens a person's immune system by destroying important cells that fight disease and infection.

IT: Information technology; anything related to technology, such has hardware, software, professionals, etc.

Intercommunication: Communication between different practices or organizations.

Intracommunication: Communication within a practice or organization.

Magnetic Resonance Imaging (MRI): A medical imaging technique used in radiology to form pictures of the anatomy and the physiological processes of the body in both health and disease.

Medicare and Medicaid: National health insurance programs in the United States.

Semi-Structured Data: Structured data that does not fully conform with the formal structure of data models associated with relational databases or other forms of data tables

Structured Data: Information that can easily be stored or formatted by a machine

Unstructured Data: Information that is not organized in any manner.

Chapter 6
The Promise of Gamification in Addressing Health Challenges of the Modern World

Taiki Nishihara
University of California – Berkeley, USA

Yagana Parwak
University of California – Berkeley, USA & University of California – San Francisco, USA

Eghosa Edogun
University of California – Santa Cruz, USA

Gia Park
University of California – Berkeley, USA

Scott Lee
University of California – Berkeley, USA

ABSTRACT

This chapter explores gamification and its potential to address leading health and healthcare issues, to promote healthy behaviors and empower patients to take charge of their own health. It discusses some of the key advantages of gamification over past iterations of technology-based behavioral health interventions, including personal informatics and serious games. The advantages discussed in this chapter include: 1) a greater emphasis on the promotion of intrinsic motivation through quality, intentional game design; 2) broader accessibility to patients through mobile technology and advancing sensor systems; and 3) broader applicability to tackle a variety of health challenges. This chapter is useful for those hoping to gain a deeper understanding of the promise that drives the excitement in gamification as a method for addressing the health challenges of the modern world, as well as the work that is still required to fulfill that promise.

DOI: 10.4018/978-1-7998-0047-7.ch006

INTRODUCTION

One of the defining health challenges facing the world today is maximizing impact of the rapidly evolving field of medical and technological innovations on promoting positive, healthy behaviors in people. According to the World Health Organization (WHO), chronic diseases such as ischemic heart disease, obstructive pulmonary disease, lung cancer, and diabetes, all of which require careful disease management, represent some of the leading causes of morbidity and mortality in the world today. The leading risk factors for these conditions, such as poor diet, physical inactivity, tobacco use, high blood pressure, high glucose level, medication non-adherence, and obesity, are linked to lifestyle choices and individual behaviors (Stevens et al., 2009). Medication non-adherence, which refers to the extent which patients fail to take medications as prescribed by their health care providers, is widely recognized as one of the biggest challenges in the chronic illness management. On average, it is estimated that approximately 30% to 50% of adults in the United States struggle to adhere to long-term medications and that half of these patients discontinue the use of prescribed medications within the first few months of therapy (DiMattero, et al., 2002). As a consequence, a substantial number of patients do not optimally benefit from the prescribed medication and course of treatment. Effective promotion of healthy behaviors not only has a significant potential to address unmet medical need, it also has significant financial implications as well; it is estimated that nearly three quarters of all healthcare costs in the United States can be attributed to poor health behavior (Woolf, 2001).

Over the past two decades, the body of research on health behavior and promotion has rapidly grown. Within this expansion, the use of gamification as a tool to incentivize healthy decision making has become an emerging trend to reduce the burden of preventable chronic illnesses and increase overall wellbeing. Gamification is defined as the use of game design elements in non-game contexts. In gamification, the game design elements, which are motivational affordances used in entertainment games of other systems, are used to enhance overall enjoyment and engagement with the desired behavior (Deterding, 2011). Intentional and quality game design can be used to target individual health behavior decision-making and empower individuals to make positive behavioral changes.

While several studies have outlined the concept of gamification in the medical field, the current literature lacks an in-depth explanation of the key advantages that gamification possesses over the past iterations of interventions aimed to promote healthy behaviors. This chapter will begin with a brief history of gamification, followed by a discussion on three key advantages, which are fueling the excitement in this field. The chapter will close with a discussion on some of the work that still needs to be done in the field to deliver on its promise.

HISTORY OF GAMIFICATION

Gamification has emerged as a hybrid method for promoting healthy behaviors, drawing from the strengths of both personal informatics and serious games. Personal informatics or "quantified self" refers to the ability to collect and track health metrics such as vitals, movement and specific health behaviors. There are generally two forms of personal informatics: physician-initiated and patient-initiated. Physician-initiated tracking allows for healthcare providers to collect continuous health information and provide health suggestions based on that data. Patient-initiated allows for individuals to self-monitor their health information and make decisions based on their personal data. (Gimpel et al., 2013) Serious games are the use of games to address more serious concerns beyond the purpose of entertainment. They generally consist of stand-alone consoles with the purpose of altering health behaviors through a specific and standardized medium. Serious games attempt to appeal to participant's intrinsic motivation by increasing engagement and enjoyment while impacting health. Concerns for personal informatics include lack of engagement. Concerns for serious games include cost of game development and cost-effectiveness. These precursors have allowed gamification to address limitations in technology and healthcare, therefore holding key advantages over its past counterparts.

ADVANTAGES OF GAMIFICATION

Promotion of Intrinsic Motivation Through Effective Gamification Design

Motivation is the main factor that drives every behavior change, from eating healthier, to increasing physical activity, to adhering to a medication regimen to better manage health. One of the most significant appeals of applying gamification to promote positive health behavior and wellness is the ability to foster a strong sense of motivation within individuals. There are two classical types of motivation that pertain to driving behavior change: extrinsic and intrinsic motivation. While extrinsic motivation deals with the desire to perform a task based on external factors such as punishments and rewards, intrinsic motivation deals with one's desire to perform a task for its own sake. Several studies have shown that intrinsic motivation has the ability to create a more sustainable, long-lasting behavior change compared to extrinsic motivation (Teixeira et al., 2012); thus, interventions that cultivate intrinsic motivation remains a high priority.

Self-Determination Theory, an established motivation theory, explains that it is necessary to satisfy three innate psychological needs of individuals including autonomy, competence and relatedness in order to maintain and foster intrinsic motivation (Ryan et al., 2006). Appealing to these core psychological needs of the user, gamification-based interventions aim to actively foster a sense of intrinsic motivation by utilizing intentional motivational affordances such as badges, personal profiles, leaderboards, social feedback, levels, and challenges. One randomized controlled trial has shown that a novel smartphone exercise game created a significant increase in intrinsic motivation for physical activity in inactive individuals with Type II diabetes. The exercise game accomplished this through the incorporation aforementioned game design elements and through providing personalized physical activity recommendations in a participant's storyline (Hochsmann et al., 2019). Further studies have indicated that there is a statistically significant positive correlation between several key design elements and the satisfaction of autonomy, competence and relatedness (Wee and Chong, 2019). To understand the theoretical explanation for these findings, the remainder of this section will discuss the various game design elements that have been linked to drive an increase in intrinsic motivation by satisfying each of the three psychological needs.

Autonomy refers to the independent will of the users in performing tasks with the freedom to make their own decisions. Design elements that empower users to exert decision-making control over their actions and strategies in the game have been theorized to enhance autonomy (Ryan et al., 2006). In line with this theoretical framework, Wee et al. (2019) have shown a significant positive correlation between game design elements such as personal profiles and non-fixed structure with feelings of autonomy in the users. Personal profiles give users the freedom to make their own decisions about how they wish to portray themselves. The freedom to make choices ranging from profile pictures and customizable avatars to interests and slogans supports the psychological need for autonomy. Non-fixed structure refers to the freedom for users to select their own strategy and movements in the game. Rather than clearly defined challenges that are laid out for users to follow in sequential fashion, non-fixed structure allows the user to select how, when and which challenges to tackle. Research has shown games that give participants the ability to make their own decisions and distinctively shape the narrative of the game are substantially more likely to enjoy the game they are participating in.

Competence refers to the ability of users to perform certain tasks. Studies have shown a significant positive correlation between game elements, such as challenges and short cycle times, and the satisfaction of the psychological need for competence (Wee et al., 2019). Whether it is remembering to take medication for seven consecutive days or meeting a weekly physical activity goal, having a sense of accomplishment leads to increased motivation and confidence in our abilities. Short cycle times of each challenge is also an important driver in meeting the need for competence, as it breaks down overall goals and missions of the application into manageable portions. Short cycles also allow users to more consistently meet the goals of their challenges and avoid the feelings of burnout, stress and fatigue.

Lastly, relatedness refers to individuals' needs to connect or relate to each other. Relatedness in gamification builds on this innate human desire to be connected to others in order to cultivate intrinsic motivation. Wee et al. (2019) have shown through their study that game elements such as chat based social networks are positively correlated with the psychological need for relatedness. In the modern world driven by constant communication via instant messaging platforms (Gemmil, E. & Peterson, M., 2006), gamification design elements such as chat features and online social support that promote relatedness within participant groups have been shown to increase motivation and patient empowerment by expanding the user's social network and feeling of community (Ahmed et al., 2015).

With the utilization of these key design elements, gamification has the potential to cultivate a strong sense of intrinsic motivation. This is one of the key advantages of gamification compared to the past iterations of health behavior change interventions such as personal health informatics which aimed to motivate behavior change in a much more passive fashion by merely providing the tools for collecting and reflecting on information about one's own health (Li et al., 2010).

Broad Accessibility Through Mobile Technology and Sensors

The unprecedented spread of mobile technologies such as cellular devices, as well as innovative advancements made in their application to healthcare has made it an effective conduit for applying the game design elements of gamification. Mobile health (mHealth) is an emerging field in healthcare that deals with the delivery of health-related services through the use of portable devices such as cellphones (Whittaker, 2012). According to the International Telecommunication Union, there are now approximately 5 billion mobile phone subscriptions in the world today, with over 85% of the world's population covered by wireless signal (MHealth: New horizons…, 2011). In the United States, nearly 90% of American adults own a mobile phone and more than 70% own a mobile phone with app capabilities (Smartphone Milestone…, 2014). This allows the health-related application of gamification on mHealth to have a significantly higher degree of accessibility compared to past behavioral interventions such as serious health games, which rely upon an independent gaming console.

Mobile health applications take advantage of internal sensors ranging from cameras, microphones, GPS, and accelerometer built into mobile phones, as well as various external sensors ranging from simple light and pressure sensors to blood glucose level monitors, which can all be transmitted to the mobile phone through the use of Bluetooth and other wireless technology. Types of sensors include smart pill bottles that detect when the bottle is opened, indigestible sensors that detect when a medication is taken, wearable sensors that detect hand to mouth movement, and computer vision that analyzes movements to record certain actions (Aldeer, et al., 2018). The use of such monitoring systems, which Aldeer et al. describes as Cyber-Physical Systems (CPS) allows healthcare professionals, family members, and individuals to effectively monitor patient health and medication adherence. Given the falling cost of physiologic sensors as well inexpensive data transmission, these sensing systems hold great promise (Dobkin, 2013). This ability to continuously and remotely monitor patient behavior, combined with the advances in data analytics show particular promise in seamlessly integrating with the key design elements of gamification discussed above. The sensors also allow for an additional level of accessibility to patients of all backgrounds, as effective health interventions from health professionals are no longer confined to the traditional walls of hospitals and medical offices.

Together, the application of gamification to mobile devices and wireless sensor systems may present the future of health-related behavioral intervention: a sensor based, data driven method for promoting wellbeing and self-care.

Broad Applicability

Gamification in health care proves a unique niche for a versatility of functions. With an increase in availability and accessibility to technology and smartphones, people are connected to resources and applications more readily. This section will explore the versatility and broad applicability of gamification related to chronic disease management, physical activity, medication adherence, and imparting health knowledge.

As reported by the CDC, an estimated 90% of the $3.3 trillion annual US health care expenditure is spent on individuals with chronic and mental health illness. Chronic diseases can range from heart disease to cancer to diabetes making it a difficult challenge to tackle. However common risk factors, such as tobacco use, poor nutrition and lack of physical activity can provide easier avenues to tackling such a large problem. Although the data is limited, the online platform "ONESELF" exhibits versatility. Randomized control trials have shown the effectiveness and applicability. Gamification and web-based social support features showed favorable outcomes of decreased utilization of healthcare and medication overuse while increasing physical activity and patient sense of empowerment in Rheumatoid arthritis patients (Ahmed et al., 2015). Another study exhibited that interactive components of an internet-based intervention developed in conjecture with physiotherapists and rheumatologists positively impacted patient empowerment and pain manifestations for chronic lower back pain (Riva, et al., 2014).

Another gamification application is for medical adherence and health monitoring, such as medication adherence and diabetes management. Pertinent applications include Mango Health, Bayer's Didget Blood Glucose Meter and MySugr. Mango Health uses a system of points, levels and rewards to incentivize medication adherence and healthy behaviors such as drinking more water and increasing steps taken throughout the day. Bayer's Didget Blood Glucose Meter and MySugr attempt to use gamification to incentivize blood glucose level management. While data is limited, a pilot study to assess mHealth applications has shown a 50% increase in the frequency of their daily measurements in a small sample of adolescent patients with Type I diabetes (Miller, et al., 2016).

Gamification can also be used for younger age groups, which allows for earlier opportunities for positive health behavior modifications and development of healthy habits. Examples include ProVitao and Zamzee. ProViTao is a gamified platform that provides obesity treatment through a nine-month program via mobile and web applications. Although research on the effectiveness of the platform is in its preliminary stages, there are strong indications for success. Zamzee, a platform designed with the intention to make physical activity fun, engaging and sustainable for children, has reported 59% more activity in Zamzee users than non-Zamzee users. For health care providers and public health practitioners, disseminating appropriate health knowledge to individuals at risk of specific diseases or afflicted with certain ailments is a critical task. These platforms also educate and disseminate health information so that participants can engage with their healthy choices in a way that would sustain the same healthy choices in the future.

DISCUSSION

Since its emergence within the past decade, gamification has garnered overwhelming attention from academia and industry alike, easily outpacing publication volume for other health behavior intervention methods such as personal informatics and serious games (Hamari et al., 2014). This groundswell of interest can be explained by some of the key advantages that gamification holds over its counterparts, including the ability to promote intrinsic motivation through intentional game design elements, broad accessibility through mobile technology and intelligent sensor systems, and broad applicability across various diseases and health promotion goals. Lastly, we will discuss some of the current limitations and suggestions for future direction with respect to the use of gamification in promoting positive health behaviors.

Key Advantages

Prior to gamification, health behavior modification initiatives allowed users to access health information and collect or monitor behaviors, which allows for limited engagement. Gamification uses intentional game design to harness internal motivation, thereby increasing engagement and encouraging increased healthy decision-making. Gamification uses individual agency (such as the use fixed and non-fixed structure) to engage users, and incentivization (such as the use of points and badges) to create a context that allows participants to exercise autonomy, rather than cultivating feelings of paternalism or shame that may be associated with making less healthy choices. Incentives provide positive reinforcement and opportunities for increasing and sustaining long-term health.

A hallmark of gamification has been its ability to integrate mobile technology and intelligent sensor systems into its platforms. Traditional methods of modifying health behaviors required purchasing additional hardware or programs, or in the case of serious games, stand alone consoles. Gamification prioritizes streamlined integration; As mobile devices and sensor technology have become increasingly accessible, available and user friendly, gamification has used this opportunity to gamification of healthcare capabilities. Individuals can more readily participate and have access to their health information without expending additional effort.

This level of accessibility to personal health data paired with intentional gamification design allows for scientifically sound and real-time personalized health information to be applied to versatile applications based on how gamification design is implemented. For the user, this translates to an easy way to record current health indicators and apply them to different aspects of health- from physical exercise to medication adherence to discontinuing bad health behaviors. These benefits can be seen through the examples such as Mango Health, MySugr and Zamzee. Preliminary studies indicate much promise in gamification, however there are limitations that need be addressed to assess the validity of its impact and potential.

Future Research Directions

With the rapidly evolving innovations in the field of technology, further research and work is needed for gamification in healthcare to keep pace. Limited empirical data on effectiveness posits gaps in knowledge and literature. Although the majority of studies indicate that gamification can lead to positive change in behavior, the legitimacy of these techniques have been called to question. Presently, there is little empirical evidence on the efficacy of health initiatives that contain the mechanics of gamification; Research conducted is generally small scale with limited sample size, and long-term behavior change and sustainability of gamification is yet to be explored.

Furthermore, studies have not clearly tested the link between specific gamification components that produce health benefits. It is unclear as to which conceptual ideas and motivational elements are responsible, for example, in increased physical activity. Future study designs should focus on differentiating different gamification aspects and analyzing correlation and causation patterns.

Assessing intrinsic motivation and changes in intrinsic motivation prove a challenging task. Current research relies on participant feedback related to feelings of autonomy and empowerment, which leads to a level of subjectivity and uncertainty. Results of these studies might also be impacted by the novelty and promotion of these platforms, which could have skewed to inflated autonomy and empowerment data. Further research is needed to determine if feelings of autonomy and empowerment, as well as healthy choices are sustained long term.

Scaling and management of gamified health initiatives creates an intersection for many sectors. While health and technology are the most obvious, it is important to consider the public and private sectors. In contrast with strategic implementation, the emergence of mHealth is occurring in many Member States through experimentation with technologies in many health settings. Policy-makers and administrators need to have the necessary knowledge to make the transition from pilot programs to strategic large-scale deployments. The question of which sector or entities are best suited for implementation and management of systems and access to health data is a conversation to be had moving forward.

A final consideration for future direction is the issue of data management and security. Large-scale data can be collected, but the analysis and management of health related and user-involved big data must be discussed carefully and thoroughly as this field continues to evolve and expand.

CONCLUSION

The application of gamification in addressing modern health challenges has been a rapidly growing field. This chapter has explored some of the key advantages the gamification holds over past iterations of technology-based behavioral health interventions such as serious health games and personal informatics. Using gamified platforms has been related to improved health-related decision making and behavior modification in chronic diseases and risk factor management. However, there is much work to be done to deliver on these promises. Although the field is growing, there is still limited knowledge and research on this topic. Future considerations include more research in the form of scientifically sound studies with larger sample sizes, implementation considerations, and issues of data management and security.

REFERENCES

Allam, A., Kostova, Z., Nakamoto, K., & Schulz, P. J. (2015). The Effect of Social Support Features and Gamification on a Web-Based Intervention for Rheumatoid Arthritis Patients: Randomized Controlled Trial. *Journal of Medical Internet Research, 17*(1), e14. doi:10.2196/jmir.3510 PMID:25574939

Deterding, S., Dixon, D., Khaled, R., & Nacke, L. (2011). From game design elements to gamefulness. *Proceedings of the 16th International Academic MindTrek Conference on Envisioning Future Media Environments – MindTrek 11*. 10.1145/2181037.2181040

Dimatteo, M. R., Giordani, P. J., Lepper, H. S., & Croghan, T. W. (2002). Patient Adherence and Medical Treatment Outcomes. *Medical Care, 40*(9), 794–811. doi:10.1097/00005650-200209000-00009 PMID:12218770

Dobkin, B. H. (2013). Wearable motion sensors to continuously measure real-world physical activities. *Current Opinion in Neurology, 26*(6), 602–608. doi:10.1097/WCO.0000000000000026 PMID:24136126

Gemmill, E. L., & Peterson, M. (2006). Technology Use Among College Students: Implications for Student Affairs Professionals. *Journal of Student Affairs Research and Practice, 43*(2). doi:10.2202/1949-6605.1640

Gimpe, H., Nißen, M., & Görlitz, R. (2013). Quantifying the quantified self: A study on the motivations of patients to track their own health. In *International Conference on Information Systems ICIS 2013*, Milan, Italy: Association for Information Systems.

Hamari, J., Koivisto, J., & Pakkanen, T. (2014). Do Persuasive Technologies Persuade? - A Review of Empirical Studies. Persuasive Technology Lecture Notes in Computer Science, 118-136. doi:10.1007/978-3-319-07127-5_11

Health and Economic Costs of Chronic Disease I CDC. (n.d.). Retrieved from https://www.cdc.gov/chronicdisease/about/costs/index.htm#ref1

Li, I., Dey, A., & Forlizzi, J. (2010). A stage-based model of personal informatics systems. *Proceedings of the 28th International Conference on Human Factors in Computing Systems - CHI 10*. 10.1145/1753326.1753409

MHealth: New horizons for health through mobile technologies. (2011). Geneva, Switzerland: World Health Organization.

Miller, A. S., Cafazzo, J. A., & Seto, E. (2014). A game plan: Gamification design principles in mHealth applications for chronic disease management. *Health Informatics Journal, 22*(2), 184–193. doi:10.1177/1460458214537511 PMID:24986104

Riva, S., Camerini, A., Allam, A., & Schulz, P. J. (2014). Interactive Sections of an Internet-Based Intervention Increase Empowerment of Chronic Back Pain Patients: Randomized Controlled Trial. *Journal of Medical Internet Research, 16*(8), e180. doi:10.2196/jmir.3474 PMID:25119374

Ryan, R. M., Rigby, C. S., & Przybylski, A. (2006). The Motivational Pull of Video Games: A Self-Determination Theory Approach. *Motivation and Emotion, 30*(4), 344–360. doi:10.100711031-006-9051-8

Stevens, G., Mascarenhas, M., & Mathers, C. (2009). Global health risks: Progress and challenges. *Bulletin of the World Health Organization, 87*(9), 646–646. doi:10.2471/BLT.09.070565 PMID:19784438

The top 10 causes of death. (n.d.). Retrieved from https://www.who.int/news-room/fact-sheets/detail/the-top-10-causes-of-death

Wee, S., & Choong, W. (2019). Gamification: Predicting the effectiveness of variety game design elements to intrinsically motivate users energy conservation behaviour. *Journal of Environmental Management, 233*, 97–106. doi:10.1016/j.jenvman.2018.11.127 PMID:30572268

Whittaker, R. (2012). Issues in mHealth: Findings From Key Informant Interviews. *Journal of Medical Internet Research, 14*(5), e129. doi:10.2196/jmir.1989 PMID:23032424

Woolf, S. H. (2008). The Power of Prevention and What It Requires. *Journal of the American Medical Association, 299*(20), 2437. doi:10.1001/jama.299.20.2437 PMID:18505953

KEY TERMS AND DEFINITIONS

Cyber-Physical Systems: Monitoring systems that allow healthcare professionals, family members, and individuals to effectively monitor patient health metrics and behaviors.

Extrinsic Motivation: The type of motivation that deals with one's desire to perform a task based on external factors such as punishments and rewards.

Game Design Elements: Motivational affordances (e.g. points, badges, leaderboards, social networks) which are used in games to enhance the overall enjoyment and engagement with a certain behavior.

Gamification: The application of typical elements of game playing (e.g. points, competitions, social networks, leaderboards) to other areas of activity, such as the promotion of healthy behaviors.

Intrinsic Motivation: The type of motivation that deals with one's desire to perform a task due to personal enjoyment in the task itself.

mHealth: The use or portable devices such as mobile phones and other wireless technology for the delivery of health-related services.

Personal Informatics/Quantified Self: The use of technology to track and reflect on one's own health metrics such as vitals, movement and specific health behaviors.

Self-Determination Theory: A macro theory of human motivation and personality that concerns people's inherent growth tendencies and innate psychological needs. It theorizes that it is necessary to satisfy the three innate psychological needs of individuals (autonomy, competence, and relatedness) in order to maintain and foster intrinsic motivation.

Serious Game: Full-fledged games that have been developed for non-entertainment purposes, such as promotion of healthy behaviors.

Chapter 7
Use of Predictive and Simulation Models to Develop Strategies for Better Access Specialists Care

Siang Li Chua
https://orcid.org/0000-0001-9494-5221
Changi General Hospital, Singapore

Wai Leng Chow
Changi General Hospital, Singapore

ABSTRACT

No-shows are patients who miss scheduled Specialist Outpatient Clinic (SOC) appointments. No-shows can impact patients' access to care and appointment lead time. This chapter describes a data-driven strategy of improving access to specialist care through first developing a stratified predictive scoring model to identify patients at risk of no-shows; second, studying the impact of a dynamic overbooking strategy that incorporates the use of the no-show prediction model using discrete event simulation (DES) on lead time. Seventeen variables related to new SOC appointments for subsidized patients in 2016 were analyzed. Multiple logistic regression (MLR) found eight variables independently associated with no-shows with area under receiver operation curve (AUC) 70%. The model was tested and validated. DES model simulated the appointment overbooking strategy as applied to the top highest volume specialties and concluded that lead time of Specialty 1 and 2 can be shortened by 27.5 days (49% improvement) and 21.3 (33%) respectively.

INTRODUCTION

No-shows are patients who miss scheduled Specialist Outpatient Clinic (SOC) appointments without informing service providers. No-shows result in wastage of limited clinic resources, affect patients' timely access to care and negatively affect appointment lead time. Lead time is the period from appointment request date to appointment date.

DOI: 10.4018/978-1-7998-0047-7.ch007

No-shows are a common problem internationally (Dantas, Fleck, Oliveira, & Hamacher, 2018) with the African continent having the highest average no show rate at 43% followed by South America at 27.8%, and Asia at 25.1%. The overall average no-show rate across 105 studies was 23%.

Non-attendance is also a pressing problem in Singapore, particularly given limited specialist healthcare resources in its public hospitals. Accessibility, quality and affordability are important characteristics of Singapore's healthcare system (Ministry of Health Singapore, 2012). Therefore, lead times of new cases to see a specialist in public hospitals are being tracked by the Ministry of Health (MOH) as a quality indicator (Ministry of Health Singapore, 2017).

A total of 4.937 million outpatient attendances occurred in Singapore's public hospitals from a population of 5.61 million in 2017 (Department of Statistics Singapore, 2013; Ministry of Health Singapore, 2018). The median lead time for non-urgent specialties was 27 days (Ministry of Health Singapore, 2017). We turn to Changi General Hospital (CGH), a public hospital providing both subsidized and private specialist services, for a specific example. It serves 1.4 million residents in the eastern region of Singapore. Internal statistics reported to the MOH revealed that CGH median and 95th percentile lead times of subsidized new consultation appointment ranged from 9 to 58 days and 14 to 260 days respectively, depending on specialties involved (Chua & Chow, 2019). Internal reports also revealed that the hospital had 26% no-shows out of 96,502 new appointments made at CGH subsidized clinics.

BACKGROUND

Predicting No-Show

Many studies concurr that a no-show does not occur arbitrarily and instead, aimed to predict it. Almost all no-show studies had analyzed the relationship between no-shows and appointment records through univariate and bivariate analysis. Multiple Logistic Regression (MLR) is the most commonly used predictive method (56 out of 105 studies) for this type of analysis (Dantas et al., 2018). Other statistical and predictive methods used include Gradient Boosting Algorithm (Elvira, Ochoa, Gonzalvez, & Mochón, 2018), stochastic programming (Samorani & LaGanga, 2011), database exploration technique (Samorani & LaGanga, 2015) and association rule mining (Glowacka, Henry, & May, 2009). Hybrid methodologies such as empirical Markov modeling with MLR (Goffman et al., 2017) and empirical Bayesian inference with MLR (Alaeddini, Yang, Reddy, & Yu, 2011) have also been used.

Overbooking: A Strategy to Reduce Wastage of Outpatient Resources From No-Shows

Many countries faces the challenges of long lead times as well. Thirteen Organisation for Economic Co-operation and Development (OECD) countries had jointly written a book on lead time policies (OECD, 2013). Systematic reviews on outpatient lead times in recent years reported on the different strategies that institutions had deployed (Naiker, FitzGerald, Dulhunty, & Rosemann, 2018). Common strategies involved realigning resources, increasing operations efficiency and improving processes. More than 50% of the studies with positive results were process improvement strategies at tactical and strategic levels. These strategies included managing overbooking through no-show prediction and patient engagement, scheduling appointment through patient profiling, efficient use of resources through capacity planning, eliminating waste, and reminding patients through text messaging. Some of these strategies require more resources than others. Several studies suggested that overbooking to compensate for no-show is a method to reduce long lead time without incurring additional resources (Alaeddini et al., 2011; Muthuraman & Lawley, 2008; Naiker et al., 2018; Samorani & LaGanga, 2011, 2015; Zeng, Turkcan, Lin, & Lawley, 2010). Overbooking refers to booking more appointments than available slots.

Currently, CGH practices overbooking in a uniform way, whereby each service provider receives the same number of overbooking slots to compensate for no-shows. Implementing an average overbooking percentage to every clinic session equivalent to overall no-show percentage is not optimal because the number of no-shows are not constant for every clinic session. On sessions where all patients including the overbooked ones turned up, the resources will be over utilized, thus resulting in long patient wait times, clinic overtime, and patient and staff dissatisfaction. During other sessions when no-shows exceed the expected average number of no-shows, resources are wasted. The performance of overbooking can be improved by predicting likelihood of no-shows when each appointment is booked. In this way, overbooking for each session varies according to the likelihood of patients not showing up and a more reliable overbooking strategy can be achieved.

The first part of this chapter discusses the development of a tool to predict the risk of no-shows among subsidized new appointments so as to implement a dynamic overbooking strategy on full sessions to improve appointment lead time.

Simulation

Simulating appointment scheduling by considering no-shows derived from a predictive model has been used to evaluate model utility and improve lead time, (Daggy et al., 2010).

Therefore, the second part of this chapter discusses use of a Discrete Event Simulation (DES) model to examine the impact of evidence-guided over-booking on appointment scheduling and appointment lead times. The results of the DES provide evidence of the effectiveness of the overbooking strategies used to guide implementation in real-world settings.

MATERIALS AND METHODS

Setting

CGH is an acute public hospital with over 1,000 beds caring for a community of 1.4 million people in eastern Singapore. CGH offers a comprehensive range of 24 medical specialties and services. CGH provides a mixed public and private outpatient specialist service whereby patients who are Singapore residents can choose to receive subsidized or private care. Care provided at subsidized clinics are heavily subsidized by the government and make up 80% of the SOC workload. Patients receiving care in the subsidized clinic are managed by a rotating team of doctors. Private patients do not receive any subsidy for the care provided and are able to receive care from their specialist of choice. The demand for private care is lower and has a shorter appointment lead time. As a public hospital, the priority is to ensure that the Singapore residents requiring subsidized care have timely access to healthcare services.

Referral and Appointment Making Process

To qualify for a subsidized case, the new case has to be referred from polyclinics, other CGH departments or other public institutions. Polyclinics are subsidized primary care centers. Patients who have not been previously managed by a particular medical specialty are considered a new case and appointments will be made on the next earliest available slot. The visit attendance type will be considered a consultation visit. Number of slots per sessions are pre-planned before they are opened up for booking in the Outpatient Appointment System (OAS). OAS is a web-based system used to manage outpatient appointments. The system allows: administrators to set up the service providers, calendar, and appointment slots; call centre operators to search for earliest appointment and book appointments; and managers to query and generate reports. Generally, about 1 or 2 slots per session are included as overbooking slots to cater for no-shows. If a session including an overbooking slot is fully booked, a forced booking slot may be created with approval by the doctor if a new case requires urgent medical service.

Analysis Plan

Data Set

The predictive tool was built using retrospective data of CGH SOC visits from January to December 2016. Outpatient and administrative data from hospital wide appointment and patient transactions systems were used. Data inclusion criteria retained actualized, no-shows, new subsidized cases and consultations visits. Cancelled, walk-ins and consultations related to pre-operations were excluded.

The model was built using 50% of 2016 data and validated using the other 50% data. It was then further tested using visit data from January to December 2017 with selection criteria similar to the model building data set.

Variables

The authors selected 17 variables in this study. The choice of variables was guided by availability of data, ease of obtaining data operationally in future using routinely captured administrative data, and significant factors related to no-shows concluded by other studies. Systematic review on no-shows had summarized significant factors from 105 studies. The factors were demographics such as age, gender, race, socioeconomic status, marital status and level of education; appointment characteristics such as lead time, prior no-show history, appointment data and time, referral source and visit type; and, other characteristics such as payment, distance between clinic and patient home zip code, provider rank/seniority, specialty, patient medical history and clinical diagnosis (Dantas et al., 2018).

The 17 variables used in this chapter's study were:

1. Patient demographics
    a. Gender
    b. Age
    c. Race
    d. Nationality
    e. Patient Address by Region

2. Appointments records
   a. Force book
   b. Overbook
   c. Specialty
   d. Appointment lead time
   e. Appointment month
   f. Appointment day of week
   g. Was preceding day of appointment a public holiday?
   h. Was preceding day of appointment a work day?
   i. Was day of appointment a school holiday?
3. Historical records
   a. Referral Source
   b. Previous Visit Type
   c. Previous Visit Status (Previous Visit referred to the latest SOC visit that the patient had to any CGH specialty during the past year).

In model building, January to December 2015 visit data were used to compute the Previous Visit. In this set of data, all visit status (actualized, no-show, cancelled, walk-ins) and visit types (new consultation, follow-up consultation, new ancillary, follow-up ancillary) were included.

Descriptive analysis was performed for each variable. Continuous variables such as age and appointment lead time were categorized for further analysis based on the findings of descriptive analysis. Patients' postal codes were grouped into Regional Health System (RHS) region.

Bivariate analysis was performed to determine the significant factors associated with no-shows. Missing data of each variable were excluded from the bivariate analysis. Due to the large data set, the level of statistical significance was set at 0.01. IBM SPSS Statistics version 22 (SPSS) was used in the analysis.

Predictive Scoring Tool

Logistic regression analysis was used to develop the predictive model as 53% of past studies on no-show modelling used this method (Dantas et al., 2018). SPSS randomly selected 50% of the training data set. The method Forward Likelihood Ratio (LR) was used and the significant factors associated with no-shows under bivariate analysis were considered as the covariates. The stepwise selection of variables was tested with the significant level of 0.01.

A total of three logistic regression models were built progressively to obtain the no-show risk stratified predictive scoring tool for ease of use operationally:

- **Model 1:** To determine the predictors by identifying the independent variables associated with no-shows
- **Model 2:** To determine the weighted scores of predictors
- **Model 3/Final Tool:** To stratify the risk scores into 5 categories for versatile use by operations team

Model 1

In the Model 1, a total of 3 LR logistic regressions were run. In 1st regression run, 1st value/category of each variable was used as the reference. Multi-collinearity of the significant variables was checked and highly correlated variables were removed. The lowest odds ratios (OR) of each variable in the 1st run was identified as the reference for the 2nd run. All the factors in this model would have positive OR. The purpose was to prepare for computation of the weighted score in a later step. The insignificant values/categories within a variable were grouped together with the reference for the 3rd run. In this way, the model was not only simplified with a reduction of values/categories but also contained only meaningful ORs from significant factors only. This step would be required in the computation of weighted score.

Model 2

The lowest OR of all variables in Model 1 was identified and used to normalize the OR of each factor into the weighted scores. The weighted scores of the predictors were computed, summed and assigned to each appointment. The score of each appointment was analysis against the actual visit status. Each score was also summarized by the population size and the actual visit status. Scores with less than 0.1% of the population were too small to be representative of a group. They were grouped together with the adjacent score to achieve population size of at least 0.1% or more. The score was then used as the single predictor to feed into logistic regression.

Model 3

The scores were grouped into 5 categories of risk level. The grouping scores were guided by similarity of OR in Model 2 and proportion of no-shows while trying to achieve equal population size of each risk category. Finally, the risk level was used as the single predictor to derive the final stratified scoring model.

Model 1 and 2 were validated against the other 50% of 2016 data. Model 3, which was the final model, was further tested using SOC visit data in 2017.

Overbooking Strategy

The number of overbooking slots was determined dynamically at the end of an operational day after all the appointment bookings were completed for the day. The predictive tool determines the number of extremely high risk no-show patients. To save time and effort, the tool applies fully-booked sessions only. Tool prediction accuracy was considered in the computation of overbooking slots in order to address the concern of wrongly predicted no-shows who turned up for the appointments.

For each fully-booked session *i*:

$$a_i = \text{rounddown int}(c_i * ns * pred_{accuracy})$$

$$t_i = c_i - b_i + a_i$$

where

a_i = additional capacity in session *i*
t_i = total available slots in session *i*
c_i = current capacity as set up in the calendar in session *i*
b_i = number of appointments booked in session *i*
ns = number of extremely high risk of no-shows
$pred_{accuracy}$ = accuracy of predictive tool

Simulation Model

A discrete event simulation model was developed to simulate the appointment making process of the top 2 highest volume specialties. Simul8 2015 Professional was used. The inputs of the models were the arrival rate and the slot capacity. The outputs were lead times of each appointment simulated.

Arrival rate of each specialty was computed using the request for appointments data during the period from January to December 2017. The daily average arrivals were summarized by days (e.g. Monday through Sunday) since requests for appointments could occur any day of the week. Weekend requests were usually from the wards and emergency department. The Day Planner feature in Simul8 was used. This worked well because Day Planner is a matrix used to specify arrivals by day of the week indexed by time of day. Therefore, the hourly arrivals during each weekday are distributed equally throughout the day. This is because lead time refers to the number of the days (not hour) from request date to appointment date.

Slot capacity was derived from 2017 resource set up data. The daily capacity of each specialty were summarized by Monday through Friday. Saturday clinics, which were unusual, were excluded. The model read the initial capacity from the spreadsheet feature of Simul8. Using Visual Logic features, the model dynamically reduced the available slots as and when appointments were being booked.

Visual Logic controls the dynamic search of earliest available slot from Monday through Friday. If no slot was found for the first week, the search continued into subsequent week(s) until a slot was found.

The simulation was run for Monday through Sunday periods. The resulting collection period was for 1 year. The simulated lead time of each appointment was exported to Excel to compute the overall median lead time and percentage of appointments that waited for more than 60 days.

The base model was validated using the current lead time. In the what-if scenarios, the increase in slot capacities were computed using the earlier described booking strategy.

RESULTS

The most pertinent results related to 8 variables, namely: age, race, patient address, specialty, appointment lead time, referral source, previous visit type and previous visit status. These were the variables that remained independently associated with no-shows in MLR model described in the next section.

The largest age group of patients were in the 55-64 years old category (20.3%). Age category 25-34 years had the highest no-show rate at 37.1% (Figure 1) and was similar to the majority of the studies examined (Dantas et al., 2018). The majority of the patients were Chinese (68.6%) and non-Chinese had a higher no-show rate (Figure 2). As CGH is located in the East, 72.1% of the patients were staying the East and had no-show rates lower than patients coming from other zones (Figure 3). No-show rates were significantly different across different specialties (Figure 4). Overall, 23% of the appointments waited for 31 to 60 days. The no-show rate linearly increased as the appointment lead time increased until the threshold of 150 days. There was a slight dip in the no-show rate here to 39.4% for 151 to 180 days before the rate shot up to 60.5% for appointments with lead time of more than 180 days (Figure 5). Most of referrals (40.4%) were from Polyclinics but referrals from Ward and A&E had higher no-show rates (Figure 6). 36.3% of the patients did not have a previous appointment with CGH during the past 1 year (Figure 7). Highest no-show rates were observed among those who were new case for their previous appointment (29.3%) and those who did not show up for their previous appointment (45.3%) (Figure 8).

Predictive Model: Bivariate Analysis

A total of 90,199 new subsidized appointments were made from January to December, 2016. Among these, 22,812 people did not turn up yielding a no-show rate of 25.3%.

Table 1 shows the bivariate analysis whereby 14 variables were significantly higher among no-shows.

Predictive Scoring Tool

Model 1

The 8 variables that remained independently associated with no-shows in MLR model were age, race, patient address, specialty, appointment lead time, referral source, previous visit type and previous visit status.

There was no multi-collinearity among the significant factors in the model as Tolerance < 0.1 or VIF > 10 (Table 2).

In the 1st regression run, 4 variables had their lowest ORs in non-reference group. The 4 factors were referral from SAF, 65-74 years old, Specialty 15, and Ancillary New Case from Previous Visit Type. These 4 factors were changed into reference group in the 2nd run. In this run, the only insignificant cat-

Figure 1. Appointment volume and no-show rate by age

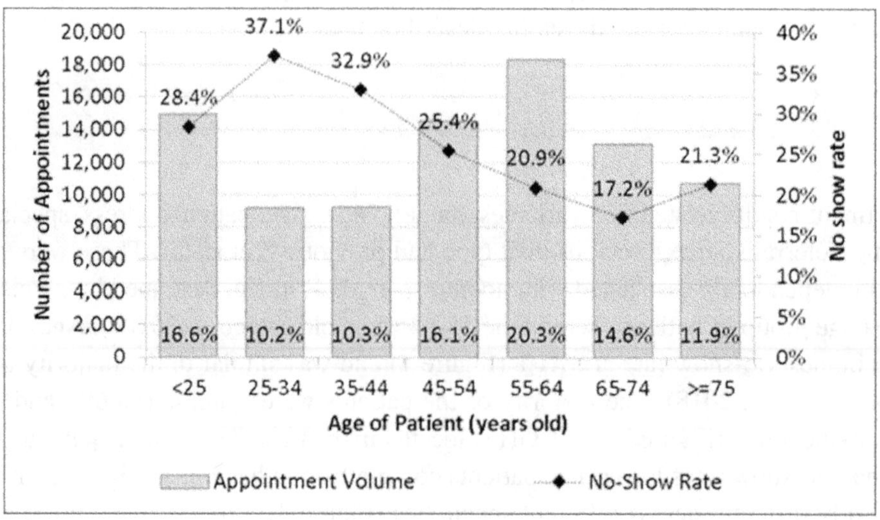

Figure 2. Appointment volume and no-show rate by race

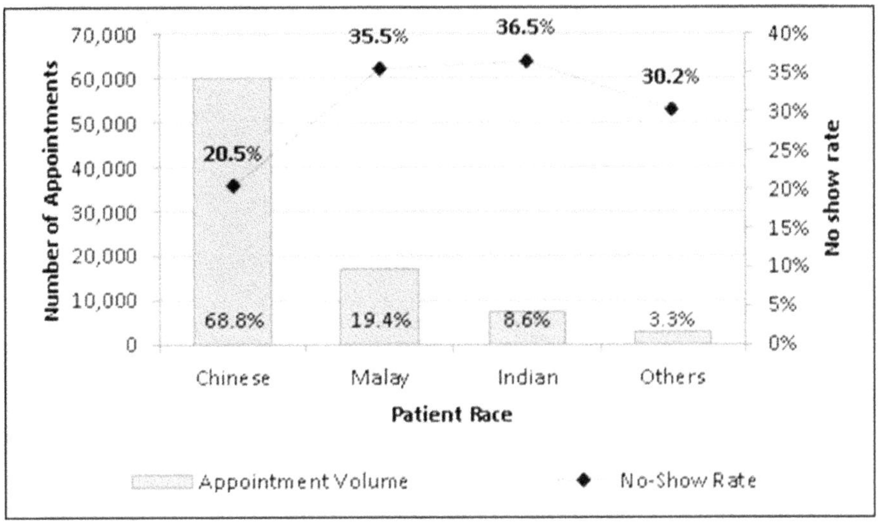

Figure 3. Appointment volume and no-show rate by patient address

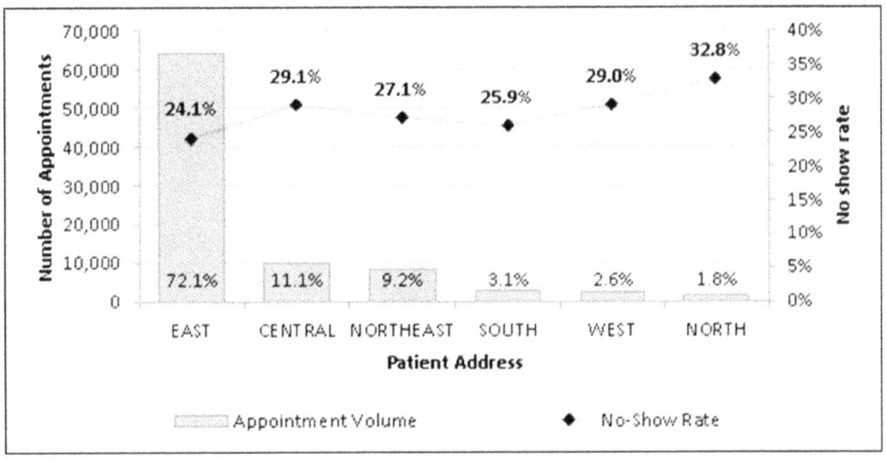

Figure 4. Appointment volume and no-show rate by specialty

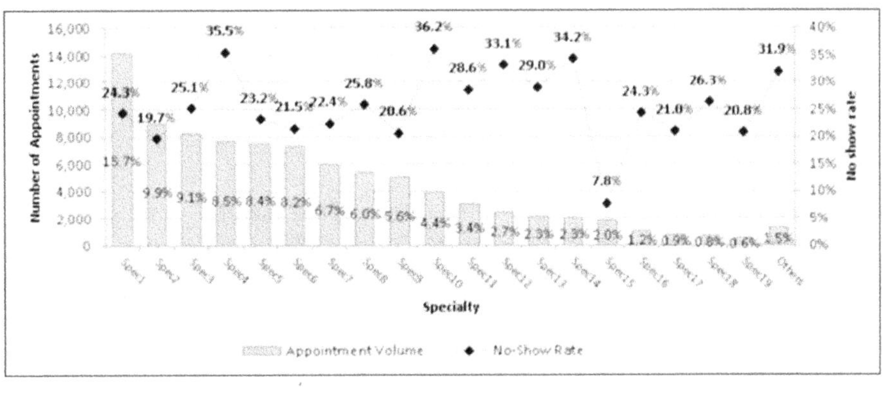

Figure 5. Appointment volume and no-show rate by appointment lead time

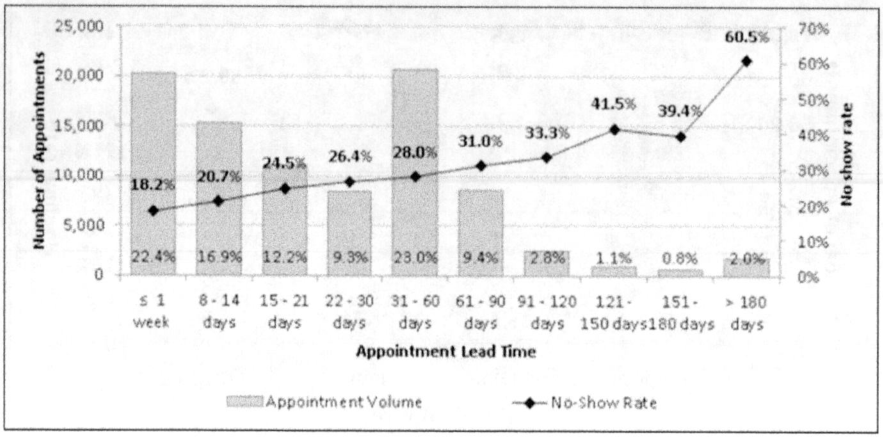

Figure 6. Appointment volume and no-show rate by referral source

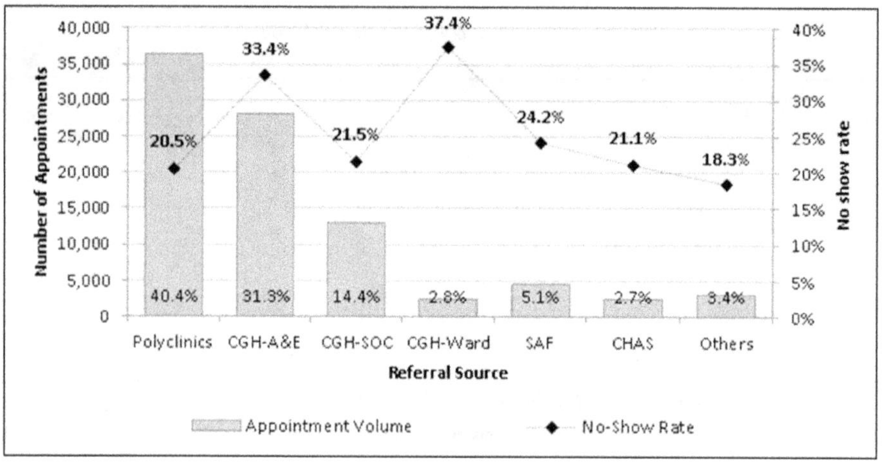

egory was Ancillary Follow-up from Previous Visit Type. It was grouped together with the reference group for the 3rd run. Table 3 shows the final run of Model 1. This model had an area under ROC (AUC) of 72.4%. At a cut-off of 0.25, which is equivalent to no-show rate, the sensitivity and specificity were 63.9% and 69.3% respectively. Applying the model to the validation data, the sensitivity and specificity were 68.8% and 64.2% respectively.

Model 2

Table 4 shows the method of deriving the weighted scores using the odds ratio generated by Model 1. The smallest Odds Ratio (OR) was found to be 1.140. The weighted score of each factor was obtained by dividing the OR by 1.140. Finally, these scores were assigned into individual variables in the original data to obtain the predictive score for each appointment. For example, a new appointment booked for a

Figure 7. Appointment volume and no-show rate by previous appointment visit type

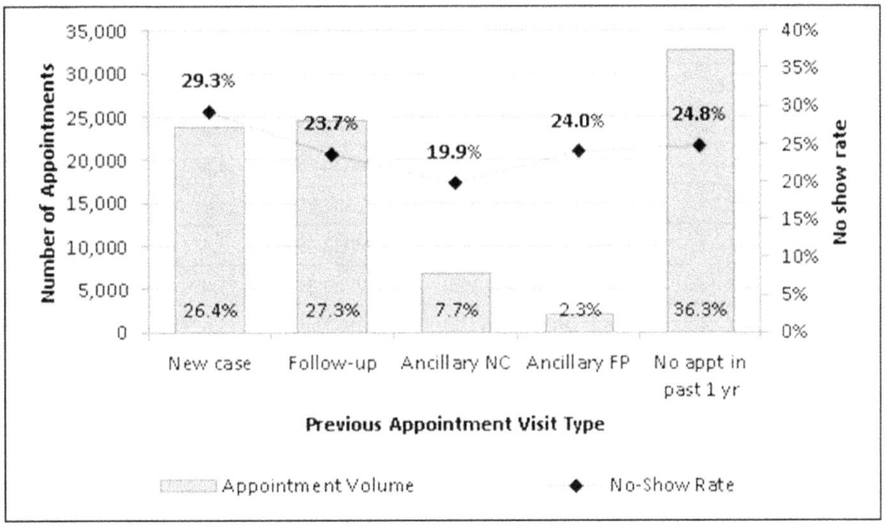

Figure 8. Appointment volume and no-show rate by previous appointment visit status

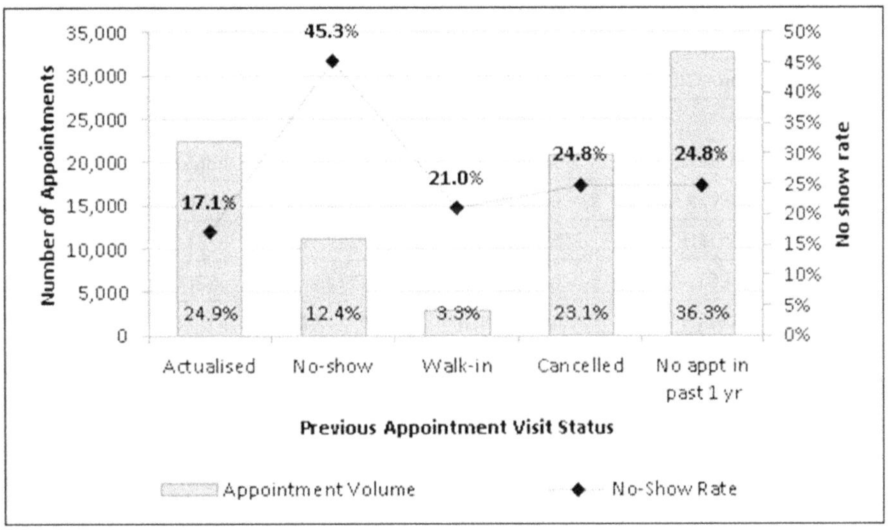

45 year old (1), Malay (2) staying at the eastern zone (0) who was referred from Polyclinic (1) to see a doctor at Specialty 4 (6), was given a slot 2 weeks later (1) and found to have a previous followed-up (1) appointment actualized (0) in any specialty, had a predictive score of 12 (1+ 2 + 0+ 1 + 6 + 1 + 1 + 0).

The derived predictive score had a range of 1 to 23 (Figure 9). It was observed that Scores 1, 2, 22 and 23 had low appointment volumes at less than 0.1% each. As having small population size is not representative of a group, Scores 1 and 2 were grouped together with Score 3 while Scores 22 and 23 were grouped with Score 21.

Table 1. Bivariate analysis

S/N	Variables		Total	Actualised	No-show	No-show%	X^2 p-value
		Total	90,199	67,387	22,812	25.3%	
1	Gender	M	50,703 (56.2%)	37,424 (55.5%)	13,279 (58.2%)	26.2%	p < 0.01
		F	39,496 (43.8%)	29,963 (44.5%)	9,533 (41.8%)	24.1%	
2	Age (years old)	<25	14,964 (16.6%)	10,716 (15.9%)	4,248 (18.6%)	28.4%	p<0.01
		25-34	9,224 (10.2%)	5,799 (8.6%)	3,425 (15.0%)	37.1%	
		35-44	9,286 (10.3%)	6,227 (9.2%)	3,059 (13.4%)	32.9%	
		45-54	14,511 (16.1%)	10,818 (16.1%)	3,693 (16.2%)	25.4%	
		55-64	18,322 (20.3%)	14,489 (21.5%)	3,833 (16.8%)	20.9%	
		65-74	13,144 (14.6%)	10,879 (16.1%)	2,265 (9.9%)	17.2%	
		>=75	10,748 (11.9%)	8,459 (12.6%)	2,289 (10.0%)	21.3%	
3	Race	Chinese	60,242 (68.8%)	47,920 (73.0%)	12,322 (56.1%)	20.5%	p < 0.01
		Malay	16,960 (19.4%)	10,939 (16.7%)	6,021 (27.4%)	35.5%	
		Indian	7,510 (8.6%)	4,766 (7.3%)	2,744 (12.5%)	36.5%	
		Others	2,859 (3.3%)	1,996 (3.0%)	863 (3.9%)	30.2%	
		Missing data	2,628	1,766	862		
4	Nationality	SG	85,845 (95.2%)	64,347 (95.5%)	21,498 (94.2%)	25.0%	p < 0.01
		non-SG	4,354 (4.8%)	3,040 (4.5%)	1,314 (5.8%)	25.3%	
5	Patient Address	EAST	64,279 (72.1%)	48,790 (73.3%)	15,489 (68.8%)	24.1%	p < 0.01
		NORTHEAST	9,919 (11.1%)	7,034 (10.6%)	2,885 (12.8%)	29.1%	
		CENTRAL	8,193 (9.2%)	5,973 (9.0%)	2,220 (9.9%)	27.1%	
		SOUTH	2,792 (3.1%)	2,068 (3.1%)	724 (3.2%)	25.9%	
		WEST	2,321 (2.6%)	1,647 (2.5%)	674 (3.0%)	29.0%	
		NORTH	1,624 (1.8%)	1,091 (1.6%)	533 (2.4%)	32.8%	
		Missing data	1,071	784	287		
6	Force book	Yes	2,550 (2.8%)	2,098 (3.1%)	452 (2.0%)	17.7%	p < 0.01
		No	87,649 (97.2%)	65,289 (96.9%)	22,360 (98.0%)	25.5%	
7	Overbook	Yes	3,565 (4.0%)	2,709 (4.0%)	856 (3.8%)	24.0%	0.038
		No	86,634 (96.0%)	64,678 (96.0%)	21,956 (96.2%)	25.3%	

continues on following page

Table 1. Continued

S/N	Variables		Total	Actualised	No-show	No-show%	X^2 p-value
8	Specialty	Specialty 1	14,154 (15.7%)	10,710 (15.9%)	3,444 (15.1%)	24.3%	p<0.01
		Specialty 2	8,965 (9.9%)	7,203 (10.7%)	1,762 (7.7%)	19.7%	
		Specialty 3	8,236 (9.1%)	6,167 (9.2%)	2,069 (9.1%)	25.1%	
		Specialty 4	7,694 (8.5%)	4,961 (7.4%)	2,733 (12.0%)	35.5%	
		Specialty 5	7,550 (8.4%)	5,802 (8.6%)	1,748 (7.7%)	23.2%	
		Specialty 6	7,353 (8.2%)	5,770 (8.6%)	1,583 (6.9%)	21.5%	
		Specialty 7	5,999 (6.7%)	4,654 (6.9%)	1,345 (5.9%)	22.4%	
		Specialty 8	5,434 (6.0%)	4,032 (6.0%)	1,402 (6.1%)	25.8%	
		Specialty 9	5,078 (5.6%)	4,031 (6.0%)	1,047 (4.6%)	20.6%	
		Specialty 10	3,931 (4.4%)	2,509 (3.7%)	1,422 (6.2%)	36.2%	
		Specialty 11	3,045 (3.4%)	2,175 (3.2%)	870 (3.8%)	28.6%	
		Specialty 12	2,434 (2.7%)	1,628 (2.4%)	806 (3.5%)	33.1%	
		Specialty 13	2,088 (2.3%)	1,482 (2.2%)	606 (2.7%)	29.0%	
		Specialty 14	2,037 (2.3%)	1,340 (2.0%)	697 (3.1%)	34.2%	
		Specialty 15	1,809 (2.0%)	1,668 (2.5%)	141 (0.6%)	7.8%	
		Specialty 16	1,043 (1.2%)	790 (1.2%)	253 (1.1%)	24.3%	
		Specialty 17	796 (0.9%)	629 (0.9%)	167 (0.7%)	21.0%	
		Specialty 18	691 (0.8%)	509 (0.8%)	182 (0.8%)	26.3%	
		Specialty 19	530 (0.6%)	420 (0.6%)	110 (0.5%)	20.8%	
		Others	1,332 (1.5%)	907 (1.3%)	425 (1.9%)	31.9%	
9	Appointment Lead Time	≤ 1 week	20,215 (22.4%)	16,543 (24.5%)	3,672 (16.1%)	18.2%	p < 0.01
		8 - 14 days	15,273 (16.9%)	12,115 (18.0%)	3,158 (13.8%)	20.7%	
		15 - 21 days	11,035 (12.2%)	8,326 (12.4%)	2,709 (11.9%)	24.5%	
		22 - 30 days	8,424 (9.3%)	6,198 (9.2%)	2,226 (9.8%)	26.4%	
		31 - 60 days	20,711 (23.0%)	14,921 (22.1%)	5,790 (25.4%)	28.0%	
		61 - 90 days	8,501 (9.4%)	5,863 (8.7%)	2,638 (11.6%)	31.0%	
		91 - 120 days	2,552 (2.8%)	1,702 (2.5%)	850 (3.7%)	33.3%	
		121 - 150 days	1,019 (1.1%)	596 (0.9%)	423 (1.9%)	41.5%	
		151 - 180 days	703 (0.8%)	426 (0.6%)	277 (1.2%)	39.4%	
		> 180 days	1,766 (2.0%)	697 (1.0%)	1,069 (4.7%)	60.5%	

continues on following page

Table 1. Continued

S/N	Variables		Total	Actualised	No-show	No-show%	X^2 p-value
10	Appointment Month	1	7,497 (8.3%)	5,625 (8.3%)	1,872 (8.2%)	25.0%	0.062
		2	6,830 (7.6%)	5,055 (7.5%)	1,775 (7.8%)	26.0%	
		3	7,368 (8.2%)	5,574 (8.3%)	1,794 (7.9%)	24.3%	
		4	7,303 (8.1%)	5,552 (8.2%)	1,751 (7.7%)	24.0%	
		5	7,349 (8.1%)	5,486 (8.1%)	1,863 (8.2%)	25.4%	
		6	7,564 (8.4%)	5,679 (8.4%)	1,885 (8.3%)	24.9%	
		7	6,904 (7.7%)	5,159 (7.7%)	1,745 (7.6%)	25.3%	
		8	8,650 (9.6%)	6,399 (9.5%)	2,251 (9.9%)	26.0%	
		9	7,585 (8.4%)	5,630 (8.4%)	1,955 (8.6%)	25.8%	
		10	7,999 (8.9%)	5,965 (8.9%)	2,034 (8.9%)	25.4%	
		11	8,053 (8.9%)	6,020 (8.9%)	2,033 (8.9%)	25.2%	
		12	7,097 (7.9%)	5,243 (7.8%)	1,854 (8.1%)	26.1%	
11	Appointment Day of Week	Mon	17,898 (19.8%)	13,181 (19.6%)	4,717 (20.7%)	26.4%	$p < 0.01$
		Tue	19,360 (21.5%)	14,614 (21.7%)	4,746 (20.8%)	24.5%	
		Wed	18,927 (21.0%)	13,880 (20.6%)	5,047 (22.1%)	26.7%	
		Thu	18,925 (21.0%)	14,201 (21.1%)	4,724 (20.7%)	25.0%	
		Fri	14,963 (16.6%)	11,416 (16.9%)	3,547 (15.5%)	23.7%	
		Sat	126	95 (0.0%)	31 (0.0%)	0.0%	
12	Was preceding day of appointment a public holiday?	No	88,109 (97.7%)	65,881 (97.8%)	22,228 (97.4%)	25.2%	0.003
		Yes	2,090 (2.3%)	1,506 (2.2%)	584 (2.6%)	27.9%	
13	Was preceding day of appointment a work day?	No	19,988 (22.2%)	14,687 (21.8%)	5,301 (23.2%)	26.5%	$p < 0.01$
		Yes	70,211 (77.8%)	52,700 (78.2%)	17,511 (76.8%)	24.9%	
14	Was day of appointment a school holiday?	No	80,174 (88.9%)	59,829 (88.8%)	20,345 (89.2%)	25.4%	0.049
		Yes	10,025 (11.1%)	7,558 (11.2%)	2,467 (10.8%)	24.6%	
15	Referral Source	Polyclinics	36,446 (40.4%)	28,979 (43.0%)	7,467 (32.7%)	20.5%	$p < 0.01$
		A&E	28,192 (31.3%)	18,764 (27.8%)	9,428 (41.3%)	33.4%	
		SOC	12,978 (14.4%)	10,187 (15.1%)	2,791 (12.2%)	21.5%	
		Ward	2,556 (2.8%)	1,601 (2.4%)	955 (4.2%)	37.4%	
		SAF	4,579 (5.1%)	3,473 (5.2%)	1,106 (4.8%)	24.2%	
		CHAS	2,395 (2.7%)	1,889 (2.8%)	506 (2.2%)	21.1%	
		Others	3,053 (3.4%)	2,494 (3.7%)	559 (2.5%)	18.3%	
16	Previous Visit Type	New case	23,812 (26.4%)	16,825 (25.0%)	6,987 (30.6%)	29.3%	$p < 0.01$
		Follow-up	24,611 (27.3%)	18,779 (27.9%)	5,832 (25.6%)	23.7%	
		Ancillary NC	6,947 (7.7%)	5,568 (8.3%)	1,379 (6.0%)	19.9%	
		Ancillary FP	2,074 (2.3%)	1,576 (2.3%)	498 (2.2%)	24.0%	
		No appointment in past 1 yr	32,755 (36.3%)	24,639 (36.6%)	8,116 (35.6%)	24.8%	

continues on following page

Table 1. Continued

S/N	Variables		Total	Actualised	No-show	No-show%	X^2 p-value
17	Previous Visit Status	Actualised	22,456 (24.9%)	18,615 (27.6%)	3,841 (16.8%)	17.1%	$p < 0.01$
		No-show	11,200 (12.4%)	6,125 (9.1%)	5,075 (22.2%)	45.3%	
		Walk-in	2,966 (3.3%)	2,342 (3.5%)	624 (2.7%)	21.0%	
		Cancelled	20,822 (23.1%)	15,666 (23.2%)	5,156 (22.6%)	24.8%	
		No appointment in past 1 yr	32,755 (36.3%)	24,639 (36.6%)	8,116 (35.6%)	24.8%	

Scores of 1 to 9 had higher proportions of actualized appointments than no shows while scores of 10 to 23 had higher proportions of no-shows than actualized appointments (Figure 10). Using the predictive score as the predictor, the logistic regression model was generated as shown in Table 5. The AUC was 70.7%.

Model 3

For ease of use, the 23 predictive scores were stratified into 5 risk groups. Considerations for the groupings were guided by the following factors: whether the percentage of no-shows was higher than actualized; statistical significant level; OR of the scores; and, population size of each group.

The first distinctive 'cut' was between Score 9 and Score 10 as illustrated in Figure 10. Next, within Scores 1 to 9, the OR were closer for Scores 1 to 7 (up to 1.35) while Scores 8 to 9 were closer (5.66 to 8.31). The population sizes for Scores 1 to 7 and Scores 8 to 9 were also the best evenly distributed with 20% and 34% respectively. Within Scores 10-23, the first distinctive 'cut' was between 13 and 14 for 2 reasons. Their ORs were vastly different at 31.39 and 44.85. Although there were vastly different ORs between Scores 17 to 23, Scores 14-23 represented only 6.8% of the population leaving 39.6% population for Scores 10-13. Thus the next cut was between 11 and 12.

Finally, Table 6 showed the 5 risk groups, namely, Extremely Low Risk, Low Risk, Medium Risk, High Risk and Extremely High Risk which is the predictive scoring tool. The AUC of the scoring tool was 69.8%. The scoring tool was validated using the other 50% of the data (Table 7). The validation data achieved an AUC of 69.7%.

The scoring tool was tested using the January to December, 2017 data set (Table 7). The results showed that the percentage of no-shows for test data remained similar to the model building data. The test data achieved an AUC of 69.7% which showed that the model was robust.

Overbooking Strategy and Simulation Model

The demand, capacity and no-show rate differ across various specialties. Therefore, the DES model evaluated one specialty at a time. The top two highest volume specialties were selected for the simulation as the improvement in their lead times contribute most to the overall CGH lead time improvement.

Table 2. Multi-collinearity test among the significant factors in the model

Model		Unstandardized Coefficients		Standardized Coefficients	t	Sig.	Collinearity Statistics	
		B	Std. Error	Beta			Tolerance	VIF
1	(Constant)	.120	.007		16.294	.000		
	AgeCat	-.023	.001	-.105	-30.503	.000	.922	1.084
	RaceCat	.067	.002	.121	36.234	.000	.988	1.013
	ClusterCat	.010	.001	.026	7.807	.000	.959	1.043
	VisitSpecCat	.001	.000	.014	4.084	.000	.952	1.051
	LeadTimeCat	.032	.001	.158	47.379	0.000	.978	1.023
	RS_Cat	-.003	.001	-.011	-3.126	.002	.932	1.073
	PrevVisitTypeCat	-.012	.001	-.045	-10.401	.000	.583	1.715
	PrevVisitStatusCat	.009	.001	.033	7.642	.000	.571	1.751
a. Dependent Variable: NoShow								

Table 3. Model 1, third run

		B	S.E.	Sig.	Odds Ratio	95% C.I.for OR	
						Lower	Upper
Previous Visit Status	Actualised	Ref					
	No-show	1.202	.042	.000	3.327	3.064	3.613
	Walk-in	.512	.080	.000	1.668	1.426	1.952
	Cancelled	.344	.040	.000	1.410	1.303	1.526
	No appt in preceding 1 yr	.664	.056	.000	1.943	1.740	2.170
Appointment Lead Time	≤ 1 week	Ref					
	8 - 14 days	.176	.043	.000	1.192	1.096	1.296
	15 - 21 days	.543	.046	.000	1.721	1.573	1.883
	22 - 30 days	.760	.050	.000	2.138	1.939	2.359
	31 - 60 days	.974	.042	.000	2.648	2.441	2.873
	61 - 90 days	1.106	.053	.000	3.023	2.727	3.352
	91 - 120 days	1.538	.077	.000	4.654	4.000	5.416
	121 - 150 days	1.846	.106	.000	6.336	5.148	7.800
	151 - 180 days	1.771	.125	.000	5.879	4.606	7.504
	> 180 days	2.400	.085	.000	11.024	9.325	13.032
Referral Source	Polyclinics	.234	.064	.000	1.263	1.114	1.433
	CGH-A&E	.941	.065	.000	2.564	2.258	2.911
	CGH-SOC	.440	.072	.000	1.553	1.348	1.789
	CGH-Ward	.977	.091	.000	2.657	2.221	3.179
	SAF	Ref					
	CHAS	.423	.097	.000	1.526	1.262	1.845
	Others	.284	.097	.004	1.328	1.097	1.607

continues on following page

Table 3. Continued

		B	S.E.	Sig.	Odds Ratio	95% C.I.for OR	
						Lower	Upper
Race	Chinese	Ref					
	Malay	.558	.030	.000	1.746	1.648	1.850
	Indian	.603	.040	.000	1.828	1.690	1.976
	Others	.386	.063	.000	1.471	1.300	1.665
Age (years old)	<25	.610	.049	.000	1.841	1.672	2.026
	25-34	.845	.051	.000	2.327	2.108	2.570
	35-44	.719	.051	.000	2.053	1.859	2.268
	45-54	.381	.047	.000	1.464	1.336	1.605
	55-64	.161	.045	.000	1.175	1.075	1.284
	65-74	Ref					
	>=75	.290	.051	.000	1.337	1.210	1.477
Speciality	Specialty 1	.570	.147	.000	1.768	1.325	2.359
	Specialty 2	.810	.149	.000	2.249	1.680	3.009
	Specialty 3	.997	.148	.000	2.710	2.028	3.622
	Specialty 4	1.846	.147	.000	6.335	4.749	8.453
	Specialty 5	1.204	.148	.000	3.333	2.493	4.457
	Specialty 6	.756	.150	.000	2.130	1.588	2.857
	Specialty 7	.903	.150	.000	2.468	1.839	3.311
	Specialty 8	.971	.150	.000	2.640	1.967	3.543
	Specialty 9	.883	.153	.000	2.419	1.791	3.267
	Specialty 10	1.216	.154	.000	3.375	2.497	4.563
	Specialty 11	1.375	.155	.000	3.955	2.918	5.361
	Specialty 12	1.297	.159	.000	3.659	2.677	5.000
	Specialty 13	1.026	.162	.000	2.789	2.031	3.829
	Specialty 14	1.189	.161	.000	3.283	2.395	4.499
	Specialty 15	Ref					
	Specialty 16	1.141	.181	.000	3.129	2.196	4.457
	Specialty 17	1.116	.196	.000	3.052	2.078	4.482
	Specialty 18	1.148	.195	.000	3.152	2.152	4.614
	Specialty 19	.791	.213	.000	2.205	1.453	3.347
	Others	1.065	.174	.000	2.900	2.063	4.077
Patient Address	EAST	Ref					
	NORTHEAST	.260	.037	.000	1.297	1.205	1.396
	CENTRAL	.131	.041	.002	1.140	1.051	1.236
	SOUTH	.203	.068	.003	1.225	1.072	1.400
	WEST	.207	.075	.006	1.230	1.061	1.425
	NORTH	.266	.084	.002	1.305	1.107	1.539

continues on following page

Table 3. Continued

		B	S.E.	Sig.	Odds Ratio	95% C.I.for OR	
						Lower	Upper
Previous Visit Type	New case	.333	.054	.000	1.396	1.256	1.551
	Follow-up	.253	.052	.000	1.288	1.163	1.426
	Ancillary Visit	Ref					
Constant		-4.641	.170	0.000	.010	0	0

Table 4. Deriving the weighted scores

		Sig.	Odds Ratio	OR/ min(OR)
Previous Visit Status	Actualised	Ref		0
	No-show	.000	3.327	3
	Walk-in	.000	1.668	1
	Cancelled	.000	1.410	1
	No appt in past 1 yr	.000	1.943	2
Appointment Lead Time	≤ 1 week	. Ref		0
	8 - 14 days	.000	1.192	1
	15 - 21 days	.000	1.721	2
	22 - 30 days	.000	2.138	2
	31 - 60 days	.000	2.648	2
	61 - 90 days	.000	3.023	3
	91 - 120 days	.000	4.654	4
	121 - 150 days	.000	6.336	6
	151 - 180 days	.000	5.879	5
	> 180 days	.000	11.024	10
Referral Source	Polyclinics	.000	1.263	1
	A&E	.000	2.564	2
	SOC	.000	1.553	1
	Ward	.000	2.657	2
	SAF	. Ref		0
	CHAS	.000	1.526	1
	Others	.004	1.328	1
Race	Chinese	. Ref		0
	Malay	.000	1.746	2
	Indian	.000	1.828	2
	Others	.000	1.471	1
Age (years old)	<25	.000	1.841	2
	25-34	.000	2.327	2
	35-44	.000	2.053	2

continues on following page

Table 4. Continued

		Sig.	Odds Ratio	OR/ min(OR)
	45-54	.000	1.464	1
	55-64	.000	1.175	1
	65-74	. Ref		0
	>=75	.000	1.337	1
Speciality	Specialty 1	.000	1.768	2
	Specialty 2	.000	2.249	2
	Specialty 3	.000	2.710	2
	Specialty 4	.000	6.335	6
	Specialty 5	.000	3.333	3
	Specialty 6	.000	2.130	2
	Specialty 7	.000	2.468	2
	Specialty 8	.000	2.640	2
	Specialty 9	.000	2.419	2
	Specialty 10	.000	3.375	3
	Specialty 11	.000	3.955	3
	Specialty 12	.000	3.659	3
	Specialty 13	.000	2.789	2
	Specialty 14	.000	3.283	3
	Specialty 15	. Ref		0
	Specialty 16	.000	3.129	3
	Specialty 17	.000	3.052	3
	Specialty 18	.000	3.152	3
	Specialty 19	.000	2.205	2
	Others	.000	2.900	3
Patient Address	EAST	Ref		0
	NORTHEAST	.000	1.297	1
	CENTRAL	.002	1.140	1
	SOUTH	.003	1.225	1
	WEST	.006	1.230	1
	NORTH	.002	1.305	1
Previous Visit Type	New case	.000	1.396	1
	Follow-up	.000	1.288	1
	Ancillary Visit	Ref		0

Table 5. Logistic regression model using predictive score

Predictive Score	# Appts	# Accumulative Appts	B	S.E.	Sig.	Odds Ratio	95% C.I.for OR	
							Lower	Upper
1-3	95 (0.3%)	139 (0.4%)	Ref					
4	311 (0.7%)	450 (1.1%)	0.303	.587	.605	1.35	0.429	4.276
5	1013 (2.3%)	1463 (3.5%)	1.103	.520	.034	3.01	1.087	8.348
6	2461 (5.7%)	3924 (9.2%)	1.285	.512	.012	3.61	1.325	9.855
7	4725 (10.9%)	8649 (20.0%)	1.362	.510	.008	3.90	1.438	10.602
8	7142 (16.5%)	15791 (36.5%)	1.733	.508	.001	5.66	2.088	15.321
9	7409 (17.1%)	23200 (53.6%)	2.118	.508	.000	8.31	3.070	22.503
10	6642 (15.3%)	29842 (68.9%)	2.412	.508	.000	11.16	4.120	30.201
11	4924 (11.4%)	34766 (80.3%)	2.836	.508	.000	17.04	6.293	46.142
12	3486 (8.0%)	38252 (88.3%)	3.048	.509	.000	21.07	7.778	57.098
13	2102 (4.8%)	40354 (93.2%)	3.447	.509	.000	31.39	11.572	85.175
14	1190 (2.7%)	41544 (95.9%)	3.803	.511	.000	44.85	16.481	122.025
15	687 (1.6%)	42231 (97.5%)	3.911	.513	.000	49.95	18.267	136.610
16	383 (0.9%)	42614 (98.4%)	3.883	.518	.000	48.58	17.606	134.062
17	246 (0.6%)	42860 (98.9%)	3.864	.524	.000	47.65	17.074	132.961
18	178 (0.4%)	43038 (99.3%)	4.272	.532	.000	71.64	25.246	203.318
19	126 (0.3%)	43164 (99.6%)	4.177	.541	.000	65.15	22.561	188.108
20	105 (0.2%)	43269 (99.9%)	5.163	.572	.000	174.71	56.900	536.414
21-23	65 (0.2%)	43334 (100.1%)	5.205	.580	.000	182.25	58.473	568.040

Table 6. The scoring tool

Scoring Algorithm	Predictive Score	% of population	Accumulation %	B	S.E.	Sig.	Odds Ratio	95% C.I.for OR	
								Lower	Upper
Extremely low risk	1 - 7	20.0%	20.0%	Ref					
Low risk	8 - 9	33.6%	53.6%	.669	.043	.000	1.952	**1.795**	**2.122**
Medium risk	10 - 11	26.7%	80.3%	1.330	.042	.000	3.779	3.481	4.103
High risk	12 - 13	12.9%	93.2%	1.929	.046	.000	6.880	6.292	7.521
Extremely high risk	14 - 23	6.9%	100.1%	2.688	.052	.000	14.697	13.266	16.282

Table 7. Validating and testing of scoring tool

Scoring Algorithm	Predictive Score	Model Building Data (50% of 2016)		Model Validation Data (50% of 2016)		Model Testing Data (2017)	
		% No show	% of population	% No show	% of population	% No show	% of population
Extremely low risk	1 - 7	9.6%	19.9%	10.1%	20.4%	10.7%	21.7%
Low risk	8 - 9	17.1%	33.6%	17.2%	33.6%	18.1%	34.9%
Medium risk	10 - 11	28.5%	26.7%	29.1%	26.2%	30.5%	25.1%
High risk	12 - 13	42.1%	12.9%	43.3%	12.8%	45.6%	11.7%
Extremely high risk	14 - 23	60.8%	6.9%	59.8%	7.0%	60.8%	6.5%

Figure 9. Histogram of predictive scores

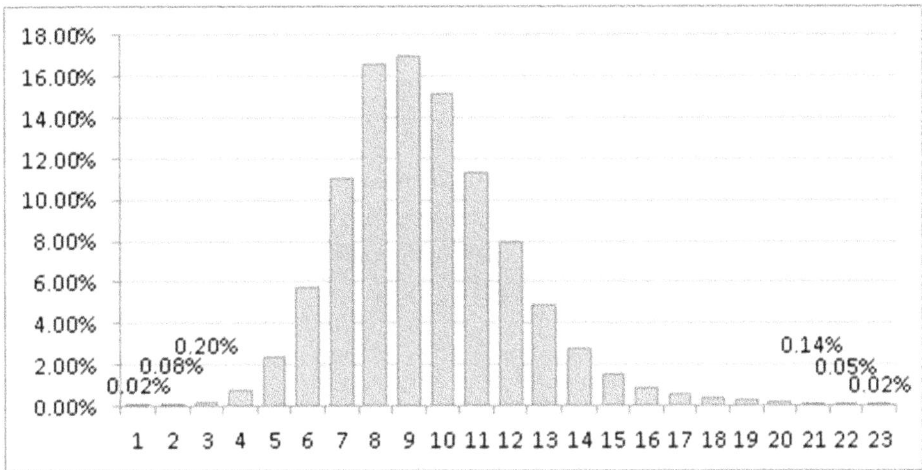

Figure 10. Distribution of predictive scores by visit status

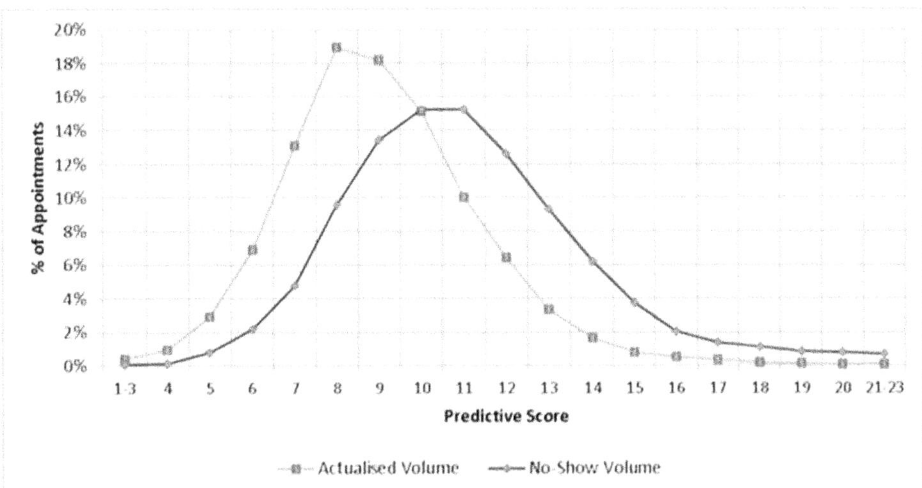

Figure 11 shows the DES model that simulated the scheduling process of appointment making in the 2 top volume specialties. The scheduler logic of Specialty 1 was duplicated in Specialty 2. Each specialty had its own set of inputs (e.g arrival rate and slot capacities). The scheduler searched for the earliest available appointment and if a slot was found, it dynamically created a link from the arrival to the server.

Specialty 1

Specialty 1 had a no-show rate of 24.3%. Table 8 listed the average daily demand of appointments and capacities. The overall what-if capacity was increased due to added capacity from no-shows and predictive model accuracy. For example, on Monday, the current 30 slots could potentially be allocated with 34 appointments instead of the current 30 appointments.

The model was verified against the actual lead times found in the January through October, 2017 data set (Table 9). With the increased capacity recommended by the predictive tool, the median lead time and percentage of lead time more than 60 days could potentially improve by 49% from 56 days to 28.5 days and 20% from 47% to 38% respectively.

Specialty 2

Table 10 listed the average daily demand of appointments and capacities of Specialty 2 which had a no-show rate of 19.7%. Using the predictive tool and artificially increase the capacity, the median lead time and percentage of lead time more than 60 days can potentially improve by 33% from 64 days to 42.7 days and 28% from 53% to 38% respectively.

Figure 11. The discrete event simulation model

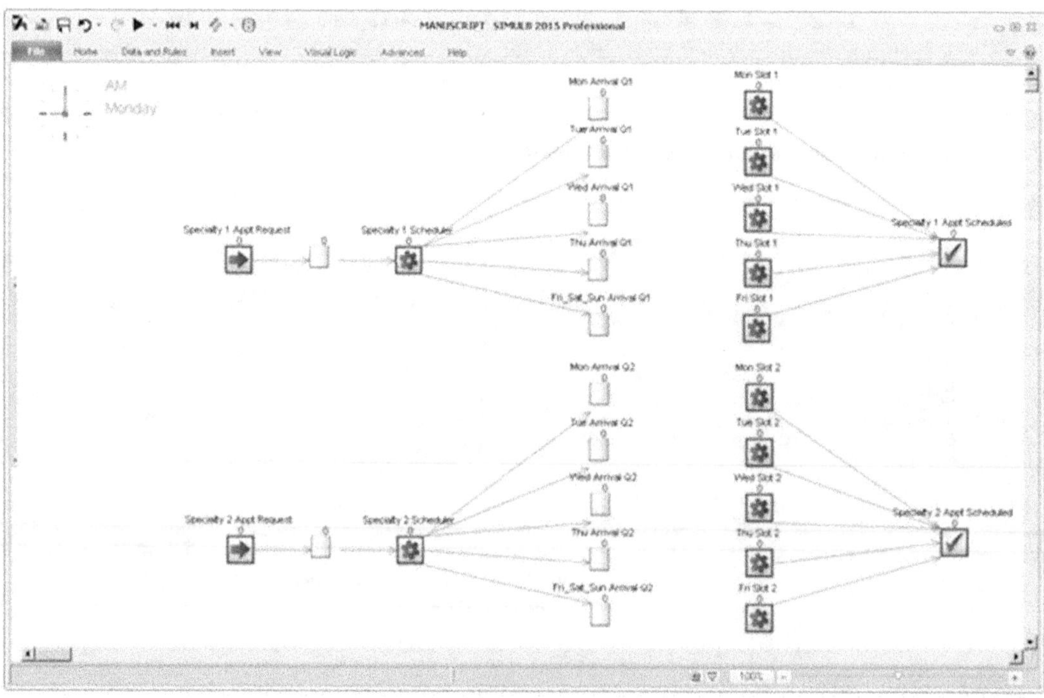

Table 8. Simulation inputs of Specialty 1

	Average Demand	Baseline Capacity	Capacity of what-if predictive tool is used
Monday	54.9	30	34
Tuesday	50.0	52	60
Wednesday	46.7	40	46
Thursday	46.2	51	59
Friday	44.5	15	17
Saturday	23.3		
Sunday	17.8		
Total	283.3	188	216

Table 9. Simulated results - lead time of Specialty 1

Scenario	Actual on Jan-Oct2017	Baseline Simulation	What-if Simulation	Absolute Improvement	Improvement %
Median	59	56.1	28.5	27.5	49%
Lead Time > 60 days	49.4%	47%	38%	10%	20%

Table 10. Simulation inputs of Specialty 2

	Average Demand	Baseline Capacity	Capacity of what-if predictive tool is used
Monday	41.5	26	29
Tuesday	41.5	32	36
Wednesday	38.7	33	37
Thursday	39.8	27	30
Friday	34.3	29	32
Saturday	15.2		
Sunday	6.4		
Total	217.3	147.0	164.0

Table 11. Simulated results - lead time of Specialty 2

Scenario	Actual on Jan-Jun2017	Baseline Simulation	What-if Simulation	Absolute Improvement	Improvement %
Median	66	64.0	42.7	21.3	33%
Lead Time > 60 days	54.6%	53%	38%	15%	28%

DISCUSSION

At 26% no-show, CGH is similar to other countries in Asia (25.1%) and close to the average no-show rates of all countries (23%) (Dantas et al., 2018). All 8 predictors of no-shows in this chapter were similarly found to be statistically-significant factors in most other studies that were included in the systematic review (Dantas et al., 2018). Payment Type, visit type and provider type were significant factors in other studies but less relevant to CGH as this study focused on only subsidized new appointments that are allocated to a rotating team of doctors. Moreover, other significant factors used in other studies such as clinical diagnosis, substance abuse and medical history were excluded in the predictive model as data for these factors may not be available for new patients. The predictive tool allows ease of operations and lower cost by using only self-contained routine administrative data and basic patient demographics data which can be gathered from the new patients by the call center during appointment booking.

The predictive model in this chapter benefitted from large sample sizes of real world appointments drawn from the hospital database. The large data set allowed for sufficient samples to be divided into data sets for training, testing and validation necessary for predictive model. The strength of the model is in the use of real world appointments data for model development unlike Samorani et al. (2011) which only used simulated data.

The authors demonstrated that it is feasible to use logistic regression to develop a risk scoring algorithm to risk stratify patients by their likelihood of no-show and develop a prediction model of good performance which is efficient for operations. Learning from best practices reported by other authors, the current study's authors chose the most common methodology, MLR, to predict no-shows for risk-free implementation operationally at hospital. This approach has been in use since 1981 and is widely accepted. Unlike other MLR models where the result was left as probability of no-shows and computation left as a black box to the users, the authors stratified the predicted no-shows by risk level. The weighted score matrix allowed users and stakeholders to understand the logic of the prediction and apply it in real-world settings.

In most studies, the overbooking strategy has been incorporated into appointment scheduling process (Alaeddini et al., 2011; Muthuraman & Lawley, 2008; Samorani & LaGanga, 2011, 2015; Zeng et al., 2010). That means that no-show prediction is applied during each appointment request. This ultimately requires additional modification to the booking process in OAS. Moreover, it is uncertain that the added step to predict no-shows will lengthen the appointment booking turnaround time during multiple concurrent requests. To mitigate this uncertainly and reduce cost to OAS modification, the authors recommend that the overbooking strategy to be applied after a session is fully booked. The script to compute the number of overbook slots using the predictive tool only needs to be run only once after the operating hours. The additional overbooking slots created overnight are also transparent to the call center operators with no change in work process nor cost in training.

In a previous study Chua and Chow (2019), similar to Elvira et al. (2018), developed the no-show predictive scoring tool without evaluating how the lead time could be improved if the tool was used. In this chapter, the authors expanded their work to develop the DES model to evaluate the predictive tool and provide evidence of its value.

CONCLUSION

The authors designed the predictive tool and overbooking strategy with the intention to implement a cost-efficient solution which would require minimal changes to the current workflow to achieve better specialist access to patient care using lead time measurement. This ultimately provides better access to patients, empowering them in a quest for better health care.

It is possible to develop a prediction model to stratify patients according to their risk of no-show for appointments using routinely collected administrative data that is available in the system with good performance parameters. The no-show risk scoring system, which derives the number of overbooking slots dynamically, was evaluated using the DES model and shown that it could improve lead time.

This chapter described an effective approach of integrating predictive modeling to estimate the number of no-shows dynamically on a daily basis to guide overbooking to reduce wastage of clinic resources followed by using DES to examine the effectiveness of the overbooking strategy before implementation in the real-world setting. Direct piloting can be challenging in this setting as the clinic is a complex system and implementation without evaluating the downstream effects beforehand could run the risk of disruption to clinic operations as well as high cost investment in technology enhancements of the appointment booking system to support a strategy that might not be effective.

On the other hand, no-show modelling is not necessary if all patients turned up for their appointments. Systematic review on text messaging (Schwebel & Larimer, 2018) reported that 56 studies used SMS appointment reminder (Schwebel & Larimer, 2018). Among these, 48 studies (86%) successfully reduced the rate of no-shows including increasing the rate of cancellation ahead of time if patients were reminded of the appointments. This suggests that patients should make more effort to remember their appointments. One possible approach would be for patients to use the reminder feature of mobile phone calendars. This would reduce dependence on hospital resources to remind patients.

FUTURE WORK

Until patients are empowered to reduce non-attendance rate to a new low, the no show predictive model continues to be a necessary tool. More work is needed and can use the current project as a starting point. Currently, the authors are working to improve the accuracy of the predictive tool by using new algorithms from R libraries instead of SPSS (Huang & Hanauer, 2014). Then, more overbooking strategies and scheduling strategies can be explored to further improve lead times. For example, the authors can study the optimal appointment time to overbook, optimal allocation of appointment slots, and scheduling multiple appointments on the same day when possible. Finally, the authors can further research the impact of consult wait time resulting from these strategies.

ACKNOWLEDGMENT

The authors would like to express their thanks to the fellow CGH colleagues: Ms. Selina Seah, Chief Operating Officer, Mr. Peter Tay, ex Chief Operating Officer, and Ms. Lee Lian Chin, Assistant Director (Specialist Clinics) for their valuable support provided in this project and granting access to anonymous attendance data, Ms. Vicki Tan, Manager (Specialist Clinics) for her valuable time and effort in sharing the clinic appointment setup to the authors.

This research received no specific grant from any funding agency in the public, commercial, or not-for-profit sectors.

REFERENCES

Agency for Integrated Care. (2016). *Introduction to Home Care*. Singapore. Retrieved from https://www.aic.sg/sites/aicassets/AssetGallery/HCIK_BOOKLET 02_FA-5(Online).pdf

Alaeddini, A., Yang, K., Reddy, C., & Yu, S. (2011). A probabilistic model for predicting the probability of no-show in hospital appointments. *Health Care Management Science*, *14*(2), 146–157. doi:10.100710729-011-9148-9 PMID:21286819

Chua, S. L., & Chow, W. L. (2019). Development of predictive scoring model for risk stratification of no-show at a public hospital specialist outpatient clinic. *Proceedings of Singapore Healthcare*, *28*(2), 96–104. doi:10.1177/2010105818793155

Daggy, J., Lawley, M., Willis, D., Thayer, D., Suelzer, C., DeLaurentis, P.-C., ... Sands, L. (2010). Using no-show modeling to improve clinic performance. *Health Informatics Journal*, *16*(4), 246–259. doi:10.1177/1460458210380521 PMID:21216805

Dantas, L. F., Fleck, J. L., Oliveira, F. L. C., & Hamacher, S. (2018). No-shows in appointment scheduling--a systematic literature review. *Health Policy (Amsterdam)*, *122*(4), 412–421. doi:10.1016/j.healthpol.2018.02.002 PMID:29482948

Department of Statistics Singapore. (2013). Waiting Time Policies in the Health Sector. Retrieved from https://www.singstat.gov.sg/find-data/search-by-theme/population/population-and-population-structure/latest-data

Elvira, C., Ochoa, A., Gonzalvez, J. C., & Mochón, F. (2018). Machine-Learning-Based No Show Prediction in Outpatient Visits. *International Journal of Interactive Multimedia & Artificial Intelligence*, *4*(7), 29–34. doi:10.9781/ijimai.2017.03.004

Glowacka, K. J., Henry, R. M., & May, J. H. (2009). A hybrid data mining/simulation approach for modelling outpatient no-shows in clinic scheduling. *The Journal of the Operational Research Society*, *60*(8), 1056–1068. doi:10.1057/jors.2008.177

Goffman, R. M., Harris, S. L., May, J. H., Milicevic, A. S., Monte, R. J., Myaskovsky, L., ... Vargas, D. L. (2017). Modeling patient no-show history and predicting future outpatient appointment behavior in the veterans health administration. *Military Medicine*, *182*(5–6), e1708–e1714. doi:10.7205/MILMED-D-16-00345 PMID:29087915

Huang, Y., & Hanauer, D. A. (2014). Patient no-show predictive model development using multiple data sources for an effective overbooking approach. *Applied Clinical Informatics*, *5*(3), 836–860. doi:10.4338/ACI-2014-04-RA-0026 PMID:25298821

Ministry of Health Singapore. (2012). MOH 2012 Committee of Supply Speech Healthcare 2020: Improving Accessibility, Quality and Affordability for Tomorrow's Challenges (Part 1 of 2). Retrieved from https://www.moh.gov.sg/news-highlights/details/moh-2012-committee-of-supply-speech-healthcare-2020-improving-accessibility-quality-and-affordability-for-tomorrow-s-challenges-(part-1-of-2)

Ministry of Health Singapore. (2017). SOC Waiting Times. Retrieved from https://www.moh.gov.sg/news-highlights/details/moh-2012-committee-of-supply-speech-healthcare-2020-improving-accessibility-quality-and-affordability-for-tomorrow-s-challenges-(part-1-of-2)

Ministry of Health Singapore. (2018). Admission and Outpatient Attendances. Retrieved from https://www.moh.gov.sg/resources-statistics/singapore-health-facts/admissions-and-outpatient-attendances

Muthuraman, K., & Lawley, M. (2008). A stochastic overbooking model for outpatient clinical scheduling with no-shows. *IIE Transactions*, *40*(9), 820–837. doi:10.1080/07408170802165823

Naiker, U., FitzGerald, G., Dulhunty, J. M., & Rosemann, M. (2018). Time to wait: A systematic review of strategies that affect out-patient waiting times. *Australian Health Review*, *42*(3), 286–293. doi:10.1071/AH16275 PMID:28355525

Samorani, M., & LaGanga, L. (2011). A stochastic programming approach to improve overbooking in clinic appointment scheduling. In *POMS annual meeting proceedings*.

Samorani, M., & LaGanga, L. (2015). Outpatient appointment scheduling given individual day-dependent no-show predictions. *European Journal of Operational Research*, *240*(1), 245–257. doi:10.1016/j.ejor.2014.06.034

Schwebel, F. J., & Larimer, M. E. (2018). Using text message reminders in health care services: A narrative literature review. *Internet Interventions*, *13*, 82–104. doi:10.1016/j.invent.2018.06.002 PMID:30206523

Zeng, B., Turkcan, A., Lin, J., & Lawley, M. (2010). Clinic scheduling models with overbooking for patients with heterogeneous no-show probabilities. *Annals of Operations Research*, *178*(1), 121–144. doi:10.100710479-009-0569-5

ADDITIONAL READING

Brandeau, M. L., Sainfort, F., & Pierskalla, W. P. (2004). *Operations research and health care: a handbook of methods and applications* (Vol. 70). Springer Science & Business Media.

Kahraman, C., & Topcu, Y. I. (2018). *Operations Research Applications in Health Care Management*. Springer. doi:10.1007/978-3-319-65455-3

Ozcan, Y. A. (2017). *Analytics and Decision Support in Health Care Operations Management*. John Wiley & Sons.

KEY TERMS AND DEFINITIONS

Appointment Center Operating Hour: 8.30am to 8pm on Monday to Friday, 8.30am to 12.30pm on Saturday and Sunday. Closed on Public Holidays.

Appointment Lead Time: Duration in days, from an appointment request till appointment date.

CHAS: Community Health Assist Scheme is a scheme by the Ministry of Health that enables Singapore citizens from lower-to-middle income households to receive subsidies for medical and dental care at participant General Practitioner and dental clinic near their home

Outpatient Appointment System: (OAS): OAS is a web-based system to manage outpatient appointments. The system allows administrators to set up the service providers, calendar, appointment slot; call center operators to search for earliest appointment and book appointments; and managers to query and generate reports.

Polyclinics: Subsidized primary care outpatient clinics fulfilled by the government.

Regional Health System (RHS): RHS were set up to strengthen partnerships across care providers in each region: both public and private, and across care settings. Each RHS is anchored by a Public hospital working closely with community hospitals, nursing homes, home care and day rehabilitation providers, as well as polyclinics and private General Practitioners (GPs) within the geographical region. The RHS functions as a coordination platform to organize service providers. It delivers patient-centric care through the integration of services and processes. Such integration helps patients navigate across providers within the same region more easily, enabling them to manage their own care needs (Agency for Integrated Care, 2016).

SAF: Singapore Armed Forces

Specialist Outpatient Clinic (SOC) operating hour: 8.30am to 6pm on Monday to Friday

Visit Status: There 4 types of visit statuses: Actualized, No-Show, Cancelled and Walk-ins. Actualized refers to a patient who attended the scheduled appointments. No-show, similar to non-attendance and missed appointments, refers to a patient who missed the schedule appointment without cancellation notice to the service provider. An appointment can be cancelled by either doctor or patient. Walk-in refers to a patient who is served without appointment.

Visit Type: There are 4 visit types: New Case (NC), Follow-up (FP), Ancillary New Case, and Ancillary Follow-up. The former 2 types required doctor services while the latter 2 types require non-doctor services.

Chapter 8
Deep Learning and Sustainable Telemedicine

Edward T. Chen
University of Massachusetts – Lowell, USA

ABSTRACT

The need for healthcare is increasing on a global scale. The lack of medical professionals available to fill this need has increased interest in deep learning and sustainable telemedicine technologies. Telemedicine has been shown to be financially beneficial to both patients and healthcare facilities, provided that government regulations and insurance companies recognize them as a reimbursable expense. Advancements in cloud computing, deep learning, and telemedicine are creating a global standard for healthcare, and at the same time increasing the need for these services.

INTRODUCTION

The use of telemedicine in the healthcare industry has been around for over a century. Since the introduction of long-distance communication methods such as the radio and the telephone, telemedicine has been used by doctors to assist patients in regions where medical personnel are scarce. As communication technology improved, so did telemedicine. The introduction of the Internet has drastically improved a person's ability to receive medical treatment without visiting a healthcare facility. As of 2016, 47% of the world's population has access to the Internet, which is a 4% increase over the previous year (Taylor, 2016). The growth of Internet capable devices such as desktops, laptops, smartphones, and tablets has drastically increased a person's ability to use telemedicine.

Telemedicine is on the rise as telehealth services are becoming increasingly available to patients across the U.S. FAIR Health, a nonprofit organization, drew on its database of over 25 billion privately billed claim records to develop the FH Healthcare Indicators resource, which evaluates changes in demographics, utilization, diagnoses, procedures and costs. The report showed that from 2011 to 2016, telehealth service use increased substantially, especially in rural areas (960 percent). In comparison, telehealth use grew by 629 percent in urban areas, and by 643 percent nationally. However, more recently urban us-

DOI: 10.4018/978-1-7998-0047-7.ch008

age has grown to match and even surpass rural usage. Between 2015 and 2016, urban areas saw a jump from just over 25 percent to over 45 percent, while rural growth increased from 35 percent in 2015 to just over 40 percent in 2016 (Fair Health, 2018).

Machine learning and artificial intelligence have many exciting applications in the medical field in general. IBM Watson Health program is able to analyze millions of pages of medical information within nanoseconds, and draw conclusions that can be used for diagnosis, comparison and recommendation. The enormous power of supercomputers to search through large volumes of data is combined with analytical and decision-making prowess in machine learning and artificial intelligence technologies (Hoyt, Snider, Thompson, & Mantravadi, 2016). Beyond just dealing with information, though, machine learning and artificial intelligence can also bring new capabilities to patient examination. For example, in radiology, machine learning algorithms can look at radiology scans and other resources to find evidence of outcomes and realities that can guide human decision-makers (Sennaar, 2019a).

There are also other formative examples of the power of machine learning and diagnosis in telemedicine. National Institute of Health provides automated analysis of retinal imaging, which can help detect certain types of sight loss linked to diabetes (Sim, Keane, Tufail, Egan, Aiello, & Silva, 2015). Google also teams up with National Health Service in UK to use Google DeepMind to help spot early signs of eye conditions that human eye care experts might miss at Moorfields Eye Hospital. Specifically, Moorfields is applying DeepMind's algorithms to 1 million anonymous OCT (Optical Coherence Tomography) scans. The aim is to determine whether the algorithms can learn to spot early signs of age-related macular degeneration and sight loss that occurs as a result of diabetes (Shead, 2017). NIH or NHS can save those diagnoses and OCT scan images in their repositories for future research and preventive treatment (Sim et al., 2015; Shead, 2017).

Recently, advancements in machine learning have brought about the creation of deep learning. The use of machine learning and deep learning with decision support tools have significantly improved a medical professional's ability to accurately diagnose and treat patients within a minimal amount of time. Combining deep learning with telemedicine will create opportunities for a vastly larger portion of the population to receive immediate healthcare without needing to enter a medical facility. Doctors will review it and sign on – instead of being only supported by videoconferencing, doctors will also be supported by key assistive technologies that are thinking and learning on their own (Sennaar, 2019b). As mentioned previously, a deep learning program is an decision support tool for physicians to provide effective healthcare services to telemedicine patients. The goal of deep learning technology is not to replace their jobs. According to a report published in the Physician Leadership Journal, physician leaders projected a 18.5% increase in telemedicine jobs in 2018, compared to 2012 (Anonymous, 2018).

The need for healthcare is increasing on a global scale. Telemedicine services have seen an increase in use to reach locations that would otherwise be unable to support the demand for healthcare professionals. Telemedicine has been shown to be financially beneficial to both patients and healthcare facilities, provided that government regulations and insurance companies recognize them as a reimbursable expense. Deep learning applications such as IBM's Watson and Google's DeepMind have paved the way for software programs to integrate with the healthcare industry. This chapter investigates the application of deep learning technology to sustainable telemedicine in the healthcare industry.

DEEP LEARNING

Deep learning is a form of machine learning that is able to learn using data representations, rather than task-specific algorithms. It consists of artificial neural networks that calculate outcomes based on the history of information that it has been provided. Raw data is entered into the system and these neural networks detect patterns and classifications through representation learning (De Cnudde, Martens, & Provost, 2018). The concept of deep learning was initially proposed by G. Hinton and co-authors in 2006, when they added deep neural networks to dimensionality reduction (Zhong, Wang, Ling, & Dong, 2016). Although deep learning still uses advanced algorithms like machine learning, deep learning is also capable of processing information from images, recognizing objects, and understanding natural language. The success of this implementation to machine learning has increased the interest in artificial intelligence and its capabilities, which is assisting in the growth of this technology (Khanna, Sattar, & Hansen, 2013).

Benefits of Deep Learning in the Healthcare Industry

The healthcare industry is one sector that has significantly benefitted from the use of deep learning and will continue to benefit as technology evolves. Machine learning depends on big data in order to operate effectively. Big data consists of large datasets that are complex, and thus require a more advanced program to manage, process, and store efficiently. As the healthcare industry continues to transition to computers for the storage of patient records, medical files, and other healthcare information, the amount of data available for machine learning algorithms increases. These algorithms are able to analyze the data and assist medical professionals with diagnosing and treating patients for various health issues (Marshall et al., 2016).

Physicians are already using this through evidence-based medicine. Evidence-based medicine is a new method of treating patients by utilizing machine-learning to review data that is collected from clinical trials, as well as other treatment options on a massive scale (Bhardwaj, Nambiar, & Dutta, 2017). The database then takes all of this information, views the results of each, and determines the best possible treatment method for the patient. This new method proves to be effective in situations such as a patient with a strain of the flu. The doctor would be able to review the data for patients within the region who have also had the flu around the same time, what treatment options they had received, and what treatments had the greatest positive result. Previous to this method, doctors would need to rely on the information that they have readily available or base their decisions on what they knew of the ailment. This method may result in a less effective form of treatment, or even misdiagnosis of a patient's issue (Saigi-Rubió, Jiménez-Zarco, & Torrent-Sellens, 2016).

The greatest benefit to using machine learning in the healthcare industry is the system's ability to process such a large amount of information in a short period of time. The myriad of medical data available is constantly increasing, and the time it would take for a person to read through, analyze, and interpret that data is astronomical in comparison with a computer's ability to do the same. The machine's ability to search through a vast amount of data and collect the information that applies to the specific case, removes the potential for information to be missed or forgotten by a person attempting to do the same work. Eliminating the possibility of human error from the equation would produce more accurate information that can be used in the diagnosis and treatment of the patient (Cohen, 2019).

The automation of tasks that would normally consume a medical professional's time allows them to focus their efforts on other aspects of healthcare such as assisting a greater number of patients. This would cause a culture shift for medical professionals, focusing less on research and more on their patients. The University of Hong Kong is already preparing for this culture shift. The new generation of healthcare professionals will perform their work differently than that of the previous generation. The younger generation is more adapted to the use of technology, and thus will be more prepared for the use of deep learning in the healthcare industry. The University of Hong Kong has created two six-year undergraduate programs for students to earn their bachelor's degree in medicine and surgery. These programs focus on the humanities, arts, and social sciences aspect of the medical field and less on the technological side (Chen, 2017). The idea behind these courses is to have these new medical professionals fill the gaps that technology will not be able to; strengthening their ability to show compassion and empathy for patients; and, working closely with them to understand their medical needs.

Increasing the number of patients that a doctor can assist within a day could potentially increase revenue for the organization. The additional income could be used to improve upon the business by investing in new medical technology, hiring more medical personnel, or making improvements in the facility. As the number of medical professionals within the business grows to fit the needs of the region and the technological improvements are added to assist them, more patients can be treated. Because of these changes, the number of patients can continue to increase, which would produce greater profits for the business, providing constant growth for the medical industry (Cohen, 2019).

Issues With Deep Learning in Healthcare

Machine learning is a new concept for the healthcare industry, and deep learning is even more recent. There are multiple issues that need to be corrected before it can be fully implemented. The biggest issue when attempting to shift processing medical information from people to machines is the machine's inability for creative thought. Information is entered into deep learning programs. The system uses that information to calculate the solution to the problem. If there are any other factors that may be detrimental to the situation and it is not entered into the data, the system will not know that it is a factor it needs to consider. It could potentially misdiagnose a patient. It has also been shown that training the system in advance does not result in more accurate information. The system needs to be fine-tuned in order to meet the needs of the data. Depending on the data provided to the system, this could consist of days of correcting processes in the system for each data set so it can accurately read the data (De Cnudde, Martens, & Provost, 2018).

A severe lack of data currently available is also an issue with deep learning. Being a recent technological advancement, there has not been enough time to create data that the systems can utilize effectively. In order for machine learning to properly function, it requires massive amounts of data. Analyzing just a small amount of information could lead to inaccurate results. An example of this is using a Support Vector Machine, which is a supervised learning model that uses special algorithms to analyze data to classify certain information into predetermined categories. If the system was analyzing samples of a disease, the system would be unable to effectively categorize the information due to the number of positive samples typically being much smaller than the negative samples (Srivastava, Soman, Rai, Srivastava, & Praveen, 2017). If there are not enough positive samples for it to gain a full understanding of the disease, it will be unable to effectively categorize samples. Fortunately, as the use of machine learning progresses and more data becomes available, this issue will be minimized (Bhardwaj et al., 2017).

The current state of technology also creates difficulty in implementing deep learning into the healthcare industry. Deep learning is still in the early stages of development. It is capable of analyzing basic information, but beyond that, the system may be incapable of understanding the data. In the healthcare industry, a significant amount of the data needed is highly complex. The added difficulty of interpreting the data may be too much for the system to process, which could lead to inaccurate results. An article by Sofie Cnudde, David Martens, and Foster Provost (2018) titled: "An exploratory study towards applying and demystifying deep learning classification on behavioral big data," discusses deep learning technology and the multiple hierarchy levels of data. The hierarchy levels are based on the complexity of the data provided. As the complexity increases, so does the hierarchy level. Their study found that deep learning is able to process data currently listed on the lowest hierarchy level, but beyond that it is incapable of accurately predicting performance (De Cnudde, Martens, & Provost, 2018). Deep learning can be used in healthcare today, but only on a basic level of information processing. As research continues with deep learning technology, its ability to understand and interpret data on higher hierarchy levels will also increase (Marshall et al., 2016).

Another issue facing deep learning is the implementation process. In order for these machines to be effective, the person operating the system must be able to correctly enter the data and interpret the results it provides. This requires a thorough understanding of statistical analysis, a trait that most physicians do not acquire through their schooling. The need for data analysts is rising as the use of machine learning across industries increases. Unfortunately, there is a lack of data scientists available. The McKinsey Global institute predicted that by 2018, there would be a shortage of 140,000 to 180,000 data scientist. To combat this issue, there have been attempts to train healthcare professionals on data analytics, but these attempts at teaching them have proven to be unsuccessful. It is difficult for them to learn this profession outside of their healthcare positions (Hoyt, Snider, Thompson, & Mantravadi, 2016). The advancements in deep learning technology is counteracted by the lack of personnel that are capable of correctly operating the system and interpreting the data. It is similar to having a plane full of passengers but no pilot. The system is capable, but if nobody knows how to operate it, it is useless.

TELEMEDICINE

Telemedicine is a medical professional's ability to provide healthcare to patients that are not in the same location through the use of technology. It has been used for over a century, beginning in the late 1800's, around the time the radio and telephone were invented. These inventions allowed doctors to treat patients that were unable to access healthcare by travelling to a medical facility. As technology advanced, so did the use of telemedicine. The biggest advancements in telemedicine occurred during the 1960's and 1970's when NASA began funding telemedicine research in order to find ways of treating astronauts while in space (Lafolla, 2017). Combining NASA's funding of these projects with the increasing use of television led to the creation of telemedicine through video.

In recent years, telemedicine has been introduced to the Internet. Healthcare websites can now provide services to customers that were previously unavailable, such as diagnosing and treating illnesses. Through these services, customers gain access to medical care through questionnaires and videoconferencing. The information provided by the user is submitted to medical professionals that are able to analyze the data, diagnose the patient's issue, and provide treatment options based on the information provided. In the event that a medical professional is unable to diagnose the issue based on this information, they may need to contact the patient through videoconferencing, which allows the doctor to further investigate symptoms. If the patient requires blood work or vaccinations, the doctor will provide them with the information needed so they can go to the nearest medical facility to have the additional treatment performed (Cohen, 2019; Panlaqui, Broadfield, Champion, Edington, & Kennedy, 2017).

Benefits of Telemedicine

Telemedicine allows access to basic healthcare for patients that may be too far away or are unable to travel to a medical facility. Advancements in technology have increased the number of methods in which a patient can access healthcare. Prior to the Internet, healthcare professionals would communicate with patients through radio and telephone. The biggest limitation was that they had to base their diagnosis solely on verbal input, since they were unable to see the patient. With the creation of the Internet came the immediate visual access that has significantly increased the effectiveness and usage of telemedicine. In a study performed on Medicaid recipients to assess the usage of telemedicine, it was found that elderly, blind, and disabled people consisted of 28.1% of telemedicine users (Daugherty Douglas et al., 2016). Patients like the ones in this study benefit from the convenience of not needing to drive themselves or burdening another person with driving them to a medical facility if they are unable to drive. Patients living further away from healthcare facilities also benefitted from telemedicine. In the same study with Medicaid recipients, the demographic information showed that although metropolitan areas had five times more enrollees than rural areas, the rural area subjects were seventeen times more likely to use telemedicine services (Daugherty Douglas et al., 2016). This could be due to the longer commute times to medical facilities in rural areas. Since rural environments tend to be lower populations and more dispersed than metropolitan areas, medical facilities could be scarce, making telemedicine the best method for patients to use.

Hospitals with a lack of healthcare professionals also utilize telemedicine to tend to patients. In regions where the need for specialty doctors and nurses is high, but the availability is scarce, hospitals will request assistance from other locations through telemedicine. Doctors are able to diagnose, treat, and monitor patients that are located in medical facilities other than their own. A study performed in Australia on 525 ICU patients between 2010 and 2015 showed that there was no significant difference in results between patients that were treated using telemedicine and those that were not. In fact, the use of telemedicine decreased the number of inter-hospital transfers (Panlaqui et al., 2017). By remotely accessing other hospitals and providing patient support, the need for intensive care specialists will lessen in areas where they are in short supply. Short staffed ICU's will be able to care for more patients, potentially keeping up with demand.

The use of telemedicine will also decrease the number of patients that visit healthcare facilities. Telemedicine is used to treat minor illnesses and issues. If a patient with a minor issue has the option to either receive medical care from their home, or go into a medical facility to receive treatment, they are more likely to choose the first option (Michaud, Zhou, McCarthy, Siahpush, & Su, 2018). Now that these problems can be solved without the need for the patient to enter a healthcare facility, the wait time to see a medical professional will be reduced. Doctors will be able to use this additional time to focus on patients that visit the hospital with more serious issues, focusing on their treatment on overall health rather than trying to assist a large number of patients as quickly as possible. This will eventually improve the healthcare quality to patients (Khanna, Sattar, & Hansen, 2013).

Medical professionals and patients are embracing the use of telemedicine. The ease of use and accessibility of its services have provided both parties with an overall positive experience. The results of a survey performed at the Echuca Regional Health High Dependency Unit, showed that the overall quality of telemedicine was satisfactory to level of care (Panlaqui et al., 2017). Telemedicine had assisted the staff in their critical care services by monitoring patients and performing tasks that the staff would normally need to do. The staff agreed that they would like to use telemedicine again should the need arise. Telemedicine services are already available in 22 US states. The Medicaid survey showed that roughly 1% of patients used telemedicine (Daugherty Douglas et al., 2016). As technology continues to improve, and awareness increases, the number of users will increase as well.

There is a financial benefit to using telemedicine as well. Accessing healthcare through telemedicine reduces the need for a physician to spend their time working with the patient, as well as the need for a physical meeting location. Since physicians are able to spend less time working with individual patients, they can provide care to an increased number of patients, reducing the cost of services per patient. This effect also occurs with hospitals using telemedicine to assist other medical facilities. In a study focused on the cost difference between using a medical doctor and a MD specialist live consultant through telemedicine, there was a $330 cost-savings per person per week for dermatology consultations through telemedicine. Another study on tele-radiology estimated that consultations via telemedicine resulted in a cost savings of $144 per reading by avoiding unnecessary CT scans (Akiyama & Byung-Kwang, 2016). These two surveys, along with many others in the article, all showed that using telemedicine is a more cost-effective way to diagnose and treat patients for minor conditions. The need for physician appointments would also decrease with the use of telemedicine, along with costs in driving to the office, and time spent during the appointment. Telemedicine removes all of these factors from the price, which significantly reduces the cost of healthcare (Chang, Savage, & Waldman, 2017; Michaud et al., 2018).

Issues With Telemedicine

Technology has shifted the use of telemedicine to computer systems using the Internet. This move has changed its focus to a broader audience. Telemedicine has increased its capability to include visuals as well as audio and allows doctors to work with patients in real-time. This form of telemedicine is still in the early stages of development. It can only be used to diagnose and treat minor illnesses. Its capabilities are extremely limited in comparison with an actual visit to a healthcare facility due to the patient not physically being in the same room as the doctor. The doctor is unable to perform any physical examinations that may increase their understanding of the patient's issue. Thus, misdiagnosis can occur. In hospital settings where doctors are using telemedicine to monitor patients, misdiagnosis or mistreatment can also occur since they are basing the majority of their conclusion on visuals and information provided to them. They are unable to work with the patient directly. So, they may miss important information that is critical to their patient's health (Addady, 2016).

Most patients do not have the medical knowledge or expertise to fully understand their illnesses, which is why they seek a medical professional for help. Telemedicine services depend on the patients to enter in their symptoms so the doctor can diagnose and treat them. If the patient incorrectly enters, or misses vital information when submitting data, the doctor may not be able to provide an accurate diagnosis. Doctors may also not ask about important information that is crucial for an accurate diagnosis. In a 2016 study of telemedicine services, Dermatologist Jack Resneck stated, "the services failed to ask simple, relevant questions of patients about their symptoms, leading them to repeatedly miss important diagnoses" (Addady, 2016). There is a major social disconnect between the doctor and patient that is created when using telemedicine. This disconnect is resulting in less opportunities for the doctor to fully examine the patient, which leads to misdiagnosis of the patient's issues.

Telemedicine usage through the Internet is a recent advancement in technology. With that comes the need to train its users so it can be properly utilized. The training that healthcare professionals receive does not consider the use of telemedicine, causing a lack of understanding of the data it provides. The majority of students in the medical field are not learning how to use telemedicine or electronic health records while in school or during their residency (Aas, 2017). During an office visit, doctors are able to use multiple forms of patient analysis such as physical exams, in-person testing, and the patient's medical history. Telemedicine can only provide limited forms of this data such as inadequate body language through the use of webcams. This information can be miscommunicated though, as webcams can have poor image resolution or lighting issues. The doctor must learn how to work with the information provided through the telemedicine software.

Patients also face a learning curve with telemedicine software. Users that are new to telemedicine may not understand how to correctly use the software or what information is necessary for them to enter. Patients may develop a negative perception of telemedicine because of their lack of understanding. The data they enter may give them undesired results such as a diagnosis different from what they wanted, or if an office visit is required for further examination. Issues such as these can also lead to patient's self-diagnosing issues or entering information that results in a diagnosis they want, rather than what they need. Proper training of telemedicine software will assist in preventing situations. For patients that are still determined to self-diagnose their issues, doctors will need to be trained on how to determine the patient's issues and how to tell the patient no when they are persistent on their incorrect self-diagnosis (Cohen, 2019).

BENEFITS OF INTEGRATING DEEP LEARNING WITH TELEMEDICINE

Combining deep learning technologies with telemedicine could significantly increase the availability of healthcare while decreasing the need for medical professionals. Medical data can be entered into deep learning programs so that they develop an understanding of medical issues that patients may have. Integrating this software with telemedicine would allow these programs to accept patient data, cross reference it with the data that has already been entered into the system, and determine what issues that patient may have, and what is the best route for treatment of that issue (Razzak, Naz, & Zaib, 2017; Srivastava et al., 2017).

There are deep learning programs that have recently been introduced to the healthcare industry. These systems are still within the initial introductory phase of learning healthcare, but they have made significant advances in the field. Neural network software such as DeepCare uses memory cells that can store, forget, update information, and manipulate data on illness experiences over certain periods of time. This software is able to read medical records and store a patient's medical history. Advancements in the technology have allowed it to use these records to determine current illnesses using a patient's data, predict the stages of disease progression in a patient, recommend treatments, and alert the patient of potential risks they may face with this disease (Pham, Tran, Phung, & Venkatesh, 2017). These computer systems are able to store massive amounts of medical data which help determine when a patient has an issue. The memory cells that these systems have are based on a human's memory cells in that they base the majority of the diagnosis on the more recent data that is entered, and they are able to forget older information or information that is not vital to the patient's diagnosis.

Using machine learning allows a more in-depth reading of the patient's information that results in an accurate diagnosis. This removes the possibility of human error through a doctor missing or forgetting vital information that may result in a misdiagnosis. The machine's ability to spot differences in images goes beyond human capability. These subtle differences can be overlooked by professionals, causing issues to go undiagnosed. Machine learning programs are being used in research labs such as the Broad Institute of MIT and Harvard in Cambridge, where cell images are scanned by the software to find subtle biological phenomena that a person may not be able to see otherwise (Maxmen, 2018). These programs can reveal issues such as cancer within a single cell and monitor the progression of diseases from the very beginning. Technological advances assist in the understanding of how diseases spread throughout the body and may help in determining preventative measures that can be taken to prevent this disease from spreading in other patients.

The need for medical professionals is an ongoing concern in the healthcare industry. The Association of American Medical Colleges performed a study that concluded by 2030, the U.S. alone will have a shortage of physicians ranging from 40,800 to 104,900 (Sweeney, 2017). Integrating deep learning with telemedicine applications would assist with diverting patients away from seeking medical professionals for basic care. Patients are able to use telemedicine programs from their home to get their issue diagnosed and be provided with treatment options. The benefits of using telemedicine versus going to the hospital could convince patients with minor illnesses to use their services rather than visit a medical professional for help. Integrating deep learning into these telemedicine programs would remove the need for a medical professional in the telemedicine program since the computer program would be able to accurately diagnose and treat the patients for their issues. Although this may not resolve the shortage of medical professionals, it will assist in decreasing the deficit. The time that deep learning telemedicine programs save these physicians will allow them to focus on more on patients with serious issues that require a medical professional's help (Michaud et al., 2018).

ISSUES WITH DEEP LEARNING AND TELEMEDICINE

Deep learning is a relatively new technology for the medical industry. In order for the software to learn, it needs to be provided large amounts of data that will help it understand the differences between healthy and unhealthy cells as well as other aspects of the human body. If customers are using telemedicine services that are operating using deep-learning technology, it is critical to the success of the system that the technology has a full understanding of patient issues. Otherwise, it may misdiagnose or completely disregard important information that the patient provides. This software requires thorough training involving datasets on different types of medical issues. Since deep learning is a new concept in the medical field, there is not a significant amount of data currently available that the software is able to use as a dataset. This creates further problems, as the only way to obtain this data is through medical experts creating the datasets, and having multiple experts examine the work to ensure accuracy (Razzak, Naz, & Zaib, 2017). The lack of data severely limits deep learning's capabilities of diagnosing medical issues for patients, so it may only be able to assist with minor issues but could not fully operate a telemedicine service.

Privacy is a concern that needs to be addressed with deep learning telemedicine programs. Providing sustainable telemedicine services through web-based applications requires a significant amount of data storage. A large portion of this data consists of patient's private medical information. Cloud data storage services, as well as mobile devices and other computer platforms are being used to store this massive amount of data (Gheorghe, 2014). Using these various storage services increases the vulnerability of data breaches by hackers. A study performed in the UK showed that most individuals are worried about the level of privacy with their health records (Srivastava et al., 2017). The sophistication of data hacks has been increasing over time. To combat this issue, there has been research into creating regulations for security in these telemedicine programs. Methods such as data encryption and restricted access for unauthorized users has been put into place to increase the level of security for this data (Jo & Chung, 2015). Ongoing research into data security will be required to keep these programs safe from hackers and prevent any loss of users' private medical information (Pegah, Mahdavi, Shahram, & Arasteh, 2018).

As with sustainable telemedicine services operated by medical professionals, deep learning telemedicine services face the issue of patient inaccuracy and lack of in-person examination. Since sustainable telemedicine services rely on patients entering in their symptoms, the deep learning program will have to determine the diagnosis based on what the patient enters. If some of the symptoms are missed or entered incorrectly, the diagnosis could end up wrong. There is also the removal of the human factor when using deep learning in sustainable telemedicine. To some extent, the doctor will use visual cues from the patient to assist in diagnosis. Since machines lack that ability, they are entirely dependent on patient input, as well as medical records and any patient lab work that may have been performed.

GOVERNMENT REGULATIONS

Government regulations play a big factor in the use of sustainable telemedicine services. If deep learning programs are to succeed in sustainable telemedicine services, they will require a large number of patients so that they receive the data they need to help them learn and grow as a more efficient service. Government regulations are slowing the growth of sustainable telemedicine. In a study on telemedicine usage with Medicaid patients, they discovered that only 22 states in the United States offered reimbursement programs for telemedicine services (Daugherty Douglas et al., 2016). There was also a limit to the services through telemedicine that were available for reimbursement, whereas in-patient visits were reimbursed. Although most of these services involved mental health issues, as deep learning programs in telemedicine increase their ability to diagnose physical issues, there may be limits to reimbursement on these as well. Reimbursement for in-patient visits disincentivizes the use of telemedicine, as patients are more likely to seek the services that are covered by their health insurance policies.

Programs such as the Affordable Care Act (ACA) did increase the usage of sustainable telemedicine services. This study on Medicaid, showed that the number of mental health issues was much greater within the Medicaid population versus the general population (Daugherty Douglas et al., 2016). Prior to the ACA, enrollees had to meet eligibility requirements in order to receive treatment for mental health conditions, which limited the number of mental health patients. The ACA removed that requirement so more people were able to seek the treatment they needed. Many of them utilized telemedicine services for this treatment. The study showed that of the 4.5 million telemedicine users, 95% of the claims were for behavioral health (Daugherty Douglas, et al., 2016). The number of telemedicine users could increase drastically if government regulations adapt to the changing healthcare environment and allow for reimbursement of these services.

FUTURE DIRECTION OF DEEP LEARNING AND TELEMEDICINE

Advancements in software programs will lead to an increase in deep learning's ability to understand medical data. Companies are already using deep learning technologies such as IBM's Watson Analytics, which is a program that is uses a practitioner approach to analyze datasets, examine that data to determine the level of quality, and find the optimal statistical approach (Hoyt, Snider, Thompson, & Mantravadi, 2016). This software is able to understand natural language and offers exploratory, predictive, and visual analytics, making it user-friendly for medical professionals that may not have a full understanding of statistical data analysis.

Watson Analytics is frequently improving its software and adding new features. One new feature that has been introduced is its four sections of data processing. The first section is *Refining*, which organizes the information based on different attributes and separates it into groups or hierarchies. Groups and hierarchies then can be manipulated based on the needs of the user. *Exploring* is the second section. Exploring allows the user to search through the data by entering questions in the tool. The results can be provided in multiple formats and are easily saved and shared for future use. The third section, *Prediction*, is a beneficial tool for the medical industry. Data is entered into the system and predictive analytics allows the user to see the potential for certain outcomes. This section could be utilized by medical professionals to determine outcomes of diseases based on the patient's current situation. The final section, *Assemble*, allows the user to create visuals and presentations with the data provided. This could be useful as a learning tool for students or healthcare practitioners looking to expand their knowledge of specific health conditions.

Watson Analytics is a helpful tool for the healthcare industry. It will be able to significantly decrease the time spent analyzing patient data. This software is still limited in its abilities. It is reliant on the data that it is provided. The results will still need to be examined by a professional to determine if it is correct. Watson Analytics can handle large datasets but may have issues when using multiple datasets. It is unable to use machine-learning methods such as data mining. As the technology progresses and more improvements are made on this software, it may no longer have these issues and could provide greater use in the healthcare industry.

Technological improvements are not the only issue that needs to be resolved in order for deep learning and sustainable telemedicine to increase in usage. Financial issues with telemedicine services will need to be resolved as well. Reimbursement for telemedicine services has been an issue in the United States. Although sustainable telemedicine services have seen remarkable success rates, programs such as Medicare are unwilling to see telemedicine as a reimbursable expense, as it is used in the home rather than a medical facility (Dinesen et al., 2016; Michaud et al., 2018). The lack of funding is not an issue on the global scale though, as other countries are working toward increasing the use of sustainable telemedicine (Chang, Savage, & Waldman, 2017; Cilliers, 2014).

The World Health Organization created a policy framework for European countries called "Health 2020" (Dinesen et al., 2016). This program is working to increase overall health of citizens in these countries through new technologies such as telemedicine, as it provides people with access to quality healthcare in regions that may not have enough medical resources. Other programs have been established as well (Cilliers, 2014). The European Union created the research program "Horizon 2020", which is an initiative to fund telemedicine projects on an international level (Dinesen, et al., 2016). Programs such as these are advancing the use of sustainable telemedicine services on a global scale. Integrated deep learning technologies into these telemedicine services will increase the number of patients that these services are able to assist as the lack of medical professionals will no longer be an issue.

Deep learning in telemedicine focuses on two aspects: empowerment of patient access to the appropriate healthcare services and improvement in the physician's treatment of the patient. Telemedicine is considered to be one of the most important tools in the healthcare industry today due to lower utilization of resources, reduced costs, better patient care, and educating patients with preventive measures. Deep learning is an emerging technology and is evolving to be integrated in many industries. The adoption of deep learning is crucial to integrating sustainable telemedicine development within the healthcare sector. Different organizational and governmental barriers, enablers, and drivers may affect the adoption of deep learning in sustainable telemedicine. Identifying these barriers, enablers, and drivers and their role in deep learning adoption is the core of successful deep learning in telemedicine. However, there is scarcity of studies applying quantitative models and combining barriers, enablers and drivers to check their effect on deep learning adoption in sustainable telemedicine. This chapter calls for more research to be conducted on the study of an effective and sustainable healthcare system such as one where deep learning is implemented in the telemedicine system to provide quality healthcare at a low cost.

CONCLUSION

Deep learning programs integrating with telemedicine will allow a greater number of patients access to healthcare from an Internet connected device. Having the patient work with a computer program decreases the demand for medical professionals. Thus, it will remove the bottleneck that the healthcare industry is currently facing. These programs will be able to review patient entered information, patient's medical history, and lab work that may have been submitted to determine an accurate diagnosis based on the previously entered medical datasets in the system. The use of cloud computing will significantly increase the effectiveness of deep learning technologies, as systems will be able to access medical data on a global scale. As the amount of data available for these deep learning systems increases, the understanding of medical issues will also increase. Sustainable telemedicine will be able to broaden the range of medical issues that it can provide patient assistance. The increasing convenience of sustainable telemedicine services will deflect patients with minor issues from visiting healthcare facilities, permitting medical professionals to focus on more serious cases.

As the medical industry integrates deep learning technologies and telemedicine into more services, the need for medical professionals to perform certain tasks may no longer be necessary. Technology may reach the point where the majority of patient services are performed by machines, such as robotic surgeons removing the need for a human surgeon. The knowledge and abilities that doctors currently are required to have will need to adapt to these changes. The University of Hong Kong understands that technology will eventually be able to perform the majority of the work that a current physician performs, so they teach students ways to bridge the gap that technology cannot fill. The program focuses on the social aspect of healthcare, teaching students to spend more time with patients, learning about them to better understand their needs. Medical students gain an in-depth knowledge of the human condition while developing critical thinking and observational skills, as well as learning to become more compassionate with their patients. Programs such as this one will spread to other colleges and universities as the use of deep learning technologies increase in the medical field.

The advancements in telemedicine, deep learning technology, wearable devices, and cloud computing are all increasing the possibility that deep learning will be utilized in sustainable telemedicine. The financial benefit of using telemedicine versus in-patient services, combined with the increasing global need for access to healthcare has created a need for this technology to integrate into the healthcare industry. Translating the laboratory data to be effectively utilized in hospital settings is one of the greatest challenges that these deep learning technologies need to overcome. Deep learning software and sustainable telemedicine services are already established. So, AI researchers can design the programming to meet the needs of the healthcare system.

REFERENCES

Aas, E. (2017). Prepare providers for telemedicine: 3 critical training areas. Retrieved from http://managedhealthcareexecutive.modernmedicine.com/managed-healthcare-executive/news/prepare-providers-telemedicine-3-critical-training-areas

Addady, M. (2016). A new study of telemedicine services finds bad diagnoses. Retrieved from http://fortune.com/2016/05/16/telemedicine-services/

Akiyama, M., & Byung-Kwang, Y. (2016). A systematic review of the economic evaluation of telemedicine in Japan. *Journal of Preventive Medicine and Public Health*, *49*(4), 183–196. doi:10.3961/jpmph.16.043 PMID:27499161

Anonymous. (2018). Screen Time. *Physician Leadership Journal*, *5*(1), 80.

Bhardwaj, R., Nambiar, A., & Dutta, D. (2017). A study of machine learning in healthcare. *Proceedings of 2017 IEEE 41st Annual Computer Software and Applications Conference*, Torino, Italy: IEEE Computer Society, 236-241. 10.1109/COMPSAC.2017.164

Chang, J., Savage, S. J., & Waldman, D. M. (2017). Estimating willingness to pay for online health services with discrete-choice experiments. *Applied Health Economics and Health Policy*, *15*(4), 491–500. doi:10.100740258-017-0316-z PMID:28290107

Chen, J. (2017). Playing to our human strengths to prepare medical students for the future. *Korean Journal of Medical Education*, *29*(3), 193–197. doi:10.3946/kjme.2017.65 PMID:28870022

Cilliers, L. (2014). Using the cloud to provide telemedicine services in a developing country. *South African Journal of Information Management*, *16*(1), 1–7. doi:10.4102ajim.v16i1.611

Cohen, J. K. (2019). CEO power panel: Patient access is next frontier for health systems. *Modern Healthcare*, *49*(20), 32. Retrieved from https://www.modernhealthcare.com/providers/ceo-power-panel-patient-access-next-frontier-health-systems

Daugherty Douglas, M., Xu, J., Heggs, A., Wrenn, G., Mack, D., & Rust, G. (2016). Assessing telemedicine utilization by using Medicaid claims data. *Psychiatric Services (Washington, D.C.)*, *68*(2), 173–178. doi:10.1176/appi.ps.201500518 PMID:27691381

De Cnudde, S., Martens, D., & Provost, F. (2018). An exploratory study towards applying and demystifying deep learning classification on behavioral big data. *University of Antwerp Working Paper*, 1-32.

Dinesen, B., Nonnecke, B., Lindeman, D., Toft, E., Kidholm, K., Jethwani, K., . . . Albert, N. M. (2018). Fair Health. FH Healthcare Indicators™ and FH Medical Price Index™: a new view of place of service trends and medical pricing. Retrieved from https://s3.amazonaws.com/media2.fairhealth.org/whitepaper/asset/FH%20Medical%20Price%20Index%20and%20FH%20Healthcare%20Indicators--white%20paper.pdf

Gheorghe, M. (2014). Mobile cloud computing for telemedicine solutions. *Informações Econômicas*, *18*(4), 50–61. doi:10.12948/issn14531305/18.4.2014.05

Han, J. J., & Nesbitt, T. (2016). Personalized telehealth in the future: A global research agenda. *Journal of Medical Internet Research*, *18*(3), 1–31. PMID:26932229

Hoyt, R., Snider, D., Thompson, C., & Mantravadi, S. (2016). IBM Watson Analytics: Automating visualization, descriptive, and predictive statistics. *JMIR Public Health and Surveillance*, *2*(2), 157–183. doi:10.2196/publichealth.5810 PMID:27729304

Jo, S. M., & Chung, K. Y. (2015). Design of access control system for telemedicine secure XML documents. *Multimedia Tools and Applications*, *74*(4), 2257–2271. doi:10.100711042-014-1938-x

Khanna, S., Sattar, A., & Hansen, D. (2013). Artificial intelligence in health – the three big challenges. *The Australasian Medical Journal*, *6*(5), 315–317. doi:10.4066/AMJ.2013.1758 PMID:23745154

Lafolla, T. (2017). *History of Telemedicine Infographic*. Retrieved from http://blog.evisit.com/history-telemedicine-infographic

Marshall, D. A., Burgos-Liz, L., Pasupathy, K. S., Padula, W. V., IJzerman, M. J., Wong, P. K., ... Osgood, N. D. (2016). Transforming healthcare delivery: Integrating dynamic simulation modelling and big data in health economics and outcomes research. *PharmacoEconomics*, *34*(2), 115–126. doi:10.100740273-015-0330-7 PMID:26497003

Maxmen, A. (2018). *Deep learning sharpens views of cells and genes*. Retrieved from https://www.scientificamerican.com/article/deep-learning-sharpens-views-of-cells-and-genes/

Michaud, T. L., Zhou, J., McCarthy, M. A., Siahpush, M., & Su, D. (2018). Costs of home-based telemedicine programs: A systematic review. *International Journal of Technology Assessment in Health Care*, *34*(4), 410–418. doi:10.1017/S0266462318000454 PMID:30058505

Panlaqui, O., Broadfield, E., Champion, R., Edington, J., & Kennedy, S. (2017). Outcomes of telemedicine intervention in a regional intensive care unit: A before and after study. *Australian Society of Anaesthetists*, *45*(5), 605–610. PMID:28911290

Pegah, N. B., Mahdavi, M., Shahram, E. B., & Arasteh, S. (2018). Security analysis of a key based color image watermarking vs. a non-key based technique in telemedicine applications. *Multimedia Tools and Applications*, *77*(24), 31713–31735. doi:10.100711042-018-6218-8

Pham, T., Tran, T., Phung, D., & Venkatesh, S. (2017). Predicting healthcare trajectories from medical records: A deep learning approach. *Journal of Biomedical Informatics*, *69*, 218–229. doi:10.1016/j.jbi.2017.04.001 PMID:28410981

Razzak, M., Naz, S., & Zaib, A. (2017). *Deep learning for medical image processing: overview, challenges and future.* Retrieved from https://arxiv.org/ftp/arxiv/papers/1704/1704.06825.pdf

Saigi-Rubió, F., Jiménez-Zarco, A., & Torrent-Sellens, J. (2016). Determinants of the intention to use telemedicine: Evidence from primary physicians. *International Journal of Technology Assessment in Health Care*, *32*(2), 29–36. doi:10.1017/S0266462316000015 PMID:27472158

Sennaar, K. (2019a). Machine learning for medical diagnostics – 4 current applications. *Emerj - Artificial Intelligence Research and Insight.* Retrieved from https://emerj.com/ai-sector-overviews/machine-learning-medical-diagnostics-4-current-applications/

Sennaar, K. (2019b). Artificial intelligence in telemedicine and telehealth – 4 current applications. *Emerj - Artificial Intelligence Research and Insight.* Retrieved from https://emerj.com/ai-sector-overviews/artificial-intelligence-in-telemedicine-and-telehealth/

Shead, S. (2017). Google DeepMind is funding NHS research at Moorfields Eye Hospital. *Business Insider*. Retrieved from https://www.businessinsider.com/deepmind-is-funding-nhs-research-2017-7?r=UK

Sim, D. A., Keane, P. A., Tufail, A., Egan, C. A., Aiello, L. P., & Silva, P. (2015). Automated retinal image analysis for diabetic retinopathy in telemedicine. *Current Diabetes Reports*, *15*(14), 577–590. doi:10.100711892-015-0577-6 PMID:25697773

Srivastava, S., Soman, S., & Rai, A., & Srivastava, P. K. (2017). Deep learning for health informatics: recent trends and future directions. *Proceedings of 2017 International Conference on Advances in Computing, Communications and Informatics (ICACCI)*, Udupi, India. 10.1109/ICACCI.2017.8126082

ADDITIONAL READING

Abbas, Q., Fondon, I., Sarmiento, A., Jiménez, S., & Alemany, P. (2017). Automatic recognition of severity level for diagnosis of diabetic retinopathy using deep visual features. *Medical & Biological Engineering & Computing*, *55*(11), 1959–1974. doi:10.100711517-017-1638-6 PMID:28353133

AlDossary, S., Martin-Khan, M. G., Bradford, N. K., & Smith, A. C. (2017). A systematic review of the methodologies used to evaluate telemedicine service initiatives in hospital facilities. *International Journal of Medical Informatics*, *97*, 171–194. doi:10.1016/j.ijmedinf.2016.10.012 PMID:27919377

Bergmo, T. S. (2015). How to measure costs and benefits of e-health interventions: An overview of methods and frameworks. *Journal of Medical Internet Research*, *17*(11), e254. doi:10.2196/jmir.4521 PMID:26552360

Bouskill, K., Smith-Morris, C., Bresnick, G., Cuadros, J., & Pedersen, E. R. (2018). Blind spots in telemedicine: A qualitative study of staff workarounds to resolve gaps in diabetes management. *BMC Health Services Research, 18*(1), 617–625. doi:10.118612913-018-3427-9 PMID:30086743

Chen, E. T. (2017). Considerations of telemedicine in the delivery of modern healthcare. *American Journal of Management, 17*(3), 20–28.

Craig, J. A., Carr, L., Hutton, J., Glanville, J., Iglesias, C. P., & Sims, A. J. (2015). A review of the economic tools for assessing new medical devices. *Applied Health Economics and Health Policy, 13*(1), 15–27. doi:10.100740258-014-0123-8 PMID:25139635

Drummond, M. F., Sculpher, M. J., Claxton, K., Stoddart, G. L., & Torrance, G. W. (2015). *Methods for the economic evaluation of health care programmes* (4th ed.). Oxford: Oxford University Press.

Dullet, N. W., Geraghty, E. M., Kaufman, T., Kissee, J. L., King, J., Dharmar, M., ... Marcin, J. P. (2017). Impact of a university-based outpatient telemedicine program on time savings, travel costs, and environmental pollutants. *Value in Health, 20*(4), 542–546. doi:10.1016/j.jval.2017.01.014 PMID:28407995

Grustam, A. S., Severens, J. L., Nijnatten, J., Koymans, R., & Vrijhoef, H. J. (2014). Cost-effectiveness of telehealth interventions for chronic heart failure patients: A literature review. *International Journal of Technology Assessment in Health Care, 30*(1), 59–68. doi:10.1017/S0266462313000779 PMID:24495581

Hansen, S. W., Gogan, J. L., Baxter, R. J., & Garfield, M. J. (2019). Informed collaboration in health care: An embedded-cases study in geriatric telepsychiatry. *Information Systems Journal, 29*(2), 514–547. doi:10.1111/isj.12218

Hatipoglu, N., & Bilgin, G. (2017). Cell segmentation in histopathological images with deep learning algorithms by utilizing spatial relationships. *Medical & Biological Engineering & Computing, 55*(10), 1829–1848. doi:10.100711517-017-1630-1 PMID:28247185

Johns, N. E., Foster, D. G., & Upadhyay, U. D. (2017). Distance traveled for Medicaid-covered abortion care in California. *BMC Health Services Research, 17*(1), 287–297. doi:10.118612913-017-2241-0 PMID:28420438

Kidholm, K., & Kristensen, M. B. D. (2018). A Scoping Review of Economic Evaluations Alongside Randomised Controlled Trials of Home Monitoring in Chronic Disease Management. *Applied Health Economics and Health Policy, 16*(2), 167–176. doi:10.100740258-017-0351-9 PMID:28871514

Kratzwald, B., Ilić, S., Kraus, M., Feuerriegel, S., & Prendinger, H. (2018). Deep learning for affective computing: Text-based emotion recognition in decision support. *Decision Support Systems, 115*, 24–35. doi:10.1016/j.dss.2018.09.002

LeCun, Y., Bengio, Y., & Hinton, G. (2015). Deep learning. *Nature, 521*(7553), 436–444. doi:10.1038/nature14539 PMID:26017442

Majtner, T., Yildirim-Yayilgan, S., & Hardeberg, J. Y. (2019). Optimised deep learning features for improved melanoma detection. *Multimedia Tools and Applications, 78*(9), 11883–11903. doi:10.100711042-018-6734-6

Mistry, H., Hyeladzira, G., & Oppong, R. (2014). Critical appraisal of published systematic reviews assessing the cost-effectiveness of telemedicine studies. *Telemedicine Journal and e-Health, 20*(7), 609–618. doi:10.1089/tmj.2013.0259 PMID:24820406

Murray, E., Hekler, E. B., Andersson, G., Collins, L. M., Doherty, A., Hollis, C., ... Wyatt, J. C. (2016). Evaluating digital health interventions: Key questions and approaches. *American Journal of Preventive Medicine*, *51*(5), 843–851. doi:10.1016/j.amepre.2016.06.008 PMID:27745684

Safdar, S., Zafar, S., Zafar, N., & Khan, N. F. (2018). Machine learning based decision support systems (DSS) for heart disease diagnosis: A review. *Artificial Intelligence Review*, *50*(4), 597–623. doi:10.100710462-017-9552-8

Seth, S., & Agarwal, B. (2018). A hybrid deep learning model for detecting diabetic retinopathy. *Journal of Statistics & Management Systems*, *21*(4), 569–574. doi:10.1080/09720510.2018.1466965

Wang, J., Wang, Y., Wei, C., Yao, N., Yuan, A., Shan, Y., & Yuan, C. (2014). Smartphone interventions for long-term health management of chronic diseases: an integrative review. *Telemedicine Journal and E-health: the official journal of the American Telemedicine Association, 20*(6), 570-583.

Yoo, T. K., Choi, J. Y., Seo, J. G., Ramasubramanian, B., Selvaperumal, S., & Kim, D. W. (2019). The possibility of the combination of OCT and fundus images for improving the diagnostic accuracy of deep learning for age-related macular degeneration: A preliminary experiment. *Medical & Biological Engineering & Computing*, *57*(3), 677–687. doi:10.100711517-018-1915-z PMID:30349958

KEY TERMS AND DEFINITIONS

Algorithms: An algorithm is a well-defined procedure that allows a computer to solve a problem. A particular problem can typically be solved by more than one algorithm. Optimization is the process of finding the most efficient algorithm for a given task.

Artificial Intelligence: The theory and development of computer systems able to perform tasks normally requiring human intelligence, such as visual perception, speech recognition, decision-making, and translation between languages.

Decision Support System: A decision support system (DSS) is a computerized information system used to support decision-making in an organization or a business. A DSS lets users sift through and analyze massive amounts of data, and compile information that can be used to solve problems and make better decisions.

Deep Learning: Deep learning is a collection of algorithms used in machine learning, used to model high-level abstractions in data through the use of model architectures, which are composed of multiple nonlinear transformations. It is part of a broad family of methods used for machine learning that are based on learning representations of data.

eHealth: An emerging field in the intersection of medical informatics, public health and business, referring to health services and information delivered or enhanced through the Internet and related technologies.

Information Accessibility: The right of a patient to seek, receive and impart information and ideas concerning health issues. This access to information, however, should not impair the right to have personal health data treated with confidentiality.

Machine Learning: Machine learning is an application of artificial intelligence (AI) that provides systems the ability to automatically learn and improve from experience without being explicitly programmed. Machine learning focuses on the development of computer programs that can access data and use it learn for themselves.

Telehealth: The delivery and facilitation of health and health-related services including medical care, provider and patient education, health information services, and self-care via telecommunications and digital communication technologies.

Telemedicine: Telemedicine is the use of telecommunication and information technology to provide clinical health care from a distance. It has been used to overcome distance barriers and to improve access to medical services that would often not be consistently available in distant rural communities.

Videoconferencing: A video conference is a live, visual connection between two or more people residing in separate locations for the purpose of communication. At its simplest, video conferencing provides transmission of static images and text between two locations. At its most sophisticated, it provides transmission of full-motion video images and high-quality audio between multiple locations.

Chapter 9
Patient-Centered Empowerment Through Evidence-Based Engagement in Sensitive Clinical Settings

Iris Reychav
https://orcid.org/0000-0001-8963-3776
Ariel University, Israel

Roger W. McHaney
https://orcid.org/0000-0001-9501-3741
Kansas State University, USA

Lin Zhu
Ariel University, Israel

Rami Moshonov
Assuta Ramat Hahaial Medical Center, Israel

ABSTRACT

Patient-centered empowerment is enhanced through evidence-based engagement in stressful medical situations. The current study provided expert-vetted educational materials in dynamic text and video formats using the 5S approach. The materials are relevant, reliable, and readable for patients with abnormal Pap test results. Findings indicated patients that understood the information better were more engaged. Engagement was measured using a coding system that kept track of explicitly shared information, requested recommendations, and tacit knowledge during patient-physician interaction. Other outcomes were that dynamic text had a greater impact on engagement in both initial and follow-up meetings. Important findings included that those who found the dynamic text relevant had their social well-being, self-esteem, optimism, and acceptance improved in initial meetings. Those who found the dynamic text reliable were more confident in the relationship with their physician in follow-up meetings and felt their social well-being was improved in both initial and follow-up meetings.

DOI: 10.4018/978-1-7998-0047-7.ch009

INTRODUCTION

Abnormal medical exam results are cause for concern, worry and stress for most patients. In the current study, the subjects were women who had been referred to a specialty gynecology clinic after having an abnormality detected in their routine Pap test results. Usually, these women were highly stressed and worried (Reychav, McHaney, Zhu, & Moshonov, 2018). They used the World Wide Web to search for information regarding their situation. They may have discovered information---perhaps accurate or perhaps out of date and wrong. In general, these women do not have access to current research-based evidence usually found in scientific journals and clinical databases. Even if they do have access to these items, they may lack the skills to interpret their findings and apply the information to their situation. They also may suffer from a lack of time needed to search for accurate and relevant information; and may not have the skills needed to identify the correct information. This can increase their fear prior to their appointment at a specialized gynecology clinic (Reychav, Parush, McHaney, Hazan, & Moshonov, 2018).

To the best of our knowledge, training in the appraisal of evidence has not been a component of most HPV educational curricula. In the current study, we used a knowledge-based evidence approach. This approach focuses on 3Rs: reliability, relevance and readability (in the case of video presentation: understandability) (Straus & Haynes, 2009). In this paradigm, evidence is reliable if it can be shown to be highly valid. The method used to generate this knowledge must be explicit and rigorous, or at least provide the best available result. To be clinically relevant, material should be distilled and indexed from the medical literature so that it consists of content that is specific to the distinct needs of well-defined groups of women dealing with HPV and arriving at the specialty clinic for the first time or as a follow-up meeting. To be readable or understandable, it must be something that makes sense to the patient considering her cultural, educational, and literacy levels.

The current study focused on making videos with information easily understood by the target audience. We asked an expert physician to evaluate and present evidence in a meaningful way. The clinic manager had a good understanding of the target audience and assumed the expert role. He became the primary speaker for the video to provide one source of information. A supporting physician and health provider team developed a dynamic presentation to reinforce his message. The presentations for both sources used friendly tones and approaches, and went into deeper but relevant details regarding HPV and other topics.

The expert team used the "5S" approach to ensure the information was evidence-based and useful (Haynes, 2007). This framework provides a model for organizing evidence-based information. To do this, information was collected based on the "moving up" strategies using the "5S" pyramid. This approach includes primary studies at the bottom and moves to the next level of detail which systematically organizes these studies (syntheses). This level is followed by synopses to further reinforce the material. More concise summaries are found in the next level to provide a comprehensive overview of evidence related to the clinical problem of HPV. At the top of the pyramid are details about systems such as electronic health records and the experiences of the team in this clinic.

The resources become more reliable, relevant and readable from the physician's perspective going up the pyramid and helped support evidence-based decision making. However, in the current situation, the patient perspective is paramount. The team's goal was to ensure the "5Ss" resulted in patients having an informed point of view and deeper understanding of the source information. It was important for them to move through the 5Ss and ultimately acquire useful knowledge in a way that helped in their current situation.

Our goal was to ensure accessibility and understandability of information in the clinic through mobile technology provided in the waiting room. We believed promoting specialized information in the clinic with high quality, relevant resources using an evidence-based information organization approach would lead to better engagement inside the clinic. Improved engagement would enhance empowerment and this would result in higher levels of patient confidence. They would ask insightful questions and, in return, receive better answers. Ultimately, a pattern of accessibility of valuable information with high potential to increase empowerment outcomes was expected to emerge.

BACKGROUND

HPV and HPVV

Human papillomavirus (HPV) is a common virus known to cause genital warts, and potentially fatal diseases such as, vaginal, vulvar, anal, and oropharyngeal cancers (Ng et al., 2017). This virus is responsible for over 600k new cases of cervical and genital cancer worldwide each year (Rimer, Harper, & Witte, 2014) including over 13k in the United State alone, with mortality of more than 50% making it a serious health concern (National Cancer Institute, 2018). HPV vaccine (HPVV) has been available globally since 2006. It is recommended by the World Health Organization (WHO) and the Centers for Disease Control and Prevention for girls aged 9 to 26. This recommendation was extended to boys in 2011 (World Health Organization, 2016). Later, the age was expanded to 45 years (National Cancer Institute, 2018). Worldwide vaccination uptake at a rate of 80% would prevent an estimated two-thirds of all new cervical cancer cases, making vaccine programs a high priority (World Health Organization, 2016). And, some researchers suggest that a goal of eliminating cervical cancer by the year 2050 is realistic (Hall et al., 2019). In spite of all these facts, the rate of vaccination in most of the world (excluding Australia and Canada) is persistently low; in fact, in parts of the United States the vaccination rate is under 20% (Hall et al., 2019; Markman, 2019). Multiple interventions to address poor vaccination rates have increased knowledge of HPV-related diseases, HPVV, and broader impact of related diseases (Kahn et al., 2007; Kester, Shedd-Steele, Dotson-Roberts, Smith, & Zimet, 2014; Mehta, Sharma, & Lee, 2014; Paiva, Lipschitz, Fernandez, Redding, & Prochaska, 2014; Perkins & Clark, 2012; Reiter, Stubbs, Panozzo, Whitesell, & Brewer, 2011).

Recent systematic reviews examining interventions to increase HPVV uptake have conflicting conclusions. Fu et al. (2014) reviewed 33 articles describing educational interventions and concluded that no specific strategy merited recommendation. In a contrary finding, Niccolai et al. (2015) reviewed 14 community and clinic interventions and found several successes (Niccolai, & Hansen, 2015). Research has shown that HPVV has high efficacy for prevention of HPV-related disease and fatal outcomes (Future II Study Group, 2007; Garland et al., 2007). Barriers to vaccination include costs, limited vaccine availability in some countries, and lack of vaccine awareness (Herzog, Huh, Downs, Smith, & Monk, 2008), and some reluctance of the population because of misleading information in the media. Women are more likely to accept the vaccination if they believe they are at risk of HPV infection and the vaccine is effective, and if a provider recommends it (Brewer & Fazekas, 2007). The most important factor concerning HPVV is safety of the vaccine. Although safety was proven in large studies and recommended by WHO and other objective medical organizations, disbelief and mistrust still persist. Higher awareness was reported in studies that only included women attending a *Well Woman* clinic which were asked to complete a questionnaire assessing HPV awareness and specific knowledge about the virus (Waller et al., 2003). In the Waller et al. (2003) study, about 30% of women (316/1032) had heard of HPV. There were significant, but generally small associations with demographic characteristics. For instance, awareness of HPV was higher in older (47%) rather than younger women (25%). Women reporting a history of genital warts had higher awareness of HPV, as did those who reported ever having an abnormal pap smear result. Not surprisingly, knowing someone who had had HPV was associated with greater awareness. Awareness was lower among smokers (22%) than nonsmokers (35%). But, even women who had heard of HPV had poor knowledge and misconceptions about the frequency of viral carrier status (50-80%) and the spread of the virus disease.

In other research, provider recommendation is a key determinant of HPV vaccine uptake (Reiter, Brewer, Gottlieb, McRee, & Smith, 2009; Rosenthal et al., 2011). Teachers and school administrators play an increasingly important role in influencing whether adolescent females and males receive HPV vaccine. As an example, researchers describe the exceptional success of school-based HPV vaccination programs in Australia and the United Kingdom (Brabin et al., 2008; Brotherton et al., 2008). This further emphasizes that it is critical for key stakeholders to possess adequate knowledge about HPV and the vaccine. Research suggests that knowledge is important in the early stages of behavior change as shown in multiple frameworks that characterize the stages of adoption of health behaviors (Glanz, Rimer, & Viswanath, 2008). Furthermore, adequate knowledge is a prerequisite for making informed decisions about vaccination and vaccine policies. For this reason, providing information (to improve knowledge) is a common component of behavioral interventions (Abraham & Michie, 2008). Given inadequate HPV and HPVV knowledge, educational interventions designed to improve knowledge levels represent a potentially important initial step toward increasing vaccination rates among adolescents. Educational interventions may also influence individuals' beliefs and attitudes about HPVV, such as the acceptability of school-based HPVV programs. Only a few intervention studies, however, have been conducted, all of which showed that simple strategies (e.g., providing written materials or verbal information) improved knowledge among parents, adult women, or students (Dempsey, Zimet, Davis, & Koutsky, 2006; Lambert, 2001; Papa, Simas, Reynolds, & Melnitsky, 2009).

Knowledge related to HPV, its relationship to cervical cancer, and cervical cancer outcomes are improving but continue to have deficits in both younger and older women (Denny-Smith, Bairan, & Page, 2006; Holcomb, Bailey, Crawford, & Ruffin, 2004; Ingledue, Cottrell, & Bernard, 2004; Jain et al., 2009).

Given the recent emphasis on HPV in the media along with the availability of the vaccine, it becomes more important than ever to gain a better understanding of women's awareness, and their knowledge about HPV. To the best of our knowledge, no studies have assessed the effectiveness of education interventions among healthcare providers. This is especially true regarding the potential to empower patients arriving at a gynecological clinic by exposing them to different sources of information vetted by expert physicians and directly measure engagement in physician-patient meetings. We believe the information must be understandable in either written or video form. This creates a challenge because the information must be both evidence-based and tailored to the non-expert. And, it has to be reliable and relevant to the patients' situations.

Sources of Information

Information regarding women's preferences and opinions about various sources of information on abnormal Pap test results and HPV has been collected in prior research. For example, McCree et al. (2006) interviewed 44 low income, high risk HPV positive women. These women responded to open ended questions addressing their preferences regarding sources of health and medical information related to HPV and abnormal Pap tests. Unsurprisingly, this study found they preferred sources that were trustworthy, accessible, and convenient.

McCree et al. (2006) used printed brochures and videotapes for the educational content. There was general consensus among the subjects that the brochures were an adequate method for delivering information about HPV. Some women preferred that brochures be placed in an accessible and frequently visited location within clinics, local health departments, or physician offices. Others preferred to receive brochures via mail from their health care providers. There was also general consensus among women that privacy was a major benefit of brochures as they can be read in a private location where women would be more able to digest the information. Further information revealed that some women expressed negative opinions about the plethora of information for their own personal circumstances. Others expressed concerns about being unable to read and/or fully understand the information and therefore felt misled.

The general opinion about the use of videotapes in the McCree et al. (2006) study as a source of information was positive. Most women suggested that videotapes were easy to follow, provided a form of entertainment that reading did not, and enabled them to better comprehend the material than printed material did. Women in the study also found videotapes to be convenient because they could be viewed in clinic waiting rooms or in their privacy of their homes. Women also suggested that videotapes increased comprehension and are particularly suited to those who are visual learners and/or unable to read. Negative opinions expressed included concerns about trust related to the source for the information presented on the videotapes. Some women felt that it was easier for them to trust their doctors than to trust an unfamiliar person on the videotape. Additionally, some women felt that interaction was an important factor and it was missing from videotapes. They expressed a need to have a one-on-one in-depth conversation with their doctor. This opinion is further supported in the literature which suggests that women participating in cervical cancer screening with HPV testing need concise information about HPV and its role in cervical cancer. Health care providers need to moderate the psychological effects of diagnosis through both the manner and mode they deliver HPV diagnoses (McCaffery & Irwig, 2005; Warren & Ebel, 2005). Others reached the same conclusions. For instance, Waller et al. (2003) report that information presentation manner is crucial in minimizing negative psychological impacts associated with testing positive for HPV. Waller et al. (2003) further suggests that this is essential to ensure women continue with future cervical cancer screenings.

Engagement

Patient engagement can take multiple forms in health care (Domecq et al., 2014). Among these is communication and interaction between patient and physician inside the medical encounter which goes beyond patient education (Gruman et al., 2010). Other research suggests patient engagement is correlated to information flow between patient and health care specialist, patient's role in health care decisions, or how involved patients and representative advocate groups are in health policies (Carman et al., 2013). Research in this area is still seeking consensus and as a result, patient engagement has been subject to a number of academic research initiatives and by all accounts is receiving increased attention (Barello, Graffigna, & Vegni, 2012). A recent study by Flickinger et al. (2013) showed that engagement in HIV patients was improved with higher quality communications and relationships between patients and physicians. The current study uses a similar approach. Empowerment

WHO suggests patient empowerment centers on processes that enable people to gain greater control over any decision or action that might impact their health. Empowerment necessitates elements at both individual and community levels in order to be effective (World Health Organization, 2009). Prior research supports this viewpoint. For instance, Gibson (1991) says that empowerment is the process used by individuals or groups to enhance their ability to meet their perceived needs and gain a sense of control over their lives. Gibson and others suggest empowerment occurs at individual, organizational, and societal levels (Gibson, 1991; D. Narayan, 2005; Zimmerman, 1990). For individuals, empowerment "includes participatory behavior, motivations to exert control, and feelings of efficacy and control" (Zimmerman, 1990). It contains elements of individual perception and behavior.

Empowerment has been investigated within the context of healthcare. In this setting, research suggests empowerment hinges on contributions to health-related decisions by both patients and health care providers (Feste & Anderson, 1995; Webb, Horne, & Pinching, 2001). For instance, Webb et al. (2001) measured empowerment by asking patients about their perceived involvement and subsequent satisfaction with treatment decisions. Roberts (1999) looked at patient empowerment through the lens of health and power with an informed, active patient being likely to feel more empowered. Health information appears to affect patient empowerment. Physician-provided information may either enhance empowerment or result in confusion. In these instances, the information must be carefully vetted to the patient's level of understanding and to avoid information overload (Hay, Coups, & Ford, 2006; Jotterand, Amodio, & Elger, 2016; Malhotra, Jain, & Lagakos, 1982).

WHO further suggests patient empowerment has important merits. They describe four components as essential to patient empowerment. These include: 1) patient understanding of his or her role; 2) sufficient patient knowledge acquisition to facilitate healthcare provider engagement; 3) patient skills; and 4) a facilitating environment. Taken holistically, WHO defines patient empowerment as, "[a] process in which patients understand their role, are given the knowledge and skills by their health-care provider to perform a task in an environment that recognizes community and cultural differences and encourages patient participation" (World Health Organization, 2009, p. 190).

Patient empowerment efforts are successful in settings that offer a potential for improving health outcomes through greater involvement and education. For instance, patients faced with immediate, life-threatening injury or disease will not have time nor capability to acquire or apply knowledge in a meaningful way. Instead, empowerment must focus on situations that offer patients a setting where their outcomes can be improved with education, communication, and a health care provider partnership. WHO suggests the following items as ways to enhance patient empowerment (World Health Organization, 2009, pp. 191–192):

- Remove key barriers such as complicated processes by redefining and communicating patients' roles;
- Enhancing patients' knowledge about their condition, various options, as well as their values and preferences;
- Enhancing patients' skills to ensure they are competent in managing required health activities;

- Facilitating an environment for patient empowerment that considers patients' rights, a menu of appropriate choices, easy access to valid information about the choice options, decision aids, and access to skilled/trained health care providers relevant to the situation;
- Ensure empowerment efforts are customized to different patient groups and promote equity across groups that consider culture, education, insurance availability, and income levels; and,
- Motivate patients to achieve more efficient health outcomes.

Empowerment has been quantified by researchers. Uden-Kraan et al. (2009) developed empowerment outcomes which support many of the characteristics for empowerment suggested by WHO. These outcomes, specifically developed for patients, include the following constructs: being better informed; feeling more confident in the relationship with the physician; improved acceptance of the illness; feeling more confident with the treatment; increased optimism and control over the future; enhanced self-esteem; and enhanced social well-being.

Van Uden-Kraan et al. (2009) developed their empowerment outcomes when they examined the influence of knowledge processes on knowledge outcomes in online patient support groups (van Uden-Kraan et al., 2008). The current study uses the items relevant to empowerment outcomes in our unique clinical setting. We believe the underlying premise of these items remains valid in the current study although we are not dealing with online patients. The evaluation of the patients remains the same. We call our outcome *patient-centered empowerment* to differentiate it and emphasize that the patient is our focus rather than ease of the providers.

METHODS

The primary purpose of this study was to evaluate patient-centered empowerment based on providing expert-vetted, knowledge content on mobile devices to women at a gynecology clinic which deals with sensitive HPV-related issues and its impact on patient engagement. The primary indicator of patient-centered empowerment was engagement in medical encounters. Better engagement was posited to lead to higher levels of patient-centered empowerment. To fully explore this area, we examined expert-vetted content provided in two different formats: dynamic text presentation and physician narrated video. The informational content was predefined by expert physicians and a health care team to fit the situation of the women arriving the clinic. The study sought to determine which information form, video or text, was more likely to result in better empowerment outcomes by examining its underlying characteristics related to enhanced communications and relationships within medical visits (Flickinger et al., 2013).

We also considered two clinic visit types which had been referred to the specialty clinic by the subjects' primary physician (e.g. first visits or follow-ups) to one of three physicians. Therefore, the dependent variable in this study was patient-centered engagement. The independent variables used to assess the quality of the information regarding patient-centered empowerment were readability (understandability for the video treatment), reliability, and relevance (3Rs). These variables were a composite of empowerment process variables from van Uden-Kraan et al. (2009). They included: Understood, Valuable, Practical, New, Related to Health Status, Reliable, Correct, Adds to Physician Information, Similar To Physician Information. These items were collected from answers to a patient survey in the waiting room prior to the physician visit. These items comprised the variables used in the analysis to reflect the following (Straus & Haynes, 2009):

- **Readability (Understandability for the Video Treatment):** Understood, Valuable, Practical;
- **Reliability**: Reliable, Correct, New;
- **Relevant**: Related to Health Status, Adds to Physician Information, Similar to Physician Information.

These items were measured to ensure there were sufficient details for the patients to understand the information, and for it to have practical value in their situations. If the presented material had too technical language it would not be understood, and therefore, would not be practical for the patient. It had to be user-friendly and of sufficient detail. That meant the information presented had to be readable, reliable, and relevant to our patients' situations. Our conceptual research model is provided in Figure 1.

Sample Characteristics and Procedure

Women who attended the clinic during the time of the study were given an opportunity to take part in the research. Those willing to participate signed a consent letter in the presence of the researcher responsible for the study which was the physician manager of the clinic. Once a woman approved her participation, she received a mobile tablet device holding the two sources of information. The participant chose which source to access. The choices included a dynamic text presentation or a video that featured the clinic manager. 64 participants selected the dynamic presentation content and 59 chose the physician video content. Average viewing time for the dynamic text presentation was 195.06 seconds. For the physician video content, subjects viewed the content for an average of 192.34 seconds.

Average age of the participants viewing the dynamic text was 38.9 years (standard deviation of 11.0). Those watching the physician video were on average 39.15 years old (standard deviation of 10.88). Family status of the patients choosing the dynamic text presentation included 18 single, 35 married, and 11 divorced women. The family status of the subjects who chose the physician video were 18 single, 31 married, and 10 divorced women. The education of the patients seeing the dynamic text presentation included eight with a high school education, two completing technical studies, and 54 with some form of higher academic education. The patients that chose to see the physician video included eight high school educated women, two with additional technical studies, and 49 with higher academic education.

Figure 1. Conceptual research model

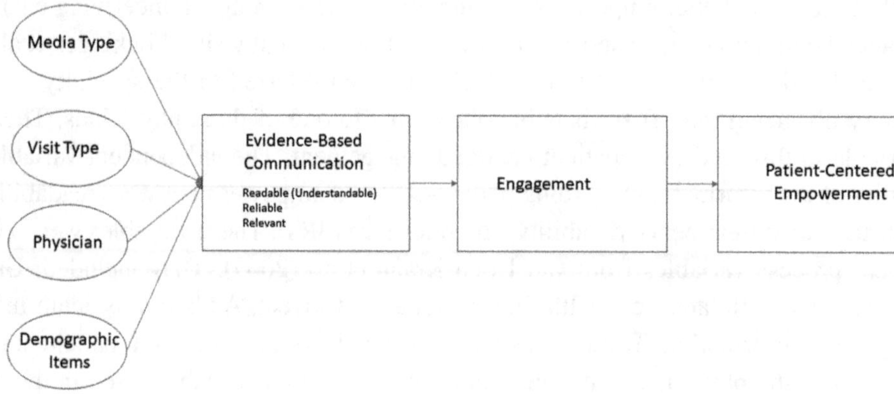

The clinic utilized three physicians during the time of the study. The distribution for the patients who watched the dynamic text presentation was 22 women for the first doctor, 15 women for the second doctor, and 27 women for the third doctor. The distribution for the patients who watched the physician video was 20 women for the first doctor, 15 women for the second doctor and 24 women for the third doctor.

Women who attended the clinic during the study period came either for the first time, for treatment, or for a follow up session. The arrival distribution of patients who watched the dynamic text presentation was 22 for a first session, five for a treatment session, and 37 for a follow up session. The distribution of patients who watched the physician video comprised 20 women for a first session, four women for a treatment session, and 35 women for a follow up session. Since the number of patients that arrived for a treatment session during the study period was low, we removed these subjects from the study and focused only on arrivals for first sessions or follow up sessions.

Source Content

As previously mentioned, two formats of information were available to the study's participants. One was a dynamic text presentation and the second was a video that featured the clinic manger. The dynamic text presentation content discussed how HPV is distributed, how to handle the situation and how to utilize the vaccine. It also discussed the side effects; how a person knows if he or she has the virus; and, what tests are used to determine infection. The presentation provided a statement emphasizing that the kind of cancer caused by HPV can be prevented and recommended that the subjects tell others about this and request help to increase the awareness. The presentation concluded with statistics about infected patients, results of the disease, and a photo of the virus.

The physician video featured the clinic manager who is a doctor himself. He explained for whom HPVV is suitable as well as describing the efficiency and advantages of taking the vaccine. The video described how HPV can attack men and women, and can influence both. The physician emphasized the vaccine is not only for women. He stressed in an easily understood way that both men and women need HPVV, and that a high frequency of this virus exists in young populations with numbers approaching the 50% level. At the end, the physician recommended that people should take this vaccine. And he added a personal touch where he described his doctor and that his father also was a doctor. His family has a history of helping society through medicine.

Two observers were stationed inside meetings between practitioners and patients. These observers recorded explicit information, recommendations, and tacit information sharing using a coding system. These logs formed the basis for evaluating the effectiveness of communication between physicians and patients, and provided a basis for understanding the impact of either video or text-based information on the patients' experiences. The composites of the coded information were used as an engagement score (Blankenburg et al., 2018).

RESULTS

Content Sources and Engagement

The 5S information content sources provided to the study subjects were evaluated through categorization of evidenced-based communication focused on engagement inside the meetings. Engagement scores were developed through meeting interactions by coding patient questions and answers that reflected their active behaviors. Regression was used to analyze the results. The following sections describe the results.

Information Acquired From Dynamic Text Presentation by Patient Attending Initial Meeting

Evidence-based communication following consumption of the 5S information significantly and positively predicted the patient-centered engagement in an initial clinic meeting for information evaluated with higher readability (β= 0.612, $p < .001$). Likewise, it significantly and negatively predicted patient engagement inside the clinic meeting for information evaluated as having higher reliability (β= -0.372, $p < .1$). Readability and reliability of the information also explained a significant proportion of variance in engagement scores ($R^2 = .414$, $F(3, 18) = 4.238$, $p < .001$).

Information Acquired From Dynamic Text Presentation by Patient Attending Follow Up Meeting

Evidence-based communication following consumption of 5S information significantly and positively predicted patient engagement inside the clinic meeting for information evaluated to possess higher readability (β= 0.123, $p < .001$). Readability of the information also explained a significant proportion of variance in engagement scores in this situation ($R^2 = .399$, $F(3, 33) = 7.314$, $p < .001$).

Information Acquired From Physician Video by Patient Attending Initial Meeting

Evidence-based communication following consumption of 5S information significantly and positively predicted patient engagement in the clinic meeting for information that was evaluated with higher understandability (β= 0.651, $p < .001$). It also significantly and negatively predicted patient engagement in the clinic meeting for information evaluated with higher reliability (β= -0.475, $p < .10$). Understandability and reliability of the information also explained a significant proportion of variance in engagement scores ($R^2 = .448$, $F(3, 16) = 4.226$, $p < .05$).

Information Acquired From Physician Video by Patient Attending Follow Up Meeting

Evidence-based communication following consumption of 5S information significantly and positively predicted patient engagement patient in clinic meetings for information evaluated as having with higher understandability (β= 0.123, $p < .001$). Understandability of the information also explained a significant proportion of variance in engagement scores ($R^2 = .401$, $F(3, 31) = 6.905$, $p < .001$).

Content Sources and Patient-Centered Empowerment

The information content sources provided to the study subjects also were evaluated through categorization of evidenced-based communication following consumption of 5S information influence on empowerment inside the meetings. Engagement scores were developed through coding patient and physician interactions, questions, and answers that reflected aspects of their meeting behavior that corresponded to items developed by van Uden-Kraan et al. (2009). Regression was used to analyze the results. The following sections describe the results.

Empowerment Achieved From Dynamic Text Presentation by Patient Attending Initial Meeting

A number of items from van Uden-Kraan et al. (2009) were found to be significantly related to evidence-based communication following consumption of 5S information. The *being better informed* item of the patient-centered empowerment items was significant (β= 0.465, $p < .1$). Evidence-based communication based on 5S information also significantly and positively predicted improved acceptance of the illness (β= 0.888, $p < .05$). Likewise, increased optimism and control over the future (β= 0.825, $p < .05$); enhanced self-esteem (β= 0.439, $p < .1$) ; and enhanced social well-being (β= 0.478, $p < .01$) were all positively and significantly related to evidence-based communication focused on 5S information.

Reliability and Relevancy of the information explained a significant proportion of variance in enhanced social well-being scores ($R^2 = .347$, $F(3, 18) = 3.187$, $p < .05$).

Relevancy of the information explained a significant proportion of variance in other items including: improved acceptance of the illness ($R^2 = .494$, $F(3, 18) = 5.850$, $p < .001$); increased optimism and control over the future ($R^2 = .372$, $F(3, 18) = 6.943$, $p < .001$); enhanced self-esteem ($R^2 = .494$, $F(3, 18) = 3560$, $p < .05$); and enhanced social well-being ($R^2 = .347$, $F(3, 18) = 3.187$, $p < .05$).

Patient-Centered Empowerment Achieved From Dynamic Text Presentation by Patient Attending Follow-Up Meeting

Evidence-based communication following consumption of 5S information significantly and positively predicted two patient-centered empowerment items: feeling more confident in the relationship with my physician (β= 1.656, $p < .1$); and enhanced social well-being ($\beta = 0.719$, $p < .1$).

Reliability of the information explained a marginal proportion of variance in feeling more confident in the relationship with my physician scores ($R^2 = .093$, $F(3, 33) = 1.128$, $p < .05$) and a significant portion of the variance in enhanced social well-being ($R^2 = .297$, $F(3, 33) = 4.645$, $p < .001$).

Patient-Centered Empowerment Achieved From the Physician Video by Patient Attending Initial Meeting

Evidence-based communication following consumption of 5S information significantly and positively predicted enhanced social well-being (β= 0.570, $p < .1$). Relevance of the information positively predicted increased optimism and control over the future (β= 0.764, $p < .1$). Reliability of the information explained a significant proportion of variance in enhanced social well-being regarding physician scores ($R^2 = .352$, $F(3, 16) = 2.896$, $p < .1$). Relevance of the information explained a significant portion of the variance in increased optimism and control over the future ($R^2 = .531$, $F(3, 16) = 6.034$, $p < .001$).

Patient-Centered Empowerment Achieved From Physician Video by Patient Attending Follow Up Meeting

No significant effects were found for evidence-based engagement following consumption of 5S information for the physician video regarding various patient-centered empowerment in this study.

DISCUSSION

The current study provides a better understanding of patient-centered empowerment and evidence-based engagement in stressful situations brought about by abnormal Pap test results. A period of time between initial test results and clinic visits may increase the likelihood of patients feeling stressed and worried about their futures. To mitigate this, the women entered a specialty clinic where they were offered carefully vetted information, based on Haynes' (2007) 5S construction recommendations. The information considered their test results, related conditions and outcomes. They could choose to view the information in either video form, with a message from the clinic director; or in a dynamic text form. Both formats were pre-loaded on tablet devices.

Data about their use of the tablet-based information was collected and their interactions with physicians in their meetings (either initial or follow-up) were carefully coded. Their questions, answers, and other forms of communication were analyzed to develop engagement scores.

The results demonstrated that in the dynamic text presentation of the 5S structured information, readability predicted more patient-centered engagement in both initial and follow-up meetings between patients and physicians. This finding supports the WHO report suggesting that enhanced patient empowerment requires that barriers be removed considering patient backgrounds. Greater readability removed barriers to understanding. The results also supported another of WHO's recommendations that patient knowledge about their condition and various options is a key element in empowerment. The findings suggest engagement is a key aspect of patient empowerment (Coulter & Ellins, 2007). Table 1 summarizes the dynamic presentation results.

When the information was communicated through the physician-narrated video, the readability construct is better described as understandability to reflect the different form of communication. Similar to the results for the dynamic text presentation, understandability enhanced patient engagement. In physician-patient meetings, both initial and follow-up, better questions and answers were provided and this supported the idea that when patients are better informed in ways that are relevant to their situation, they are more likely to interact in positive ways. Again, higher levels of engagement are important to empowerment (Coulter & Ellins, 2007) and are believed to increase the likelihood for positive health outcomes (Wallerstein, 2006). Table 2 illustrates.

The results of the study demonstrate that engagement was enhanced when the information was more readable or more understandable. It becomes important to better understand the nature of the impact on patient-centered empowerment items. We investigated items described by van Uden-Kraan et al. (2009) related to several different attributes. First, we found that information provided in the dynamic text

Table 1. Dynamic text presentation outcomes

	Engagement	
Dynamic Presentation	**Initial Meeting**	**Follow-up Meeting**
Readable	+	+
Reliability	NS	NS
Relevant	NS	NS

Table 2. Physician video engagement outcomes

	Engagement	
Physician Video	**Initial Meeting**	**Follow-up Meeting**
Understandability	+	+
Reliability	-	NS
Relevant	NS	NS

presentation correlated with more confidence in patient's relationship with her physician in follow-up meetings when the information was considered reliable. This was not the case for those educated with the video presentation. Likewise, when information was considered reliable for either video or text formats, patients felt their social well-being was enhanced in the initial meetings. This feeling persisted into the follow-up meeting for those viewing information in the text format but not in the video format. Finally, those that viewed the dynamic text presentation, when information was considered relevant, were more likely to accept their illness better, were more optimistic and had better feelings of social well-being. All these feelings were present immediately after the initial meeting but were not always the same in follow-up meetings. For those receiving information through the video presentation, those in initial meetings felt increased optimism for the future. Furthermore, we believe the findings show that adequate knowledge is a prerequisite for making informed decisions about vaccination and vaccine policies. For this reason, providing information to improve knowledge is a necessary component of behavioral interventions (Abraham & Michie, 2008). We know that in general, inadequate HPV and HPVV knowledge exists in the public. Therefore, education interventions designed to improve knowledge levels are an important initial step toward increasing vaccination rates among adolescent females. We also believe that educational interventions will influence individuals to accept school-based HPVV programs and other initiatives (Dempsey et al., 2006; Lambert, 2001; Papa et al., 2009).

Our ideas regarding empowerment were influenced by the concept of informed decision making which is about presenting opportunities and encouraging active participation between physician and patient. The current methodology enabled the technology to become an important component of the informed decision making process. Inside the meeting, engagement represented the shared decision making role. In the past, physicians specifically chose an option for a patient. Now, the focus is more on active participation through engagement. The accessibility of knowledge through mobile technology in the waiting room plays an important role in informed decision making (Reychav, Najami, Raban, McHaney, & Azuri, 2018).

Passing on medical information is a complex process. In these complicated situations, there may be a big difference in patient perception and potential for understanding health information. It is important to present it at a level relevant to the patient. While patients exposed to news that indicates they have a severe health issue may find the information reliable and correct, it might scare them or cause them to become passive. So medical information presented to the patient must be controlled and presented at a level that enables the patient to cope. The 5Ss can help structure information in a way that personalizes it to the individual. Saying hard things to a patient with all the details may not increase engagement. The current results indicate this research result.

Patient empowerment efforts are successful in settings that offer a potential for improving health outcomes through greater involvement and education. For instance, patients faced with immediate, life-threatening injury or disease will not have time nor capability to acquire or apply knowledge in a meaningful way. Instead, empowerment must focus on situations that offer patients a setting where their outcomes can be improved with education, communication, and a health care provider partnership.

CONCLUSION

The current study demonstrates that patient-centered empowerment is enhanced through evidence-based engagement in stressful situations brought about by abnormal Pap test results. The study provided educational materials in dynamic text and video formats that were developed using the 5S approach to structure the information to be relevant, reliable and readable for patients. In general, those that understood the information better, were more engaged in consultations with their specialist doctors. Engagement was measured on direct observation using a coding system that kept track of explicitly shared information, requested recommendations, and tacit knowledge during patient-physician interaction. The dynamic text presentation had a greater impact on patient engagement in both initial and follow-up meetings. Other important findings included that those who found the dynamic text relevant had their social well-being, self-esteem, optimism, and acceptance improved in initial meetings. Likewise, those who found the dynamic text reliable were more confident in the relationship with their physician in follow-up meetings and felt their social well-being was improved in both initial and follow-up meetings. Those viewing the video presentation that found it reliable were more likely to have a sense of enhanced social well-being in their initial meetings. Those that found the video reliable experienced increased optimism during their initial meeting.

PRACTICAL IMPLICATIONS

In a practical sense, this study demonstrates that carefully structuring material according to the 5S approach can result in enhanced patient education that makes information more readable, reliable, and relevent to those in stressful medical situations. It further demonstrates that carefully vetted material can be used in waiting rooms to help improve a patient-physician encounter and enhance engagement. This can have a greater impact when someone with knowledge regarding the patients' profiles and backgrounds is involved in creation of the materials. That was the situation in the current study with the clinic manager's direct involvement. Prior research as summarized by Coulter (2012) suggests that engagement leads to improvements in patients' knowledge and understanding of their condition, an increased sense of empowerment, greater ability to cope with the effects of illness, and improved patient satisfaction. In the longer term, these may lead to improved health behaviors and outcomes. This current study supports this view but takes it one step further through direct observation in a real-world clinical setting. In general, we believe that patient education can contribute to social well being. This means that patients may be more likely to encourage others and promote the importance of being vaccinated against HPV. This can have a broader impact in the general population.

THEORETICAL IMPLICATIONS

Current study measured real engagement, not just reported perceptions as in prior research. For instance, Webb et al. (2001) measured empowerment by asking patients about their perceived involvement and subsequent satisfaction with treatment decisions. The current study collected this information through coded direct observation in real world clinical encounters between physicians and patients. The current study also suggests that physician-provided information may either enhance empowerment or result in confusion. Information must be carefully structured to avoid issues. Likewise, information must be vetted to the patient's level of understanding to avoid information overload (Hay et al., 2006; Jotterand et al., 2016; Malhotra et al., 1982).

LIMITATIONS

The current research does have limitations. It was conducted at a single medical facility for women with abnormal Pap test results. The results may not be generalizable to other situations without further research. Likewise, it was dependant on the technology used and the doctors employed by the clinic.

FUTURE RESEARCH

A number of areas for future research exist. Alternate forms of information could be provided to patients. Other meeting approaches and types could be investigated. Age, culture, and other factors could be considered. We believe this study provides a good starting point for additional work in this area.

REFERENCES

Abraham, C., & Michie, S. (2008). A taxonomy of behavior change techniques used in interventions. *Health Psychology*, *27*(3), 379–387. doi:10.1037/0278-6133.27.3.379 PMID:18624603

Barello, S., Graffigna, G., & Vegni, E. (2012). Patient engagement as an emerging challenge for healthcare services: mapping the literature. *Nursing Research and Practice, 2012*. Retrieved from http://www.ncbi.nlm.nih.gov/pmc/articles/PMC3504449/

Blankenburg, R., Hilton, J. F., Yuan, P., Rennke, S., Monash, B., & Harman, S. M., … Huynh, E. (2018). Shared Decision-Making During Inpatient Rounds: Opportunities for Improvement in Patient Engagement and Communication. *Journal of Hospital Medicine*, *13*(7), 453–461. PMID:29401211

Brabin, L., Roberts, S. A., Stretch, R., Baxter, D., Chambers, G., Kitchener, H., & McCann, R. (2008). Uptake of first two doses of human papillomavirus vaccine by adolescent schoolgirls in Manchester: Prospective cohort study. *BMJ (Clinical Research Ed.)*, *336*(7652), 1056–1058. doi:10.1136/bmj.39541.534109.BE PMID:18436917

Brewer, N. T., & Fazekas, K. I. (2007). Predictors of HPV vaccine acceptability: A theory-informed, systematic review. *Preventive Medicine*, *45*(2–3), 107–114. doi:10.1016/j.ypmed.2007.05.013 PMID:17628649

Brotherton, J. M., Pitcher, H., Passaris, I., Deeks, S. L., Webby, R., & Campbell-Lloyd, S., … Watson, M. (2008). Interim estimates of human papillomavirus vaccination coverage in the school-based program in Australia. *Communicable Diseases Intelligence Quarterly Report*, *32*(4), 457–461. PMID:19374275

Carman, K. L., Dardess, P., Maurer, M., Sofaer, S., Adams, K., Bechtel, C., & Sweeney, J. (2013). Patient and family engagement: A framework for understanding the elements and developing interventions and policies. *Health Affairs*, *32*(2), 223–231. doi:10.1377/hlthaff.2012.1133 PMID:23381514

Coulter, A. (2012). Patient engagement-What works? *The Journal of Ambulatory Care Management*, *35*(2), 80–89. doi:10.1097/JAC.0b013e318249e0fd PMID:22415281

Coulter, A., & Ellins, J. (2007). Effectiveness of strategies for informing, educating, and involving patients. *BMJ (Clinical Research Ed.)*, *335*(7609), 24–27. doi:10.1136/bmj.39246.581169.80 PMID:17615222

Dempsey, A. F., Zimet, G. D., Davis, R. L., & Koutsky, L. (2006). Factors that are associated with parental acceptance of human papillomavirus vaccines: A randomized intervention study of written information about HPV. *Pediatrics*, *117*(5), 1486–1493. doi:10.1542/peds.2005-1381 PMID:16651301

Denny-Smith, T., Bairan, A., & Page, M. C. (2006). A survey of female nursing students' knowledge, health beliefs, perceptions of risk, and risk behaviors regarding human papillomavirus and cervical cancer. *Journal of the American Academy of Nurse Practitioners*, *18*(2), 62–69. doi:10.1111/j.1745-7599.2006.00100.x PMID:16460412

Domecq, J. P., Prutsky, G., Elraiyah, T., Wang, Z., Nabhan, M., & Shippee, N. … Erwin, P. (2014). Patient engagement in research: a systematic review. *BMC Health Services Research, 14*(1), 89. Retrieved from https://bmchealthservres.biomedcentral.com/articles/10.1186/1472-6963-14-89

Feste, C., & Anderson, R. M. (1995). Empowerment: From Philosophy to Practice. *Patient Education and Counseling*, *26*(1), 139–144. doi:10.1016/0738-3991(95)00730-N PMID:7494713

Flickinger, T. E., Saha, S., Moore, R. D., & Beach, M. C. (2013). Higher quality communication and relationships are associated with improved patient engagement in HIV care. *Journal of Acquired Immune Deficiency Syndromes*, *63*(3), 362–366. doi:10.1097/QAI.0b013e318295b86a PMID:23591637

Fu, L. Y., Bonhomme, L.-A., Cooper, S. C., Joseph, J. G., & Zimet, G. D. (2014). Educational interventions to increase HPV vaccination acceptance: A systematic review. *Vaccine*, *32*(17), 1901–1920. doi:10.1016/j.vaccine.2014.01.091 PMID:24530401

Future II Study Group. (2007). Quadrivalent vaccine against human papillomavirus to prevent high-grade cervical lesions. *The New England Journal of Medicine*, *356*(19), 1915–1927. doi:10.1056/NEJMoa061741 PMID:17494925

Garland, S. M., Hernandez-Avila, M., Wheeler, C. M., Perez, G., Harper, D. M., Leodolter, S., ... Koutsky, L. A. (2007). Quadrivalent vaccine against human papillomavirus to prevent anogenital diseases. *The New England Journal of Medicine*, *356*(19), 1928–1943. doi:10.1056/NEJMoa061760 PMID:17494926

Gibson, C. H. (1991). A Concept Analysis of Empowerment. *Journal of Advanced Nursing, 16*(3), 354–361. doi:10.1111/j.1365-2648.1991.tb01660.x PMID:2037742

Glanz, K., Rimer, B. K., & Viswanath, K. (2008). *Health behavior and health education: theory, research, and practice*. Hoboken, NJ: John Wiley & Sons.

Gruman, J., Rovner, M. H., French, M. E., Jeffress, D., Sofaer, S., Shaller, D., & Prager, D. J. (2010). From patient education to patient engagement: Implications for the field of patient education. *Patient Education and Counseling, 78*(3), 350–356. doi:10.1016/j.pec.2010.02.002 PMID:20202780

Hall, M. T., Simms, K. T., Lew, J.-B., Smith, M. A., Brotherton, J. M. L., Saville, M., ... Canfell, K. (2019). The projected timeframe until cervical cancer elimination in Australia: A modelling study. *The Lancet Public Health, 4*(1), e19–e27. doi:10.1016/S2468-2667(18)30183-X PMID:30291040

Hay, J., Coups, E., & Ford, J. (2006). Predictors of Perceived Risk for Colon Cancer in a National Probability Sample in the United States. *Journal of Health Communication, 11*(S1), 71–92. doi:10.1080/10810730600637376 PMID:16641075

Haynes, B. (2007). Of studies, syntheses, synopses, summaries, and systems: The "5S" evolution of information services for evidence-based healthcare decisions. *Evidence-Based Nursing, 10*(1), 6–7. doi:10.1136/ebn.10.1.6 PMID:17218282

Herzog, T. J., Huh, W. K., Downs, L. S., Smith, J. S., & Monk, B. J. (2008). Initial lessons learned in HPV vaccination. *Gynecologic Oncology, 109*(2), S4–S11. doi:10.1016/j.ygyno.2008.01.018 PMID:18482557

Holcomb, B., Bailey, J. M., Crawford, K., & Ruffin, M. T. (2004). Adults' knowledge and behaviors related to human papillomavirus infection. *The Journal of the American Board of Family Practice, 17*(1), 26–31. doi:10.3122/jabfm.17.1.26 PMID:15014049

Ingledue, K., Cottrell, R., & Bernard, A. (2004). College women's knowledge, perceptions, and preventive behaviors regarding human papillomavirus infection and cervical cancer. *American Journal of Health Studies, 19*(1), 28.

Jain, N., Euler, G. L., Shefer, A., Lu, P., Yankey, D., & Markowitz, L. (2009). Human papillomavirus (HPV) awareness and vaccination initiation among women in the United States, National Immunization Survey: Adult 2007. *Preventive Medicine, 48*(5), 426–431. doi:10.1016/j.ypmed.2008.11.010 PMID:19100762

Jotterand, F., Amodio, A., & Elger, B. S. (2016). Patient education as empowerment and self-rebiasing. *Medicine, Health Care, and Philosophy, 19*(4), 553–561. doi:10.100711019-016-9702-9 PMID:27179973

Kahn, J. A., Slap, G. B., Bernstein, D. I., Tissot, A. M., Kollar, L. M., Hillard, P. A., & Rosenthal, S. L. (2007). Personal meaning of human papillomavirus and Pap test results in adolescent and young adult women. *Health Psychology, 26*(2), 192–200. doi:10.1037/0278-6133.26.2.192 PMID:17385971

Kester, L. M., Shedd-Steele, R. B., Dotson-Roberts, C. A., Smith, J., & Zimet, G. D. (2014). The effects of a brief educational intervention on human papillomavirus knowledge and intention to initiate HPV vaccination in 18--26 year old young adults. *Gynecologic Oncology, 132*, S9–S12. doi:10.1016/j.ygyno.2013.12.033 PMID:24384459

Lambert, E. C. (2001). College students' knowledge of human papillomavirus and effectiveness of a brief educational intervention. *The Journal of the American Board of Family Practice*, *14*(3), 178–183. PMID:11355049

Malhotra, N. K., Jain, A. K., & Lagakos, S. W. (1982). The Information Overload Controversy: An Alternative Viewpoint. *Journal of Marketing*, *46*(2), 27–37. doi:10.1177/002224298204600204

Markman, M. (2019). 16% HPV Vaccination Rate Among US Adolescents "Inadequate." Retrieved from https://www.medscape.com/viewarticle/908885

McCaffery, K., & Irwig, L. (2005). Australian women's needs and preferences for information about human papillomavirus in cervical screening. *Journal of Medical Screening*, *12*(3), 134–141. doi:10.1258/0969141054855238 PMID:16156944

McCree, D. H., Sharpe, P. A., Brandt, H. M., & Robertson, R. (2006). Preferences for sources of information about abnormal Pap tests and HPV in women tested for HPV. *Preventive Medicine*, *43*(3), 165–170. doi:10.1016/j.ypmed.2006.04.001 PMID:16701815

Mehta, P., Sharma, M., & Lee, R. C. (2014). Designing and evaluating a health belief model-based intervention to increase intent of HPV vaccination among college males. *International Quarterly of Community Health Education*, *34*(1), 101–117. doi:10.2190/IQ.34.1.h PMID:24366025

Narayan, D. (2005). Conceptual Framework and Methodological Challenges. In D. Narayan (Ed.), *Measuring Empowerment* (pp. 3–38). Washington, D.C.: The World Bank.

National Cancer Institute. (2018). Cervix Uteri Cancer.

Ng, J. H., Sobel, K., Roth, L., Byron, S., Lindley, M. C., & Stokley, S. (2017). Supporting human papillomavirus vaccination in adolescents: Perspectives from commercial and medicaid health plans. *Journal of Public Health Management and Practice: JPHMP*, *23*(3), 283–290. doi:10.1097/PHH.0000000000000440 PMID:27798527

Niccolai, L. M., & Hansen, C. E. (2015). Practice-and community-based interventions to increase human papillomavirus vaccine coverage: A systematic review. *JAMA Pediatrics*, *169*(7), 686–692. doi:10.1001/jamapediatrics.2015.0310 PMID:26010507

Paiva, A. L., Lipschitz, J. M., Fernandez, A. C., Redding, C. A., & Prochaska, J. O. (2014). Evaluation of the acceptability and feasibility of a computer-tailored intervention to increase human papillomavirus vaccination among young adult women. *Journal of American College Health*, *62*(1), 32–38. doi:10.1080/07448481.2013.843534 PMID:24313694

Papa, D., Simas, T. A. M., Reynolds, M., & Melnitsky, H. (2009). Assessing the role of education in women's knowledge and acceptance of adjunct high-risk human Papillomavirus testing for cervical cancer screening. *Journal of Lower Genital Tract Disease*, *13*(2), 66–71. doi:10.1097/LGT.0b013e31818a53f0 PMID:19387125

Perkins, R. B., & Clark, J. A. (2012). What affects human papillomavirus vaccination rates? A qualitative analysis of providers' perceptions. *Women's Health Issues*, *22*(4), e379–e386. doi:10.1016/j.whi.2012.04.001 PMID:22609253

Reiter, P. L., Brewer, N. T., Gottlieb, S. L., McRee, A.-L., & Smith, J. S. (2009). Parents' health beliefs and HPV vaccination of their adolescent daughters. *Social Science & Medicine*, *69*(3), 475–480. doi:10.1016/j.socscimed.2009.05.024 PMID:19540642

Reiter, P. L., Stubbs, B., Panozzo, C. A., Whitesell, D., & Brewer, N. T. (2011). HPV and HPV vaccine education intervention: Effects on parents, healthcare staff, and school staff. *Cancer Epidemiology and Prevention Biomarkers*, *20*(11), 2354–2361. doi:10.1158/1055-9965.EPI-11-0562 PMID:21949110

Reychav, I., McHaney, R., Zhu, L., & Moshonov, R. (2018). Media Impact on Patient Empowerment in Complicated Medical Situations: A TREO Talk Paper. In *Twenty-fourth Americas Conference on Information System*. New Orleans, LA: AIS. Retrieved from https://aisel.aisnet.org/amcis2018/TREOsPDS/Presentations/8/

Reychav, I., Najami, I., Raban, D., McHaney, R., & Azuri, J. (2018). The impact of media type on shared decision processes in third-age populations. *International Journal of Medical Informatics*, *112*, 45–58. doi:10.1016/j.ijmedinf.2018.01.004 PMID:29500021

Reychav, I., Parush, A., McHaney, R., Hazan, M., & Moshonov, R. (2018). The use of mobile technology in waiting rooms to leverage women's empowerment: A conceptual context. *Health Informatics Journal*, *24*(3), 277–292. doi:10.1177/1460458216671561

Rimer, B., Harper, H., & Witte, O. (2014). *Accelerating HPV vaccine uptake: urgency for action to prevent cancer. A report to the President of the United States from the President's Cancer Panel*. Bethesda, MD: National Cancer Institute.

Roberts, K. J. (1999). Patient Empowerment in the United States: A Critical Commentary. *Health Expectations*, *2*(2), 82–92. doi:10.1046/j.1369-6513.1999.00048.x PMID:11281882

Rosenthal, S. L., Weiss, T. W., Zimet, G. D., Ma, L., Good, M. B., & Vichnin, M. D. (2011). Predictors of HPV vaccine uptake among women aged 19--26: Importance of a physician's recommendation. *Vaccine*, *29*(5), 890–895. doi:10.1016/j.vaccine.2009.12.063 PMID:20056186

Straus, S., & Haynes, R. B. (2009). Managing evidence-based knowledge: The need for reliable, relevant and readable resources. *Canadian Medical Association Journal*, *180*(9), 942–945. doi:10.1503/cmaj.081697 PMID:19398741

van Uden-Kraan, C. F., Drossaert, C. H., Taal, E., Shaw, B. R., Seydel, E. R., & van de Laar, M. A. (2008). Empowering Processes and Outcomes of Participation in Online Support Groups for Patients with Breast Cancer, Arthritis, Or Fibromyalgia. *Qualitative Health Research*, *18*(3), 405–417. doi:10.1177/1049732307313429 PMID:18235163

Van Uden-Kraan, C. F., Drossaert, C. H. C., Taal, E., Seydel, E. R., & van de Laar, M. A. F. J. (2009). Participation in online patient support groups endorses patients' empowerment. *Patient Education and Counseling*, *74*(1), 61–69. doi:10.1016/j.pec.2008.07.044 PMID:18778909

Waller, J., McCaffery, K., Forrest, S., Szarewski, A., Cadman, L., & Wardle, J. (2003). Awareness of human papillomavirus among women attending a well woman clinic. *Sexually Transmitted Infections*, *79*(4), 320–322. doi:10.1136ti.79.4.320 PMID:12902585

Wallerstein, N. (2006). *What is the evidence on effectiveness of empowerment to improve health?* Copenhagen Denmark World Health Organization [WHO] Regional Office for Europe Health Evidence Network. Retrieved from https://www.popline.org/node/175634

Warren, T., & Ebel, C. (2005). Counseling the patient who has genital herpes or genital human papillomavirus infection. *Infectious Disease Clinics*, *19*(2), 459–476. PMID:15963883

Webb, D. G., Horne, R., & Pinching, A. J. (2001). Treatment-Related Empowerment: Preliminary Evaluation of a New Measure in Patients with Advanced HIV Disease. *International Journal of STD & AIDS*, *12*(2), 103–107. doi:10.1258/0956462011916875 PMID:11236098

World Health Organization. (2009). *WHO guidelines on hand hygiene in health care: A summary. First global patient safety challenge. Clean care is safer care.* Geneva, Switzerland: World Health Organization. Retrieved from http://www.who.int/gpsc/5may/tools/who_guidelines-handhygiene_summary.pdf

World Health Organization. (2016). *Human Papillomavirus (HPV) and Cervical Cancer Fact Sheet.* Retrieved from http://www.who.int/mediacentre/factsheets/fs380/en/

Zimmerman, M. A. (1990). Taking Aim on Empowerment Research: On the Distinction between Individual and Psychological Conceptions. *American Journal of Community Psychology*, *18*(1), 169–177. doi:10.1007/BF00922695

ADDITIONAL READING

Anderson, R. M., & Funnell, M. M. (2010). Patient empowerment: Myths and misconceptions. *Patient Education and Counseling*, *79*(3), 277–282. doi:10.1016/j.pec.2009.07.025 PMID:19682830

Balapour, A., Reychav, I., Sabherwal, R., & Azuri, J. (2019). Mobile technology identity and self-efficacy: Implications for the adoption of clinically supported mobile health apps. *International Journal of Information Management*, *49*, 58–68. doi:10.1016/j.ijinfomgt.2019.03.005

Holmström, I., & Röing, M. (2010). The relation between patient-centeredness and patient empowerment: A discussion on concepts. *Patient Education and Counseling*, *79*(2), 167–172. doi:10.1016/j.pec.2009.08.008 PMID:19748203

KEY TERMS AND DEFINITIONS

3Rs: Measures for quality of the information including readability, reliability, and relevance. **5S**: This is a framework that organizes evidence-based information and it includes: primary studies at the bottom, systematic organization of the studies called syntheses, followed by synopses, concise summaries and finally details about systems.

Empowerment: Implies power or authority is provided to an individual.

HPV Vaccine (HPVV): A vaccine meant to prevent HPV. It has been available globally since 2006 and is recommended by the World Health Organization and the Centers for Disease Control and Prevention.

Human Papillomavirus (HPV): A common virus known to cause potentially fatal diseases such as, vaginal, vulvar, anal, and oropharyngeal cancers. It is responsible for over 600k new cases of cervical and genital cancer worldwide each year.

Patient-Centered Empowerment: While very similar to patient empowerment, patient-centered empowerment takes the process further and seeks to ensure the techniques used focus on the patient rather than ease of the provider team.

Patient Empowerment: A process to help patients gain (or regain) control over issues that impact their healthcare with a sense of confidence.

Patient Engagement: Represents the combination of medical patient's knowledge, capabilities, skills, and inclination to collaborate in their healthcare management via communications with their care givers. Engaged patients want to be healthier and are willing to work with those seeking to improve their health.

Sensitive Clinical Settings: A health care facility that caters to medical treatment that could cause embarrassment to patients due to the intimate nature of their condition.

Section 3
Cases With Empowerment Through IT

Chapter 10
Using Technology to Empower People With Multiple Sclerosis (MS) to Make Shared Decisions About Managing Their Own Healthcare:
A UK Case Study

Helen King
Independent Researcher, UK

Darina M. Slattery
University of Limerick, Ireland

ABSTRACT

In 2014, the UK National Health Service (NHS) 'Five Year Forward View' plan set out key objectives to reform the NHS, which included empowering the population as a whole (particularly those with long-term health conditions) to take more responsibility for managing their own healthcare and introducing initiatives to use technology to improve services and reduce costs. The "Long Term Plan" explains how the 2014 initiatives will be further developed. This chapter presents a review of literature on digital health information and information usability. It presents the key findings from a mixed methods study that explored how people with MS (PwMS) access and use health digital information when trying to manage their MS. While the study found that there is much good quality digital health information available for PwMS, and that this facilitates shared decisions, some necessary information is still missing. The chapter concludes with recommendations for digital health information providers.

DOI: 10.4018/978-1-7998-0047-7.ch010

INTRODUCTION

The Internet has changed the way many people around the world search for information about healthcare. Governments, healthcare providers, and agencies have been quick to move to providing a range of digital health services and resources, which continue to expand at a rapid pace. Eysenbach (2001, para. 3) offered the following definition of e-health:

e-health is an emerging field in the intersection of medical informatics, public health and business, referring to health services and information delivered or enhanced through the Internet and related technologies.

Rapid developments since Eysenbach's definition mean that there is now a confusing array of seemingly interchangeable terms used to describe health information that is provided on a digital platform (examples include telemedicine, digi-health, health informatics, and e-health). The increasing use of mobile devices has itself generated several new terms (such as health-app and m-health).

In this chapter, the term "digital health information" is used to refer to health information that can be accessed online or in some other electronic format.

This chapter will provide some background to multiple sclerosis (MS) and to various National Health Service (NHS) policies and initiatives, before discussing some literature on digital and health literacies and the usability of information. Finally, the chapter will present findings from a case study that explored if, and how, people with MS (PwMS) use technology to access health information and engage in shared decision making with clinicians. The chapter will conclude with recommendations for digital health information providers and suggestions for future research.

BACKGROUND TO MULTIPLE SCLEROSIS

MS is a neurological condition of the central nervous system. The name derives from the scars (sclerosis) that usually form in multiple sites of the nerves in the brain and spinal cord. It is an autoimmune disease, which means that the body's immune system attacks itself instead of attacking germs or infections. In MS, these attacks damage myelin, which coats the nerves in the central nervous system. The damaged nerves cause a wide range of physical and cognitive symptoms in people with MS (PwMS).

There is no universally accepted theory defining the cause of MS and there is no cure for it. MS is not hereditary, contagious, or infectious. Worldwide, there are many clinical studies and trials researching potential causes of and treatments for MS.

Twice as many women have MS than men (MS Trust, 2019). The typical age of onset and diagnosis is 20-40. It is rare in children, but childhood cases have increased in recent years (perhaps due to better diagnostic technology).

There is no universal consensus on how many different types of MS there are, and neurologists continue to debate the criteria for diagnosing the different types of MS, particularly benign MS. However, the National Health Service (NHS), MS Trust, and MS Society in the UK agree that there are four types of MS: relapsing remitting (RR), secondary progressive (SP), primary progressive (PP), and benign MS.

Although there are some patterns and trends in MS and its progression, the unique and diverse course of MS for each individual means that providing relevant information and services to support PwMS can be a challenge.

MS is a long-term health condition. The life expectancy of those with MS is improving as new drugs and treatments for it are developed. This means that many people will live with MS for most of their adult lives and need different types of information to help them understand and manage their MS as it changes, they grow older, and new treatments emerge.

The MS International Federation's (MSIF) 2013 Atlas of MS recorded that 2.3 million people around the world have been diagnosed with MS. This shows a 2.4% increase in the number of cases of MS since the previous record was published in 2008. The MSIF findings show that MS is most prevalent in North America and Europe.

The UK has one of the highest prevalence rates of MS per level of population in the world (MS Trust, 2019). Despite this prevalence, there is no mandatory NHS register for MS and no comprehensive data on the exact number of people living with MS in the UK and the types of MS that they have. The lack of accurate data has serious implications for healthcare planning and provision, policy making, and assessing the economic impact of MS in the UK. The MS Society and University of Swansea established a UK register in 2011 as part of a collaborative study. Although the data has grown since its establishment, some PwMS and clinicians are unaware of it, or prefer not to register details in it.

McKenzie et al. (2013) conducted a descriptive study based on the General Practitioner's Research Database (GPRD) to determine the number of people living with MS in the UK between 1990 and 2010. They concluded that in 2010, 126,669 people in the UK had MS. The study also reported a 2.4% increase in the number of people diagnosed each year and that people with MS were living longer. In 2016, the MS Society conducted further research using the McKenzie et al. methodology and incorporated new population data from the Office of National Statistics. Their 'MS in the UK' report concluded that in January 2016, 107,740 people in the UK had MS and 89,030 lived in England. The MS Society's totals are lower as the McKenzie et al. report included *possible* as well as confirmed cases of MS. However, the Society's data also confirms the number of people diagnosed and living with MS is increasing each year in England.

HEALTH POLICIES IN THE UK

The NHS was one of the early adopters of digital health information and continues to pioneer and trial a wide range of digital health projects. The NHS has ambitious plans to increase the use of technology in healthcare (NHS, 2014). In 2014, the UK's House of Commons Health Select Committee advised that the management of long-term health conditions (LTCs) was one of the greatest challenges to the NHS in England. Their 2014 report found that 70% of healthcare expenditure in England was on the 15 million people living with LTCs (House of Commons, 2014). With the expectation that this number would rise to 18 million by 2025, the Committee called for an urgent review of the co-ordination and management of this care and called for a systematic and cultural shift towards greater personalization of healthcare and services.

Consequently, NHS England established its 'Five Year Forward View' (2014) project to implement the required changes. The project set many targets for the NHS including targets for improving and integrating health and social care models, reducing hospital and particularly accident and emergency admissions, and ensuring availability of sufficient staff in the NHS trained to support the significant changes that the plan will introduce.

A key provision in the plan was to empower people with LTCs to manage their healthcare by:

- Improving both the information, and access to information, for those with ltcs
- Improving education for those with ltcs to help them manage their condition, make treatment choices, and use technology in healthcare
- Increasing the use of technology to allow all patients to access (and input into) their own digital health records.

Simultaneously, NHS England was charged with making significant financial savings across its services and reducing expenditure on LTCs. It believed the targets it set out (in 'Five Year Forward View') would change the management and care of people with LTCs, lead to improved services, and reduced costs. For example, people with diabetes would spend less time in hospital if they learned to recognize and deal with their insulin problems quickly.

The MS 'Forward View' (MS Trust, 2016a, p. 6) acknowledged that the success of the 'Five Year Forward View' project relies on organizations for specific LTCs (e.g. the MS charities) supporting the targets to make them a reality. The report identified a number of MS specific issues that must be addressed to *empower all people with MS* to access information and contribute to managing their care. The MS Trust argues that the current provision of funding, information, care and services for PwMS is heavily biased to relapsing remitting MS (RR), to the detriment of other types of MS (secondary progressive SP, primary progressive PP, and benign MS). Worryingly, a survey undertaken by the MS Trust (2016b) found that "people with progressive MS, *who make up almost half of the total MS population in the UK*, are seeing their key specialist health professionals far less often than people with relapsing remitting MS, and often failing to receive the proactive, continuing care that can make all the difference to living well with the disease" (p.2, emphasis added). There is no typical course of MS, but many people move from RR to SP and PP over time. PwMS are now living longer, so more of them are likely to develop one of the progressive forms of the disease and will need to make decisions about managing the changes it brings. During the progressive stages of MS, there are less relapses, but disability increases, which means that people with progressive forms of MS have vastly different information, care and treatment needs to those with RR MS. The bias towards RR MS results in unequal access to the personalized information needed to meet the 'Five Year Forward View' objectives, and limits the potential for people with *other* types of MS to engage in shared decision making, as the authors will explore later in this chapter.

In 2017, the NHS 'Next Steps on the Five Year Forward View' interim report provided a "balanced but not comprehensive" summary of progress towards the objectives in the original 'Five Year Forward View' plan (NHS, 2017, p. 9). The report (favorably) summarized a number of successful initiatives that were underway to meet some of the financial targets and improvements in integrating health and social care services to provide more individualized care to patients.

The interim report also set out the next steps in the phased technology program of work aimed at "simplifying access to care, in the most appropriate location, while supporting people in managing their own health" (2017, p. 64). It focused on making more services available online to patients, increasing patients' access to their own medical records online, and the introduction of NHS approved library of health apps to help patients manage their own conditions. Many of the technology and digital projects, set out in the 2014 and 2017 reports, have been taken forward by NHS Digital, a public body in the Department of Health, which was launched in April 2017.

The 'Long Term Plan' (LTP) provides examples of some of the successful digital projects that have been completed since 2014 (NHS, 2019). However, it acknowledges that there is still much work to do to reach the 'digital first' options it plans to implement for all types of patient contact with the NHS. Eventually, NHS patients will be provided with digital options for everything from booking a GP appointment, accessing their own records, ordering prescriptions, to consultations with specialists. The 'digital first' agenda will reduce costs, take much of the complex administration out of the NHS, and better enable staff to focus on clinical care.

Since 2014, NHS Digital has driven technology projects, which are now embedded in the NHS. It has:

- Led on improvements to the NHS website (formerly known as NHS Choices and NHS Direct)
- Introduced Artificial Intelligence (AI) into the NHS to help with clinical decision making and triage activities
- Led on integrating patient NHS records and care plans to ensure healthcare professionals and patients have access to their full records
- Overseen the development of the NHS apps library. The library, now part of the NHS website, hosts 70 approved apps targeting a range of conditions (e.g. anxiety) and general topics (e.g. how to access health data). There are no MS specific apps in the library, but some apps may help to manage some of the symptoms of MS (e.g. anxiety). Many apps have been developed in association with charities and patient organizations, which has been welcomed by the Patient Information Forum (PIF, 2019).

The LTP contains bold statements setting out the ambition to transform health and social care by improving access to NHS digital tools. It aims to become a "trustworthy" source of information and health apps (p. 93). Perhaps because of previous criticisms from the Kings Fund, Patient Information Forum, and health charities, the LTP plan includes a new objective to work with the wider health sector and voluntary groups and individuals as it takes forward the digital agenda. This objective has been welcomed by the PIF (2019) and Kings Fund (2019), although both organizations express concerns about the lack of funding and resources needed to deliver the work to schedule.

The commitment to involve patients, their carers, and lay members of the public in NHS projects was initiated in 2014, and continues to expand across a range of projects and technology developments to ensure products better meet user needs. The LTP states that by 2020, every person with a long-term health condition will be supported to manage it, by interoperability of data, monitoring devices, and home use technology. Furthermore, all secondary care providers must be fully digitized by 2024 to support their patients and ensure health and social care records are seamlessly integrated.

The Patient Information Forum and the Kings Fund have long criticized the Government's record on delivering health technology reform projects on time and within budget. The Kings Fund (2019) believes there are still a number of risks that will affect delivery of the LTP digital objectives, which include:

- The end of the technology funding in 2021
- The ongoing delay of deadlines for digitization (for health and care organizations, the deadline has moved from 2020 to 2024)
- Severe staff shortages across the NHS
- High dependence on the digital infrastructure (also acknowledged in the LTP itself)
- Lack of training and capacity building for staff and patients to use and understand technology.

PwMS now have access to a vast range of regulated and unregulated digital healthcare information on the internet (a Google search for 'multiple sclerosis information' on March 6, 2019 gave about 41, 000,000 results). Given the unprecedented pace of change, PwMS face significant choices about the quality, validity, and reliability of information available and need to determine if it can empower them to participate in making decisions about their healthcare.

DIGITAL HEALTH INFORMATION

This section will present some relevant literature on digital and health literacies, the usability of digital health resources, the information and communication needs of patients and healthcare providers, and technology for patient empowerment and shared decision making.

Digital and Health Literacies

It is important to consider the impact of making more health information available online to all potential users. 'The Real Digital Divide?' (Good Things Foundation, 2017) analyzed the level of access to the internet in the UK and found that 15.2 million people are either non-users or limited users of the internet. 11.5 million users lack basic digital skills. The report's sociodemographic data shows that those with limited or no access to the internet are likely to be from disadvantaged groups, with lower levels of employment, income, and education. 47.7% of the low or non-user group had a disability or long-term health condition.

There is no universal definition of health literacy. However, Health Literacy UK (2019) describe it as "the personal characteristics and social resources needed for individuals and communities to access, understand, appraise and use information and services to make decisions about health".

The ability to not just understand, but to act on information about health, is becoming increasingly important as the NHS (and other providers) implement policies that require the population at large to be active participants in their own healthcare. Health Literacy UK report that England has very poor levels of functional health literacy, and that 43% of the adult population cannot understand much of the health information provided. If the health information includes numerical information, this rises to 61%. This figure is significant as it implies that 61% of people may not be able to follow a prescription dosage correctly, which is not only a danger to health, but costs the NHS millions of pounds in wasted medications each year. As health information is increasingly provided in digital format, the population needs to become digitally literate to access and search for information.

Moccia et al. (2015) found that people with MS are very active users of digital health information. However, their study analyzing the readability of 10 MS websites in the UK and US found that most websites failed to meet the US Institute of Health Readability Guidelines and were therefore difficult for PwMS to read and use. They concluded that PwMS would need help from clinicians to interpret some of the complex MS digital information provided. By contrast, Lejbkowicz et al. (2010) found that many PwMS do not use the internet at all and argued that other forms of health information must be provided to avoid disadvantaging this group. Marrie et al. (2014) conducted literacy tests with 13,020 PwMS and concluded that most (68%) performed well in both digital health and functional literacy tests. They noted that there is a need to expand research to cover the less literate PwMS. Importantly, they also state that research is needed to establish links between health literacy and adherence to healthcare treatment plans.

Patients will only make use of new NHS services, such as information sent by email and telephone support lines, if it is presented in a format that is appropriate for their needs and clearly signposted to them (Patient Information Forum, 2018). The Patient Information Forum (PIF) report stresses that the literacy issues identified by Health Literacy UK must not be ignored if the benefits of new NHS digital services are to be accessible to all.

The Usability of Digital Health Resources

At a time when traditional healthcare systems struggle to cope with demand for services, providing digital health information and data can be an effective cost-saving strategy for governments and a source of revenue for commercial providers. However, as websites become larger and more complex, the cost of building, testing, and maintaining their infrastructure also increases, and the complexity of some products means they can fail to meet their users' needs. In addition, many users now expect to access digital health information from different types of devices at any time of day and from phones when mobile (m-health). Additional usability testing is required to ensure information design for m-health meets user expectations and engages the audience.

Usability and readability are particularly important for digital health information, as there is potential for harm, and even danger, if users cannot locate and understand information about their healthcare.

Studies by Chaudhry et al. (2006) and Hinchcliffe and Mummery (2008) found that lack of user engagement in the design of health websites reduced their effectiveness as they failed to provide relevant information to users.

Powell et al. (2011) agreed website designers must understand how and why users search for digital health information. A mixed method survey of 792 users categorized reasons for using the NHS Direct website (the forerunner of the current NHS Choices), and found that people wanted to find trustworthy information that they could use to develop their own understanding and to prepare for discussions with clinicians. Powell et al. concluded the NHS Direct website could attribute its high usability satisfaction to the NHS commitment to user engagement in the design.

Changes in both technology and the type of information presented on health websites means users now have more choice of information than ever. Ziebland et al. (2016) conducted an extensive study examining whether usability of websites is improved if they include patient experience (Pex) information. Although their study concluded Pex information was valuable to many (and it is indeed now a common feature on many health websites), the MS sub-group within the study reported major concerns that sharing such information could frighten many PwMS and provide a very negative user experience. This study, in particular, highlights how different users may have very different preferences for information. Dennison et al. (2016) conducted a small qualitative study of PwMS and identified that some PwMS prefer not to know about their full prognosis or likely outcomes. Thorne (2009) questions the trend for using experience narratives to explain health issues. She notes it can be an effective communication method, but needs to be used carefully with qualitative research into the validity of the narrative and its potential impact on readers.

Synott et al. (2016) found that relatively little research had been conducted to establish what exactly MS users need from digital health information. They conducted a qualitative research project investigating how PwMS find and use information. They noted that while some PwMS felt empowered to search for information, others could find the search results upsetting. Participants expressed a need for information about the *practicalities* of living with MS (which was not always available) as well as medical data. Over time, participants developed strategies for identifying trustworthy sources of information, and became more selective in their searches than they were at diagnosis.

Kopke et al. (2014) carried out a study reviewing the importance and preferred formats of information for PwMS in 10 different treatment trials. They found that the information provided resulted in PwMS learning and retaining more about MS medical *issues* than managing the practical aspects of life with MS. Unlike studies by Synott et al. (2014), Thorne (2009), and Ziebland (2016), Kopke et al. found that information for PwMS did not cause any negative or upsetting reactions.

Marrie et al. (2013) also studied the information preferences of 8,464 PwMS in a review of MS projects around the world. Their study found that the three most trusted sources of MS specific information in the cohorts of PwMS were doctors, the internet, and patient advocacy groups. Preferences for the format and perceived quality of the information varied, with the age and sociodemographic of the participants affecting their preferences.

Colombo et al. (2014) conducted qualitative research into how PwMS and their families search for and use online information. They reported an increase in use of social media sites (e.g. Facebook, YouTube, and MS Association Discussion Forums) to find information, particularly among the younger cohorts of PwMS. They noted participants trusted sources affiliated to MS associations more than other sites (these sources were often moderated) and included links to further relevant information endorsed by the associations. Riel et al. (2017) studied the impact of internet searches carried out by 936 patients and their GPs and found that two thirds of patients search the internet to prepare for consultations with clinicians, and often did so to be better informed and to facilitate discussions with their clinicians. In this study, clinicians did not feel threatened by internet information and some clinicians reported that relatives' opinions had more impact on patients than online search results.

Sbaffi and Rowley (2017) conducted a systematic literature review of health information to identify factors that affect users' perception of the trustworthiness and credibility of web-based information. They found that the authority of the website owner and content authors, clear design, and interactive features had a positive impact on the user, and that advertisements had a negative impact. This study, and those by Colombo et al. (2014) and Marrie et al. (2014), agree that there is merit in conducting more research into understanding how PwMS select, use, and evaluate the credibility of online information.

The Information and Communication Needs of Patients and Healthcare Providers

The PIF report (2018) identifies key times when patients need good communication with their healthcare professionals and information to help them manage their long-term condition. The report stresses that information at diagnosis is crucial, yet notes that many patients were not provided with any information at diagnosis. Others were given information they could not understand. Diagnosis can stress and overwhelm patients but the combination of patient appropriate information and strong communication from healthcare professionals can mitigate this to some extent.

Edwards et al. (2008) carried out a qualitative study of PwMS in the UK and found that 43% of PwMS had not been given any information at diagnosis. However, when PwMS were provided with information and clinicians explained it to them, it reduced patient anxiety and depression. Furthermore, not only did support from healthcare professionals help PwMS through the often-lengthy diagnosis stage, it set the tone for how many people coped with MS in the longer term and how they sought information and communicated with their healthcare professionals in future.

Solari (2014) conducted an informal literature review of the experiences of people at the time of their MS diagnosis. She also noted that the process for making a definitive MS diagnosis can be lengthy and cause anxiety and stress for the patients. In interventions where PwMS were provided with additional clinical communications, stress and anxiety were reduced.

Thorne et al. (2004) also reported that communications with healthcare professionals can shape the way PwMS perceive treatment options and self-management. In their qualitative study, PwMS felt dependent on healthcare professionals for information. When information was too generalized, further communications with healthcare professionals were crucial to relate it to the specific needs of each person – this was particularly important to manage fear at diagnosis.

The PIF report explains that over time information needs change for those living with long-term conditions, to the point where patients often consider themselves experts on their condition. Corrie and Finch (2015) report that the expert patient will demand better information and communication from the NHS in future and is willing to use technology to both seek information and communicate with healthcare professionals. Bodeheimer et al. (2002) recognized there is a paradigm when both the patient and doctor are both experts: the doctor is an expert in medicine, but the patient is the expert in how their medical condition affects their life. Good communication between both parties with doctors adding information to the knowledge the patient has already gained, can lead to good shared decision making, better adherence to treatment plans, and patient empowerment.

Technology for Patient Empowerment and Shared Decision Making

Shared decision making (SDM) is driving health authorities to introduce SDM-specific programs and initiatives and is shaping the ways clinicians are trained to communicate with patients. In some countries (notably the US), technology is enabling clinicians and patients to use new communication and monitoring applications to share decision making and to empower patients to take more responsibility for their own healthcare.

The European MS Platform's Code of Good Practice in MS (2014) calls for MS organizations in all European states to provide appropriate information to empower PwMS to take part in the decision making "that ultimately affects their lives" (p. 9). Increasing SDM between patients and clinicians is one of the key objectives of the NHS 'Five Year Forward View' (2014).

There are many benefits and challenges associated with shared decision making. Corrie and Finch (2015) found that patients engaged in shared decisions are more likely to adhere to treatment plans and need less urgent care, thus contributing to cost savings. Ruddell et al. (2016) recommended the use of an MS SDM healthcare app, which helped PwMS monitor and track aspects of living with MS. The app facilitated communication between clinicians and PwMS and led to improved management of fatigue, as PwMS and clinicians could identify and manage fatigue triggers.

Heesen et al. (2007) noted the potential for good health outcomes and improved patient clinician relationships, *provided* decisions were made jointly. McMullan (2006) found that some clinicians felt threatened by the SDM process as it enables patients to challenge their decisions; other clinicians felt frustrated that patients brought digital health information to meetings, which contradicted their clinical decisions. The 'Implementing Shared Decision Making' report (Health Foundation, 2013) recommends ensuring staff buy in to the SDM projects so that they do not feel threatened if their decisions are challenged and concludes that most patients need support from healthcare staff to make decisions; in other words, information alone is not enough. Kvedar et al. (2015) reviewed the impact of a wide range of apps and telemedicine products in the US and noted that successful products ensure patient and clinician input in design and support communications for SDM, rather than trying to replace face-to-face appointments and meetings.

Heesen et al. (2007) reviewed the role preferences of PwMS when making decisions with doctors. They found that the majority (79%) of PwMS wanted to make shared and informed decisions, and have an active role in the decision. However, others did not want to take part in SDM at all; some preferred to have an autonomous role and make their own decision, and others wanted their doctors to have a paternalistic role and make decisions for them. Heesen et al. found that PwMS were more likely to adhere to treatment plans when their preferences were accommodated.

There are also times when PwMS prefer not to know at all about prognosis and likely outcomes of their MS, particularly if the outcomes are deteriorating health and disability (Dennison et al. 2006). Although, prognostication techniques offer opportunities for shared decision making about future beneficial management and treatments, there are complex ethical concerns for healthcare staff working with PwMS who do not want to know about prognosis, let alone share decisions about it. For some PwMS, the prognosis forecasting can be emotionally distressing or have negative psychological effects.

Furthermore, the 'Falling Short' report (Neurological Alliance, 2017) notes fewer people with neurological conditions feel they can contribute to making choices about their own healthcare (63% of the 3,328 surveyed in 2016, compared to 71% in the same study in 2014). They attribute lack of access to neurological specialists, particularly clinical nurse specialists, and barriers to accessing information, to some of this dissatisfaction. The report recommends that NHS trusts and staff should work closely with patient groups, particularly at diagnosis, to ensure better access to condition specific information. It further recommends clinicians work with patient groups to ensure letters and patient information includes signposting to sources of help and information, rather than leaving patients to conduct their own research into information that they can find frightening and confusing.

A reliance on providing information over the Internet can create barriers for PwMS (Lebjkowicz et al., 2010), as they might not have Internet access and/ or the necessary digital skills, as discussed earlier. However, when PwMS and clinicians *jointly search* for web-based information, it can overcome some of these barriers, by increasing user search confidence and directing PwMS to reliable and patient specific sources of information.

The 'Acute Neurology Survey' (Association of British Neurologists, 2017) reports that a serious shortage of neurologists means there are huge regional variations in access to specialist neurology centers and support for all neurological patients across England. The 'Long and Winding Road' report (Marie Curie, 2016) found that, even though the NHS has many digital and non-digital SDM tools and resources at its disposal, the NHS is struggling to implement SDM in many regions of England, as some staff have not received adequate training to support it. The report also notes that the fall in number of clinical specialist nurses across many disciplines is having a detrimental effect, as they are often the experts in SDM and the key link between patients, other clinicians, and community service providers. The 'Forward View' report confirms that the staff shortages and reduced patient access to neurology specialists are having a detrimental effect on both PwMS, and the staff working with them, to make shared decisions (MS Trust, 2016a). The NHS has acknowledged that its staff and those working with the NHS need more training in communications to support SDM. The 'Person Centred Approaches Framework' will support training and development for staff working towards SDM in future (Health Education England, Skills for Health, and Skills for Care, 2017).

CASE STUDY

This case study presents the findings from a mixed methods study conducted between June and August 2017. The purpose of the study was to determine if technology and digital health information empowers PwMS to make shared decisions about managing their own healthcare.

The study received approval from the University of Limerick (UL) Research Ethics Committee.

Data Collection

Participants for the PwMS cohort were recruited from a small number of online and face-to-face support groups for PwMS in England. Two of the support groups were established by national MS charities and both groups are moderated by charity staff and have clear terms of reference. The other group is an informal Facebook group originally established as a self-help forum, which is administered by two PwMS. Participants in the PwMS cohort were from a number of different Clinical Commissioning Groups in England. The participants had different types of MS, and had lived with MS for different lengths of time.

Six information providers from the two major MS charities, as well as one NHS clinician, also participated in the study. Table 1 summarizes the methods used to collect primary data for the case study and how many people participated in each stage of the research.

Table 1. Summary of data collection methods and participants

Data Collection Methods	Notes
Qualitative semi-structured interviews with PwMS	Six interviews were conducted with PwMS (either face-to-face or by Skype). Interviews were audio recorded and transcribed for analysis.
Focus group for PwMS	One focus group was attended by three PwMS. A record of the key themes discussed at the meeting was produced.
Online questionnaire for PwMS	A further 17 PwMS completed an online questionnaire. This method provided a broader sample of PwMS in the short time permitted for the study. It allowed further perspectives to be collected on the key topics identified during the literature review.
Online questionnaire for clinicians working with PwMS	One MS clinician completed a questionnaire.
Online questionnaire for information providers	Six staff at charities producing MS information completed questionnaires.

Data Analysis

Given the small scale of the study, data from the interviews and focus group was transcribed and coded into themes using a simple coding system, as recommended by Mason (2002). Curry (2015) suggests using an integrated method for coding to produce a starter list of themes derived from the literature review, and adding sub-codes to the starter list as the researcher becomes more familiar with the data content, and when an extra level of coding would be helpful to the analysis. In this case study, a starter list of themes was produced from the literature and sub-codes were added to the themes. The coding system was then tested and amended after the first interview and focus group. Table 2 presents the themes and sub-codes discussed in this chapter.

Results

This section presents the results from our case study, focusing specifically on health and digital literacy and information usability.

Table 2. Themes and sub-codes from data analysis

Theme	Sub-codes
Health and digital literacy	Sources of digital health information Accessibility Proactive use of information
Information usability	Trustworthiness Currency Importance of other PwMS experiences Missing information

Health and Digital Literacy

NHS Digital continues to upgrade existing digital information (e.g. the NHS Choices website) and introduce new online healthcare initiatives to meet the objectives of the 'Five Year Forward View' plan (NHS, 2014).

Although the nine participants from the interviews and focus groups said they have reliable internet connections and consider themselves regular and proficient users of technology, they were largely unaware of the current and future changes to NHS services. None of them had access to their own online healthcare records or knew how to request access to online services. Only one participant was aware of the plans to digitize services such as booking appointments, requesting prescriptions, and obtaining test results.

These nine participants used a range of devices to access digital health information—nine used a laptop or desktop computer; three of them also used a tablet. One participant said that she did not like to use a smartphone, as her MS meant that she sometimes had problems with her grip and a static larger keyboard was easier to use than a phone.

All the PwMS in this study (n=26) confirmed that they use digital health information. When asked to list the sources they use, they reported as follows (see Figure 1).

Each participant used several different types of digital health information. Use of MS apps was low, with only one participant using an app to record taking medications.

Five of the six information providers reported that they provide information to PwMS in a range of formats that include hard copy information leaflets, websites, blogs, and social media sites. "We sometimes have to print out webpages to send to those PwMS that have no access to the internet." (IS5) One clinician said she only provided hard copy information leaflets from the MS Trust and MS Society charities, to PwMS.

A number of participants gave examples that demonstrated their ability to act on health information and how they use it to help manage their MS. One participant described a long struggle with an MS nurse, as she tried to withdraw from a drug that made her feel worse.

Figure 1. Sources of digital information used by PwMS in this study

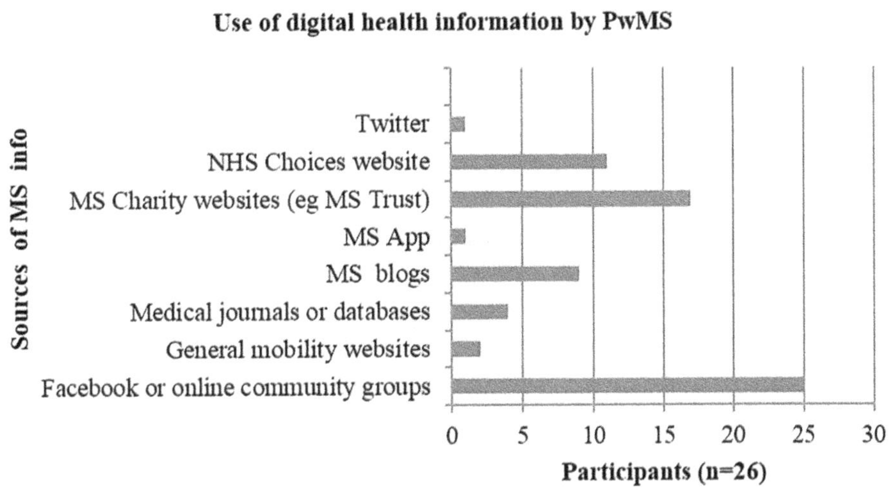

It was a really big research job for me, but eventually, I had enough evidence and my GP accepted I was right. Even then, the MS nurse was still dismissive, saying my side effects were very rare. I told her winning the lottery was rare but someone wins every week! But seriously, it was so frustrating that so many people just wouldn't listen to me. (P5)

Others felt they had to be proactive and use information to resolve problems to influence the outcomes of decisions about managing their care. Further examples included using funding information for an appeal when (successfully) re-applying for aids a doctor had refused to authorize (P1, P8) and taking information to appointments to make the most of time with healthcare staff: "doctors expect you to do some research before you arrive and to be prepared these days." (P2)

Information Usability

Nine participants indicated why they use digital health information, by selecting all applicable reasons from a list of options (see Table 3).

Three PwMS said the currency of digital health information was important. They thought that digital health information was more likely to be up to date than hard copy information sheets available in healthcare centers. One participant (P3) noted that her local neuroscience center was issuing an old edition of an information sheet about types of MS that had been updated several times by the charity that produced it. "And that's what our hospital was giving to people who had just been told they've got MS." (P2)

PwMS use digital sources not only to search for facts about MS and treatment options, but also to learn about the experiences of others living with MS. This partly accounts for the high use of social media sites. "I like to see how other people manage and if their ideas can help me." (P2); "Facebook can be a great and quick way to get advice from others." (P1) The convenience of being able to find information when travelling and at any time of day from social media was important to some. (P6, P9) "*Social media is the way now and the NHS just isn't there so I use the MSS site.*"(P9) Three participants (P3, P5, P8) said they did not like to use Facebook, but felt it was becoming an important source of MS information so they would need to use in future.

Reduced access to healthcare professionals also increases the use of social media, as PwMS search for answers to questions they would have previously directed to their healthcare team. "People start to rely on social media more if you can't find out what you are supposed to do and need help between appointments." (P4)

Table 3. Reasons why PwMS use digital information

Reasons for using digital health information	Participant responses (n=9)
To keep myself informed about new MS developments.	7
To help me make shared decisions about how to manage my MS with healthcare professionals and others (e.g. family).	3
If my MS changes and I need advice.	7
To feel as if I am being proactive in managing my MS.	6

Eight of the nine participants felt that their methods for searching for information to help to manage their MS had changed since they were diagnosed. They had become more proactive in using the internet and social media to find information about treatments and living with MS. "I mostly look online now rather than wait to be given information. I know what I am looking for now and what works for me." (P6)

Participants also described how they decide whether health information is trustworthy and reliable. The reasons they provided are summarized in Table 4.

One comprehensive response on how to decide if information is trustworthy summarizes several reasons (some also offered by other PwMS) for determining if information is reliable:

I look at the content and decide the value and authenticity by looking at what authority the source has in putting forward MS information. I look at the history of the source and feedback from others. A biggie for me is that the source is speaking from an understanding viewpoint (experience of or personally or emotionally invested in MS) rather than a knowledge of MS. (P15)

Several participants preferred information that included experience of other PwMS: "I tend to trust people that have it [MS] more than general health websites." (P7); "I value sites where other people with MS can advise me and personal experience of it is very important." (P6)

Five participants said that they carry out their own research before deciding if a source is trustworthy or not. This included following links from MS website data to the corresponding full research reports and medical databases: "I do my own academic research and follow up more than most people do. I read the full reports and it's better than stuff on the general websites." (P7); "I look for evidence based and accredited sources." (P18) Research experience also helps PwMS decide when not to use a source: "I am sceptical (sic.) about a lot of it as I know the research is just based on case notes." (P8)

Nine of the 26 participants said that they trust information provided by the MS Society and MS Trust more than other sources. "I probably shouldn't say this, but I never look at the NHS MS info! I trust the MS Trust and MS Society info as I know it is peer reviewed, professionally written, evidence based and up to date. I've never been given any NHS info or directed to the website by my healthcare team so now I just go straight to the MS Trust and MS Society stuff." (P4)

Four participants commented that moderated social media sites (particularly the MS Trust forum) were helpful as they combine personal experience of others with MS with suggestions from the forum moderators and links to more detailed reliable information.

Table 4. Reasons for deciding information is trustworthy and reliable

Reasons given by PwMS for deciding whether information is trustworthy and reliable	Participant responses (n=26)
Use information recommended by healthcare staff	2
Trust and use the NHS information	2
Use own personal judgement/ want to make own decisions	3
Look for information based on personal experience from other PwMS	3
Use official sources (sources not specified)	2
Conduct own research	5
Use information from the MS Trust or MS Society	9

Over time, some PwMS become more confident in choosing sources of information that they trust and think are relevant to their own needs: "I know a great deal about my condition and that helps me recognise information that is not trustworthy. This was not always the case!" (P12); "I have learned to choose trusty websites and now stay away from the strange ones - you know, the (sic.) you can be cured if you only drink goats' milk sites." (P8)

The staff at the charities providing information (used by the clinician and PwMS) refer to a number of sources to ensure the information they produce is evidence based and reliable. One charity uses the Oxford Centre for Evidence-based Medicine levels for assessing and weighing evidence before it is incorporated into information given to PwMS (IS2). Staff also refer to peer reviewed scientific and medical sources (IS5, IS4) and involve clinicians and PwMS in their authoring and editing process. (IS3)

Despite the wealth of MS information available online, nine participants reported that they had been unable to find information on some topics that they believe hinders them when trying to manage their MS. Some felt that there is not enough information about local services (n=2/9) and others wanted information on aids and equipment for living with MS (n=4/9): "I need info about adaptations and equipment and things that would make life easier, safer and better for me and my career." (P5) They felt that there is little information about making life changing decisions about moving home due to disability (n=2/9) and opportunities for respite care. Others (n=3) felt there is a lack of information about places accessible to disabled people, but noted that this did not just apply to PwMS. There is less information available about SP and PP than RR MS (n=4/9), "It's all about DMDs and RR, and it's so unfair!" (P7) Some participants (n=3/9) said they thought information specifically for carers and relatives of PwMS is needed. "There's stuff written for children, but nothing to tell other relatives about how MS will impact on everyone - not just the one that gets the MS, and how to cope with all that." (P1)

Information staff generally thought there was a good range of information available, but did identify some gaps. They agreed more information about how local services could help PwMS would be useful (n=2/6). Information on coordinating symptomatic treatments (n=1/6) and explanations of how to access healthcare staff (n=2/6) could reduce the number of queries they receive on these topics. "We take a number of calls from PwMS who don't want to trouble the MS team, or know who to contact for help between appointments." (IS5)

Asked how healthcare staff could help to improve the use of digital information to make shared decisions, nine PwMS felt that the healthcare team could signpost them to information about local MS services (n=2) and reliable digital information (n=3) "so that I don't spend two hours searching MS information that can scare me to death." (P4)

Some participants suggested that providing digital information in shorter, bite-sized easy to read formats, podcasts, and infomercials would be helpful. Some (n=3) thought the NHS was lagging behind in using technology to improve access to healthcare staff and that NHS staff should consider offering forums for questions from PwMS and Skype or smartphone appointments with clinicians.

DISCUSSION

The majority of PwMS described in our case study have access to the internet and are capable of searching for their own digital information. However, the results from charity staff and volunteer participants concur with a study by Lebjkowicz et al. (2010), which found that some PwMS do not use the internet at all and need information in other formats. Indeed, in our study, the focus group felt that providing information in different formats (such as podcasts and infomercials) would be helpful. This finding aligns with the 'Perfect Information Journey' report (PIF, 2018) that says information should be provided in a variety of formats to meet all users' needs (recommendation #1).

Our study also found the majority of PwMS (including those who are proactive users of health information) had little knowledge of plans to digitize many services (e.g. online health records) that may affect how they communicate with healthcare staff and manage their MS in future. For example, NHS Digital is currently developing an NHS Apps Library, and other healthcare apps are already available for purchase. While the participants in this study stated that they are not interested in using many of the apps that are on offer, some participants had experience of technology-based reviews or appointments with healthcare staff (e.g. Skype and conference telephone calls with doctors and MS nurses) and believed expanding this provision could improve use of staff resources. However, the NHS (and other providers) should be mindful of the analyses by Rudell et al. (2016) and Kvedar et al. (2015) that show that PwMS and clinicians will only engage with and use new technology if the benefits of using it are clearly outlined to them (recommendation #2).

On a positive note, our study aligns with the results of previous studies by Powell et al. (2011) and Riel et al. (2017) that found people use digital healthcare information as they want to both improve their understanding of their condition and to prepare for discussions with clinicians. On a negative note, however, our findings suggest that lack of access to, and perceptions of poor support from, healthcare specialists left some PwMS feeling that they had no choice but to be proactive and search for their own health information. Echoing findings in the 'Long Winding Road' (Marie Curie, 2017), 'Forward View' (MS Trust, 2016a) and 'Falling Short' (Neurological Alliance, 2017) reports, our study found almost a quarter of participants do not have access to neurology experts that can help them make decisions to manage their MS. As discussed earlier in this chapter, there is a bias towards providing people with RR MS with access to healthcare specialists, at the detriment of people with other types of MS (MS Trust, 2016b). Consequently, people with other types of MS will have fewer opportunities for SDM. If the NHS is serious about empowering everyone to engage in SDM, it will need to readdress this imbalance (recommendation #3).

Our study found that participants value health information that includes experiences of other PwMS. These findings correlate with previous studies by Ziebland et al. (2016), Marrie et al. (2013), and Colombo et al. (2014) attributing the use of social media sites to the need to learn from and communicate with other PwMS but also the need for communication forums moderated by trusted MS organizations. Several participants in this study expressed serious concerns about the ability of other PwMS to understand information to manage their MS. In addition, they expressed concerns about advice from non-clinicians (to PwMS) about medications and treatments that could be dangerous. Those expressing such views sometimes contribute to social media forums, discussions and blogs as a way of helping the PwMS that they are concerned about. Given the NHS plans to develop additional digital services, associated social media forums will need to be moderated by experts (recommendation #4).

Although there is a vast range of MS information available, the results of our study concur with others by Synott et al. (2014) and Kopke et al. (2014) who found that PwMS perceive there is far more *clinical* information available than guidance about the *practicalities* of living with MS and its impact on PwMS, their carers, and families. However, once the participants in the study find sources of information they trust, they tend to return to those sources again, which could mean they miss updates from, and improvement to, other sources. For example, most interviewees in our study did not know that the NHS Choices site includes a searchable (by postcode) directory of MS health, care and mobility services that provides some of the practical information they believe is missing. To fully engage PwMS with digital health information, there needs to be appropriate guidance, signposting to, and orientation for users of that information (recommendation #5).

FUTURE RESEARCH DIRECTIONS

Future research could review the impact of digitization of the NHS with larger cohorts of PwMS to determine whether technology really does empower people to make shared decisions. The proposed study could also analyze which particular tools and technologies empower PwMS and which tools they find useful. As the NHS digital programme expands, the study could review the full impact of the new digital service model on PwMS and wider aspects of their care and management.

It would also be interesting to study the needs of PwMS who are not digitally literate or are less digitally literate, and consider the implications of shared decision making for this cohort of PwMS. While younger "digital natives" are familiar with using technology in their day-to-day lives, there is still a large cohort of people who do not have access to technology, or who do not possess skills to use technology to manage their healthcare effectively.

Finally, researchers could examine digital healthcare initiatives in other countries, to determine best practice for using technology for shared decision making.

CONCLUSION

This chapter presented a review of literature on digital health information and information usability. It presented some findings from a mixed methods study that explored how people with MS (PwMS) access and use health digital information when trying to manage their MS. While our study found that there is much good quality digital health information available for PwMS, and that this facilitates shared decisions, PwMS report that some necessary information is still missing, such as practical details about living with MS (for PwMS, their carers, and families). The chapter concludes with some recommendations for providers of digital health information for PwMS and suggestions for future research.

ACKNOWLEDGMENT

This research received no specific grant from any funding agency in the public, commercial, or not-for-profit sectors.

This research was facilitated by volunteer participants from The MS Trust, The MS Society, and members of the MS community in England.

REFERENCES

Association of British Neurologists. (2017). Acute Neurology Services Survey. Retrieved from http://www.theabn.org/media/docs/ABN%20publications/ABN%20acute%20neurology%20survey%20final%2013%20March%202017.pdf

Bodenheimer, T., Wagner, E. H., & Grumbach, K. (2002). Improving primary care for patients with chronic illness. *Journal of the American Medical Association*, *288*(14), 1775–1779. doi:10.1001/jama.288.14.1775 PMID:12365965

Chaudhry, B., Wang, J., Wu, S., Maglione, M., Mojica, W., Roth, E., ... Shekelle, P. G. (2006). Systematic review: Impact of health information technology on quality, efficiency, and costs of medical care. *Annals of Internal Medicine*, *144*(10), 742–752. doi:10.7326/0003-4819-144-10-200605160-00125 PMID:16702590

Colombo, C., Mosconi, P., Confalonieri, P., Baroni, I., Traversa, S., Hill, S. J., ... Filippini, G. (2014). Web search behavior and information needs of people with multiple sclerosis: Focus group study and analysis of online postings. *Interactive Journal of Medical Research*, *3*(3), e12. doi:10.2196/ijmr.3034 PMID:25093374

Dennison, L., Smith, E. M., Bradbury, K., & Galea, I. (2016). How do people with multiple sclerosis experience prognostic uncertainty and prognosis communication? A qualitative study. *PLoS One*, *11*(7). doi:10.1371/journal.pone.0158982 PMID:27434641

European Multiple Sclerosis Platform. (2014). Defeating MS together: The European code of good practice in MS. Retrieved from http://www.emsp.org/wp-content/uploads/2015/06/140824-Revised-Code-of-Good-Practice.pdf

Eysenbach, G. (2001). What is e-health? *Journal of Medical Internet Research*, *3*(2), e20. Retrieved from http://www.ncbi.nlm.nih.gov/pmc/articles/PMC1761894/. doi:10.2196/jmir.3.2.e20 PMID:11720962

Good Things Foundation. (2017). The Real Digital Divide? Retrieved from https://www.goodthings-foundation.org/sites/default/files/research-publications/ofcom_report_v4_links.pdf

Health Education England, Skills for Health, and Skills for Care (2017). Person-Centred Approaches: Empowering people in their lives and communities to enable an upgrade in prevention, wellbeing, health, care and support. Retrieved from http://www.skillsforhealth.org.uk/images/pdf/Person-Centred-Approaches-Framework.pdf?s=form

Health Foundation. (2013). Implementing Shared Decision Making. Retrieved from http://www.health.org.uk/sites/health/files/ImplementingSharedDecisionMaking.pdf

Health Literacy, U. K. (2019). Why is Health Literacy Important? Retrieved from http://www.healthliteracy.org.uk/index.php/about-health-literacy

Heesen, C., Kaspar, J., Kopke, S., Richter, T., Segal, J., & Mulhauser, I. (2007). Informed shared decision making in multiple-sclerosis – inevitable or impossible? *Journal of the Neurological Sciences*, *259*(1-2), 109–117. doi:10.1016/j.jns.2006.05.074 PMID:17400253

Hinchliffe, A., & Mummery, W. K. (2008). Applying usability testing techniques to improve a health promotion website. *Health Promotion Journal of Australia: Official Journal of Australian Association of Health Promotion Professionals*, *19*(1), 29–35. doi:10.1071/HE08029 PMID:18481929

House of Commons. (2014). Managing the care of people with long term health conditions. Retrieved from https://www.publications.parliament.uk/pa/cm201415/cmselect/cmhealth/401/401.pdf

Kings Fund. (2016). A Digital NHS? Retrieved from https://www.kingsfund.org.uk/sites/default/files/field/field_publication_file/A_digital_NHS_Kings_Fund_Sep_2016.pdf

Kings Fund. (2019). The NHS long-term plan explained. Retrieved from https://www.kingsfund.org.uk/sites/default/files/field/field_publication_file/A_digital_NHS_Kings_Fund_Sep_2016.pdf

Köpke, S., Solari, A., Khan, F., Heesen, C., & Giordano, A. (2014). Information provision for people with multiple sclerosis. *Cochrane Database of Systematic Reviews*, *4*. PMID:24752330

Kvedar, J. C., Colman, C., & Cella, G. (2015). The internet of healthy things. Boston, MA: Partners Connected Health.

Lejbkowicz, I., Paperna, T., Stein, N., Dishon, S., & Miller, A. (2010). Internet usage by patients with multiple sclerosis: Implications to participatory medicine and personalized healthcare. *Multiple Sclerosis International*, *2010*. doi:10.1155/2010/640749 PMID:22096625

Marie Curie. (2017). The Long and Winding Road. Retrieved from https://www.mariecurie.org.uk/globalassets/media/documents/policy/campaigns/the-long-and-winding-road.pdf

Marrie, R. A., Salter, A. R., Tyry, T., Fox, R. J., & Cutter, G. R. (2013). Preferred sources of health information in persons with multiple sclerosis: Degree of trust and information sought. *Journal of Medical Internet Research*, *15*(4), e67. doi:10.2196/jmir.2466 PMID:23635393

Mckenzie, I. S., Morant, S. V., Bloomfield, G. A., MacDonald, T. M., & O'Riordan, J. (2013). Incidence and prevalence of multiple sclerosis in the UK 1990–2010: A descriptive study in the general practice research database. *Journal of Neurology, Neurosurgery, and Psychiatry*, *85*(1), 76–84. doi:10.1136/jnnp-2013-305450 PMID:24052635

Moccia, M., Carotenuto, A., Massarelli, M., Lanzillo, R., & Brescia Morra, V. (2016). Can people with multiple sclerosis actually understand what they read in the Internet age? *Journal of Clinical Neuroscience*, *25*, 167–168. doi:10.1016/j.jocn.2015.10.003 PMID:26526382

Multiple Sclerosis International Federation. (2013). Atlas-of-MS. Retrieved from https://www.msif.org/wp-content/uploads/2014/09/Atlas-of-MS.pdf

Neurological Alliance. (2017). Falling short: How has neurology patient experience changed since 2014? Retrieved from http://neural.org.uk/store/assets/files/668/original/Neurological_Alliance_-_Falling_Short_-_How_has_neurology_patient_experience_changed_since_2014.pdf

NHS. (2014). Five year forward view. Retrieved from https://www.england.nhs.uk/wp-content/uploads/2014/10/5yfv-web.pdf

NHS. (2017). Next steps on the NHS five year forward view (2017). Retrieved from https://www.england.nhs.uk/wp-content/uploads/2017/03/NEXT-STEPS-ON-THE-NHS-FIVE-YEAR-FORWARD-VIEW.pdf

NHS. (2019). The long term plan. Retrieved from https://www.longtermplan.nhs.uk/wp-content/uploads/2019/01/nhs-long-term-plan.pdf

Patient Information Forum. (2017). Perfect patient information journey: Phase 1 summary report. Retrieved from https://www.pifonline.org.uk/wp-content/uploads/2017/05/PIF-PPI-Journey-4May17-final.pdf

Patient Information Forum. (2018). Perfect patient information journey: 7 steps for health services to improve information for people with long term condition. Retrieved from https://www.pifonline.org.uk/wp-content/uploads/2014/11/PIF-PPI-Journey-Final-25Jun18-1-website-version.pdf

Patient Information Forum. (2019). NHS plan promise empowered and informed patients via digital tools. Retrieved from https://www.pifonline.org.uk/blog/nhs-plan-promises-empowered-informed-patients-via-digital-tools/

Powell, J., Inglis, N., Ronnie, J., & Large, S. (2011). The characteristics and motivations of online health information seekers: Cross-sectional survey and qualitative interview study. *Journal of Medical Internet Research*, *13*(1), e20. doi:10.2196/jmir.1600 PMID:21345783

Register, M. S. (2019). Let's make sense of MS. Retrieved from https://ukmsregister.org/

Riel, N. V., Auwerx, K., Debbaut, P., Hees, S. V., & Schoenmakers, B. (2017). The effect of Dr Google on doctor–patient encounters in primary care: A quantitative, observational, cross-sectional study. *BJGP Open*, 1(2), 1-10. Retrieved from https://bjgpopen.org/content/1/2/bjgpopen17X100833.abstract.

Rudell, E., Peterson, P., Pulim, S., Griffin, A. L., & Bowen, J. D. (2016). Connecting healthcare providers with patients through mobile technology: Formula for shared decision making and improved patient outcomes. *Iproceedings*, *2*(1), e3. doi:10.2196/iproc.6224

Sbaffi, L., & Rowley, J. (2017). Trust and credibility in web-based health information: A review and agenda for future research. *Journal of Medical Internet Research*, *19*(6), e218. doi:10.2196/jmir.7579 PMID:28630033

Solari, A. (2014). Effective communication at the point of multiple sclerosis diagnosis. *Multiple Sclerosis Journal*, *20*(4), 397–402. doi:10.1177/1352458514523061 PMID:24503056

Synnot, A. J., Hill, S. J., Garner, K. A., Summers, M. P., Filippini, G., Osborne, R. H., ... Mosconi, P. (2016). Online health information seeking: How people with multiple sclerosis find, assess and integrate treatment information to manage their health. *Health Expectations*, *19*(3), 727–737. doi:10.1111/hex.12253 PMID:25165024

Thorne, S., Con, A., McGuinness, L., McPherson, G., & Harris, S. R. (2004). Health care communication issues in multiple sclerosis: An interpretive description. *Qualitative Health Research*, *14*(1), 5–22. doi:10.1177/1049732303259618 PMID:14725173

Thorne, S. E. (2009). Is the Story Enough? *Qualitative Health Research*, *19*(9), 1183–1185. doi:10.1177/1049732309343951 PMID:19690200

Trust, M. S. (2016a). MS forward view: A consensus for the future of MS services. Retrieved from https://www.mstrust.org.uk/sites/default/files/Future%20of%20MS%20Services%20WEB%20FINAL.pdf

Trust, M. S. (2016b) Is MS care fair? Retrieved from https://www.mstrust.org.uk/file/ms-care-media-reportpdf/download?token=R8dXTbMB

Trust, M. S. (2019). Prevalence and incidence of multiple sclerosis. Retrieved from https://www.mstrust.org.uk/a-z/prevalence-and-incidence-multiple-sclerosis

Ziebland, S., Powell, J., Briggs, P., Jenkinson, C., Wyke, S., Sillence, E., . . . Farmer, A. (2016). Examining the role of patients' experiences as a resource for choice and decision-making in health care: A creative, interdisciplinary mixed-method study in digital health. Retrieved from http://www.ncbi.nlm.nih.gov/books/NBK401199/

KEY TERMS AND DEFINITIONS

Digital Health Information: Health information that can be accessed in electronic form.

E-Health: Health services and information delivered using digital technologies.

Health Literacy: Personal characteristics and social resources needed by an individual to access, evaluate, and use health-related information.

Long-Term Condition (LTC): Term used to describe chronic health conditions.

Multiple Sclerosis (MS): A neurological condition of the central nervous system.

National Health Service (NHS): The body responsible for policies, priorities and directions of health and care in England.

Person or People With MS (PwMS): A neutral (and non-offensive) term used to describe someone who has MS.

Shared Decision Making (SDM): An initiative to encourage patients and their healthcare staff to share responsibility for health decisions.

Chapter 11
The Design and Evaluation of an Intelligent Pain Management System (IPMS) in Cancer Patient Care

Y. Ken Wang
University of Pittsburgh at Bradford, USA

Juan J. Gu
Roswell Park Comprehensive Cancer Center, USA

Yunheng Sun
Xinhua Hospital Affiliated to Shanghai Jiao Tong University School of Medicine – Chongming, China

Feng Jiang
Xinhua Hospital Affiliated to Shanghai Jiao Tong University School of Medicine – Chongming, China

Hongwei Hua
Xinhua Hospital Affiliated to Shanghai Jiao Tong University School of Medicine – Chongming, China

Jing Li
Xinhua Hospital Affiliated to Shanghai Jiao Tong University School of Medicine – Chongming, China

Zhijun Cheng
Xinhua Hospital Affiliated to Shanghai Jiao Tong University School of Medicine – Chongming, China

Zhijun Liao
Xinhua Hospital Affiliated to Shanghai Jiao Tong University School of Medicine – Chongming, China

Qian Huang
Xinhua Hospital Affiliated to Shanghai Jiao Tong University School of Medicine – Chongming, China

Weiwei Hu
Xinhua Hospital Affiliated to Shanghai Jiao Tong University School of Medicine, China

Gang Ding
Shanghai International Medical Center, China

DOI: 10.4018/978-1-7998-0047-7.ch011

ABSTRACT

This case study reviews the design and development of a mobile-based intelligent pain management system (IPMS) app in cancer patient care and pain management in a rural hospital in China. Healthcare professionals were involved throughout the design to the evaluation stages. The IPMS facilitated real-time pain recording and timely intervention among cancer patients with pain. To evaluate the effectiveness of the IPMS, a clinical trial was administrated under the supervision of healthcare professionals. The result confirmed that the IPMS was a feasible, effective, and low-cost pain management tool for cancer patients and healthcare professionals. This case provides preliminary data to support the potentials of using IPMS in cancer pain management and emphasized that the involvement of healthcare professional throughout the system development lifecycle is crucial to the successful implementation of the IPMS.

INTRODUCTION

Cancer represents a group of diseases characterized by uncontrolled growth and spreading of neoplasm cells in part of the body (Mathur, Nain, & Sharma, 2015). The World Health Organization (WHO) estimated that 14 million new cancer patients were diagnosed worldwide every year and cancer resulted in 8.2 million deaths in 2012 (World Health Organization, 2017). As a leading cause of human death globally, cancer, as well as cancer treatment became a focus of medical research for many decades.

Typical symptoms of cancers include weight loss, unexplained bleeding, and pain (Linder et al., 2015). Cancer patients, especially at their terminal stages, often experienced cancer pain. Prior research found that over one-third of cancer patients experienced cancer pain (Deandrea, Montanari, Moja, & Apolone, 2008). Cancer pain has been considered a major reason that caused a lower quality of life of the patients (Lesage & Portenoy, 1999; Portenoy & Lesage, 1999). Under-treatment of cancer pain has been a worldwide problem (Deandrea et al., 2008; Greco et al., 2014). Effective management and further mitigation of cancer pain requires an accurate and precise assessment of the pain (Forbes, 2011; Jacobsen et al., 2009; Kuzeyli Yildirim & Uyar, 2006; Kwon, 2014).

Conventional paper-based, self-reported pain questionnaires are limited in terms of efficiency and accuracy. Ward et al. (1993) surveyed 270 patients with cancer and found that patients were reluctant to share their pain information in self-reported questionnaires due to privacy and other concerns. Paper-based pain reporting methods are prone to potential biases in the collected data due to patients' lack of relevant knowledge. Ward et al. (2014) reported that elderly, less educated, and low-income patients are more likely to have concerns at pain reporting and the levels of concerns were correlated to the levels of pain. Particularly, under-medicated patients had significantly higher concerns to report their pain possibly due to anxiety. Such limitations call for a more efficient and accurate method in pain reporting and management. Modern technology, such as visual interactivity and touch screens may help those patients better understand the reporting procedures and provide effective guidance for them to report pain.

Rapidly growing mobile technology use gave rise to the emergence of more advanced electronic pain reporting and assessment systems (Agboola, Ju, Elfiky, Kvedar, & Jethwani, 2015; Heinonen, Luoto, Lindfors, & Nygard, 2012; Jan et al., 2007; Marceau, Link, Jamison, & Carolan, 2007; Mulvaney, Anders, Smith, Pittel, & Johnson, 2012; O'Reilly & Spruijt-Metz, 2013; Stone & Broderick, 2007). Such systems, often in the form of smartphone applications (apps), sometimes referred to as intelligent pain management systems (IPMS), can be more effectively capturing, transferring, and analyzing the pain data (Sun et al., 2017). Marceau et al. (2007) introduced PDA (personal digital assistant) devices to pain management. Over the two weeks experimental period, chronic pain patients were asked to monitor their pain, mood, activity interference, medication use, and pain location on paper or on PDA devices. The participants reported that the use of PDA devices was more convenient, time-saving, and easier to report data.

Mobile-based pain management apps provide a low cost, conveniently implemented solution to facilitate real-time pain recording and timely intervention among cancer patients. Such apps often have multiple features depending on the smartphone's operating system (e.g., Android, iOS, BlackBerry, etc.) to evaluate real-time pain along with other data, such as the Karnofsky Performance Status (KPS) scores for the assessment of quality of life, and possibly generate an action plan to visit the physician or to adjust pain medication dosage when the pain threshold is reached (Schag, Heinrich, & Ganz, 1984).

Smartphones and mobile apps have been introduced to pain management since Apple's iPhone became available and popular in the world. Wallace and Dhingra (2014) reviewed 220 Android, BlackBerry, and iPhone applications associated with features on pain management in the U.S. The majority of applications were operating on Apple's iPhones. About half of the applications focused on chronic pain, and the other half focused on back pain, neck pain, and other pains. Although most of the pain management applications offered features on pain education, pain self-management, or both, the majority (65%) of the applications did not involve healthcare professionals (Wallace & Dhingra, 2014). Wallace and Dhingra (2014) found that few evidence-based pain management features were implemented in those applications due to the lack of professional involvement in the design and development stages.

Rosser and Eccleston (2011) reviewed 111 mobile applications with generic pain management features. Although most of those applications incorporated some pain management features such as daily tracking of pain variables, few were designed with the involvement of healthcare professionals. The effectiveness promised by those applications was established on a very weak clinical basis posing significant potential risks to the misled patients (Rosser & Eccleston, 2011).

Reynoldson et al. (2014) assessed the interface design, clinical content, usability, and overall quality of two mobile applications for self-management of pain. Lack of user and clinician engagement in the development stage was found to be a major issue. End-user requirements were generally overlooked causing unsatisfactory delivery of key features. Some basic details in user interface design, such as the color scheme and text fonts, could have been improved with early involvement of clinical users in the process of development (Reynoldson et al., 2014).

A recent systematic review studied the use of mobile-based pain management apps in both in-clinic and out-clinic settings (Thurnheer, Gravestock, Pichierri, Steurer, & Burgstaller, 2018). Among 15 studies being reviewed, most supported the conclusion that pain management apps were able to help decrease the severity of pain through patient empowerment. Patient empowerment prepared patients with the knowledge and skills of pain management and life management. Empowered patients were able to self-manage their chronic pain and effectively communicate with healthcare professionals for assistance.

Overall, mobile-based pain management apps have been found to be able to effectively alleviate the pain of patients. An appropriately designed pain management app requires the involvement of healthcare professionals at the planning, design, development, implementation, and evaluation stages.

Healthcare professionals may offer important advice to the engineering team on pain assessment including validated multidimensional tools to describe pain (intensity, quality, and location of the pain) and to evaluate pain interferences (emotional effects and daily activities) (Dalal & Bruera, 2012; Jibb et al., 2014; Kuzeyli Yildirim & Uyar, 2006; Palermo, 2009).

This case study will review the design and development of a mobile-based intelligent pain management system (IPMS) app in cancer patient care and pain management in a rural hospital in China. To evaluate the effectiveness of the IPMS, a clinical trial will be reported to test the effectiveness of the designed IPMS mobile app.

SYSTEM DEVELOPMENT

Cancer Pain Management in China

The original demand for designing and developing this IPMS came from healthcare practitioners in rural China. Although China has become the second largest economy in the world, the country is facing a wide resource gap across age groups and geographic areas. Compared to western developed countries, China has very limited medical resources to cure and care cancer in underdeveloped rural areas. There is a shortage of medical doctors, nurses, and other healthcare professionals in rural China. A 2011 study shows that China has the doctor-to-resident ratio of 2.8 doctors per 1,000 residents in large cities, whereas in the rural areas such ratio declines to 0.95 doctors per 1,000 rural residents (O'Reilly & Spruijt-Metz, 2013).

Another serious social problem China is facing is the unstoppable trend of population aging. China is becoming an aged nation and soon will become a super-aged nation due to its historical one-child policy. Although China's one-child policy was officially terminated in 2016, the elderly dependency ratio, defined as the ratio between the elderly population and the working age (15-64 years) population, keeps growing (Rapoza, 2017). China's fast-growing economy and the rising cost of childcare and development are discouraging the young generations to consider having more children. As society inevitably grows older, China's elderly people in the cities and rural areas are more and more dependent on social medical attention. Therefore, home care and mobile care are believed to be future solutions to such a gap of medical resources in China's urban and underdeveloped rural areas.

Cancer has become increasingly prevalent in China over the past few decades. In China, the diagnosis rate of cancer increased rapidly over the past few decades. A review of the literature showed that China reported approximately 3.07 million new cases of diagnosed cancer in 2012, which represented 21.8% of the global total (Agboola et al., 2015; Edwards et al., 2014; Goss et al., 2014). Despite the prevalence of cancer, advancement in diagnostic methods and therapeutic medicines have been able to extend the life of cancer patients beyond what was previously possible. For doctors and other healthcare providers, maintaining cancer patients' quality of life becomes increasingly important and challenging.

Among symptoms related to the quality of life of cancer patients, pain commonly has been recognized as a most critical factor that may also result in ineffective treatment of cancer. More than one-third of cancer patients in China have experienced cancer pain. Among possible solutions to better pain management for cancer patients, smartphone based IPMS apps may be the low hanging fruit. A Chinese research team developed and tested a mobile app named Pain Guard. This mobile app was designed to provide treatment information to discharged cancer patients with pain (Yang et al., 2019). The mobile app involved features of pain management, pain evaluation, and patient acceptance of the app. A study showed that patients with the Pain Guard mobile app reported higher medication adherence and higher global quality of life scores (Yang et al., 2019).

Feature and Interface Design

Mobile-based IPMS apps should be designed with the advantages of easy access, low cost, and quick response to patients' needs. In addition, the ability to instantly communicate with healthcare providers is also a very welcoming feature for cancer patients. A well-designed pain management mobile app should incorporate rich interactive features between the human and the computing machine. The app should not only be used to report and evaluate patients' pain status (self-management) but also to be a tool facilitating doctor-patient communication and decision making. Thus, healthcare professionals needed to be involved in the early stages of the system design and development.

A group of healthcare professionals took leadership in the design of this IPMS mobile app. Physicians and researchers from a rural hospital in China proposed the system prototype. Based on their experiences with cancer patients, they communicated the requirements for basic features and interactivity to the engineering contractor and requested a prototype of the app to be developed for evaluation. Upon the request of the leading physician, the engineering contractor designed a prototype that operates on the Android mobile operating system in order to provide an affordable, portable, and easy to use environment for rural patients.

The healthcare professionals conducted a pilot study in 2015 to estimate the potential effectiveness of the prototype. The result showed that patients who used the IMPS app reported significant more pain-under-control days compared to the control group (Hu & Ding, 2015). Feedback opinions on the improvement of the user interface were collected from pilot users. Confirmed by the pilot study data, the engineering team decided to move forward with interface design and further incorporated user satisfaction and quality of life surveys into the app deliverable.

The design team adopted a modularity approach consisting of several functional subsystems to facilitate speedy development by multiple teams. The core system consisted of four modules: Life Quality Self-evaluation, Cancer Pain Self-evaluation, Real-time Messaging, and Standard Medication. After system architecture design, the engineering team including the programming and system integration personnel took over to complete the development and simulation test before the clinical trial.

Life Quality Self-Evaluation

Figure 1 shows a screenshot of the running IPMS app. The life quality self-evaluation module consisted of two submodules. One is a questionnaire based on the KPS scale to measure the level of patient activity and medical care requirements (Schag et al., 1984). The KPS scale measures to what extent a patient can independently perform daily life activities on a scale of 100. A KPS score of 100 means normal, no complaints, and no evidence of disease. A KPS score of 0 means the patient is dead. For the convenience of Chinese cancer patient users, the KPS scale was translated into Chinese for display in the IPMS mobile app.

Figure 2 shows the actual look of the KPS questionnaire screen. The English translation is provided for readers' convenience only. No English was displayed in the mobile app.

Figure 3 shows a 12-item questionnaire in a flow chart format used to assess the Quality of Life (QOL) of the cancer patients. These questions covered a wide range of life aspects.

1. Appetite
    a. Almost no food intake
    b. Food intake is less than ½ normal amount
    c. Food intake is about ½ normal amount
    d. Food intake is less than normal
    e. Food intake is normal
2. Spirit
3. Sleep
4. Fatigue
5. Pain
6. Family members' understanding and cooperation
7. Peers' understanding and cooperation
8. Knowledge about cancer
9. Attitude towards treatment
10. Daily life
11. Side effect from treatment
12. Facial expressions

Figure 1. Screenshot of the intelligent pain management system (IPMS) mobile app home screen: Life quality self-evaluation (upper left), cancer-pain self-evaluation (upper right), real-time message (lower left) and medication reminder (lower right). (English translation is provided for readers' convenience)

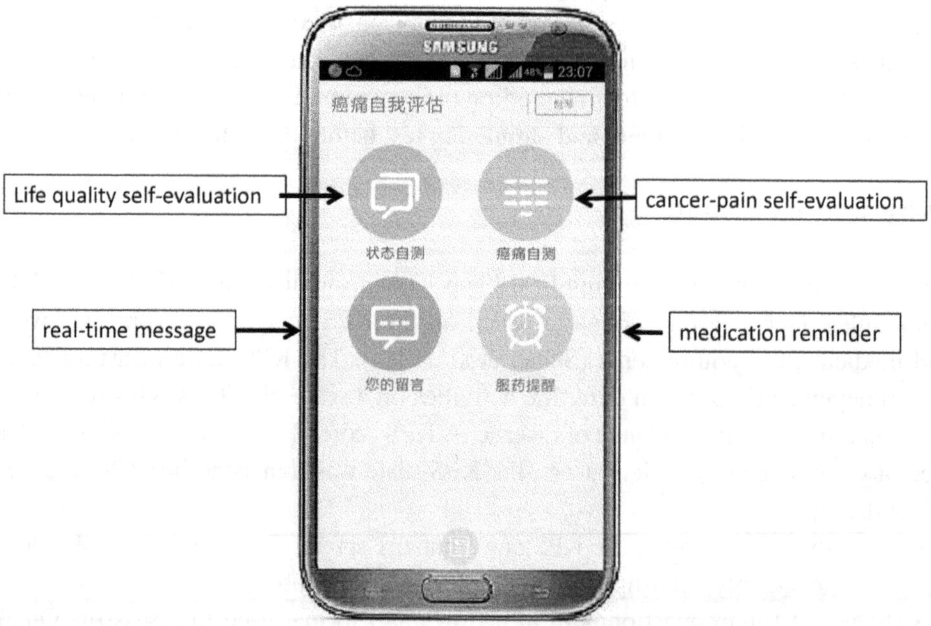

Figure 2. Screenshot of Karnofsky Performance Status (KPS) in the life quality self-evaluation module (English translation is provided for readers' convenience)

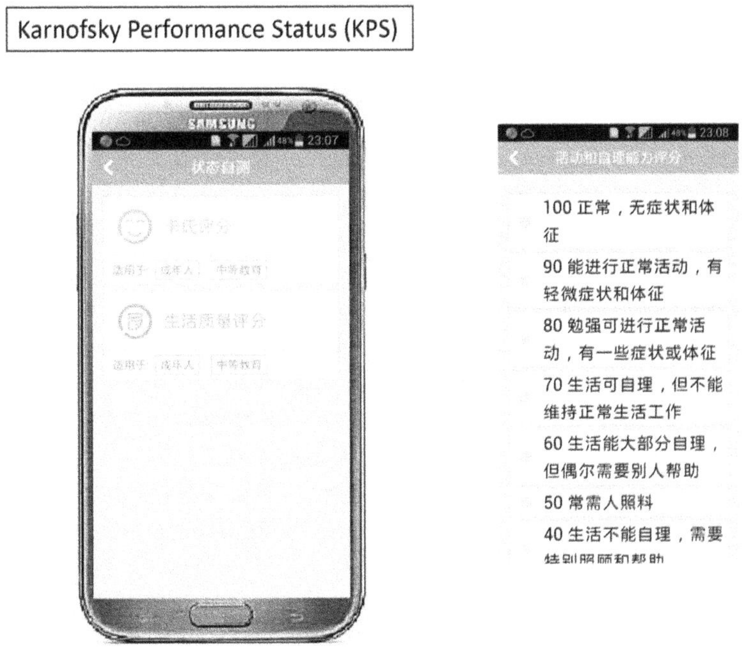

Figure 3. The questionnaire flow chart in the life quality self-evaluation module (English translation is provided for readers' convenience)

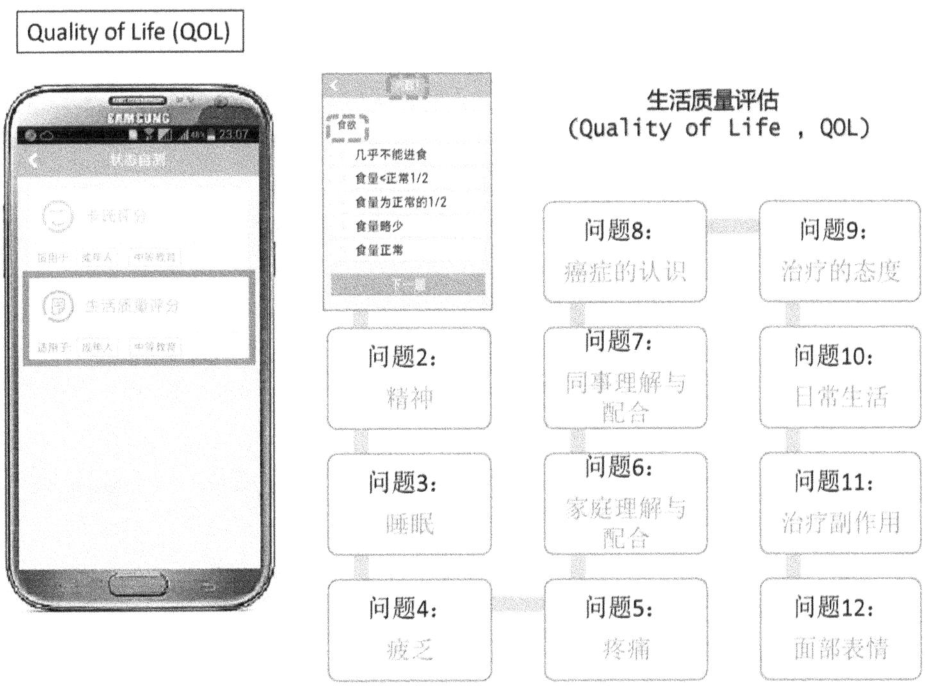

Cancer Pain Self-Evaluation

The cancer pain self-evaluation module is the core module of the IPMS app designed to track patients' self-reported pain data. This module contained two submodules: a daily pain assessment submodule and an instant pain assessment submodule.

The daily pain assessment submodule (Figure 4) displayed a body map on the smartphone screen allowing the patient to choose the precise position of a recently occurred cancer pain (picture 1). Feedback from the pilot study indicated that patients preferred an intuitive visual interface in pain assessment. The body map helped patients accurately illustrate the positions of their pain in the body.

The pain assessment questionnaire was developed based on the numerical rating scale (NRS) from 1 to 10 as an assessment vehicle, with 1 being no pain and 10 being the worst extreme pain. The patients were asked to assess the most (picture 2), least (picture 3), and average pain (picture 4) in NRS scores in the past 24 hours and the current pain score (picture 5) as well.

In addition, a list of pain medication was displayed to allow the patients to report their current medication (picture 6) and the effectiveness of the pain medicine (picture 7).

Lastly, a final pain assessment questionnaire consisted of 8 aspects (14 questions) to investigate the additional cancer pain influence in daily life, such as movement, hobby, the relationship between family members, etc. (picture 8).

Figure 5 shows the instant pain assessment submodule, in which NRS was used to evaluate the patient's current pain scores. The interface was designed to be user-friendly for patients who suffered from variable intense pain (breakthrough pain). In this section, if a patient's self-evaluated pain score reached a high level (> 7), an automated message would be sent to the patient that he or she will be contacted by a physician soon.

Figure 4. Screenshots of daily pain assess sub-module in cancer-pain self-evaluation module (English translation is provided for journal readers)

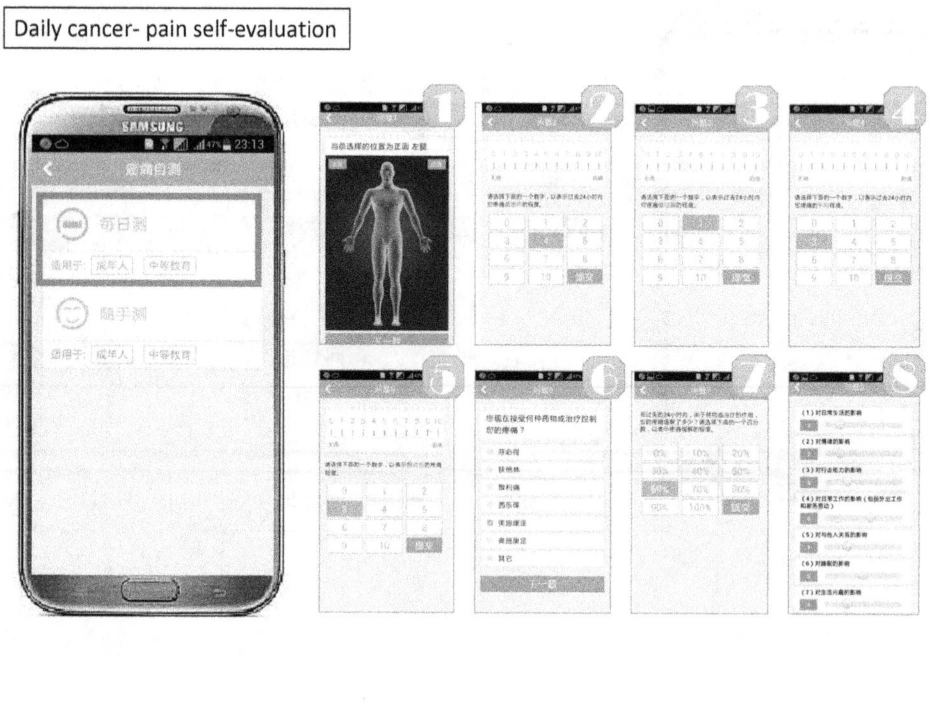

Figure 5. Screenshots of instant pain assess sub-module in cancer-pain self-evaluation module (English translation is provided for journal readers)

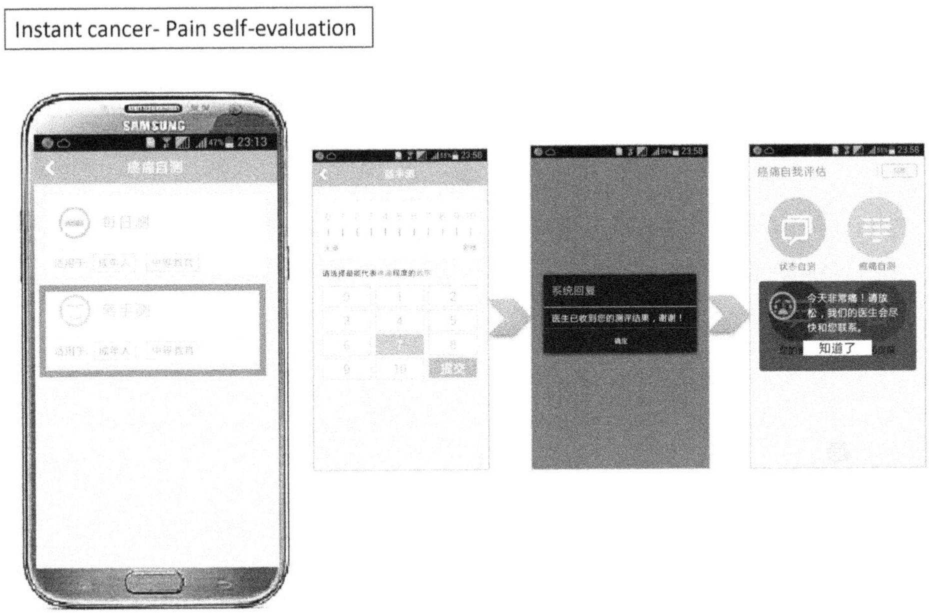

Real-Time Instant Messaging

This module was designed to assist patients to initiate a real-time consultation session on pain management with the healthcare professionals (Figure 6). The screenshot shows a transcript of the conversation between a patient and his doctor.

Logged in
Dr. Huang: *Hello. The System shows you have pain today.*
Dr. Huang: *Your pain seems to be moderate. Is it getting worse?*
Li Bin: *Doctor, today is worse than yesterday.*

Medication Reminder

This module was designed to remind patients of their medication schedule (Figure 7) so that they would be assured to take the pain medicine on a regular basis.

SYSTEM EVALUATION

To evaluate the effectiveness of this IPMS app, a randomized controlled clinical trial was implemented. The clinical trial involved two groups: a trial (intervention) group and a control group.

Figure 6. Screenshots of the real-time messages (left) and example (right) (English translation is provided for journal readers)

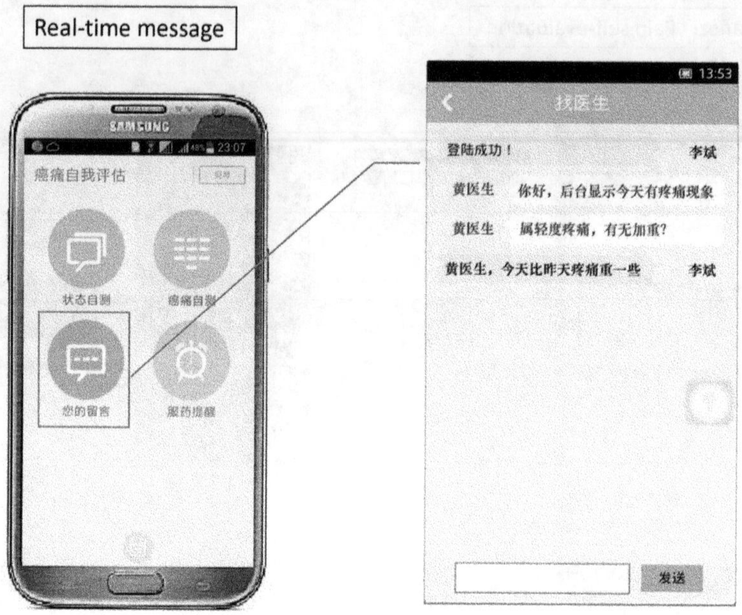
Real-time message
癌痛自我评估
状态自测
您的留言
服药提醒
13:53
找医生
登陆成功！
李斌
黄医生
你好，后台显示今天有疼痛现象
黄医生
属轻度疼痛，有无加重?
黄医生，今天比昨天疼痛重一些
李斌
发送

Figure 7. Screenshots of standard medication reminder module (English translation is provided for journal readers)

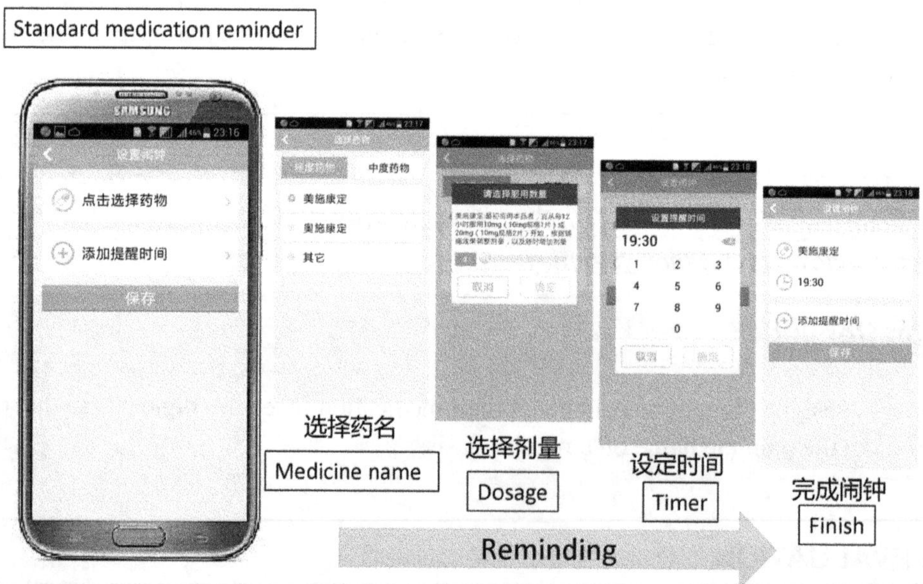

Group Assignment

The participants in the trial group were asked to complete the first day's pain assessment questionnaire and the quality of life questionnaire on the provided smartphones. Participants were then encouraged to use the IPMS app as much as possible to record their pain status at least once every day for 14 days. They were asked to report the pain scores through the IPMS only. All other measurements were conducted by self-report questionnaires without face-to-face assessments.

Every day in the 14-day trial period, the control group was communicated with through conventional telephone calls or door-to-door visits to report their pain assessment data.

Measurement

The primary objective was to assess feasibility by observing the number of daily pain assessments recorded among patients. The secondary endpoint was to evaluate the effectiveness of pain management, changes in the quality of their lives and users' satisfaction.

The IPMS satisfaction evaluation questionnaire was completed by participants at the end of the study. Each questionnaire involved multiple 5-point Likert scores to rate among the options from "extremely like it" (5 points), "like it" (4 points), "okay" (3 points), "dislike it" (2 points) and "extremely dislike it" (1 point). The data generated after the survey were used to evaluate the satisfaction of IPMS usage. The questionnaire also contained an open-end question where participants were encouraged to put in any other suggestions about the IPMS app that they felt needed improvement.

A baseline pain assessment and a KPS evaluation were conducted using a numerical rating scale (NRS) in both groups. After obtaining consent, nurses conducted a standardized education session using a booklet to teach participants proper pain-related and rating system knowledge. At the end of the trial, the pain assessment and KPS evaluation were repeated in both groups.

All participants were asked to complete a general information questionnaire on pain management containing five questions upon registration. Each question was a 3-point Likert type response anchored from "well-known", "known", to "unknown". The same questionnaire was repeated at the end of the trial. Data generated at the beginning and the end of the trial were used to evaluate the participants' change of pain knowledge in the IPMS app or the conventional communication conditions.

Clinical Trial

To test the effectiveness of this designed IPMS app, a randomized, controlled clinical trial was conducted in a rural hospital in China from April to May 2016. Healthcare professionals in the rural hospital designed and supervised the processes of random group allocation, participant enrollment, and clinical intervention.

Enrollment of the Participants

The healthcare professionals, i.e., clinical physicians, recruited an original sample of 60 patients from the list of office or hospital visits to this rural hospital. Several selection criteria were set up to determine the eligibility of the participants. The patients must:

1. Be able to read Chinese and use smartphones;
2. Be between 45 and 70 years old;
3. Have been diagnosed with cancer and have self-reported cancer pain within a month prior to the study;
4. Have been seen on a regular basis by the oncology team;
5. Be under standard analgesia treatments;
6. Be estimated to have over 3 months of survival time.

To exclude possible confounding pain effects, eligible participants who self-reported to have severe cognitive impairments or major comorbid illnesses that would interfere with pain assessment were removed from the final list. For example, patients who received radiation therapy were excluded due to possible burning pain from the therapy. A total of 46 qualified cancer patients (14 females and 32 males) were finally included in the clinical trial.

Participant Characteristics

Included participants were randomly allocated to either the trial group or the control group. The random allocation (simple randomization) of the participants was automatically performed by a computer-generated random number table.

The participants were then randomly assigned into two groups: the trial group (25) and the control group (21). The trial group had six (24%) females and the control group had eight (38%) females. Each participant in the trial group was provided with an Android mobile phone with the IPMS loaded free of charge. They were given a demonstration and training by nurses and physicians on how to operate the smartphone and the IPMS app.

Data Analysis

The clinical trial was a double-blind experiment in which both the outcome assessors and participants were blinded to the procedure and data collection. The collected data were analyzed in the R Statistical Software Package 3.1.3. Independent Student's t-test and the Chi-square (χ^2) test were used to analyze the differences (NRS, AGE, KPS) in pain-controlled duration and breakthrough pain between the trial group and the control group. The significant difference was determined by $p < .05$.

IPMS Feasibility Testing

The compliance rate was consistently high over the course of the trial with no statistical difference ($p > .05$) in total numbers of daily pain assessment between week 1 ($M = 16.72$, $SD = 5.95$) and week 2 ($M = 18.36$, $SD = 6.35$). The total numbers of pain assessment differed between the day times ($M = 1.82$, $SD = 0.43$) and the night times ($M = 0.56$, $SD = 0.18$), respectively. There was no significant difference ($p > .05$) between the usage times in weekdays ($M = 2.45$, $SD = 0.6$) and weekends ($M = 2.15$, $SD = 0.18$).

Pain Management and KPS Evaluation

At the beginning of the trial, there was no significant difference ($t = 1.95, p = .06$) in the baseline pain scores between the trial group ($M = 3.28$, $SD = 0.68$) and the control group ($M = 2.90$, $SD = 0.62$). Over the 14-day trial period, the average pain score of the trial group was 2.53 ($SD = 0.42$), compared to 2.81 ($SD = 0.47$) of the control group with a significant difference ($t = -2.14, p = .04$). At the end of the trial period, the average pain score of the trial group was 2.20 ($SD = 0.50$), compared to 2.95 ($SD = 0.59$) of control group with a significant difference between the two groups ($t = -4.64, p < 0.001$).

To compare the pain score changes within each experiment group, a pair-wise t-test was conducted. For the trial group, there was a significant change of the pain score (t = 7.69, df = 24, p < .001) over the 14-day trial period. For the control group, the pain score change over the 14-day trial period was not significant (t = -0.27, df = 20, p = 0.789).

As to the evaluation of the acquired pain management knowledge after 14 day's IPMS interaction, there was a 2.96 ($SD = 0.61$) increase in the knowledge score of the trial group after using the IPMS for two weeks, compared a 0.81 ($SD = 0.67$) increase of the control group. Although both groups demonstrated increased pain management knowledge, the trial group indicated a higher score increase in pain management knowledge than did the control group ($t = 6.19, p < .001$).

Another feature of the app was the education and evaluation of quality of life through KPS. There had been no significant difference in the baseline KPS ($t = -0.07, p = .94$) between the trial group ($M = 50.80$, $SD = 7.02$) and the control group ($M = 50.95$, $SD = 7.40$) before the participants entered into the trial. At the end of the trial, the KPS was re-evaluated in the two groups. There was a significant difference ($t = 5.80, p < .001$) between the trial group (M = 68.80, SD = 7.23) and the control group (M = 56.19, SD = 7.40). Both groups increased the mean KPS scores significantly from the baseline, but the mean increase in the IPMS trial group ($M = 18.00$, $SD = 7.68$) was significantly larger ($t = 6.19, p < .001$) than the mean increase in the control group ($M = 5.23$, $SD = 5.11$).

Satisfaction

A post-trial evaluation was conducted to measure the participants' satisfaction toward using the IPMS. On the ease of use of the IPMS, of the 25 participants in the trial group, 9 (36%) indicated "very much like it (the IPMS)" and 16 (64%) indicated "like it (the IPMS)". No participant indicated dislike of the IPMS. On the helpfulness of the IPMS, 20 (80%) responded "very helpful" and 5 (20%) responded "helpful". On the software technical support, (18) 72% indicated "very much like it" and 7 (28%) indicated "like it". On the consultant and training course, a majority of participants 18 (72%) reported "very much like it" and (7) 28% reported "like it". On the prompt response for help, 7 (28%) indicated "very much like it", 11 (44%) indicated "like it", and 7 (28%) indicated "okay". The data suggested a high level of user satisfaction towards the IPMS.

DISCUSSION

Cancer has long become a threat to human health and well-being. Cancer pain originating from the tumor or the treatment thereof, is one of the most common and troublesome problems for patients with cancer. Psychologically, cancer pain affects the attention, memory and verbal ability of the majority of cancer patients. Cancer pain also causes depression, anxiety, fear, and anger. Chronic pain reduces the patients' physical function and overall quality of life, which demoralizes and debilitates the patients and their caregivers. Multiple pieces of evidence show that cancer pain also involves the endocrine, immune and nervous system, thus controlling cancer pain becomes increasingly imperative.

The clinical trial of this IPMS app indicated that pain management mobile apps could gain a high rate of compliance and satisfaction among cancer patients. Similar mobile pain management apps have been reported in the literature with regard to the use of technology without clinical intervention on cancer pain. Stinson et al. reported the development and testing of a multidimensional iPhone-based pain assessment application for youth cancer patients (Stinson et al., 2013). Their application was a game-based program to assess pain, which was specially designed for adolescent cancer patients with no healthcare professional intervention (Jibb et al., 2014; Stinson et al., 2013). Patients were prompted twice a day to complete a questionnaire on the status of pain. Although the usage data showed high compliance and satisfaction rates, no effect on the change or control of pain was reported (Stinson et al., 2013).

Compared to apps designed and operated without healthcare professionals involved, this IPMS app demonstrated the potential to improve pain management and patients' quality of life with its unique features of synchronized and asynchronized communication with healthcare professionals for clinical intervention. Patients were able to consult with healthcare professionals in real time about their pain control needs. Through the clinical trial data, this case indicated that timely healthcare professional intervention is the key to the success of similar pain management apps. The real-time communication feature provided in this mobile app was very limited. Only a few short text messages were allowed. A more feasible solution, particularly in China, is to incorporate such features in popular social networking apps, such as WeChat, which provide rich choices of communication channels, including text-based, audio, video and group communication.

The data collected from the clinical trial indicated that patients were more frequently using their IPMS app during night times than day times. Such convenience was made available across time and location, such as outside of normal business hours or in the rural areas where professional pain assistance was traditionally very rare or almost unavailable. In addition, this usage pattern suggested a potential advantage of the IPMS for collecting pain data at night times which was always a challenge for conventional methods. Real-time pain assessment data have been valuable for researchers and healthcare providers. With such a powerful tool like the IPMS, healthcare professionals and researchers may be able to better understand pain burst out patterns and provide timely responses to patients' needs, allowing for improved pain management and higher quality of pain treatment.

The clinical trial offered useful feedback on the feature offerings and the user interface of the IPMS. The patient satisfaction rate was high indicating patients' approval of the app's ease of use, as well as its value in medical consultation and training courses. Future improvements may include prompt responses to help requests and advanced features with new technology, such as voice control and machine learning.

This case revealed that the IPMS app also helped patients improve their knowledge of pain management and quality of life. In the clinical trial, patients in both groups were exposed to the same levels of clinical care, educational program, and pain management knowledge training. The patients in the intervention group reported better improvement in their knowledge of pain management and quality of life after the trial. These patients were more beneficial possibly due to the interactive learning mechanism that gave the trial group patients more confidence and knowledge to deal with their pain management. A similar phenomenon has also been observed and reported by Jan et al. (2007).

FUTURE RESEARCH DIRECTIONS

The currently available pain management apps do not directly measure pain, instead, they rely on patients' self-reported data to indirectly assess the level of pain. Self-reported data are inaccurate and subject to biases and errors. Researchers are working on new methods to assess the level of pain. A recent breakthrough on pain assessment is that certain blood gene expression biomarkers may be used to predict the state of pain (Niculescu et al., 2019). If future blood tests or other forms of physical examinations are able to objectively measure the severity of pain, healthcare professionals will have new ways to treat and care patients who are in pain.

The advancement of information and computer technology provides novel solutions to future pain management. For example, machine learning is expected to play a more active role in medical data analysis. Compared to traditional inferential statistics, which test hypotheses with data from a sample in order to draw conclusions about the population based on a series of preset statistical rules, machine learning, however, learns from currently available data without the necessity of previous knowledge (Lotsch & Ultsch, 2018). Machine learning algorithms can be used to identify and recognize patterns in complex data sets, such as a large volume patient and clinical data. With the assistance of machine learning algorithms, healthcare professionals will be able to reveal hidden relationships in pain data, identify the possible cause of pain, and be alerted of potential pain risks in patients.

Artificial intelligence (AI) is another emerging technology that may transform the future horizon of pain management and even the field of medicine. Compared to machine learning, which lets computers learn by themselves without human intervention, AI goes a step further by enabling computers to think and make decisions on behalf of a human. A recent study found that an AI-based smartphone app, ePAL, reduced the severity of patients' self-reported pain and the hospital admission rate (Kamdar, Centi, Fischer, & Jethwani, 2018). The AI algorithm was able to automatically pick out urgent issues from non-urgent issues in real time, and thus improved the efficiency of pain identification and response.

CONCLUSION

The rapid adoption of mobile devices worldwide provided a promising future for IPMS in cities and rural areas. This case presented an IPMS app that incorporated multidimensional features, including a fundamental pain assessment feature, along with other supplemental features such as KPS evaluation, medication reminders, real-time messaging consultation, and pain management education. The real-time messaging feature played a key role in patients' pain management. This IPMS app allowed patients to be able to instantaneously assess and report pain, thus healthcare professionals were able to provide prompt advice on the dosage change of pain control medication, which effectively reduced the pain. Compared to the control group which implemented a conventional method (i.e., telephone-based intervention) for pain communication and clinic intervention, the clinical trial group experimented with the IPMS app and reported more effective pain control results and better satisfaction. It is expected that the IPMS will become a popular communicating vehicle between the healthcare professionals and the cancer patients in the near future.

In conclusion, this case underscored the feasibility and acceptability of IPMS as a novel and effective pain assessment tool for patients with cancer pain. The clinical trial found that the IPMS system was considered easy to use and helpful by patients and it was beneficial for pain management, quality of life and pain management education among cancer patients. The IPMS has the potential to change the current atlas of pain management, especially in underdeveloped rural areas with improved efficiency and effectiveness of pain management and interactions between cancer patients and healthcare professionals.

ACKNOWLEDGMENT

This project was supported by the National Nature Science Foundation of China (81572859); Chinese National Program on Key Basic Research Project (973 Program) (2014CB910303); Shanghai Collaborative Innovation Center (TM201521). Registration: Clinicaltrials.gov NCT02765269, http://clinicaltrials.gov/ct2/show/ NCT02765269. Part of this project has been published in JMIR mHealth uHealth (Sun et al., 2017).

REFERENCES

Agboola, S. O., Ju, W., Elfiky, A., Kvedar, J. C., & Jethwani, K. (2015). The effect of technology-based interventions on pain, depression, and quality of life in patients with cancer: A systematic review of randomized controlled trials. *Journal of Medical Internet Research, 17*(3), e65. doi:10.2196/jmir.4009 PMID:25793945

Dalal, S., & Bruera, E. (2012). Assessing cancer pain. *Current Pain and Headache Reports, 16*(4), 314–324. doi:10.100711916-012-0274-y PMID:22585314

Deandrea, S., Montanari, M., Moja, L., & Apolone, G. (2008). Prevalence of undertreatment in cancer pain. A review of published literature. *Annals of Oncology: Official Journal of the European Society for Medical Oncology, 19*(12), 1985–1991. doi:10.1093/annonc/mdn419 PMID:18632721

Edwards, B. K., Noone, A. M., Mariotto, A. B., Simard, E. P., Boscoe, F. P., Henley, S. J., ... Ward, E. M. (2014). Annual report to the nation on the status of cancer, 1975-2010, featuring prevalence of comorbidity and impact on survival among persons with lung, colorectal, breast, or prostate cancer. *Cancer, 120*(9), 1290–1314. doi:10.1002/cncr.28509 PMID:24343171

Forbes, K. (2011). Pain in patients with cancer: The World Health Organization analgesic ladder and beyond. *Clinical Oncology (Royal College of Radiologists (Great Britain)), 23*(6), 379–380. doi:10.1016/j.clon.2011.04.016 PMID:21636259

Goss, P. E., Strasser-Weippl, K., Lee-Bychkovsky, B. L., Fan, L., Li, J., Chavarri-Guerra, Y., ... Chan, A. (2014). Challenges to effective cancer control in China, India, and Russia. *The Lancet Oncology, 15*(5), 489–538. doi:10.1016/S1470-2045(14)70029-4 PMID:24731404

Greco, M. T., Roberto, A., Corli, O., Deandrea, S., Bandieri, E., Cavuto, S., & Apolone, G. (2014). Quality of cancer pain management: An update of a systematic review of undertreatment of patients with cancer. *Journal of Clinical Oncology, 32*(36), 4149–4154. doi:10.1200/JCO.2014.56.0383 PMID:25403222

Heinonen, R., Luoto, R., Lindfors, P., & Nygard, C. H. (2012). Usability and feasibility of mobile phone diaries in an experimental physical exercise study. *Telemedicine Journal and e-Health, 18*(2), 115–119. doi:10.1089/tmj.2011.0087 PMID:22283356

Hu, W., & Ding, G. (2015). The application of intelligent pain management system in cancer pain patients. *Chinese Journal of Pain Medicine, 21*(2), 107–110.

Jacobsen, R., Liubarskiene, Z., Moldrup, C., Christrup, L., Sjogren, P., & Samsanaviciene, J. (2009). Barriers to cancer pain management: A review of empirical research. *Medicina (Kaunas, Lithuania), 45*(6), 427–433. doi:10.3390/medicina45060055 PMID:19605961

Jan, R. L., Wang, J. Y., Huang, M. C., Tseng, S. M., Su, H. J., & Liu, L. F. (2007). An Internet-based interactive telemonitoring system for improving childhood asthma outcomes in Taiwan. *Telemedicine Journal and e-Health, 13*(3), 257–268. doi:10.1089/tmj.2006.0053 PMID:17603828

Jibb, L. A., Stevens, B. J., Nathan, P. C., Seto, E., Cafazzo, J. A., & Stinson, J. N. (2014). A smartphone-based pain management app for adolescents with cancer: Establishing system requirements and a pain care algorithm based on literature review, interviews, and consensus. *JMIR Research Protocols, 3*(1), e15. doi:10.2196/resprot.3041 PMID:24646454

Kamdar, M. M., Centi, A. J., Fischer, N., & Jethwani, K. (2018). A randomized controlled trial of a novel artificial-intelligence based smartphone application to optimize the management of cancer-related pain. Paper presented at the *2018 Palliative and Supportive Care on Oncology Symposium*, San Diego, CA. 10.1200/JCO.2018.36.34_suppl.76

Kuzeyli Yildirim, Y., & Uyar, M. (2006). Barriers to effective cancer pain management. *The Journal of the Turkish Society of Algology, 18*(3), 12–19. Retrieved from https://www.ncbi.nlm.nih.gov/pubmed/17089225 PMID:17089225

Kwon, J. H. (2014). Overcoming barriers in cancer pain management. *Journal of Clinical Oncology, 32*(16), 1727–1733. doi:10.1200/JCO.2013.52.4827 PMID:24799490

Lesage, P., & Portenoy, R. K. (1999). Trends in cancer pain management. *Cancer Control, 6*(2), 136–145. doi:10.1177/107327489900600202 PMID:10758542

Linder, L. A., Ameringer, S., Baggott, C., Erickson, J., Macpherson, C. F., Rodgers, C., & Stegenga, K. (2015). *Measures and Methods for Symptom and Symptom Cluster Assessment in Adolescents and Young Adults with Cancer, 31*(3), 206–215.

Lotsch, J., & Ultsch, A. (2018). Machine learning in pain research. *Pain, 159*(4), 623–630. doi:10.1097/j.pain.0000000000001118 PMID:29194126

Marceau, L. D., Link, C., Jamison, R. N., & Carolan, S. (2007). Electronic diaries as a tool to improve pain management: Is there any evidence? *Pain Medicine, 8*(suppl_3), S101-S109. doi:10.1111/j.1526-4637.2007.00374.x

Mathur, G., Nain, S., & Sharma, P. K. (2015). Cancer: An overview. *Academic Journal of Cancer Research, 1*(1), 01-09.

Mulvaney, S. A., Anders, S., Smith, A. K., Pittel, E. J., & Johnson, K. B. (2012). A pilot test of a tailored mobile and web-based diabetes messaging system for adolescents. *Journal of Telemedicine and Telecare, 18*(2), 115–118. doi:10.1258/jtt.2011.111006 PMID:22383802

Niculescu, A. B., Le-Niculescu, H., Levey, D. F., Roseberry, K., Soe, K. C., Rogers, J., ... White, F. A. (2019). Towards precision medicine for pain: Diagnostic biomarkers and repurposed drugs. *Molecular Psychiatry*. doi:10.103841380-018-0345-5

O'Reilly, G. A., & Spruijt-Metz, D. (2013). Current mHealth technologies for physical activity assessment and promotion. *American Journal of Preventive Medicine, 45*(4), 501–507. doi:10.1016/j.amepre.2013.05.012 PMID:24050427

Palermo, T. M. (2009). Assessment of chronic pain in children: Current status and emerging topics. *Pain Research & Management, 14*(1), 21–26. doi:10.1155/2009/236426 PMID:19262912

Portenoy, R. K., & Lesage, P. (1999). Management of cancer pain. *Lancet, 353*(9165), 1695–1700. doi:10.1016/S0140-6736(99)01310-0 PMID:10335806

Rapoza, K. (2017). China's aging population becoming more of a problem. Forbes. Retrieved from https://www.forbes.com/sites/kenrapoza/2017/02/21/chinas-aging-population-becoming-more-of-a-problem/#25c770ac140f

Reynoldson, C., Stones, C., Bennett, M. I., Jones, R., Allsop, M., Gardner, P., . . . Knapp, P. (2014). Assessing the quality and usability of smartphone apps for pain self-management. *Pain Medicine, 15*(6), 898-909. doi:10.1111/pme.12327

Rosser, B. A., & Eccleston, C. (2011). Smartphone applications for pain management. *Journal of Telemedicine and Telecare, 17*(6), 308–312. doi:10.1258/jtt.2011.101102 PMID:21844177

Schag, C. C., Heinrich, R. L., & Ganz, P. A. (1984). Karnofsky performance status revisited: Reliability, validity, and guidelines. *Journal of Clinical Oncology, 2*(3), 187–193. doi:10.1200/JCO.1984.2.3.187 PMID:6699671

Stinson, J. N., Jibb, L. A., Nguyen, C., Nathan, P. C., Maloney, A. M., Dupuis, L. L., ... Orr, M. (2013). Development and testing of a multidimensional iPhone pain assessment application for adolescents with cancer. *Journal of Medical Internet Research, 15*(3), e51. doi:10.2196/jmir.2350 PMID:23475457

Stone, A. A., & Broderick, J. E. (2007). Real-time data collection for pain: Appraisal and current status. *Pain Medicine, 8*(Suppl 3), S85–S93. doi:10.1111/j.1526-4637.2007.00372.x PMID:17877531

Sun, Y., Jiang, F., Gu, J. J., Wang, Y. K., Hua, H., Li, J., ... Hu, W. (2017). Development and testing of an Intelligent Pain Management System (IPMS) on mobile phones through a randomized trial among Chinese cancer patients: A new approach in cancer pain management. *JMIR mHealth and uHealth, 5*(7), e108. doi:10.2196/mhealth.7178 PMID:28743681

Thurnheer, S. E., Gravestock, I., Pichierri, G., Steurer, J., & Burgstaller, J. M. (2018). Benefits of mobile apps in pain management: Systematic review. *JMIR mHealth and uHealth, 6*(10), e11231. doi:10.2196/11231 PMID:30348633

Wallace, L. S., & Dhingra, L. K. (2014). A systematic review of smartphone applications for chronic pain available for download in the United States. *Journal of Opioid Management, 10*(1). doi:10.5055/jom.2014.0193 PMID:24604571

Ward, S. E., Goldberg, N., Miller-McCauley, V., Mueller, C., Nolan, A., Pawlik-Plank, D., ... Weissman, D. E. (1993). Patient-related barriers to management of cancer pain. *Pain, 52*(3), 319–324. doi:10.1016/0304-3959(93)90165-L PMID:7681557

World Health Organization. (2017). Cancer Fact Sheet. Retrieved from http://www.who.int/mediacentre/factsheets/fs297/en/

Yang, J., Weng, L., Chen, Z., Cai, H., Lin, X., Hu, Z., ... Liu, M. (2019). Development and testing of a mobile app for pain management among cancer patients discharged from hospital treatment: Randomized controlled trial. *JMIR mHealth and uHealth, 7*(5), e12542. doi:10.2196/12542 PMID:31144672

KEY TERMS AND DEFINITIONS

Cancer Pain: Cancer pains are usually caused by tumors pressing on bones, nerves or other organs in the body or cancer treatment such as chemotherapy or radiotherapy. Cancer pains include nerve pains, bone pains, soft tissue pains, phantom pains, and referred pains. Chronic cancer pain, often due to nerve changes, may cause mild to severe pain for a long period of time. Controlling cancer pain is a critical part of cancer patient care, especially for patients at the terminal stages.

Clinical Trial: Clinical trials are experiments conducted in clinical research and practice to discover the effect of particular treatments or interventions. Clinical trials are usually conducted with at least an intervention group and a control group, in order to identify the true effect without interference from uncontrolled variables.

Intelligent Pain Management Systems (IPMS): An intelligent pain management system (IPMS) is a computer system that can effectively capture, transfer, store, and analyze patients' pain data with minimum intervention from the healthcare providers. A recent IPMS often includes a module to support mobile devices. It is expected that future IPMS will incorporate new advancements from the research of artificial intelligence, cloud computing, and the fifth generation of mobile communication system (5G).

Karnofsky Performance Status (KPS): The Karnofsky Performance Score (KPS) was developed by Dr. David A. Karnofsky and his colleagues to evaluate patients' health status. The KPS ranking describes patient's health status from 0 to 100, with 0 being patient death to 100 being patient in perfect health condition. In practice, the KPS scores are often evaluated in an interval of 10.

Life Quality: Life quality (also known as quality of life) is an overall assessment of the important aspects of patients' life, including the status of patients' cognitive, emotional, physical, social, and spiritual aspects as well as the patients' health care and personal autonomy aspects.

Machine Learning: Machine learning is a technology that relies on computer algorithms and statistical methods to automatically generate patterned models from sample data sets without human intervention. The sample data sets, also known as the *training data*, may be *labeled* (containing both inputs and known outputs) or *unlabeled* (only containing inputs without outputs). If a patterned model is generated from *labeled* data sets, the process is called *supervised* learning. If a patterned model is generated from *unlabeled* data sets, the process is called *unsupervised* learning.

Mobile Applications: Mobile applications (also known as mobile apps) are software programs that operate on mobile devices, including smartphones, tablets, wearable devices, etc. Mobile apps are often optimized for mobile devices to offer location-based, personalized, and time-sensitive features. Examples of mobile apps include social networking, maps and navigation, communication, shopping, personalized education, etc.

Numerical Rating Scale: The Numeric Rating Scale is a quantitative measure of patients' pain intensity. In practice, patients are often surveyed with questions related to their perceived level of pain. A patient selects a whole number (from 1 to 10) that best reflects the intensity of his or her pain.

Pain Management: Pain management employs a combination of medical, physical, and psychological approaches to ease the painful feeing of patients and to improve their quality of life. Pain management methods involve medication, psychological counseling, physical therapies, nursing care, etc. Effective management of chronic pain is important for cancer patients.

Chapter 12
Promises and Challenges of Medical Patient Healthcare Portals in Underserved Communities:
The Case of Einstein Medical Center Philadelphia (EMCP)

Diane C. Lee
Drexel University, USA

David Gefen
Drexel University, USA

ABSTRACT

As a safety-net medical center that serves many underserved communities, Einstein Medical Center Philadelphia (EMCP) faces many challenges in providing healthcare to its communities. To improve those services, EMCP has released a new IT healthcare portal (app). This chapter describes some of the promises and challenges EMCP is currently facing in their attempts to convince communities in its catchment area to adopt that healthcare portal. The challenges are discussed in the contexts of poor social determinants of health (SDOH), unique social factors, as well as the importance of managing community trust in EMCP within the broader contexts of underserved communities of which the new portal is only part of the story. This is not a typical case of IT adoption. The challenges at hand are not only technical but to a large degree social, dealing in part with issues of cultural diversity, perceived lack of respect, and poor health literacy.

DOI: 10.4018/978-1-7998-0047-7.ch012

INTRODUCTION

There is growing interest among medical service providers in the social factors that influence the quality and provision of medical services. These social factors, such as income and social status, education, employment, often called social determinants of health (SDOH), are the topic of this chapter. For the urban medically underserved, SDOH influences health profoundly and hinders access to medical care (Anderson, Hsieh, & Alter, 2016). Indeed, dialogue and policy surrounding health reform suggests that SDOH problems might account for nearly one third of annual deaths in the United States despite provisions in the Affordable Care Act to address SDOH (Anderson, Lippert, et al., 2016; Galea, Tracy, Hoggatt, DiMaggio, & Karpati, 2011). There is consensus that in order to address such problems healthcare providers must initiate new practices at what is often the first entry point of care to the medical system, namely the Emergency Department (ED). If the ED is the only consistent source of medical care and medical information for this vulnerable population, as it often is, then technologies such as patient portals could be of much help in enabling patients' self-management. Self-management could offset some of the strain on medical centers, a point of much importance to EDs, which are dealing with an increasing load of impoverished patients with unmet social needs across the country. Significant disparities exist in access to care and health outcomes across the United States (Wallace, Angier, Huguet, Gaudino, Krist, Dearing et al., 2016). Underserved patient populations experience barriers to accessing and engaging within the complex health system and electronic portals have been proposed as a viable solution to overcome health disparities by offering a potential new way for patients to become more active participants in their healthcare (Wallace et al., 2016).

Yet, studies specific to underserved patients suggest that underserved populations may have difficulty accessing these electronic engagement resources, which will reduce portal adoption rates (Wallace et al., 2016). A study conducted by Ancker, Barrón, Rockoff, Hauser, Pichardo, Szerencsy et al. (2011) in a large cohort of underserved patients in New York, identified significant racial and ethnic barriers among patients receiving an access activation code and subsequently using the electronic patient portals. Other studies reported more encouraging results. A study conducted by Zarcadoolas, Vaughon, Czaja, Levy, and Rockoff (2013) using focus groups found users reported finding great value in patient portals that positively impacted communication with providers, and improved knowledge, empowerment, and self-care. In another study, focus group participants were positive about online access to medical records but did express concern about potential loss of privacy and interference with the patient–provider relationship (Dhanireddy, Walker, Reisch, Oster, Delbanco, & Elmore, 2014).

A patient portal provides a secure online website that provides convenient access to personal health information. They are distinct from electronic health records that are owned, maintained and updated by healthcare organizations. Patient portals allow patients to interact with their own personal health information. Portals allow patients to securely perform a multitude of tasks that includes: scheduling appointments, retrieving laboratory results, managing medications, and accessing medical history data and other patient education or health information, and communicating with their healthcare provider to answer health questions. The asynchronous patient-provider communication may potentially improve the efficiency healthcare communications and potentially reduce the demand on provider resources (Ammenwerth, Schnell-Inderst, & Hoerbst, 2012).

Of the barriers cited impacting portal adoption, building trust and avoiding distrust are crucial in the successful adoption of IT, including medical IT portals. The importance of trust and its influence on portal adoption was examined through ethnographic experiences from *Einstein Medical Center Phila-*

delphia (EMCP), an urban medical center, focusing on patients utilizing the ED as the main source for medical care. First, the Chapter presents the importance of addressing the social determinants of health from the ED through Social Emergency Medicine. Emergency physicians caring for an underserved population, who are complicated medically and socially, may need to consider the social determinants underlying health and illness in developing systemic interventions and collaborative partnership with community resources to improve the health of this patient population. Next, social factors and the role of trust is examined as important constructs impacting portal adoption. An overview of *Einstein Medical Center*, an urban safety net hospital providing the study setting, is described to give context to the culture of the organization and the community served. The remainder of the chapter details the ethnographic experiences that highlight the promises and challenges faced by *Einstein Medical Center* as it seeks to encourage adoption and use of a patient portal. Patient portals have been shown to have potential for great utility and may be valuable in improving the health of an underserved population through greater engagement in healthcare through online access (Zarcadoolas et al., 2013). For *Einstein*, increased portal adoption may reduce the overburden of the ED adapting to a more complex patient acuity level while moving in parallel with their primary mission to provide acute and emergency care to all patients who come through their door.

BACKGROUND

Social Emergency Medicine and the Social Determinants of Health (SDOH)

Research has shown that there is reduced portal adoption by medically underserved patients (Wallace et al., 2017). Given that social factors are posited to negatively impact user acceptance of portal technology for patients using the ED as the primary source of medical care, it is important to examine these factors and the impact on the ED environment in closer detail. The social determinants of health are economic and social conditions that affect a wider range of health risks and outcomes. Socioeconomic status (SES), an important component of SDOH, is a composite measure that incorporates economic status, measured by income, social status measured by education, and work status measured by occupation (Adler et al., 1994). Circumstances shaped by the distribution of money, power, and resources influence the risk for disease or vulnerability to a disease or injury. The World Health Organization says that "This unequal distribution of health-damaging experiences is not in any sense a 'natural' phenomenon but is the result of a toxic combination of poor social policies, unfair economic arrangements [where the already well-off and healthy become even richer and the poor who are already more likely to be ill become even poorer], and bad politics" (WHO, 2008). Central to community health as an access point to the medical system, emergency medicine is a specialty born of a societal need for equal access to medical care for patients regardless of their socioeconomic status (Anderson, Hsieh, et al., 2016). Thus, the modern ED must consider the interplay between social forces and the emergency care system. A collaborative approach is needed to develop cost-effective interventions to influence the health of individuals and their communities in providing equal access to medical care for all patients regardless of their socioeconomic status. Hence, Social Emergency Medicine creates a framework for emergency medicine as society's medical and social safety-net (Anderson, Hsieh, et al., 2016).

The Social Factors in Portal Adoption

The social context influences portal adoption by placing barriers such as language and cultural differences on initiatives that are key to forging trusting relationships. People build trust with others who they perceive to be like them (Zucker, 1986). Language may function as an indicator of shared identity and may emphasize in-group versus outgroup dynamics. The language of a diverse patient population is derived from experiences and personal connections in their community which may differ from the environment where they are being treated. As trust is culture-dependent, the role of trust in a specific IT for a vulnerable population will be impacted by the perceived cultural similarity that exist between the users and the urban healthcare environment, much as it is in other contexts of IT adoption (Gefen & Ridings, 2003). But this goes both ways: cultural choice of words used by either the provider or the patient, touching, or gestures may also be misinterpreted and hinder building trust. Due to the complexity of the social factors affecting the health of medically underserved patients, physicians may consider using a variety of communication narratives to temper the SDOH barriers in understanding and treating patients that come from different backgrounds with a multitude of problems. If trust is built with underserved patients dependent on ED services where their medical and social issues are addressed, then the opinions of the provider and healthcare organization may be viewed as important in their decision process influencing user behavior towards adopting the IT healthcare portal.

In examining IT adoption, Social Identity Theory (SIT) can also be applied as it relates to focusing on how identification with groups affects individuals' beliefs and behavior. SIT recognizes that people's self-identity comes from their perception of what social group they feel they belong to and thus may add insight into individual decision-making processes. Gefen and Ridings (2003) show how user acceptance of IT increased based on a belief that the intergroup boundary between them and the IT group was reduced, and they shared the same values. The importance of social identity and its extension to trust underscores the importance of people's perceptions that they share the same values as the individuals providing the services in making those services more effective. A social emergency medicine agenda that takes an expansive view of the coordinated care of an underserved population may result in a level of understanding and relatedness that positively resonates with patients. The perception that the organization consists of "people like me" or is perceived as willing to embrace diverse backgrounds where values and objectives seem matched to "me" increases trust which in turn is associated with increases in levels of other factors that may contribute to the intention to adopt technology (Warkentin, Sharma, Gefen, Rose, & Pavlou, 2018). As such, the role of trust is important as an antecedent of the acceptance, use of and loyalty towards technology, making it a key factor across the healthcare sector (Abbas, Carroll, & Richardson, 2018).

Managing Trust (and Avoiding Distrust) in Portal Adoption

Trust is the belief that another person or organization on whom one depends will behave in a socially acceptable manner and thus, fulfill the trusting parties' expectations (Gefen, Rose, Warkentin, & Pavlou, 2005; Mayer, Davis, & Schoorman, 1995). Trust has behavioral implications because it is one of the determinants of the behavioral extent to which people are willing to rely on others. In an Internet environment, trust is especially important because visual and social cues that people in other contexts may rely on are missing. Supporting this proposition, Gefen (2000) and Gefen, Karahanna, and Straub (2003), explain that trust is crucial as an enabler of social interactions because it reduces down to manageable levels the otherwise overwhelming social complexity and uncertainty involved in assessing others' possible future behaviors, behaviors that cannot always be controlled or anticipated. Research has shown trust-based antecedents are strong predictors that influence user behavior in IT adoption (Benbasat, Gefen, & Pavlou, 2008), including governmental initiatives (Warkentin et al., 2018).

To better understand the impact of trust as it relates to IT adoption involves a closer examination of the antecedents of trust. These antecedents are important in understanding trust and its link to user behavior in the context of an underserved patient population that the medical center hopes will adopt their new medical healthcare portal, a new technology. There are two aspects of user behavior to consider in applying these trust beliefs. First, is the trust belief in the provider. The trust that develops between patient and provider is paramount. Patients with medical conditions seek treatment at the ED with the expectation and trust of receiving care from well-meaning and experienced medical providers. This implies the providers are essentially given the benefit of trust in the absence of a history of interaction.

However, information asymmetry must be taken into account when considering the physician-patient dyad, where there is an imbalance with the physician presumably knowing a lot and the patient knowing little by comparison. Power and status differences may have important and far reaching implications for perceptions, motivations, and behavior (Bunderson & Reagans, 2011). These differences may also help contextualize strain to the physician-patient dyad. When applied to a vulnerable population, the unequal distribution of power and status between the physician and patient has the potential to adversely affect forming a trust relationship. As a result, during the medical encounter, the patient may not fully understand the information being conveyed about their health condition but may not feel it is safe to question the provider or fear that doing so might lead to negative evaluation affecting their treatment plan. The perceptions of lack of psychological safety and a perceived power differential may cause patients to behave in a more tentative and inhibited way. Without questions raised by the patient, the physician may assume a trusted relationship, when under conditions of unequal power and status the patient and family leave with a lack of understanding about prognosis, resources, and post-discharge care plans.

Having trust in the patient portal is another user behavior consideration in the adoption of a healthcare patient IT portal. Regardless of the healthcare communication that may develop to influence use of the portal as a tool for self-management, the specific IT portal must be perceived to be beneficial, easy to use, and include trust building mechanisms. Thus, familiarity or knowledge-based trust with the healthcare organization is an important trust antecedent. That is the case in many business contexts too, such as outsourcing, where the client often gives strong preference to a provider with whom it had had a previous relationship (Gefen & Carmel, 2008; Gefen, Wyss, & Lichtenstein, 2008; Gulati, 1995). In that regard, EMCP is well known in the community. In addition to medical care, patients utilize the hospital for a variety of services. EMCP has demonstrated a dedicated mission to improved quality of life within the community through balanced investments in healthcare and social services. In building trust in the portal, another important consideration is institutional based trust. Institutional based trust refers to a sense of security resulting from guarantees or safety-net reassurances (McKnight, Cummings, & Chervany,1998). If the portal can match patients' expectations of a typical online tool, there is a greater chance for a high propensity for trust in the IT provider (Gefen et al., 2003).

Related to institutional based trust is structural assurances, ie, safeguards built into the website that provides users with a level of perceived security. Patients, similar to online buyers in this context (Gefen et al., 2003), may be more likely to trust an online tool that provides assurances of being reliable and credible for disclosing highly sensitive personal health information (Bansal, Zahedi, & Gefen, 2007, 2010). Studies conducted by Van Velsen, Wildevuur, Flierman, Van Schooten, Tabak, and Hermens (2015) examined trust in telemedicine, another type of e-health technology, through use of a portal. Results showed trust to be an important factor to users for both the healthcare professionals and the portal technology. The competency level of the healthcare professional contributed to a trusted relationship that developed as early as the initial face-to-face encounter. Trust in the vendor was based on reputation, and trust in the technology formed when the patient perceived control and privacy of the data (Van Velsen et al., 2015).

When considering the importance of the antecedents of trust in online environments such as patient portals, distrust is also an important consideration. While trust is built gradually, it can be broken due to an adverse circumstance and replaced with distrust (Pavlou & Gefen, 2005). Negative outcomes may cause distrust even when they are not directly related to the patient such as other patients, or even someone identified as part of the same social group, who came to the ED with a medical problem but left dissatisfied. Hospitals attempt to negate perceived broken trust by seeking feedback about the patient's experience and responding in a timely manner to expressed concerns when they perceive patient expectations have not been met. In their research on the nature and role of trust in a banking environment, Gefen et al. (2008) posit that trust and distrust are not two sides of the same continuum. Rather, trust is about giving the trustee credit of behaving in an acceptable manner, and in doing so ignoring vulnerabilities. Distrust, on the other hand, is about responding to perceived danger (Dimoka, 2010). Indeed, research shows that the positive impact of trust is attenuated by the effects of psychological contract violation, an occurrence where one party perceives another party has acted opportunistically (Pavlou & Gefen, 2005). Just as a patient's trust may encourage them to use the new portal, distrust of the physician or the medical center may detract them from doing so.

Research studies have shown trust, privacy, and user perceptions to be important elements of online technology adoption (Gefen, Karahanna, & Straub, 2003; Gefen & Straub, 2000). Durkan, Durkin, and Gillen (2003) describe online trust as an association of networked relationships between the parties involved where all partners in the network must be seen as trustworthy for members to willingly assume risk. Extending this network of trust to e-health, in the patient-provider exchange, the provider's e-health system, e.g. patient portal, can provide structural assurance that the online technology environment is safe and under control. A patient's willingness to engage in online transactions depends upon users trusting each other and the systems they use to meet, communicate, and conduct transactions (Riegelsberger, Sasse, & McCarthy, 2005). In considering why a given party will have a greater or lesser amount of trust for another party warrants examining the attributes of the trustee. As a set, ability, benevolence, and integrity are the three characteristics that appear to explain a major portion of trustworthiness (Mayer, Davis, & Schoorman, 1995). Individually, each contributes a unique perspective from which to consider the trustee while collectively providing a solid foundation for the empirical study of trust of another party (Mayer et al., 1995). The trustee is deemed to be trustworthy if all three characteristics are high. Yet, trustworthiness should be considered a continuum where all three factors can vary along this continuum. Thus, high trust may be a result of high levels of all three factors but can vary independently of the other (Mayer et al., 1995).

Managing trust is a key factor in the ethnographic experiences presented. Consider portal adoption and the influence of the community. Underserved populations may have specific needs and reasons for using technology but may feel left out of providing input into the process of selecting and implementing technologies. Trust becomes important in ensuring the primary focus is on what will be of benefit to the communities rather than perhaps a priority that benefits the organization. As communities become more involved in use of technology, it may be a way of providing people with access to information and resources that encourages self-management and meets their everyday needs.

An important cultural barrier cited in patient-physician communication has been race and ethnicity. Problems in the patient-provider communication due to cultural differences may contribute to a disparity in the understanding of the diagnosis and associated treatment plan. For the underserved patient population, the "code of the street" takes precedent in the communication process. A provider that shows respect is more likely to be trusted than one who, while not deliberately, appears condescending or "invades" the personal space, making the patient feel like they have been disrespected or uncomfortable and therefore cannot be trusted.

African Americans and other ethnic minority patients in race-discordant relationships, such as the environment at *Einstein* with a predominantly minority population being treated by primarily non-minority providers, report less involvement in medical decision making, less partnership with physicians, lower levels of trust, and lower levels of satisfaction with care (Cooper-Patrick, Gallo, Gonzales, Vu, Powe, Nelson et al., 1999; Doescher, Saver, Franks, & Fiscella, 2000). Therefore, communication and cultural competency programs with implementation of tools such as AIDET that emphasize patient centeredness is an important mechanism by which quality of care for all patients might be improved. Focusing on affective dimensions of communication versus emphasizing instrumental behaviors (information giving and medication counseling) may be more advantageous in building a trust relationship to influence patient behaviors (Cooper-Patrick et al., 1999). Effective communication enables a patient and physician to find points of commonality that in turn may build trust and satisfaction (Street, O'Malley, Cooper, & Haidet, 2008). Studies conducted by Street et al. (2008) that examined perceived personal similarity suggested the physician-patient relationship is strengthened when patients see themselves as similar to their physicians in personal beliefs, values, and communication. Findings reported higher ratings of trust satisfaction, and intention to adhere associated with perceived personal similarity.

A patient's trust in institutions that may develop various health information technologies (HIT), such as healthcare organizations, may influence their likelihood of adopting HIT and could be associated with health literacy levels (Mackert, Mabry-Flynn, Champlin, Donovan, & Pounders, 2016). Studies conducted by Mackert et al. (2016) included trust as a construct in assessing the relationship between health literacy and health information technology application adoption and usage. Results from the study showed patients with lower health literacy were more likely to place trust in healthcare providers. These findings suggest organizations implementing new HIT among lower health literate users should consider partnering with trusted healthcare providers to help ensure adoption (Mackert et al., 2016).

Similar arguments that underscore the importance of trust and its influence on portal adoption can be made for portal readiness, access to care and care coordination, and other initiatives needed to ensure that users receive full benefits from technological advances, e.g. patient portal, as a result of engaging with organizations and providers they trust.

Einstein Medical Center Philadelphia: A Safety-Net Hospital

A safety-net hospital or health system is defined as those institutions providing care to all patients regardless of their ability to pay. EMCP is a private healthcare safety-net, serving a proportionately higher number of patients regardless of race, religion, national origin, or ability to pay. Most patients are uninsured or receive government insurance, such as Medicaid, Medicare SSI, or Children's' Health Insurance Program (CHIP). EMCP, the flagship hospital in the *Einstein Healthcare Network*, is an academic community medical center situated in North Philadelphia, serving a diverse and disadvantaged community. EMCP's long-standing commitment to providing medical services meets with their recognized responsibility to use resources to elevate the health status of the communities served.

Safety-net hospitals play an important role in the nation's healthcare system, yet often encounter difficult financial positions due to the vulnerable financial state of the patients and lack of sufficient Federal, Commonwealth, and local funding as well as policy changes. As such, EMCP relies on gifts from grateful patients and families, alumni, employees, the community, and other donors that support EMCP's mission.

The culture of the hospital is largely defined by its history. The *Albert Einstein Healthcare Network* was founded in 1865 in Philadelphia as "The Jewish Hospital". It was an important institution in the history of the Jewish people in Philadelphia, providing care for the suffering poor of all religions. One of the core missions at that time was the care of Jewish veterans of the Civil War. In addition, during that era, Jewish physicians had difficulty getting admitting privileges at most hospitals. These core values extend to the mission of the organization today to "serve with humanity, humility, and honor, to heal by providing exceptionally intelligent and responsive healthcare and education to a community in need". To carry out its mission, EMCP offers a wide range of healthcare programs and services, ranging from community-based education programs and preventive medicine to complex care, requiring advanced technology and expertise (www.einstein.edu/about/einstein-legacy).

As is a standard practice at most major health systems, the *Einstein Health Portal* has been deployed to allow patients to be more actively involved in their own health care. However, like other safety-net institutions, EMCP is faced with the challenges of increasing portal adoption for a vulnerable population that is presented with social factors that are barriers to wellness. It means not only addressing questions on how to encourage portal adoption but also addressing social issues that might contribute or hinder portal utilization. Research on the challenges of deploying the portal due to social factors may provide practical value by providing insight into knowing what barriers to expect for targeted support that may increase patient engagement.

The *Einstein Health Portal* provides options for appointment scheduling, review of medications, lab results and clinical summaries from medical visits and the ability to send and receive messages. Figures 1 through 5 show screenshots of the portal interface. The homepage for *MY Einstein Health Patient Portal* provides a capsule view for user navigation, headings for portal content, and highlights value and security assurances of portal use (Figure 1). Once a patient logs into their personal health information homepage, a summary of records that can be accessed is displayed (Figure 2). In addition to a concise display of visit elements, each topic can be accessed to display more detailed clinical information. Appointments can be scheduled and communication with physicians through messaging is available (Figure 3). The clinical summary documents are archived visits with the physician that can be referenced as needed. Detailed information about a particular clinical element, such as laboratory results are available to view and displayed with reference ranges (Figure 4). Values outside the range are shown highlighted to indicate abnormal values (Figure 5). A link to obtain more information about a specific measure is also included.

Although designed with all the key features to support patient engagement, the challenges for an underserved population with health literacy issues may be expressed as difficulties in understanding and in interpreting the clinical information as it is presented. For example, lab results are reported in scientific terms with reference ranges. A link is provided as an option for more detail, but patients with lower education levels and low literacy may not find the information useful if they do not understand how it impacts their health. Clinical summaries are available. However, a message in small print indicates that a PDF reader is required, making it difficult for the elderly or for those with disabilities, such as suffering from sight impairment, to access the information. Assistance with using the site is provided through FAQs, but those assume that the user can understand and follow the instructions as written.

RESEARCH OBJECTIVE

The research objective was to bring, through ethnographic experiences as an Emergency Medicine Healthcare Administrator, an examination of the social disparities in health and healthcare and the significance those have on influencing patients' participation in their healthcare management and related decisions to adopt technology that may provide value in improving their health outcomes. The value of the knowledge gained may benefit the organization in providing insight into the factors influencing increased patient engagement and technology acceptance to improve health outcomes.

Figure 1. Homepage for MY Einstein Health Patient Portal

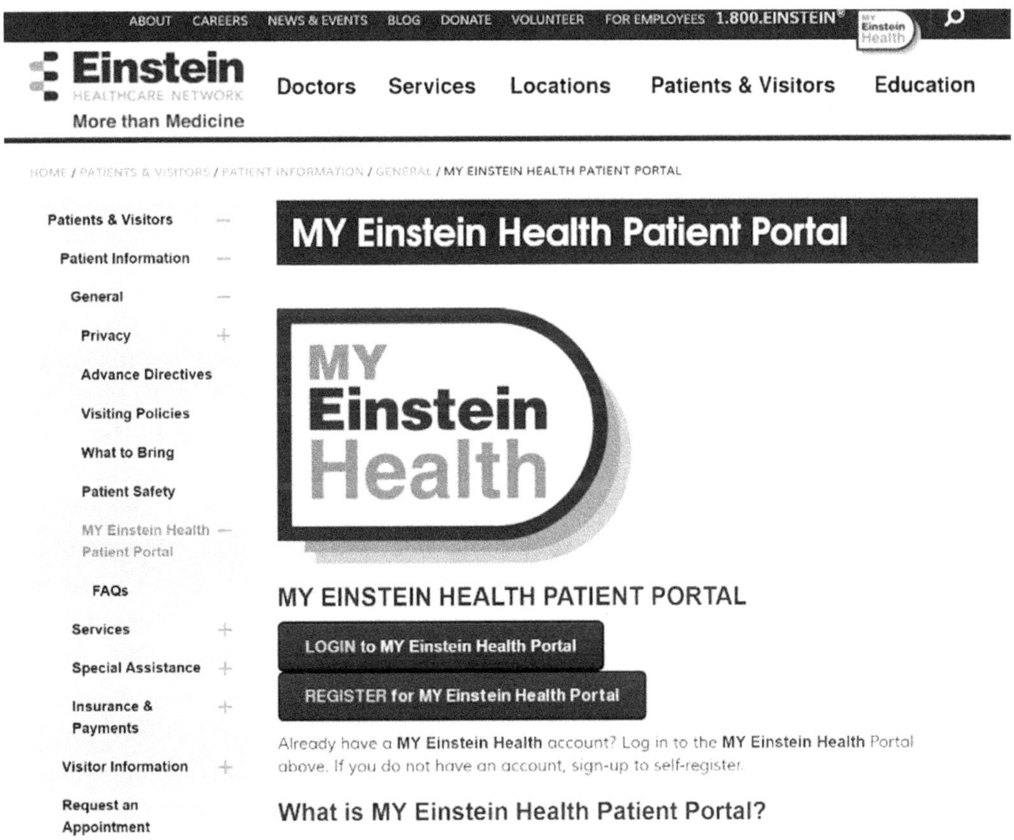

Figure 2. Summary of records

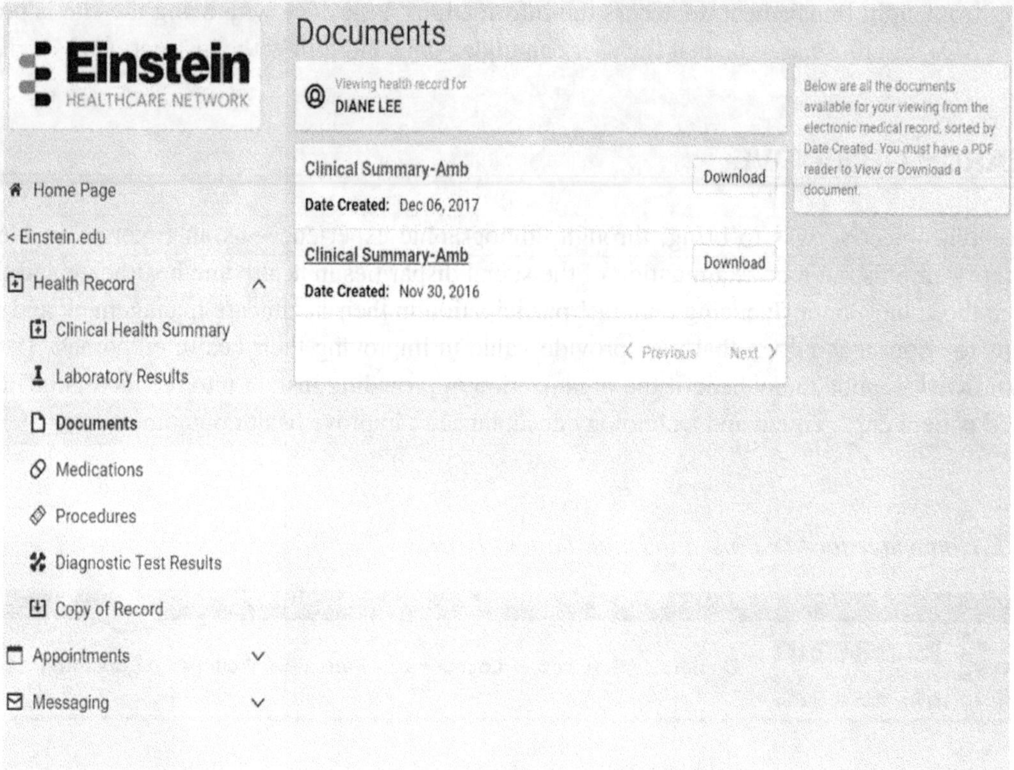

Research Methods

The methodology applied in this study was ethnography. Ethnographic research is a kind of qualitative research where the researchers immerse themselves in the organization as a way of better understanding hands-on the issues, culture, and challenges at hand over extended periods of time. This methodology is based on cultural anthropology and counts on the social understanding of the experience gained by the researcher rather than interviews or surveys of others. Ethnography is a process by which a culture group is studied as well as an outcome of research as the final written product. Ethnography relies on the participant views that are filtered through the researcher's scientific perspective to develop an overall cultural interpretation (Creswell & Poth, 2017). The cultural interpretation describes the groups and themes related to the theoretical concepts being explored in the study. The ethnography analysis results in an understanding of how the culture sharing group works, the essence of how it functions, and the group's way of life (Creswell & Poth, 2017).

As a healthcare administrator, practice operations, patient flow, and patient satisfaction dictate close interactions with the patients. Through participant observation, the challenges this patient population faces that impact their care on a daily basis is witnessed first-hand, and that allows for full immersion by the researchers enabling them to describe and interpret the shared and learned patterns of values, behaviors, beliefs, and language and the interaction among members of the culture sharing group under examination (Harris, 2001). It is in the observation of these cases and how patients respond that provides context to their challenges and behaviors that may impact the potential use of a portal and self-management.

Figure 3. Appointments and communication through portal

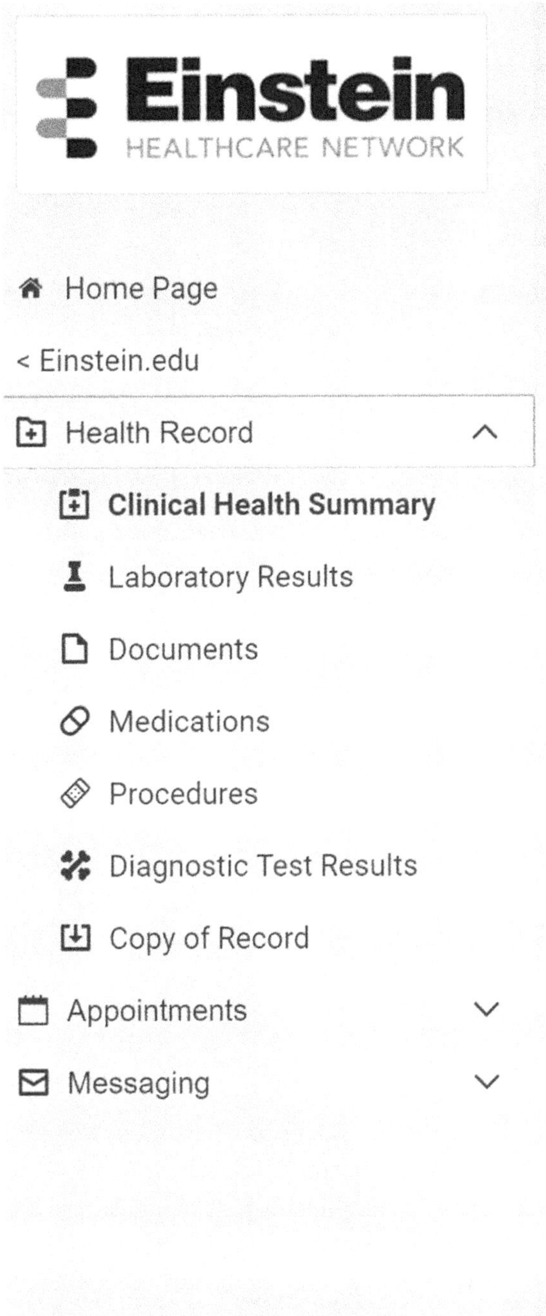

Figure 4. Laboratory results through portal

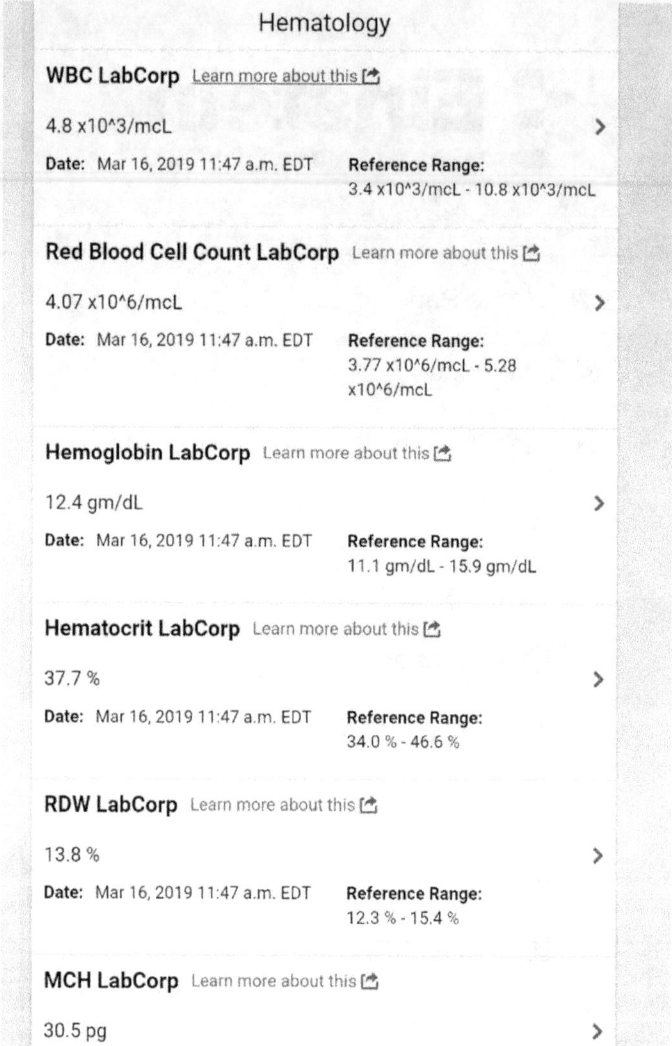

Through observation, the impact of limited resources is seen. For example, the patient who calls 911 for an ambulance to bring them to the hospital but lacks transportation to return home. Behaviors resulting from undereducated and poor health literacy may manifest in prescribed medications not taken correctly because the patient did not understand labeling instructions. Low socioeconomic status may result in patients failing to see their primary care doctor for preventive care or get the recommended diagnostic study because they lack the necessary insurance copay. Other behaviors are observed due to trauma informed care. Many patients are victims of adverse childhood experiences such as physical abuse, verbal abuse, sexual abuse, physical neglect, emotional neglect, or other trauma resulting from violence in their community. Since *Einstein* is located in a diverse community of disadvantaged patients, often they are seeking medical care from the same place where a relative or friend may have been treated without a positive outcome. Acknowledging the effect these circumstances may have had may change the initial provider question from "what's wrong with you" to "what happened to you" to understand the

Figure 5. Values outside range highlighted in portal

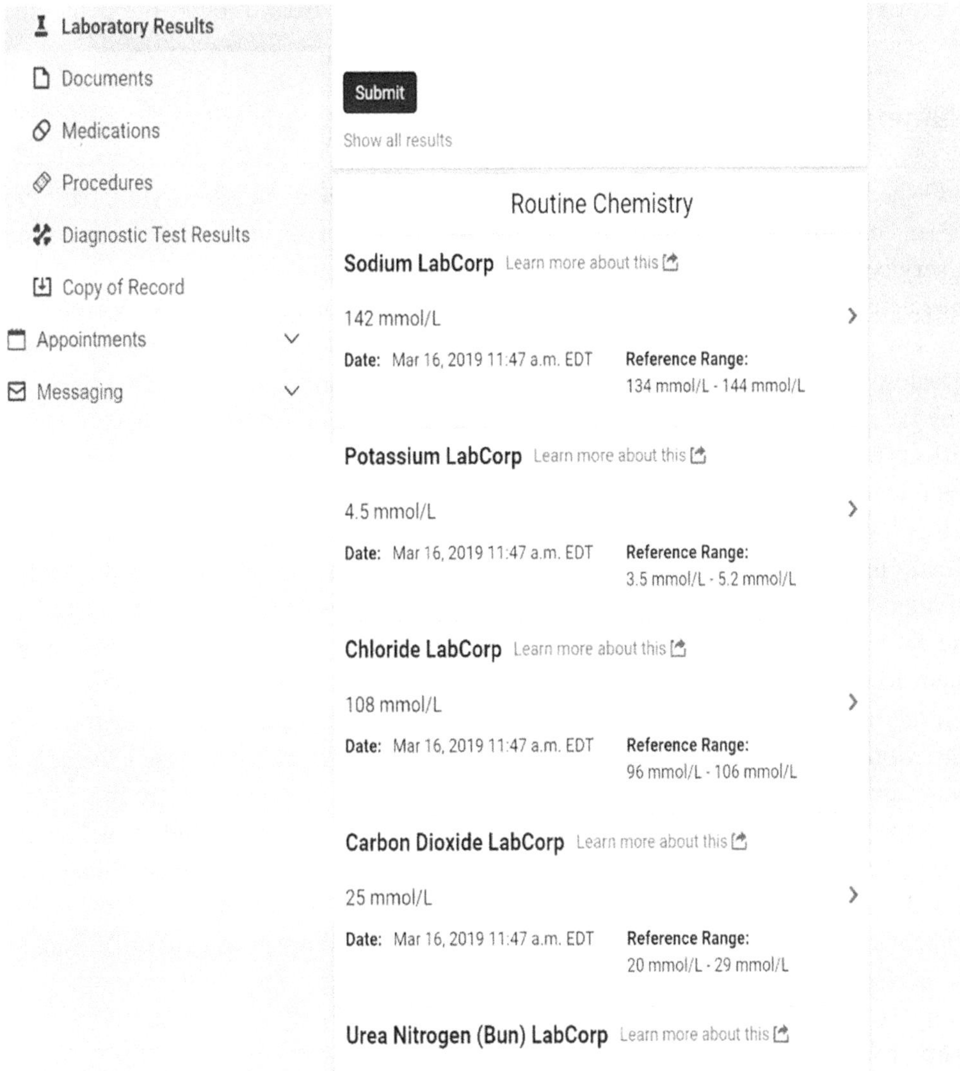

best approach to treatment and the potential need for additional social service support. For example, an ED nurse communicated to the physician before seeing a patient seeking treatment in the ED that the patient was being uncooperative. When questioned, the patient shared that the treatment room was the same as the one where her relative had died. The provider now had a different context for dealing with her medical condition and recognized her need for a referral for social service support.

Ethnographic Experiences from EMCP

The vignettes described next are short ethnographic episodes encountered by the researcher. These are brought with the intent of providing short examples that enable the reader to examine the social behaviors of an identifiable group of people by looking for patterns of social organization and worldview systems (Creswell & Poth, 2017). Patient comments for each section are included to support the discussion. The next sections will discuss the value of a healthcare portal in addressing the needs of SDOH populations served by EMCP in the context of the importance of managing trust through the deployment of the EMCP healthcare portal.

Social Vulnerability in Healthcare

King Jr and Wheeler (2007) provide clarity and distinction in referencing social vulnerability in healthcare. The term "underserved patients" refers to patients whose barriers to healthcare are due to lack of accessible services; while also "vulnerable", these patients' impediments to care are social or medical that may be related to culture, education, transportation, and language (King Jr & Wheeler, 2007). The inverse care law referenced by Fiscella and Shin (2005) provides context that suggests those patients with the greatest healthcare needs often receive the least adequate healthcare. This phenomenon has implications for healthcare and outcomes for vulnerable populations. Among these populations, the resulting effects of inverse care are greatly amplified due to increased risk factors associated with needing care combined with having poor access to it (Fiscella, 2005; Fiscella & Shin, 2005). Vulnerability factors such as low income, limited education, unemployment, minority status, lack of health insurance, residence in an underserved community, and chronic physical or mental illness collectively converge within individuals, families, and communities that are associated with poorer health and reduced access to adequate care (Fiscella, 2005). Clark (2005) uses the term "underserved" to describe people who lack adequate access to resources, e.g. technology, because of their geographic location, income level, education level, race, ethnicity, or physical capability. Vulnerable populations are also often described as racial and ethnic minorities, low income, undereducated, immigrants, and those lacking English proficiency (Zarcadoolas et al., 2013). Furthermore, such vulnerable populations are more likely to have low literacy as well as low health literacy. There is also strong evidence that links low literacy and low health literacy to poorer health behaviors, disease management skills, and health outcomes (Zarcadoolas et al., 2013). Thus, social vulnerability in healthcare refers to vulnerable patients affected by multiple chronic medical, behavioral, and social problems that interact in complex ways to undermine health that amplify the barriers to care (Fiscella & Shin, 2005).

The Broader Community IT Needs Perspective

Studies show that patient portals are an effective tool for actively engaging patients in managing their healthcare (Wallace et al., 2017). Literature shows that among medically underserved patients presenting to the ED, it is important to diagnose and treat the medical problem, but in order to improve the health of this population, there needs to be an expanded role to also diagnose and treat their social determinants (Anderson, Lippert, Newberry, Bernstein, Alter, & Wang, 2016). Therefore, when it comes to adopting a portal technology, it should not be only about giving patients what the healthcare institutions feel is best but should also address social needs.

Understanding the technology needs of the community begins with identifying the primary needs of the community. The daily lives of patients in an underserved community may be impacted by lack of money, power, resources, housing, healthcare, childcare, financial assistance, education, and community unity. Given these needs, can technology be used to meet them? Are the residents in the community aware of available resources to help them meet these needs? Important for community residents are the ability to locate relevant medical information, having basic literacy levels, and having localized community information organized and structured in a way that makes it easy for access. EMCP has gone to great lengths in addressing such needs through its corporate social responsibilities' programs. Through partnerships with community organizations, EMCP sponsors several programs as part of the organization's commitment to the health of the communities it serves, such as providing fresh fruits and vegetables to the community in the summer and fall seasons. In addition, during the summer months, EMCP takes the opportunity to highlight the importance of education by providing books to the children who are standing in line with their parents while the food is being distributed. *Einstein* delivers heart health education through community wellness events that features free health screenings and cooking demonstrations for heart healthy living as well as sponsoring organized youth sports programs. ED physicians were able to help out a local girls high school that needed physicians to perform health physicals that would allow the students to participate in sports.

Limited resources may not permit in-person visitation. Thus, having access to a computer to communicate with family and friends would be of benefit for sharing feelings or happenings about everyday situations. Collaborative efforts with nonprofits in the community (e.g. libraries, community centers, and churches) could also create centralized locations that provide information to solve social problems or make everyday life decisions.

Technology has the potential to transform underserved communities because it provides a way for people to gain access to information and resources needed to meet their everyday needs. The patient portal can be a valuable self-management tool for helping an underserved population to help themselves as active participants in their own healthcare. Effective deployment of the portal begins with focusing on the needs of the community that may build trust and then the implementation of the technology to improve health outcomes. Further, the importance of the provider-patient communication cannot be minimized. High levels of provider/patient trust have been found to be conducive to more effective healthcare (Abbas et al., 2018). The following comments highlights how this population self identifies with the community,

Yeah, honestly people are scared of using a portal. Because if I go to the doctor, what if something is wrong. How do I deal with that? Financially how do I deal with that? Mentally how do I deal with it? What about my job, can't lose my job? If you don't know about it, then it's not going to hurt you. That's not a good way to deal with things, if you don't think about it, it's not going to happen. I don't agree but that's the way people in the community think.

Often times I search the internet to give a friend advice. Say a friend says my toes been bothering me, I may look that up. Or it may be a symptom I'm having like knee pain and I may look up just to get an idea of what it might be. We look out for people in our community to help each other out.

The influence of the community holds particular significance. People in the community value the opinions of others in the community. Social identity and subjective norms where this population self-identifies with their community affects individual beliefs and behaviors and are important in their perceptions in dealing with situations that affect their everyday life. To build trust in a community where individuals have a close connection with each other, the trustee must demonstrate trustworthiness through a high degree of benevolence. The community must believe EMCP wants to do good by helping to improve their health status and the portals will be a way of achieving those positive outcomes.

Provider-Patient Communication Challenges

Healthcare communication is critical in establishing trusting professional relationships to enhance patient health. Communication concentrates on sharing medical information as well as recognizing the emotional needs of the patient exploring concerns, opinions, and potential barriers to care. Patient-centered care seeks to place the patient at the center of the healthcare spectrum that promotes self-management. The Institute of Medicine (IOM) defines patient-centered care as: "Providing care that is respectful of, and responsive to, individual patient preferences, needs and values, and ensuring that patient values guide all clinical decisions" (OneView, 2019). A communication strategy that connects patients with their health information and fosters the patient-healthcare provider relationship may contribute to increased overall patient satisfaction and utilization of healthcare tools that support engagement for safe quality healthcare. Secure Internet based communication portals are being used to enhance asynchronous communications with patients outside of face-to-face interactions. However, it is possible that the low adoption rates observed for an underserved population could be attributed to the fact that a face-to-face encounter with a provider is their preferred method of communication. It may be that it is the flexibility of the interaction where the patient develops a personal relationship with the physician through accessibility, delivery of care in a supportive way, and a unique approach to each patient's needs that enriches their communication.

Conversations the lead author had with two patients recently treated in the ED clearly articulated the feeling of having received better care because of the connection to the physician and the ability of the physician to understand them on a personal level in delivering quality healthcare. One patient shared:

it is the personal relationship that I have developed with my primary care physician that is most important that makes me a satisfied patient. I sometimes use the Internet for online health searches to find health information but wait to see my physician to ask if the information is true. The Internet is okay but not as a replacement for talking to my doctor face to face.

Another patient said:

seeing my doctor is how I find out about my health and if my medications are working. I trust her [be] cause she listens to me and cares about me and knows my personal situations and what I need. I don't own a computer but even if I did, I still want to talk to my doctor to tell me what I should do.

Developing a personal physician-patient relationship may be one of the most compelling aspects that serves as the core of effective healthcare communication for patients, and, therefore, managing its partial replacement through a healthcare IT portal is a major challenge. Among other challenges, vulnerable patients may be concerned that web access to records would change and potentially harm their relationship with their doctors. Patients fond of their providers may not want the role of the provider to be diminished by a portal where online care replaces face-to-face interactions. Instead, patients may prefer the benefit of having a basic understanding of their thoughts and intentions as well as the opportunity to expand on their narrative by being comfortable to ask relevant questions in an open and supportive environment. It is the flexibility, accessibility, and quality of the interaction that may influence the development of a shared collaborative relationship. Any effort to engage consumers through technology innovations begins with personalized care that is valued in meeting tailored healthcare needs. The results of a positive patient-physician relationship may lead to greater communication, better understanding, improved diagnostic accuracy, increased feelings of care, and increased trust with their physician. If provider endorsement is one of the most influential factors impacting patient's adoption as well as continued portal use, then the communication process that builds trust is vital for patient participation and active engagement in their healthcare management. This is evidenced in comments shared by patients about the influence of the relationship with their provider in their considering portal adoption.

I can't really tell you because I don't access it, don't use it. So, what's easier, you're talking to the wrong person in that respect. I say that because I don't use it like that. I have a personal relationship with the docs. On the other hand, I'm sure my sons would rather talk to the doctor on the television or go through a portal. I'm sure that's what they do. I'm sure they look things up in the portal. Not me. I just don't.

It's important to understand and have the doctor explain it in way that I can understand. A portal can't do that. It's also the office staff. They know me by name, not just a number. Communication is very important. I can relate to my doctor and trust her because she has my best interest at heart. If it seems I don't understand, she takes the time to go to next level of explanation, explain in a better way.

No need to access on my own. I have a trusted physician who knows what I need so I'm comfortable with my primary doctor providing my health information.

Do not need to use them. Open and upfront with my doctor who sorts out what's important and what's not. Helps to sort out baggage. I'm open to helping mind and body to achieve peace of mind.

While technology may be a way of providing this population with access to information and resources, it needs to occur through a trusted mechanism, namely the physician with whom they have a longstanding relationship. When the physician is perceived as competent, the level of trustworthiness is increased. The comments expressed imply that because physicians are perceived to be skilled and knowledgeable about the patient's medical condition, that the patients trust their opinions and are willing to adhere to their prescribed treatment. Therefore, as trusted pillars in the community, physicians play a key role in influencing behaviors that may make patients more accepting of portal adoption. Incorporating such trusted communication sensitivity into an IT portal is a challenge.

And, the Need to Acknowledge Cultural Diversity

EMCP is located in the North Philadelphia section of the city where the service area encompasses zip codes with a high percentage of medically underserved patients. The ED population is primarily African-American. The team of ED providers is primarily Caucasian. Does the lack of a diverse physician workforce affect the communication and quality of care delivered to a predominantly minority patient population utilizing the ED? The ED faculty recognized this disparity and have tried to address it through improvements in communication. The lead author questioned during a faculty discussion on improving patient-physician communication, the possibility of a need for a cultural competence course. The Medical Director was optimistic about getting faculty comfortable with communication needing to be a starting point. EMCP has embraced AIDET as a communication metric to be utilized at each patient visit: Acknowledge, Identify, Duration, Explain, Time (Braverman, Kunkel, Katz, Katona, Heavens, Miller et al., 2015; Studer, Robinson, & Cook, 2010). However, as beneficial as AIDET is as a communication tool, cultural differences may still impact the patient-physician communication, and, ultimately, medical care. For example, a physician asked a patient his social history about smoking. The patient responded by saying he did "loosies". Not understanding what was meant by "loosies", the provider inquired further and learned "loosies" is a colloquial term often used in urban communities to indicate loose cigarettes from a pack. Now a discussion with the patient about smoking cessation may be appropriate. If there are language barriers between the patients and treating providers, does it impact the treatment plan? In this case, the physician was concerned enough to inquire further, but every provider is different in their approach to the care plan. Potential biases and unfavorable interaction dynamics resulting from a lack of understanding about a patient's self-reported health conditions due to cultural language barriers has the potential to have significant consequences.

While attending a retirement function at Lankenau Hospital, the lead author encountered a nurse who previously worked in the ED at EMCP. She lamented how glad she was to no longer be employed in that "environment" with "those" patients. When asked to explain what she meant, she indicated because of the challenges with an urban patient population the culture was very different from the culture at Lankenau. That is an interesting observation because Lankenau's location is considered a suburban hospital that also serves an urban community due to its close proximity to patients from West Philadelphia with similar socioeconomic backgrounds as patients in North Philadelphia who utilize the ED as their primary source of care. These experiences highlight the need for ensuring diversity and cultural competence for healthcare professionals as a priority agenda item to address any perceived inequalities in health and healthcare.

Patient comments help to understand why the connection to their physician is so important.

I can really relate to my doctor. She speaks my language. She always listens to my issues and knows what I need.

I didn't get along with my last doctor at all. He didn't understand me or try to get into the nitty gritty of my problem.

Just find not all doctors are positive or on the same page so that I feel comfortable talking to them.

Communication training programs for physicians and other health professionals of all ethnic backgrounds should include an emphasis on understanding and addressing the needs of a culturally diverse patient population. The patient-provider connection is especially significant when there is race concordance. In this case, cultural similarity becomes even more of a trustworthiness factor. Patients expressed feeling of relatedness and a certain comfort level from the collective set of characteristics, a high degree of ability, benevolence, and integrity, that contributes to a strong trusting relationship that may be different if the patient-physician relationship was race discordant. Incorporating such cultural sensitivity into an IT portal is another compelling challenge.

PORTAL READINESS CHALLENGES

EMCP, like other healthcare organizations, has deployed portals as secure communication tools to enhance patient care via improved patient-provider communications. A potentially false assumption is that once a portal has been deployed, patients will use it as intended. The literature seems to suggest the opposite for a medically underserved population (Wallace et al., 2017). In fact, reduced rates of portal adoption have been observed among underserved populations. Studies have also identified several barriers to portal adoption: low socioeconomic measures, access, health literacy, and privacy concerns. Even if organizations can overcome these barriers, are the patients prepared to use a portal in managing their care?

Managing care through use of a portal is more than learning to navigate an online tool. Complimentary skills are needed to allow for effective management of the underlying activities associated with the information being accessed and record keeping for tracking purposes. Has the patient had experience in maintaining a calendar, setting dates for regular monitoring and noting key milestones? What involvement has there been in their participation in their healthcare? Are they able to manage information regarding treatment and care? If a patient has not been involved in these activities in the context of consumer-focused health information technology, developing and maintaining a system of record keeping of health-related activities may be challenging (Nambisan, 2017). Furthermore, the same factors, namely lack of education and health literacy, impacting this population on the intent to adopt may also play a role as antecedent barriers to portal adoption readiness. That is not to say it cannot be learned. However, the expectation that one can begin this kind of activity without first having some guidance and assistance, may be overly optimistic. On the other hand, experience and involvement in managing personal health records may prove beneficial and even appealing when preparing for and potentially adopting new healthcare portal technology (Nambisan, 2017).

Taking an organized approach to record keeping is also important for management of health records. A patient needs to be vested in wanting to keep health records as a proactive way of understanding their health status. A patient may not be inclined to maintain health records through a portal if records have not been maintained electronically or on paper, feeling it is not their responsibility. From the patient's perspective, once they see a doctor, he or she records the information and updates the patient at each visit on their health status. Such a scenario may be perceived as less stressful and creates fewer worries for patients than owning the task themselves. Patients may view taking on these additional tasks as burdensome, especially given the difficulty in managing daily responsibilities for necessary care. As a result, managing health records through a portal becomes less of a priority, resulting in a potentially lower incentive for self-management.

Finally, searching the Internet for general information and using the Internet for health information seeking are not the same activity. However, if a patient has access to the Internet and actively seeks information on diseases, treatments, and other health related concerns, the potential exists for developing positive perceptions about the value of a patient portal (Nambisan, 2017). Just as support may be needed for other portal readiness preparation, addressing health literacy through education and training could serve to influence the attitudes of patients in portal adoption. Patient comments suggest additional preparation may be needed for portal readiness.

I can never remember how to get into the portal. I think you need your medical record number and I have no idea what that is.

Don't know much about them. The doctor's office staff was not well versed about it; they only provided pamphlets about using a portal. Getting questions answered is most important; I like personal communication with my doctor to get those answers.

Education and training are not only important but essential in preparing this population for portal adoption. Building that trust begins with patients feeling confident because they have acquired the skills necessary in preparing to navigate the proposed technology tool. It needs to be a process that recognizes the need to assess cognitive ability and information retrieval as key components in designing training and support programs to enhance portal readiness. Benevolence and integrity are important to a lesser degree, but it is gaining confidence in their ability through targeted training programs that may contribute more significantly to trustworthiness. Making the IT portal able to address such problems, including low levels of technology literacy, is yet another challenge to IT portal adoption.

Addressing the Health Literacy Obstacle

Another context in which a healthcare portal could partly alleviate current obstacles concerns health literacy. Research shows that health status is influenced by individual characteristics and lifestyles (Wallace et al., 2017). However, the unique health literacy issues of an underserved population may also significantly impact their health status (Mackert et al., 2016). While the relationship between social factors and health may be easy to observe, understanding and acting upon these issues is often much more difficult (Nutbeam, 2000). A comprehensive approach to health promotion should recognize the importance of social and environmental influences on lifestyle choices, and partly address these issues through improved communication enabled by a healthcare portal. A healthcare portal could come into play in the context of health interventions that seeks to link health promotion activity, the determinants of health, and the resulting health outcomes. An IT portal could be especially important in the context of health literacy (Mackert et al., 2016). Health literacy refers to a set of skills that people need to function effectively in the healthcare environment. These skills include: 1) basic/functional-sufficient basic skills in reading and writing to be able to function in everyday situations; 2) communicative/interactive more advanced cognitive and literacy skills which together with social skills can be used to actively participate in everyday activities to extract information and to derive meaning from different forms of communication; and, 3) critical literacy even more advanced cognitive skills which together with social skills can be applied to critically analyze information and to use that information to exert greater control over life events and situations (Nutbeam, 2000). Health literacy has been cited as a barrier for a medically underserved population, and low levels of it may subsequently have adverse effects on care processes and health outcomes (Irizarry, Dabbs, & Curran, 2015). A healthcare portal could partly alleviate such problems.

Another impact of a healthcare portal is clarifying the reason patients come to the ED. Patients with low health literacy may present to the ED with a medical condition perceived as urgent when it may simply be a case of not understanding healthcare instructions or how to take their medication. When the lead author worked in a primary care office, patients were told to bring their medications to the visit so that the doctor could verify their medication regimen. It was not unusual for patients to bring in multiple medication bottles without understanding the appropriate dosage or what diagnosis the medication was being used to treat. The family doctor that the lead author worked for would take the time to fill up pill boxes for a week, sometimes two, of medications the patient was instructed to take because they were not health literate in understanding their medication regimen. In situations such as this, without education and social support regarding taking medications as prescribed, often these patients may end up in the ED. A healthcare portal could play a key role here too.

Likewise, the portal may not be considered easy to use if the population accessing it doesn't understand what's being reported or misinterprets what's being reported. The *Einstein Health Portal* contains documented visit summaries written using clinical terminology. The laboratory results reflect the actual clinical tests. A person with knowledge of healthcare terminology may not have a problem, but a patient with low health literacy may have difficulty understanding the medical terminology. Will they understand the tests listed under the heading Immunol/virology and the purpose of the reference ranges or that breast tomosynthesis is an advanced type of mammogram for better cancer detection? A healthcare portal that factors literacy into design features could go a long way towards simplifying how medical information is presented in a way that patients can understand.

With the other social factors faced by this population, stress resulting from knowing too much medical knowledge may play a role in patients not wanting to actively engage in their healthcare. Having a provider share information is one thing. Seeing it in writing may make it real in reminding them of their health problems and their poor quality of life. The reality of knowing about a disease may not work to a patient's advantage if instead of seeing the potential positive side of treatment, dwelling on the negative consumes their thoughts. Take the following patient experience. A malignant lump was discovered on a patient who went for a routine mammogram. She was told "it was the best cancer one could have with a negative and positive marker" since it was caught early. She was given a good prognosis following surgery and follow up radiation treatment. Upon completion of her radiation treatment, she became very depressed. Not because the surgery and treatment did not go well, but because she learned additional information that the best cancer is one where both markers would be negative and felt that's what the doctors should have told her prior to treatment. So instead of focusing on the positive outcomes, she was allowing this additional medical knowledge to negatively impact her recovery. A healthcare portal could be programmed to present such information in a manner more appropriate for that population.

Improving health literacy in a population will involve health education as well as helping people to develop confidence to act on healthcare knowledge and the ability to work with and support others. If we are to impact this population, asking a patient to use a portal may not immediately translate into self-management. Adding a trust-building mechanism into social emergency medicine practices of systemic interventions must address training and must include more personal forms of communication and collaborative partnership for a community-based educational outreach. These comments reflect unfavorable attitudes towards portal adoption due to potential literacy challenges faced by this population.

Portals, not sure what that is. Not everybody, number one, can afford a computer. I know a lot of people have cell phones but maybe they are worried about minutes on their cell phone and things of that nature. Also, education wise. Not everybody has a higher level of education so it might be something that is confusing.

Do not like new changes. Not personal, just no connection and confusing and not able to navigate system. Would need to make them easier to use. People in their 60s, 70s, and 80s are harder to teach modern tech. They might be slower to learn with no real interest.

For me fine but may not be best for an older crowd who don't have a computer and unable to work with a patient portal. My generation and younger are technology based and into our cell phones and computers, so it's a lot easier to use technology to get things done.

Portals may not be best for older generation who can't afford or know how to use a computer. Younger generation's use of cell phones and computers makes them more adaptable to technology.

Patients may not be willing to admit it, but health literacy is a real issue. Even though a younger generation may be able to adapt more easily to the technology, low health literacy may still impact individual's ability to find and use health information. An "on your own model" may not provide the needed support to help patients understand and navigate a portal effectively. Portal readiness assumes that a skill level health literacy must be obtained. This may be accomplished through partnerships with community centers or on-site kiosks that may be an option for training programs in a supportive environment. In this way, the organization builds trust in helping patients to gain the necessary skills (ability) to effectively navigate within a portal, demonstrate care for the patient's health and well-being (benevolence), and promote the value of a technology designed to improve health outcomes (integrity). Elevating the technology literacy level of the population is yet another challenge to IT portal adoption.

The Potential of a Healthcare Portal to Improve Access to Care and Care Coordination

The potential benefits from a healthcare portal are highlighted by the experiences that patients have. EMCP has a Patient Advocate Department that is charged with allowing patients to raise concerns about their care during their EMCP hospital visits. One of the issues cited with a medically underserved population is their access to care because of financial reasons, which is one of the reasons the ED is used as the primary source of treatment for complex medical and social problems (Shaw, Howard, Clark, Etz, Arya, & Tallia, 2013). Many of the patients have a government plan such as Medicaid or Medicare or are uninsured. Unfortunately, not all physicians participate in the government plans. This means certain services may not be covered, resulting in out of pocket expenses. Moreover, lack of physician participation often means higher associated co-pays, co-insurance, and deductibles. ED treats patients regardless of their ability to pay, which may take care of the immediate medical conditions. However, ongoing chronic disease management or specialty care becomes problematic. A healthcare portal could partly alleviate these cost issues by being a low-cost/free alternative to at least some aspects of care.

The ED is notified of complaints in two ways. First, every patient receiving treatment is surveyed to comment on their experience. Written comments, positive, negative, or both are sent to the Department for review. The Department can then make decisions how best to approach the issues including implementing processes for improving the delivery of care. In addition, patient complaints made directly to the Patient Advocate office are reviewed by the Medical Director to determine if the standard of care was followed and to respond to the patient directly about their concerns. Many of the complaints filed indicate patients felt the amount of time they have to wait before being treated was too long. While it may be an unrealistic expectation that a visit to the ED means expedited care, patients routinely share length of time as a dissatisfier in rating their ED experience. One patient shared "when I was finally looked at by a new Dr, I waited 4 hours until I was finally given my prescription and told what to do." A translated Spanish comment from a patient "when I arrived, they only took my vitals and sent me to the room to wait. Then after 1½ hours, I still had not been seen by a doctor." Another shared, "I know the ER was very busy that night, but I waited a long time. I even witnessed people leave the ER due to the long wait." In this regard too, a healthcare portal could partly alleviate these waiting time issues by being an alternative to at least some aspects of ED care.

In ongoing efforts to improve the delivery of care, the ED responds by continually assessing patient flow operations to identify areas for process improvement and efficiencies. Two of the operational approaches that the ED has implemented to address timeliness of care issues in handling the high patient volume are the implementation of *Fast Track* and *Rapid Assessment* processes. In *Fast Track,* a dedicated provider is assigned to patients presenting with non-urgent conditions to expedite treatment time during peak hours. *Rapid Assessment* moves the sickest patients to triage to quickly diagnose problems and determine next steps for treatment such as ordering labs or diagnostic studies. In addition to dedicated physicians, use of physician extenders, e.g. physician assistants and nurse practitioners, are utilized to support patient care. Positive patient comments are an indicator the processes are working. Comments from a patient survey said "Fast Track is outstanding. It removes the least serious out of the way by treating [them] in a separate area so that more attention can be given to the serious emergency patients." Patients care about EMCP acknowledging that wait time is a problem and actively addressing ways to improve on it. Continuous process improvement to enhance the patient's overall experience is an ongoing strategy that may reinforce the formation of a trusting relationship between patients and EMCP providers. In this regard too, a healthcare portal could play a key role by informing patients.

Nonetheless, access to care remains an issue often due to limited financial resources. Patient comments provide context to why the ED continues to be a point of entry to the healthcare system.

People don't go to the doctor, let alone use a portal. I find that people shy away from doctors because it cost money. So, if you cannot afford it, a lot of times you reach out to these clinical websites such as Web MD to diagnose yourself.

That's what Health Fairs do to help people who don't have any money to do screenings. On one hand, yes, the patient needs to be responsible. But not everybody has the ability to do that because it cost money. When you don't have any money, you don't do screenings. They don't even have insurance or the insurance they do have is not good enough because they have to spend too much money for these tests.

The lack of health insurance limits access to care. Without insurance, families may experience worse health and medical debt, which may also result in the costly use of inappropriate care, such as the ED and avoidable hospitalizations (Fiscella & Shin, 2005). Low income patients are disproportionately affected by rising healthcare costs and a trend toward greater burden of costs to the patient. Therefore, emergency physicians may continue to face the daunting task of providing care to a large volume of vulnerable patients seeking care in the emergency room (Anderson et al., 2016). However, by developing systemic interventions, collaborating with community partners and advocating for policies that will improve the health of patients may contribute to building patient trust. The ED may not be able to solve all problems, but through collaborative relationships that serve to expand access, enabled in part by an IT portal, increased trust may be gained to influence patient behavior toward acceptance of technology designed for greater self-management.

Addressing the Respect Obstacle to Healthcare Portal Adoption

A patient's social status should not dictate the type of treatment one can expect to receive. One of the most serious offenses, for the medically underserved patient, may be what is perceived as disrespect by the provider not listening or taking for granted the seriousness of their medical condition. Patients want empathy, acknowledgement of their concerns, and to be treated with respect regardless of their socioeconomic status. Note the following quotes that highlight patient concerns. "They weren't willing to listen to my situation at all unless I immediately went into triage which they explained was only about taking my temperature and blood pressure. I explained this was done twice in the ambulance". Others commented, "During my visit while passing the nurses station in the ER, I could hear the nurses and doctors talking about my reason for visit", or "after telling the doctor my symptoms, I expected her to come back to say what her findings were, not wait until I was being discharged." A patient's husband from another culture for religious reasons insisted that his wife should be seen by a female physician but felt like he was getting pushback from the treating physician. These are realities that need to be addressed in a way where the patient and family members feel respected and accommodated to the best ability of the institution or provided with reasons or alternatives if it cannot be met. Allowing patients to specify their needs and clearly communicating what services can be offered may help to alleviate such problems, and a healthcare portal could be part of that solution.

The belief that somehow a patient should be grateful for the care given and accept any type of behavior by medical personnel while being treated has been a pervasive perception for a population that feels they have limited options. EMCP understands the changing healthcare environment and the need for more focus on delivering high quality care and a consistently great experience when interacting with patients. This means holding the organization accountable for behaviors or actions that can be improved or need to change. It also means holding employees accountable to create and maintain a culture where excellence is expected from everyone. To that end, EMCP has developed uniform *Standards of Behavior* to define what it means to deliver a great patient experience. These *Standards of Behavior* include Respect, Empathy, Responsibility, Affinity, and Integrity. Listening was recently added as the newest standard in practice. Although physicians and medical personnel think they listen well, given the many demands of a busy ED, it may be perceived by the patient that the doctor is rushing through a conversation without appearing to listen carefully. Developing the standards is the first step, but it entails putting ideals into actions which echoes the sentiment, actions speak louder than words. The *Standards of Behavior* are concrete examples of how every EMCP employee should act. Respect is about valuing others and recognizing diversity within the patient population to be sensitive to age, color, culture, disability, education, gender, gender identity, nationality, race, religion, and all other forms of diversity. Front line employees from across EMCP who consistently model great behavior and have repeatedly shown how they can help to drive change were instrumental in developing the *Standards of Behavior*. These standards are key to EMCP's continued growth and success and the foundation for efforts in providing the best possible patient experience and respect for the population being treated. For example, these comments highlight situations where patients perceive lack of respectful behavior.

A lot of times people get nervous when they go to the doctors because of all the questions they have to answer. Then if you don't know the answers, the doctor talks down to you and you don't want to come back. Or they hardly ask you any questions at all, like going through the motion but not really caring.

Not everybody goes to college but that doesn't mean you don't understand what's going on.

I needed to see a specialist because of my heart problem but I couldn't get an appointment because the doctor didn't take my insurance. I work hard like everybody else but because of my insurance, the receptionist acted like I wasn't good enough to be seen.

Patients want to have a positive clinical experience. The comments shared inherently demonstrate factors that may cause patients to have a lack of trust in the health systems. That, in turn, may make it harder for them to access care as well as increase their concerns about not being in control as a result of their social position. Compassion, empathy, and connection with their provider are important to that interaction where the patient is made to feel like they are equal. The factors that pose barriers for underserved patients, such as low income, education, low health literacy may also result in physician biases that undermine constructive communication. Trust is based upon expectations on how another person will behave, based on their actions (Mayer et al., 1995). If this population does not judge the physician or systems to be trustworthy due to their social conditions, they may not feel the relationship is in their best interest and may not be as receptive to a message that encourages self-empowerment in their healthcare.

What Else Needs to Be Done to Ensure Healthcare Portal Adoption

Research shows that across IT types, perceived usefulness and perceived ease of use (Davis, 1989) are significant predictors of IT adoption, and this applies to portal adoption too (Dou et al., 2017). More specifically, perceived ease of use influences perceived usefulness, and both combine to affect adoption intentions which is highly correlated with subsequent actual use of an IT (Taylor & Todd, 1995). The EMCP portal design has all the elements for patient self-management but could be enhanced with "bells and whistles" to make the site more visually appealing. Perceptions of simplicity in navigating the portal may pose challenges as well. Since navigating through the site may not be very intuitive, it may be useful to have kiosks in key EMCP hospital areas where patients may be able to access the tool and have available staff who can observe the mechanics of use, provide education, instruction, and answer questions about things that the patients may not understand. It would also be a good opportunity to obtain feedback about how patients view the portal and how easy they find it to use. That may be valuable in customizing design features for a vulnerable population needing support.

Increased marketing is another strategy to promote the healthcare IT portal. The lack of awareness and access of the *Einstein Health Patient Portal* has been challenging for the organization. EMCP recognizes that patient portals are a standard practice as a tool to help patients be more actively involved in their own healthcare. However, there needs to be clear direction about portal registration and its continued use as a means of accessing their medical records and communicating with EMCP physicians and office staff.

EMCP conducted a patient enrollment campaign a couple years ago. Patients registered, but there has been continued concern about adoption rates and tracking of usage frequency patterns. A major concern expressed by patients was difficulty in accessing the system after registration because of the need for the patient's medical record number (MRN), date of birth, and the last 4 digits of their Social Security Number. Since MRN is not information a patient is likely to remember after a medical visit, many patients simply did not continue use. In addition, it was also not clear how patients were invited to participate. Some patients were told they could self-register by going online or downloading the app.

Others were advised to ask their healthcare provider about self-registration. Front office staff had no way of knowing who had already registered, so they also did not ask patients if they had an interest in registering. EMCP has recently initiated another marketing effort with improved access. The MRN is no longer needed, just an email address. An icon has been placed in the system so that staff can easily identify if a patient has an account. In the event that the front office staff did not ask the patient about signing up for the portal, the Medical Assistant has been instructed to reinforce the message when the patient is having vitals taken. Systems are not in place to register patients presenting to the ED for the health portal. However, leadership is aware that since the ED is often the primary source of entry into the healthcare system, inviting portal registration at the time of an ED visit is an opportunity to promote linkage to primary care where they can receive ongoing monitored care and keep them connected within the *Einstein* network. ED patients who are aware of the portal have expressed interest as shared in some of their comments.

Portals make it easier to communicate, like making appointments and updating personal information.

I might use it if more appealing. I mean, nice to look at, colorful and easy to find the information you want.

The less that you have to do when you go into the office the better. You can fill out information before you get there, you can do that in your home in a relaxed environment. If you don't bring your pill bottles with you, maybe taking multiple medications and don't bring them all, maybe you forgot, running late, things happen when you're going to the office, patient portals are a lot more helpful because you can sit at your pace, upload your information. You can put in your medical history, can put in past medical surgical family history, medication history right then and there to take away that worry you may be going into the office with.

I like it the way it is for me. For somebody else, I'm sure there would be a lot of good options. What if my doctor left and went somewhere else? Now I would be forced to do the portal and maybe not call my doctor anytime I want to and get information. Well, I suppose the portal would probably be a good thing. Anything that's not the same. If you give me a ton of options, some would be better, some would be over my head, a little too easy. I think as long as I have options, then that's probably the key. Just being able to have options.

Despite the challenges, this population shows interest in portal adoption provided that its use and ease of use are demonstrated to be of value. However, patients must perceive a high degree of ability, benevolence, and integrity to consider the organization to be trustworthy. Through encouraging and supportive initiatives that will meet the needs and wants of users, there is potential in building trusting relationships for developing a framework to serve underserved communities with instructional technologies.

The Case of John

Even with the passage of healthcare reform, anticipated increases in ED visits are projected, especially among low income groups presented with medical and unmet social needs (Anderson et al., 2016; Medford-Davis, Eswaran, Shah, & Dark, 2015). Anderson, Lippert, et al. (2016) describe the ED as the window into the community which fully frames the contributions of the social determinants underlying health and illness. Consider the following example. John's (a pseudonym) last visit to the ED was due to prolonged dizziness and headaches symptoms resulting from his uncontrolled hypertension. Other medical conditions included being on oxygen for chronic obstructive pulmonary disease, ambulatory dysfunction (amputee), and a recovering drug addict. In preparing for his discharge, John indicated he had housing problems but would rather be homeless than return to the residence of his brother where the living conditions were not suitable. Medically, John was stable to be discharged but his social circumstances dictated a coordinated intervention for transition to a more appropriate outpatient setting where his medical condition could be monitored on an ongoing basis. The provider decided to admit John to the observation unit for 24 hours to monitor his blood pressure, consult physical therapy to address his mobility, and request social services to find him suitable temporary housing.

Cases like John's, treated routinely at EMCP, are similar to those treated in other urban EDs across the country. Still, there remains a need for process efficiency, costs savings and improved health outcomes in the delivery of quality healthcare. Patients impacted by SDOH may sometimes be mistakenly labeled as "frequent flyers" who are non-compliant. That is not always a fair description. Often, SDOH patients may visit the ER frequently because they are seeking not only medical care but may need a social support system to address housing instability, poor access to care, food insecurity, and refuge. Addressing issues related to SDOH means recognizing that barriers exist for a marginalized population, and consequently the need to develop systemic interventions to engage patients as active participants in their healthcare. But doing so requires the development of trust. Such a level of trust may be created when the patient realizes that the hospital is acting in their best interest, and this might consequently influence their attitude and behavior towards portal technology adoption too.

LIMITATIONS

The conclusions drawn should be considered in the context of a few limitations worth noting. First, the research is limited by the geographic location of EMCP, the healthcare providers, and the patients. The culture and characteristics of the urban setting of the Philadelphia medical center may be different than that of other cities. Second, the study was limited to patients who were seen in the ED at *Einstein Medical Center* Philadelphia for discreet encounters. Even though EMCP serves a predominantly underserved population, the results may not be generalizable to the entire patient population since the experiences of patients utilizing other hospital services may have established ongoing provider relationships that influence their experiences differently. Within this context there may also be unique characteristics of the underserved population EMCP is treating that may be different than those encountered by other strata such as the elderly or disabled. While visually appealing and color formats may be desired for the study population, inappropriate font sizes, low contrast, cluttering of web page and use of dynamic and flashing objects are barriers for disabled patients. Computer literacy and anxiety, cognitive impairment (memory), health literacy, and physical limitations present a different set of challenges for an elderly population that may impact their use of a patient portal differently.

SUMMARY

There are many benefits to be gained from a healthcare IT portal, especially in the case of medically underserved populations. Patient portals provide a potential opportunity to engage patients to become more active in their healthcare. And yet, there are numerous issues that make its adoption challenging, especially for underserved populations. In addition to the technical challenges, social issues are a major factor where issues of cultural diversity, perceived lack of respect, and poor health literacy provide a complexity that is not easily resolved. As the ethnographic experiences imply, the social determinants of health, underlying health, and illness may warrant adapting a new perspective as to how to influence downstream health outcomes. These social factors and a trust building process are essential components affecting the shared patterns of behavior, beliefs, and language on this cultural group. The trustworthiness of EMCP influenced each aspect examined. The interrelationship of ability, benevolence, and integrity are important to trust in ensuring a community-focus when considering a pathway for implementing a new technology. The strength of the provider-patient relationship requires also considering issues of cultural competence, physician-patient race discordance, training, and support initiatives to ensure portal readiness and health literacy. Meeting patients at their need, valuing input, personal forms of communication, and collaborative community partnership are strategies that may help to pave the way for educating and preparing patients for portal adoption. This may be achieved by providing "community technology centers" where patients can access the Internet, participate in literacy and other educational programs as well as utilize other resources such as assistance with insurance enrollment. Finally, adhering to the "Code of the Street" levels the playing field from the patients' perspective which makes them feel respected and builds trust that may make patients more receptive to the message of the value of adopting a portal as a tool for managing their healthcare.

REFERENCES

Abbas, R. M., Carroll, N., & Richardson, I. (2018). in technology we trust: Extending TAM from a healthcare technology perspective. Paper presented at the *2018 IEEE International Conference on Healthcare Informatics (ICHI)*. 10.1109/ICHI.2018.00051

Adler, N. E., Boyce, T., Chesney, M. A., Cohen, S., Folkman, S., Kahn, R. L., & Syme, S. L. (1994). Socioeconomic status and health: The challenge of the gradient. *The American Psychologist*, *49*(1), 15–24. doi:10.1037/0003-066X.49.1.15 PMID:8122813

Agar, M. H. (1996). *The professional stranger: An informal introduction to ethnography*. New York, NY: Academic Press.

Ammenwerth, E., Schnell-Inderst, P., & Hoerbst, A. (2012). The impact of electronic patient portals on patient care: A systematic review of controlled trials. *Journal of Medical Internet Research*, *14*(6), e162. doi:10.2196/jmir.2238 PMID:23183044

Ancker, J. S., Barrón, Y., Rockoff, M. L., Hauser, D., Pichardo, M., Szerencsy, A., & Calman, N. (2011). Use of an electronic patient portal among disadvantaged populations. *Journal of General Internal Medicine*, *26*(10), 1117–1123. doi:10.100711606-011-1749-y PMID:21647748

Anderson, E. S., Hsieh, D. M., & Alter, H. J. (2016). Social emergency medicine: Embracing the dual role of the emergency department in acute care and population health. *Annals of Emergency Medicine*, *68*(1), 21–25. doi:10.1016/j.annemergmed.2016.01.005 PMID:26921967

Anderson, E. S., Lippert, S., Newberry, J., Bernstein, E., Alter, H. J., & Wang, N. E. (2016). Addressing social determinants of health from the emergency department through social emergency medicine. *The Western Journal of Emergency Medicine*, *17*(4), 487–489. doi:10.5811/westjem.2016.5.30240 PMID:27429706

Bansal, G., Zahedi, F. M., & Gefen, D. (2007). The impact of personal dispositions on privacy and trust in disclosing health information online. In *Proceedings of the AMCIS, Keystone, Colorado.*

Bansal, G., Zahedi, F. M., & Gefen, D. (2010). The impact of personal dispositions on information sensitivity, privacy concern and trust in disclosing health information online. *Decision Support Systems*, *49*(2), 138–150. doi:10.1016/j.dss.2010.01.010

Bansal, G., Zahedi, F. M., & Gefen, D. (2016). Do context and personality matter? Trust and privacy concerns in disclosing private information online. *Information & Management*, *53*(1), 1–21. doi:10.1016/j.im.2015.08.001

Benbasat, I., Gefen, D., & Pavlou, P. A. (2008). Introduction to the JMIS special issue trust in online environments. *Journal of MIS*, *25*(1), 5–12.

Braverman, A. M., Kunkel, E. J., Katz, L., Katona, A., Heavens, T., Miller, A., & Arfaa, J. J. (2015). Do I buy it? How AIDET™ training changes residents' values about patient care. *Journal of Patient Experience*, *2*(1), 13–20. doi:10.1177/237437431500200104 PMID:28725811

Bunderson, J. S., & Reagans, R. E. (2011). Power, status, and learning in organizations. *Organization Science*, *22*(5), 1182–1194. doi:10.1287/orsc.1100.0590

Clark, K. (2005). Serving underserved communities with instructional technologies: Giving them what they need, not what you want. *Urban Education*, *40*(4), 430–445. doi:10.1177/0042085905276388

Cooper-Patrick, L., Gallo, J. J., Gonzales, J. J., Vu, H. T., Powe, N. R., Nelson, C., & Ford, D. E. (1999). Race, gender, and partnership in the patient-physician relationship. *Journal of the American Medical Association*, *282*(6), 583–589. doi:10.1001/jama.282.6.583 PMID:10450723

Creswell, J. W., & Poth, C. N. (2017). Qualitative inquiry and research design: Choosing among five approaches. Thousand Oaks, CA: Sage.

Davis, F. D. (1989). Perceived Usefulness, Perceived ease of use and user acceptance of information technology. *Management Information Systems Quarterly*, *13*(3), 319–340. doi:10.2307/249008

Dhanireddy, S., Walker, J., Reisch, L., Oster, N., Delbanco, T., & Elmore, J. G. (2014). The urban underserved: Attitudes towards gaining full access to electronic medical records. *Health Expectations*, *17*(5), 724–732. doi:10.1111/j.1369-7625.2012.00799.x PMID:22738155

Dimoka, A. (2010). What does the brain tell us about trust and distrust? Evidence from a functional neuroimaging study. *Management Information Systems Quarterly*, *34*(2), 373–396. doi:10.2307/20721433

Doescher, M. P., Saver, B. G., Franks, P., & Fiscella, K. 2000. Racial and ethnic disparities in perceptions of physician style and trust. *Meyers Primary Care Institute Publications and Presentations, 553.*

Dou, K., Yu, P., Deng, N., Liu, F., Guan, Y., Li, Z., ... Duan, H. (2017). Patients' acceptance of smartphone health technology for chronic disease management: A theoretical model and empirical test. *JMIR mHealth and uHealth*, *5*(12), e177. doi:10.2196/mhealth.7886 PMID:29212629

Durkan, P., Durkin, M., & Gillen, J. (2003). Exploring efforts to engender on-line trust. *International Journal of Entrepreneurial Behaviour & Research*, *9*(3), 93–110. doi:10.1108/13552550310476184

Fetterman, D. M. (2009). Ethnography: Step-by-step. Thousand Oaks, CA: Sage.

Fiscella, K. (2005). Health vulnerability. *Journal of the American Medical Association*, *293*(15), 1924–1925. doi:10.1001/jama.293.15.1924

Fiscella, K., & Shin, P. (2005). The inverse care law: Implications for healthcare of vulnerable populations. *The Journal of Ambulatory Care Management*, *28*(4), 304–312. doi:10.1097/00004479-200510000-00005 PMID:16172559

Galea, S., Tracy, M., Hoggatt, K. J., DiMaggio, C., & Karpati, A. (2011). Estimated deaths attributable to social factors in the United States. *American Journal of Public Health*, *101*(8), 1456–1465. doi:10.2105/AJPH.2010.300086 PMID:21680937

Gefen, D. (2000). E-commerce: The role of familiarity and trust. Omega. *International Journal of Management Sciences*, *28*(6), 725–737.

Gefen, D., & Carmel, E. (2008). Is the world really flat? A look at offshoring in an online programming marketplace. *Management Information Systems Quarterly*, *32*(2), 367–384. doi:10.2307/25148844

Gefen, D., Karahanna, E., & Straub, D. W. (2003). Trust and TAM in online shopping: An integrated model. *Management Information Systems Quarterly*, *27*(1), 51–90. doi:10.2307/30036519

Gefen, D., & Ridings, C. (2003). IT acceptance: Managing user - IT group boundaries. *ACM SIGMIS Database*, *34*(3), 25–40. doi:10.1145/937742.937746

Gefen, D., Rose, G. M., Warkentin, M., & Pavlou, P. A. (2005). Cultural diversity and trust in IT adoption: A comparison of potential e-voters in the USA and South Africa. *Journal of Global Information Management*, *13*(1), 54–78. doi:10.4018/jgim.2005010103

Gefen, D., Wyss, S., & Lichtenstein, Y. (2008). Business familiarity as risk mitigation in software development outsourcing contracts. *Management Information Systems Quarterly*, *32*(3), 531–551. doi:10.2307/25148855

Gulati, R. (1995). Does Familiarity Breed Trust? The implications of repeated ties for contractual choice in alliances. *Academy of Management Journal*, *38*(1), 85–112.

Harris, M. (2001). The rise of anthropological theory: A history of theories of culture. Thousand Oaks, CA: AltaMira Press.

Irizarry, T., Dabbs, A. D., & Curran, C. R. (2015). Patient portals and patient engagement: A state of the science review. *Journal of Medical Internet Research*, *17*(6), e148. doi:10.2196/jmir.4255 PMID:26104044

King, T. E., Jr. & Wheeler, M. B. (2007). Medical management of vulnerable and underserved patients: principles, practice, and populations: New York, NY: McGraw-Hill Medical Publishing Division.

Mackert, M., Mabry-Flynn, A., Champlin, S., Donovan, E. E., & Pounders, K. (2016). Health literacy and health information technology adoption: The potential for a new digital divide. *Journal of Medical Internet Research, 18*(10), e264. doi:10.2196/jmir.6349 PMID:27702738

Mayer, R. C., Davis, J. H., & Schoorman, F. D. (1995). An integrative model of organizational trust. *Academy of Management Review, 20*(3), 709–734. doi:10.5465/amr.1995.9508080335

McKnight, D. H., Cummings, L. L., & Chervany, N. L. (1998). Initial trust formation in new organizational relationships. *Academy of Management Review, 23*(3), 473–490. doi:10.5465/amr.1998.926622

Medford-Davis, L. N., Eswaran, V., Shah, R. M., & Dark, C. (2015). The Patient Protection and Affordable Care Act's effect on emergency medicine: A synthesis of the data. *Annals of Emergency Medicine, 66*(5), 496–506. doi:10.1016/j.annemergmed.2015.04.007 PMID:25976250

Nambisan, P. (2017). Factors that impact Patient Web Portal Readiness (PWPR) among the underserved. *International Journal of Medical Informatics, 102*, 62–70. doi:10.1016/j.ijmedinf.2017.03.004 PMID:28495349

Nutbeam, D. (2000). Health literacy as a public health goal: A challenge for contemporary health education and communication strategies into the 21st century. *Health Promotion International, 15*(3), 259–267. doi:10.1093/heapro/15.3.259

OneView. (2019). The eight principles of patient-centered care. Retrieved from https://www.oneviewhealthcare.com/the-eight-principles-of-patient-centered-care/

Pavlou, P. A., & Gefen, D. (2005). Psychological contract violation in online marketplaces: Antecedents, consequences, and moderating role. *Information Systems Research, 16*(4), 372–399. doi:10.1287/isre.1050.0065

Riegelsberger, J., Sasse, M. A., & McCarthy, J. D. (2005). The mechanics of trust: A framework for research and design. *International Journal of Human-Computer Studies, 62*(3), 381–422. doi:10.1016/j.ijhcs.2005.01.001

Shaw, E. K., Howard, J., Clark, E. C., Etz, R. S., Arya, R., & Tallia, A. F. (2013). Decision-making processes of patients who use the emergency department for primary care needs. *Journal of Health Care for the Poor and Underserved, 24*(3), 1288–1305. doi:10.1353/hpu.2013.0140 PMID:23974399

Street, R. L., O'Malley, K. J., Cooper, L. A., & Haidet, P. (2008). Understanding concordance in patient-physician relationships: Personal and ethnic dimensions of shared identity. *Annals of Family Medicine, 6*(3), 198–205. doi:10.1370/afm.821 PMID:18474881

Studer, Q., Robinson, B. C., & Cook, K. (2010). *The HCAHPS handbook: Hardwire your hospital for pay-for-performance success*. Dover, AR: Fire Starter Pub.

Wallace, L. S., Angier, H., Huguet, N., Gaudino, J. A., Krist, A., Dearing, M., ... DeVoe, J. E. (2016). Patterns of electronic portal use among vulnerable patients in a nationwide practice-based research network: From the OCHIN Practice-based Research Network (PBRN). *Journal of the American Board of Family Medicine: JABFM*, *29*(5), 592–603. doi:10.3122/jabfm.2016.05.160046 PMID:27613792

Wallace, L. S., Angier, H., Huguet, N., Gaudino, J. A., Krist, A., Dearing, M., . . . DeVoe, J. E. (2017). Patterns of electronic portal use among vulnerable patients in a nationwide practice-based research network: From the OCHIN Practice-based Research Network (PBRN). *HHS Author Manuscripts*. Retrieved from https://www.ncbi.nlm.nih.gov/pmc/articles/PMC5341130/

Warkentin, M., Sharma, S., Gefen, D., Rose, G. M., & Pavlou, P. A. (2018). Social identity and trust in internet-based voting adoption. *Government Information Quarterly*, *35*(2), 195–209. doi:10.1016/j.giq.2018.03.007

WHO. (2008). Commission on Social Determinants of Health - Final Report. Retrieved from https://www.who.int/social_determinants/thecommission/finalreport/en/

Zarcadoolas, C., Vaughon, W. L., Czaja, S. J., Levy, J., & Rockoff, M. L. (2013). Consumers' perceptons of patient accessible electronic medical records. *Journal of Medical Internet Research*, *15*(8), e168. doi:10.2196/jmir.2507 PMID:23978618

Zucker, L. G. (1986). Production of trust: Institutional sources of economic structure, 1840-1920. In B. M. Staw, & L. L. Cummings (Eds.), *Research in Organizational Behavior* (Vol. 8, pp. 53–111). Greenwich, CT: JAI Press.

ADDITIONAL READING

Gefen, D., & Pavlou, P. A. (2012). The boundaries of trust and risk: The quadratic moderating role of institutional structures. *Information Systems Research*, *23*(3), 940–959. doi:10.1287/isre.1110.0395

Gefen, D., & Reychav, I. (2014). Why trustworthiness in an IT vendor is important even after the vendor left: IT is accepting the message and not just the messenger that is important. *Omega*, *44*(C), 111–125. doi:10.1016/j.omega.2013.11.002

Pavlou, P. A., & Gefen, D. (2005). Psychological contract violation in online marketplaces: Antecedents, consequences, and moderating role. *Information Systems Research*, *16*(4), 372–399. doi:10.1287/isre.1050.0065

KEY TERMS AND DEFINITIONS

Code of the Street: Behaviors considered acceptable in urban communities that demonstrate respect for individuals.

E-Health: Healthcare practices supported by electronic processes.

Ethnography: Methodology based on cultural anthropology that counts on the social understanding of the experience gained by the researcher in studying a culture group rather than interviews or surveys of others.

Health Information Technologies (HIT): Technology applied to health and healthcare supporting health information management across computerized systems and the secure exchange of health information between healthcare stakeholders, e.g. consumers, providers, payers.

Health Literacy: How people obtain, understand, use, and communicate about health information to make informed decisions ad follow instructions for treatment.

Patient Portal: A secure online website that provides convenient access to personal health information. Portals allow patients to securely perform a multitude of tasks that includes scheduling appointments, retrieving laboratory results, managing medications, accessing medical history data and other patient education or health information, and communicating with their healthcare provider.

Portal Readiness: Focus on activities that prepare patients towards using patient portals and identified individual level constructs focused on perceived need involved for which technology will be used.

Race Concordant: Race/ethnicity of the patient and provider is the same.

Safety-Net Hospital: A hospital that has a legal obligation to provide healthcare for individuals regardless of their insurance or ability to pay.

Social Determinants of Health (SDOH): Economic and social conditions resulting from circumstances in which people are born, grow up, live, work, and age that influence individual and group differences in the quality and provision of medical services.

Social Emergency Medicine: Addressing the social determinants of health from the Emergency Department by considering the social determinants underlying health illness and developing systemic interventions, measuring their effects, establishing collaborative community partnerships, and advocating for policies to improve the health of patients.

Social Identity Theory: Theory formulated by the late Henri Tajfel that predicts certain intergroup relations and group processes where group behaviors develop from a shared sense of social category membership.

Social Vulnerability (Healthcare): Social circumstances affecting vulnerable patients whereby multiple chronic medical, behavioral, and social problems interact in complex ways to undermine health that amplify the barriers to care.

Subjective Norms: One of the predictors of behavioral intentions in the Theory of Planned Behavior that refers to perceived social pressure to perform or not to perform the behavior.

Chapter 13
Challenges Implementing Telemedicine at Children's Hospital of Philadelphia (CHOP)

Christopher E. Gantz
Drexel University, USA

David Gefen
Drexel University, USA

ABSTRACT

This chapter discusses the challenges faced by one pediatric medical institution as it worked in partnership with a local school district to provide access to pediatric care through a telemedicine unit embedded in the nurse's office of the various schools within the district. The chapter touches on perceptions the community had about sharing sensitive personal health information in a school setting using mobile technology, fears related to immigration status, and operational issues encountered when deploying a new technology across multiple sites. Despite the challenges, potential benefits to the health and well-being of the community far outweighed the difficulties faced during these early days of telemedicine adoption.

INTRODUCTION

Telemedicine represents a game-changing opportunity to increase access and empower parents and caregivers who might otherwise face significant challenges accessing healthcare for their children. This chapter explores the potential of the technology to profoundly improve the lives of the children, their parents, and the larger community – and the role that trust plays in the acceptance of the technology within a specific community where the program is being piloted in a school nurse office setting. An overview of a currently underway research study, the objective of which is to understand the social context of the interaction of trust on the well-studied Theory of Planned Behavior as it relates to the communities' willingness to embrace a novel approach to healthcare delivery, will also be discussed. That study is looking into the consequences of the lack of empowerment that parents feel related to the health care

DOI: 10.4018/978-1-7998-0047-7.ch013

of their children and the factors that are theorized to be affecting their decisions related to signing up to take advantage of the new telemedicine program. These factors include the perception that the government is actively working to identify and remove undocumented members of their community and may use information shared with the school or pediatric institution to identify and deport family members, that the school or pediatric institution themselves may not be promoting the program for truly altruistic reasons, and that sensitive information about their child's health might be viewed by school staff.

The following paragraphs explore the challenges encountered by the groups working to deploy the service within the school district of an urban community and the design of a research project looking to gain insight into why parents would choose to *not* participate. The initial thinking when the service was conceptualized was that it would be extremely popular and well received, however, the staff of both the school district and the pediatric hospital were surprised to find that very few parents signed up and that the program was not embraced. The hypothesis that was developed to explain the tepid response focused on the idea that trust in the students' school district, the pediatric medical center offering the service, and more broadly, the government, was having a moderating effect on the likelihood that parents will be willing to have their children enrolled in the program. Of particular interest to the research team conducting the study is how the large undocumented population that resides in the community perceives the government's intentions towards them and how those perceptions lead them to make decisions about accessing services when they are offered. The objective of the study described in this chapter was to gather an initial understanding within a theoretical framework of challenges to the adoption by parents of this telemedicine implementation project.

The chapter summarizes the justification for the research model and the crucial role that trust plays in it. The insights that led to the development of the study are based on questions asked by parents and concerns they raised during outreach events where the Children's Hospital of Philadelphia (CHOP) presented information about the program to families. The recurring themes are presented in this chapter, including concerns about potential exposure to ICE (U.S. Immigration and Customs Enforcement). In the interest of eliciting honest and open answers, and especially in view of parents' concerns about ICE, no recordings were made. Rather, the lead author summarized his impressions shortly after each information session.

CHOP is well known to the local community and is the oldest pediatric hospital in the United States. The hospital started with only 12 beds and in its first year had only 67 inpatients and just a little over 300 clinic patients. It has since grown to be a world-renowned hospital with 546 beds and conducts more than a million visits annually (Philadelphia, 2018). A key part of the hospital's mission is to provide the highest level of health care to the community it serves. To support that mission, and in recognizing the successes of telemedicine in developing countries, CHOP decided to create its own telemedicine initiative. That telemedicine service is seen as a way to provide expanded access to care through its digital health team to schools within its service area. To that end, CHOP initiated the telemedicine pilot during the 2017/2018 school year. The telemedicine initiative is being conducted in partnership with the Norristown Area School District located in Norristown, Pennsylvania which has 7,468 students in grades K-12.

While the study discussed in this chapter focuses on this one group's experience with implementing telemedicine within a public school system in an urban setting and may not be representative of how the technology is received by other communities, the pilot and the public's response to it have offered insights into the challenges of telemedicine in a school setting, as well as how the broader community views the technology. The challenges identified could potentially inform both the ongoing attempts to increase utilization of the service within the Norristown area school district and other attempts to implement digital health solutions in other parts of the country. In that regard, this initiative also presents an opportunity to learn best practices for engaging the public and successfully rolling out new telemedicine technologies.

Background

In the Norristown area and across the country many children receive medical care for illnesses first reported during the school day in the Pediatric Emergency Department (ED) that could be more effectively delivered in a primary care setting. Parents face a variety of challenges when seeking care for their children that may lead them to seek care in the ED. Waiting times for appointments with a pediatrician can create a significant obstacle for parents as they try to find times that work for them. Parents may have to take whatever appointment time is available and may wait until the following day before being seen, which is not always a viable option when trying to juggle school and work schedules. There are also significant financial implications to using the ED that must be factored into any evaluation of impact of not seeking care of a primary care provider. Looking at the average cost of using the ED, Janet Hunt found that patients with insurance would have a copay of between $50 and $100 while individuals without insurance could face bills that range from $150 to $3,000 depending on the reason for the visit (Hunt, 2019). Without the need for a referral, parents with limited time and resources might feel like they are saving steps by visiting the ED rather than going to a primary care doctor who may refer them out to specialists requiring more time and resources.

The decision to seek care in the ED rather than visiting a pediatrician can have profound consequences for the family. The need to seek care outside of office hours with medical professionals who do not have an established relationship with the family can lead to poor outcomes and has been linked to the lack of resources some families must contend with. This reality is another prime example of how access to pediatric care in the school setting would empower families by creating a stable environment where high quality pediatric care can be accessed without having a support system in place to assist with the logistics of seeking medical support for a sick child while balancing other commitments.

The implications for reducing unnecessary ED visits are a tangible benefit of telemedicine that could be extended to communities across the country. Looking at the phenomenon of low-acuity (colds, headache, abdominal pain) ED visits, Cabey et al. (2018) found that children under the age of 18 had significantly higher levels of ED utilization with as many as half of the visits occurring in pediatric Emergency Departments being for low-acuity issues. That research also showed that lower-income minorities were frequent users of the ED and had higher rates of repeat visits. Cabey et al. (2018) learned that parents who tended to use the ED for low acuity health issues were likely to also leverage sick visits with the primary care provider in the same way. Moreover, many frequent users of the ED described themselves as the only ones in their household that provided care for the child or the children in their household. They also revealed that they lacked social networks that could provide the type of support that would reduce barriers to seeking care outside of an ED setting. These barriers include not having someone who could bring their child to a pediatrician's office during the day so that they don't have to miss work.

At the other end of the spectrum, parents and caregivers of children who were not frequent users of an ED for low-acuity health concerns were able to readily identify a strong support network, that Cabey et al. (2018) noted, helped them evaluate health care options and provide support that aided in gaining access for their children. As one can imagine, Cabey et al. (2018) found that the social support network generally included the child's other family members and trusted members of their community. The support structure these other individuals provided helped the parent make decisions about care and about evaluating options about accessing resources.

In determining the reasons for so many low-acuity visits to the ED, Cabey et al. (2018) concluded that caretakers who relied on the ED did so because they felt that the tradeoff in the relationship was worth the increased speed of getting in front of a provider. Parents did express that they preferred long term relationships with their physicians, but that changes to how many practices were now operating reduced their ability to form those relationships and created frustration. Cabey et al. concluded that caretakers were less inclined to rely on alternatives such as walk-in clinics and after-hours advice lines or even just other clinicians they were unfamiliar with. Trust in the ED's ability to treat their children effectively and the belief that the MD's there are considered specialists emerged as a key criterion in choosing the ED as the medical provider. In contrast to caretakers who used the ED for low-acuity visits, caretakers who had private insurance, while also reporting frustrations with the team approach to healthcare that many practices are now implementing, had greater trust in the overall health system. Cabey et al. also noted that the caretakers in this group relied on their social networks and the advice of trusted others for both decision-making and transportation support as well as other logistics regarding the children. Work done by Farion et al. (2015) sheds additional light on the complex issues influencing the increasing use of Pediatric EDs for low-acuity problems. Responses to the survey his team deployed showed that many of the respondents did have primary care physicians. The survey revealed that despite this fact many of the low-acuity ED visits happened during regular office hours during the week when a primary care physician would presumably be available. The respondents expressed doubt that a primary care provider would have the resources to treat their child's condition which often led them to choose an ED for care.

Parental responses to the survey conducted by Farion et al. (2015) suggested that parents chose to visit the ED because of a high level of concern over the symptoms their child was experiencing; leading them to choose a location they felt would be able to provide the highest level of care that their child's situation might require. However, despite the high level of anxiety, Farion et al. noted that almost half of the patients seen wound up not needing interventional care – and even when a patient did need an intervention, in most cases the treatment could have been delivered in a primary care setting. Lastly, the survey revealed that three-quarters of the parents did not even attempt to make an appointment with their primary care provider before deciding to take their child to the ED (Farion et al. 2015).

THE TELEMEDICINE INITIATIVE AT CHOP

As Farion's Study shows, *Children's Hospital of Philadelphia* (CHOP) is not unique in the phenomenon of parents using the ED for minor illnesses. And, while caregivers have expressed interest in the idea of telemedicine (Cabey et al. 2018), it may be difficult for families who have become accustomed to using the ED as their primary source of healthcare to become comfortable with the idea of their child receiving care without them being present and receiving the feedback from the treating physician at that moment. It may seem counterintuitive, but when faced with the option to change how they have become accustomed to receiving care, families may reject what they see as a less robust option. They might also not be motivated to sign up for a service offered to them when their child is well.

CHOP is not the first hospital in the country to implement a program aimed at providing care through a partnership with local schools via telemedicine. In a July 2017 article, Samuel (2017) writes that *Children's Health System* in Dallas had built a robust telemedicine offering with several of the schools in the area. She goes on to note that initially the program conducted telemedicine visits in only two schools but over the course of a few years has grown to support nearly 100 schools with several thousand visits happening over a four-year period. The article reveals that their approach is similar to what CHOP is doing. In addition to the robust program initiated in Texas, there are other programs in states across the country that are being established. It is worth noting that the second largest school district in the country located in Los Angeles has implemented telemedicine in a few of their schools (Wicklund, 2016).

School-based telemedicine programs are growing in popularity throughout the United States, mainly because of their potential to improve the health of children in both rural and urban settings. An embedded telemedicine program can be incredibly beneficial for reducing the number of missed school days for students and the burden for parents of having to take time off from work. In the model adopted by CHOP, the service consists of a telemedicine unit installed in the nurse's office which allows the school nurse to initiate a virtual office visit with a CHOP pediatrician when he or she deems it appropriate. Similarly to how the service is deployed in Texas, nurses use a Telemedicine unit that has a computer monitor with a camera for video conferencing with the physician and a number of smart medical tools which can relay information back to the physician in real-time. The unit allows the physician to complete most screening procedures they would conduct if the student were in their office. An encrypted HIPAA-secure connection adds a layer of protection for the student's health information.

How it Works

There are now several companies that can provide FDA approved, low cost, HIPAA-compliant telemedicine devices such as the ones being deployed in Norristown that, along with high-speed internet access, allow a health care provider to examine patients and interact with the school nurse virtually. Remote providers (ED physicians in CHOP's pilot) get clear views of the ears, throat, and skin, and can hear heart and lungs sounds. Providers can use Electric Health Records (EHR) to ePrescribe medications for parents to pick up after work and can provide the school nurses written orders upon which they can act to administer over-the-counter medications when deemed appropriate. School telemedicine students/patients may or may not choose to have their primary care provided by CHOP. Regardless, the use of the EHR allows CHOP providers to electronically send both CHOP and non-CHOP PCPs (Primary Care Physician) the visit summary to ensure the child's continuity of care.

With the clear value proposition presented by having the technology embedded in a school, the CHOP digital health team and the school district believed there would be high demand for a service which would reduce the barriers that families faced in having their child seen by a pediatrician, while reducing the number of missed days of school for the student and work for the parent. However, during the first year that the service was offered very few parents signed up. The digital health team reviewed their approach, evaluated the timing of the initial rollout which occurred during the middle of the school year rather than at the start and consulted with community engagement experts about how to move forward. Together they discussed strategies to increase enrollment while trying to better understand where parents or caregivers' reluctance might come from and the reasons why families in the school district might not take advantage of the service.

A Theoretical Perspective

While the team was able to identify what they believed to be barriers to enrollment, it was decided that the best course of action would be to work with an investigator to conduct a research study that would provide insight into how to proceed. A thorough literature review was conducted to determine which theoretical framework would be most suited to shedding light on the factors affecting the decisions of parents who were offered the chance to enroll their children in the telemedicine program. The Theory of Planned Behavior (TPB) (Ajzen, 1991) was selected because it is a highly researched theory that looks at the factors which affect people's decisions to act. TPB has been applied to many scenarios and has proven to be a reliable way to evaluate behavioral intentions across a large number of settings.

TPB posits that an individual's behavior will be determined by their intention to perform the behavior, and that that intention is affected by three factors: attitude towards the behavior, subjective norms, and perceived behavioral control. Attitude is the individual's negative or positive feelings regarding the behavior. Subjective norms are beliefs about whether significant people in the individual's life think she or he should perform the behavior. Perceived behavioral control is the individual's perception that they are in control. TPB expands on the Theory of Reasoned Action (TRA) (Fishbein & Ajzen, 1975) which has been shown to successfully predict and explain behavior in several areas related to IT (Taylor & Todd, 1995).

The importance of subjective norms in contexts such as this telemedicine one has been highlighted by an anecdote shared by a coordinator working on a study in another local school district. That program succeeded solely by a word of mouth advertising that was conducted by a mom who took it upon herself to promote the study to her social network by posting about it on social media. Teams looking to implement a strategy such as this in a school setting need to be aware that this type of grass-roots advertising cuts both ways. If that mom had criticized the study, the researchers, or the school district for allowing the programs into the school then it is likely that that study would not have succeeded. The same is likely for the successful integration of this program into the schools and its acceptance by the parents.

Integrating the inhibitors discussed above into TPB suggests the model in Figure 1. As with many other behaviors predicted by TPB, intention to adopt telemedicine is assumed to depend on the decision makers' behavioral beliefs about its benefits and the subsequent attitude those create. This is combined with the word of mouth and recommendations of other people important to the decision maker and the subjective norms the decision maker makes accordingly, as well as by perceived behavioral control on the situation. Adding to those standard elements of TPB, the model highlights how trust in the school system, the pediatric institution, and government entities could potentially have a moderating effect on the parent or caregivers' intention to enroll in the program. Some of the potential moderations of behavior include gender, immigration status, zip code, and Socio-Economic Status (SES).

The model proposes that trust in the school district, in CHOP, and in the government will each for its own reasons moderate the attitude to intentions path. The reason is based on the observations of Gefen and Pavlou (2012) that when people have very high degrees of trust in those controlling the context, i.e. the three targets of trust above, they will be more inclined to adopt the behavior and that if they have very low degrees of trust they will just refrain from it regardless of their behavioral beliefs about its potential benefits. Thus, highly trusting potential adopters of the telemedicine system might adopt it just because the authorities in charge – be that the school district, CHOP, or the government – suggest they should. Presumably, those adopters would believe that doing so would benefit them through improved services that the school district, CHOP, or the government, respectively, will be able to provide them

Figure 1. An adapted theory of planned behavior perspective to telemedicine adoption

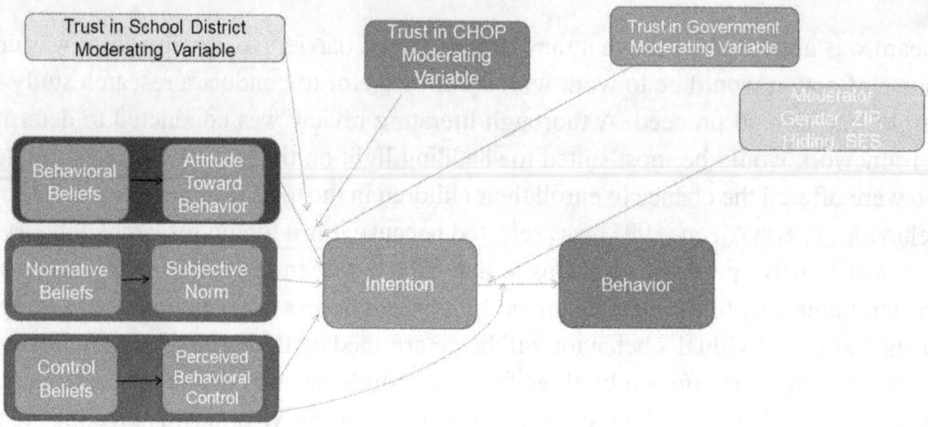

through such a telemedicine system. Trusting those authorities, the adopters would expect magnified benefits and little risk. Or, contrariwise, low trusting potential adopters may outright refuse to even try the telemedicine system precisely because those authorities in charge suggest they should, as implied by the context of suspicion that ICE may be informed about them through such activities. SES, gender, and other demographics are predicted to moderate the intentions to behavior path because of access to the technology as well as because of how such demographics change how people understand electronic messages (e.g. Gefen and Straub (1997)).

The importance of behavioral control is related in this context also to security concerns. With the frequency and size of data breaches being discussed in the news, potential telemedicine users may feel that using a service which requires information about their child to be transmitted over the internet to be too risky of a proposition and choose to refrain from participating. Data breaches have exposed the information of hundreds of millions of people within the past few years, and even well-known companies have appeared reticent to reveal that their security has been compromised and the private data of their customers has been accessed. In this climate, it would seem to be a difficult task to instill confidence in technologies where one is sharing extremely sensitive information. Many people may remember that one of the largest data breaches in recent years was at *Anthem*, a healthcare insurance company. In 2015 *Anthem* revealed that a data breach affected 75 million of their customers (Yakasai & Jusoh, 2015).

The Inhibitor to Success: The Need to Build Trust

While telemedicine offered in a school setting would seem like an ideal way to expand the reach of medical services and alleviate many of the barriers of finding effective care for their children faced by parents, it is unknown how trust in healthcare organizations, the government, or the school system is affecting parents' decisions to not take advantage of the services being offered. Indeed, across the country, there are urban legends and rumors about healthcare organizations whose alleged behavior, if true, would not be conducive to maintaining trust.

In Philadelphia, for example, there is a belief in some communities that patients and their families are screened by hospital staff for outstanding legal issues, and if any are identified the hospital would call the police on the family member. This, of course, is false. And, while it may seem ridiculous to imagine that a pediatric institution dedicated to improving the health and welfare of the children they serve and their families would do such a thing, the rumor nonetheless persists and has been fueled by the work of a former University of Pennsylvania graduate student. Knowing that for some this rumor would seem very credible, it is not hard to imagine the difficult decisions that some parents may feel forced to make when acting out of an abundance of caution.

Dan McQuade in his 2015 article in *Philadelphia Magazine* discussed a former graduate student Alice Goffman's ethnographic work while she was a student at the University of Pennsylvania, and notes that she wrote about the supposed practice as if it were in fact real. He concludes that her work has likely solidified a fallacy and contributed to a lack of trust within the local community. Citing an essay by Northwestern law professor Steven Lubet, McQuade writes that Goffman has reinforced the idea that this is occurring and created a situation where it is repeated as if it were a known fact. He also notes that Lubet, in his criticism of the work, laments that many young African American men may decide against getting care because of her reinforcing this rumor and that this effect on seeking healthcare is unfortunate (McQuade, 2015). That is an understatement, as the impact on the community has likely been profound and may affect families for generations to come (Politi, 2018).

Early in the rollout of the telemedicine pilot in the Norristown school district a team from CHOP attended a back-to-school event to discuss the program with families. While most parents took flyers, asked a few questions, and listened to the team provide information, one parent became visibly upset when one of the team indicated that there would be a need to sign up for the program and provide some information before their child would be eligible to participate in the program. He indicated that providing any type of information to a school or CHOP was unacceptable and walked off without offering any further explanation. It can be assumed from that parent's reaction that he did not feel that he could trust sharing his child's personal information. Teams that wish to be successful in engaging with the community will need to recognize that there may be individuals who need to be reassured of their positive intentions and address any misconceptions that they might have. Many parents might have misgivings but may not express them to the school or to CHOP staff. As mentioned above, many of the parents at the back-to-school event took flyers and engaged with CHOP staff. However, only a very small number of parents enrolled in the program.

Another Inhibitor: Fear of Deportation

Additionally, with a large Hispanic population in the Norristown area, it has been proposed that many undocumented immigrants living in the area may be fearful that opting into the service will lead to their Personal Health Information (PHI) as well as their undocumented status being shared with ICE, leading to dire consequences for their family members. With the current climate towards immigration being what it is, there is a strong fear of deportation along with other concerns about how immigrants might be treated regardless of their actual immigration status. It is that fear that could cause parents to avoid seeking treatment for themselves and their children. They may feel that in seeking medical help, they are putting their family at risk. These concerns about ICE are not unfounded. Stories of ICE agents making arrests at courthouses and other sensitive locations have become frequent. Jeff Gammage in his 2019 article in the Philadelphia Inquirer writes that the frequent arrest of people who have come to courthouses has caused people to stay away (Gammage 2019).[2] Similarly, last summer the arrest of a man who was driving his wife to the hospital made national news and reinforced the perception that ICE is aggressively seeking to identify and deport any person who is undocumented (Politi 2018).

Jefferies (2014), in discussing the issues faced by immigrants, notes that individuals who were not born in the United States and came here as children without permission of the government face a myriad of challenges in many areas of their life including the school system. He goes on to say that a Supreme Court case from 1982, the *Plyler v. Doe* ruling, determined that public schools could not have their funding reduced for accepting students who are undocumented. This has allowed access for students to attend elementary, middle, and high school regardless of their immigration status. The article discusses how this ruling, which was intended to help improve access to educational resources, created a disconnect between schools and the immigrant community by creating a "don't ask, don't tell" scenario where administrators do not inquire about immigration status.

Without strong communication between schools and undocumented populations, there will be challenges to building trust. In order to better understand the mindset of undocumented individuals, one need go no further than the evening news to see images of children separated from their parents and being held in detention centers. These images along with the experiences of other community members could solidify the idea that the government is actively seeking to create hardships for undocumented families. The risk that a school could be used as an access point for organizations like ICE to determine the status of the student population may not only seem reasonable but could seem likely.

Hacker et al. (2011), in a study using focus groups, found that fear of deportation increased stress levels and left people feeling more alone. She noted that there was an "overarching belief among focus group participants that those in positions of authority police, health care personnel, and health insurers had power to interact with ICE and initiate the deportation process." Hacker et al. claim that this belief was a key reason for a lack of trust that both legal and illegal immigrants felt for the communities where they reside. The lack of trust felt by these individuals created a chronic sense of insecurity and reduced their willingness to seek care when needed.

Likewise, the *2018 Nation's Progress on Children's Health Coverage* report by Joan Alker and Olivia Pham revealed that "[u]ninsured children are more likely to have unmet health needs and lack a usual source of care." The lack of consistent health care can result in missed school and lower performance. Unfortunately, their report reveals that efforts amongst both political parties to reduce the number of uninsured people in the country has been affected by the new Trump administration (Pham, 2018). A *National Public Radio* (NPR) coverage of the report notes that years of progress reducing the number of children in the U.S. without health insurance was halted in 2017 as the numbers increased during the first year of Donald Trump's presidency (Galewitz, 2018). Currently, the average number of uninsured children across the country hovers at about 5%, but in some places, it can be much higher (Galewitz, 2018). The article goes on to reveal that the Trump administration's effort to crack down on immigration (both legal and illegal) has caused people to make decisions about seeking medical care for their children. Parents often feel the risk is too great. Even in situations where a parent is going through the process of getting a Green Card, they may still be reticent to seek help for their children for fear of them being perceived as a burden on the system and therefore less eligible for a Green Card.

Along the same lines, a *Washington Post* article discussing illegal immigration and the experience of Pulitzer Prize-winning journalist Jose Antonio Vargas states that in the current climate illegal immigrants face a high chance of being deported to a country they may have only lived in as a small child. The Trump administration has shown that their immigration policies are much more severe than the previous administration's strategy of having ICE focus their efforts on deporting illegal immigrants who had a criminal background. The Trump administration has empowered immigration authorities to go after anyone who they determine to be living in the country without the proper authorization regardless of when they came or their contribution to their community (Waters, 2018).

Other Potential Inhibitors: Lack of Innovation

One of the biggest challenges to the expansion of a telemedicine program is the novelty of the approach. The most dangerous phrase uttered by medical professionals, school administrators, school nurses, and parents is that traditional in-person visits are "how it's always been done." A colleague recounted recently attending an informational session for physicians and other medical professionals where the benefits of telemedicine were described, and the need to be a first mover in the space to remain competitive in the marketplace was discussed. She was surprised that during the question and answer portion of the event there was a strong opposition to the use of the technology amongst some of the physicians who were in attendance.

The physicians lamented the fact that they would not be able to "lay hands" on the patient and the quality of care would suffer. The speaker pointed out that there has already been a long history of physicians conducting exams over the phone by asking the patient or caregiver a few questions and moving forward with a course of treatment based on that phone interaction. He went on to point out that the telemedicine approach does have some limitations but that in nearly 90 percent of his and his medical team's interactions they are able to provide a level of care that is comparable to what is received during face-to-face encounters. In situations where there is a full telemedicine unit in place, such as in a school setting, the interactions are even closer to what can be achieved with an in-person visit. With devices that can be used to listen to the heart and lungs, take temperature, and look into both the ears and mouth, treating physicians are able to approximate nearly the entirety of the information available in an in-person visit. That coupled with the time saved and the increased access provided to both patients and medical staff makes it a clear choice for health systems to support.

An additional advantage discussed was the reduction or removal of the no-show. With patient wait times reduced to minutes rather than hours, they have less of a reason to not appear for a scheduled visit. In cases where a patient does not show up for an in-person appointment, the physician is able to spend that time seeing patients virtually rather than being left idle waiting for their next patient. Pushback from medical professionals was not initially identified as a barrier to the success of the Norristown pilot, but being aware that it could be an internal challenge as the program expands to other regions may be valuable insight and may help the team be able to readily address concerns voiced by the physicians.

Other Potential Inhibitors: Bandwidth

While the Norristown school district has nurses available at the different schools throughout the district, the number of telemedicine visits they can conduct is limited by the fact that each session may take 10-15 minutes, which at certain times may not be feasible. In a conversation with the team conducting the telemedicine study, one of the potential challenges that emerged was the limited time available to the school nurse at the site of treatment. There is awareness that during certain times of the year there would be higher than normal volume of children seeking care from the nurse. During these peak times, the need for telemedicine visits would also increase, but the ability of the nurse to facilitate them would be reduced. There might be times when a student comes to the nurse, and she initiates a visit with a pediatrician, but during that visit another student may come in seeking immediate care, inhibiting the ability to conduct a thorough telemedicine examination. If the nurse is unable to triage the other students adequately, he or she might opt to not begin a visit that takes 10-15 minutes. Missteps like this with families who have signed up for the program but were unhappy with the service they received or who feel that the promise of improved care failed to materialize may lead caregivers to share their dissatisfaction with other parents and could have a chilling effect on future adoption. In the early years of the program when the technology is still not entirely mainstream, parents may take a "try it before you buy it" approach.

The same scenario could potentially play out on the hospital side of the interaction too. The physicians who have been supporting the telemedicine pilot have indicated that they currently have adequate bandwidth to conduct telemedicine visits between clinical cases. While this is true now, the ultimate goal of the research being conducted by the lead author is to dramatically increase the number of families utilizing the service and to expand the program to support the public and private schools in Philadelphia. This would be an increase from roughly 7,500 students in the current pilot to nearly 400,000 across all the schools. Without an adequate plan in place to accommodate peak visit times, the system could easily become overwhelmed, with students not receiving the care they need despite being enrolled in the program.

Looking Ahead

Looking to areas outside of the pediatric healthcare space seems like a viable approach to addressing the problems associated with engaging patients and families in the pursuit of telemedicine. Taking cues from behavioral economics, marketing and IT are potential strategies to reducing poor enrollment. One such example can be found in a paper by VanEpps, Volpp, and Halpern (2016). VanEpps, et al. discussed behavioral economic-based nudges that could facilitate enrollment and cohort retention in clinical research studies. Many of those approaches may map onto this work and allow us to examine their value in increasing engagement. Their description of how social norms can influence behavior and provide the analogy of how a friend's recommendation of a service or restaurant can affect one's behavior (VanEpps et al., 2016). This belief is in line with TPB and reinforces the idea that to win community support for the program will require advocates to clearly define the benefits of telemedicine while building a strong foundation of trust with parents and caregivers.

CONCLUSION

This chapter has provided an overview of some of the myriad challenges faced by one group working to deploy a telemedicine intervention aimed at improving access to care to a community. The fear that the government will gain access to the information of an undocumented family and use it to deport them may well present the greatest challenge to the team, as the consequences to the family would be so great that they may feel that it is in their best interest to not share any information and remain insular. With this realization in mind, both the school and CHOP might be able to gear their outreach towards addressing the concerns of families in allaying their fears. This work must be done by connecting with trusted community organizations who can advocate on behalf of the program. Having a clearly spelled out privacy policy that is correctly translated is another step that can build confidence. The team has also already taken the step of ensuring that there are Spanish-speaking employees at any outreach event. This is critically important in providing evidence that the immigrant community is valued and is not being contacted as an afterthought.

CHOP must also work to identify any rumors or misconceptions about their intentions and actively work to educate the public. The example noted above of the belief that Philadelphia hospitals, and CHOP specifically, are working with the authorities to identify and arrest adults who have any type of legal issues is particularly problematic. While false and counter to the ideals of the hospital, the story has been in the news and will show up when searched online. Even if the articles point out that this is not a policy, it may seem more likely to be true. Much like with the undocumented population this rumor might give people pause. The work that needs to be done cannot happen remotely. CHOP will need to have a continued presence within the district. Staff and hospital leadership need to continue to attend events, present the mission of the hospital, listen to concerns raised by community members, and provide thoughtful answers so that all parties will view the program as a partnership.

Across the school district, principals, school nurses, and counselors, who may have had challenging interactions with some families may need to reevaluate their experiences and work to ensure that parents know that they are motivated by the best interest of all their students. This will not happen overnight, and challenges may continue to arise, but with consistent messaging from both the district and CHOP the parents who could most benefit from the program can be educated on its true value. There must be efforts made to understand why the parents, such as the one encountered at the back-to-school event, reacted so negatively to the idea of the school nurse being present during the telemedicine visit, and if those beliefs are shared by others or if this experience is unique.

While the focus on one community could be seen as a limitation of the chapter, the challenges described are not unique to this example and will likely be faced many more times, as telemedicine is integrated in other parts of the country and throughout the world. It is hard to imagine a scenario where a new approach to providing care does not encounter challenges within the community, and hence requires teams to build trust, even while clearly providing tremendous value. The barriers to success are significant and will require teams to stay focused on how impactful their success will be for everyone who is touched by the school system. The results Ronis, McConnochie, Wang, and Wood (2017) showed in their eye-opening case study about a well-implemented program in Rochester, NY show that it is worthwhile for everyone involved to find ways to overcome the barriers to successful implementation. In their study acute care utilization increased by an astounding 75%.

The promise of successful implementation of telemedicine in the school setting is the empowerment of parents and caregivers to provide high quality healthcare for their children while also reducing their need to make difficult decisions that might jeopardize their employment by missing days of work and their children's educational experience by having to miss school. Telemedicine is the promise of a fundamental shift in how families access care. For the parent who would have agonized over decisions about seeing care or protecting their employment or immigration status this new technology and its deployment in the school levels the playing field and empowers them to make informed decisions about their child's healthcare without having to compromise. With the potential impact of successfully overcoming the obstacles that exist in the rollout of this program, it is vital that groups such as CHOP's telemedicine team keep pushing this work forward and sharing their learnings so that children and their families everywhere can be afforded the opportunity to live happier and healthier lives.

REFERENCES

Ajzen, I. (1991). The theory of planned behavior. *Organizational Behavior and Human Decision Processes*, *50*(2), 179–211. doi:10.1016/0749-5978(91)90020-T

Cabey, W. V., Shea, J. A., Kangovi, S., Kennedy, D., Onwuzulike, C., & Fein, J. (2018). Understanding Pediatric Caretakers' Views on Obtaining Medical Care for Low-acuity Illness. *Academic Emergency Medicine*, *25*(9), 1004–1013. doi:10.1111/acem.13436 PMID:29741232

Farion, K. J., Wright, M., Zemek, R., Neto, G., Karwowska, A., Tse, S., ... Barrowman, N. (2015). Understanding Low-Acuity Visits to the Pediatric Emergency Department. *PLoS One*, 10. PMID:26083338

Fishbein, M., & Ajzen, I. (1975). *Belief, Attitude, Intention and Behavior: An Introduction to Theory and Research*. Reading, MA: Addison-Wesley Publishing Company.

Galewitz, P. (2018). Number Of U.S. Kids Who Don't Have Health Insurance Is On The Rise. Retrieved from https://www.npr.org/sections/health-shots/2018/11/29/671666280/number-of-u-s-kids-who-dont-have-health-insurance-is-on-the-rise

Gammage, J. (2019). Philly sheriff tells feds: ICE agents must now identify themselves to deputies in city Courtrooms. Retrieved from https://www.philly.com/news/ice-immigrant-immigration-philly-sheriff-jewell-williams-20190402.html

Gefen, D., & Pavlou, P. A. (2012). The Boundaries of Trust and Risk: The Quadratic Moderating Role of Institutional Structures. *Information Systems Research*, *23*(3), 940–959. doi:10.1287/isre.1110.0395

Gefen, D., & Straub, D. W. (1997). Gender Differences in Perception and Adoption of E-mail: An Extension to the Technology Acceptance Model. *Management Information Systems Quarterly*, *21*(4), 389–400. doi:10.2307/249720

Hacker, K., Chu, J., Leung, C., Marra, R., Pirie, A., Brahimi, M., ... Marlin, R. P. (2011). The impact of Immigration and Customs Enforcement on immigrant health: Perceptions of immigrants in Everett, Massachusetts, USA. *Social Science & Medicine*, *73*(4), 586–594. doi:10.1016/j.socscimed.2011.06.007 PMID:21778008

Hunt, D. (2019)Average Cost of an ER visit. Retrieved from https://www.thebalance.com/average-cost-of-an-er-visit-4176166

Jefferies, J. (2014). Fear of Deportation in High School: Implications for Breaking the Circle of Silence Surrounding Migration Status AU - Jefferies, Julián. *Journal of Latinos and Education*, *13*(4), 278–295. doi:10.1080/15348431.2014.887469

McQuade, D. (2015). Alice Goffman's Book on "Fugitive Life" in Philly Under Attack. Retrieved from https://www.phillymag.com/news/2015/06/11/alice-goffman-book-philadelphia-on-the-run-criticism/

Pham, J. A. O. (2018). Nation's Progress on Children's Health Coverage Reverses Course. Retrieved from https://ccf.georgetown.edu/wp-content/uploads/2018/11/UninsuredKids2018_Final_asof1128743pm.pdf

PhiladelphiaC. H. O. (2018). About Us. Retrieved from https://www.chop.edu/about-us/about

Politi, D. (2018). ICE Officers Arrest Man Who Was Driving Pregnant Wife to Hospital for C-Section. Retrieved from https://slate.com/news-and-politics/2018/08/joel-arrona-arrested-ice-detains-man-who-was-driving-wife-to-hospital-for-c-section.html

Ronis, S. D., McConnochie, K. M., Wang, H., & Wood, N. E. (2017). Urban Telemedicine Enables Equity in Access to Acute Illness Care. *Telemedicine Journal and e-Health, 23*(2), 105–112. doi:10.1089/tmj.2016.0098 PMID:27383822

Samuel, L. (2017). At a growing number of schools, sick kids can take a virtual trip to the doctor. [July 19]. *Stat.*

Taylor, S., & Todd, P. (1995). Understanding Information Technology Usage: A Test of Competing Models. *Information Systems Research, 6*(2), 144–176. doi:10.1287/isre.6.2.144

VanEpps, E. M., Volpp, K. G., & Halpern, S. D. (2016). A nudge toward participation: Improving clinical trial enrollment with behavioral economics. *Science Translational Medicine, 8*(348), 348fs313. doi:10.1126citranslmed.aaf0946 PMID:27440726

Waters, M. C. (2018). An undocumented immigrant's life of fear and activism. Retrieved from https://www.washingtonpost.com/outlook/an-undocumented-immigrants-life-of-fear-and-activism/2018/10/18/2ab5fb86-a572-11e8-97ce-cc9042272f07_story.html?utm_term=.5cc14827604e

Wicklund, E. (2016). Factors Behind the Adoption of School-based Telehealth. Retrieved from https://mhealthintelligence.com/features/factors-behind-the-adoption-of-school-based-telehealth

Yakasai, A. B. M., & Jusoh, W. J. W. (2015). Testing the Theory of Planned Behavior in Determining Intention to use Digital Coupon among University Students. *Procedia Economics and Finance, 31*, 186–193. doi:10.1016/S2212-5671(15)01145-4

KEY TERM AND DEFINITIONS

Attitude: The degree to which an individual has a positive or negative evaluation of a behavior.

Emergency Department (ED): The department within a medical treatment facility specializing in acute care of patients who arrive without prior appointment.

Ethnographic: The scientific description of peoples and cultures with their customs, habits, and mutual differences.

Healthcare delivery: The manner in which healthcare services are provided to an individual or community.

Perceived Behavioral Control: A person's perception of the ease or difficulty of performing the behavior of interest.

Personal Health Information (PHI): Also referred to as Protected Health Information, refers to demographic information, medical histories, test and laboratory results, mental health conditions, insurance information, and other data that a healthcare professional collects to identify an individual and determine appropriate care.

Primary Care Provider (PCP): A medical professional who is the practitioner who oversees and coordinates or helps a patient access a range of health care services.

Social Norms: The customary codes of behavior in a group.

Subjective Norms: A person's beliefs about whether peers and people of importance to the person think he or she should engage in the behavior.

Telemedicine: The remote diagnosis and treatment of patients by means of telecommunications technology including video chat and internet connected medical devices.

Theoretical Framework: The theoretical framework introduces and describes the theory that explains why the research problem under study exists.

Theory of Planned Behavior(TPB): The theory states that attitude toward behavior, subjective norms, and perceived behavioral control, together shape an individual's behavioral intentions and behaviors.

Undocumented: A foreign-born person living in the United States without U.S. citizenship or other legal immigration status.

Chapter 14
Doctor-Patient Social Networking to Improve Specialist Care Coordination

Jeremy S. Kagan
https://orcid.org/0000-0003-2202-1526
CardioLync, Israel

ABSTRACT

Effective communication and coordination among medical doctors, specialists, and other caregivers could mean the difference between life and death for patients. This chapter presents a new digital health technology paradigm based on social networking that improves care coordination and communication among medical specialists. This technology integrates data across diagnostic modalities to simplify the process of accessing information, and reporting medical interpretations and treatment recommendations. This model can help care providers improve patient outcomes by facilitating initial risk stratification and remote consults with experts, thereby reducing admissions and readmissions, and making patient care more effective. Additionally, this technology can address the lack of specialists in underserved areas, and ease accessibility for aging populations.

INTRODUCTION

Effective communication and coordination among medical doctors, specialists and other caregivers could mean the difference between life and death for patients. This chapter presents a discussion on the implications of the current pitfalls in health care coordination with a review of key technological attempts to address them and introduces a new technology paradigm to resolve their shortcomings. Medical diagnostic technologies have made advances in recent years ranging from consumer devices and smartphone monitoring apps to artificial intelligence and more accurate imaging systems for hospitals. However, the availability of specialists to wade through all this data, interpret the results, and translate all of this information into actionable patient treatment plans has not increased. As fewer doctors specialize and

DOI: 10.4018/978-1-7998-0047-7.ch014

as populations age, more patients need to travel more often and over longer distances to see already overloaded and overworked specialists. Furthermore, health literacy declines with age, and decision-making processes change (Finucane et al., 2002; Kutner et al., 2006).

Tools to communicate effectively across settings and providers are lacking, as health care systems around the world are fragmented, with many providers, settings, and clinical and nonclinical staff involved with each patient's episode of illness. Fragmentation on its own may not be harmful, if clinical information is communicated across settings and providers. However, there is significant evidence that communication across providers and settings is poor (Bodenheimer, 2008). Important instructions are often not received before patients have their first visit with the care provider. For example, one study found that two-thirds of physicians treated a patient for the first time after being discharged from the hospital but before the physician received the hospital's discharge summary (Kripalani et al., 2007).

Similar incompleteness was found in transfers between primary and specialty physicians and between community physicians and hospital-based physicians (Forrest et al., 2000; Gandhi et al., 2000; Schoen et al., 2005). Even providers with robust information technology systems are often unable to use them to communicate easily with other providers because their systems are not interoperable (Elhauge, 2010). Communication between primary care physicians (PCPs) and specialists regarding patient referrals and consultations is required in order to improve patient outcomes. Communication inter-specialty is increasingly important because increasing medical sub-specialization and technological advances further split care across numerous physicians in a variety of settings. Yet, inter-specialty communication occurs inconsistently (O'Malley et al., 2011). Lack of effective clinical coordination leads to poor quality of care and inefficiency and is a health policy priority. As patients experience transitions in care, there is an even more acute need to share information between care providers in an accurate and timely manner (Health Quality Ontario 2013). Research has found that the tools that contribute most to clinical coordination are those that allow doctors to exchange information and communicate (Aller et al., 2017).

Patients who suffer from chronic disease often have multiple concurrent chronic conditions and complications that require regular visits with a number of different specialists in addition to their primary care physician (PCP). They also may have intermittent interactions with emergency rooms and other care settings. This puts them at increased risk for severe adverse events if information does not flow between health care settings in timely and accurate ways.

Aging populations add another level of medical complexity as patients are taken in charge by a continuously increasing number of different care specialties. The resulting quantity and variety of information generated are exploding. Distribution of consolidated patient information between departments is therefore a critical point and sets a new challenge for information systems. We can expect that better information in terms of quality and quantity will provide new perspectives: it will ultimately improve the outcome for the patient, and it will foster a collegial approach among clinicians (Bandon et al., 2005).

Telemedicine offers promise to improve care for aging populations, chronic patients and remote regions. Using internet technology, specialty medical outsourcing where a licensed doctor performs an existing medical practice over a distance using technology is gaining traction. Around the world, specialists are now increasingly available to interpret diagnostic images for even the smallest hospitals on a fee-per-study basis - skills that they would not be able to recruit or otherwise afford. The impact can be enormous, as telemedicine becomes a multibillion-dollar industry worldwide.

In the November 2017 Report on EU State of Play on Telemedicine Services and Uptake Recommendations, the Joint Action Group found "countries are using telemedicine, mainly with local or regional scope, comprising interactions provider-to-patient and provider-to-provider and linking the different levels of care, although mainly between primary and hospital care. Several pairs of type of service and specialty are being provided, but the wider activity is in radiology tele-diagnosis, radiology teleconsultation, cardiology tele-monitoring, cardiology teleconsultation, ... For the majority of countries telemedicine services are below 10% of total healthcare services" (Carrasqueiro et al., 2017, p. 8).

With low telemedicine penetration, a lot is at risk. According to the OECD, EU and WHO: In the European Region, health workforce imbalances and shortages are a major concern and they are concerned that their healthcare systems will remain stable and sufficient to cover the needs of ageing populations. On top of that, consistent with the findings of the Centers for Disease Control in the USA, they recognize that heart diseases are a leading cause of hospitalization and death in Europe and that cardiovascular diseases accounting for 40% of all deaths across EU constituting the main cause of mortality (European Commission, 2012; OECD/EU, 2018; WHO, 2016; euro.who.int, 2019). The solution they propose is Integrated Care (WHO, 2016): "eHealth systems and services with strong user involvement, focusing on inter-operability and the integration of emerging patient-centric technologies for cost-effective healthcare." (WHO, 2016, p. 4)

Despite modern advances in medicine and diagnostic technologies available to doctors, there are still many worrying statistics about the state of affairs in medical care. According to the Centers for Disease Control, there is a growing shortage of specialists, and access to specialists is limited as more than 118 million Americans do not live in cities (US Census Bureau, March, 2015). The use of telemedicine in the USA has seen spectacular growth with encouragement from federal and state governments as well as health insurers due to the value it brings to patients and society. Europe is not far behind in recognizing these benefits and encouraging use.

The EU eHealth Stakeholder Group on the Widespread Deployment of Telemedicine Service in Europe reports "key drivers have already been identified: 1) relative rise in patients with (multiple) chronic conditions; 2) increasing size of the elderly population, combined with a relative decrease in the resources paid by fewer taxpayers (healthcare expenditures growing faster than economies); and, 3) decreasing work force of health care professionals in European Member States" (EU eHealth Stakeholder Group, 2014, p. 4).

Like the USA, Europe is experiencing a resulting uptake of radiology outsource services from companies like TeleConsult Europe, TBS Group, and TELUS International whose businesses are growing. As the founder of TeleConsult Europe, Erik de Grijs says, "If your on-site radiologist is there for the necessary on-site work, you can use them almost 100%, but the other work you can have done remotely and basically pay per study." He says further, "We have sub-specialty radiologists on our team. You can have neuro, thorax, or musculoskeletal radiologists who we make available for even the smallest hospitals. Clients can therefore get radiologists with specialist knowledge that they wouldn't be able to recruit of afford otherwise" (Practical-patient-care.com, 2019). The new paradigm for expert care coordination technology at point of care presented in this chapter addresses the shortcomings outlined above and improves the penetration and uptake of telemedicine services as well.

BACKGROUND

The growth of computer and internet technologies has been tapped by medical caregivers who continually seek to improve the exchange of clinical information across care levels. Health care providers have deployed information systems that facilitate rapid resolution of queries, increase the response capacity of PC doctors, speed up access to secondary care, and ultimately speed up diagnosis and treatment.

EMR and PACS Technology Solutions

The EMR/EHR (electronic medical record/electronic health record) system constitutes the main route by which primary care doctors consult with certain specialists, who decide which cases can be resolved by virtual means and which ones require the patient's physical presence; and secondly, via email, which is used more sporadically. However, EMRs are mostly institution-specific and are designed for information management rather than interpretation and diagnosis. Recent research highlights difficulties with the use of shared EMRs, which points toward the need to improve EMR functionality to facilitate orderly data entry as well as to promote doctors' information technology skills (Morton et al., 2015), but also reveals some professionals' limited awareness of the concept that the EMR is a tool for collective use rather than a personal tool (Callen et al., 2013).

The primary personal tool used by specialists to access, review and interpret diagnostic imaging studies is the PACS (picture archiving and communication system). Availability of access to the same PACS across an institution and even more so from outside the institution is severely limited by function specific workflows and their associated technical challenges. Medical institutions who can invest in strong IT capabilities make sure to integrate their various PACS systems with their EMR system. Every physician, nurse practitioner, physician assistant, nurse and imaging technologist in a health organization needs to review and manipulate images, image metadata, and associated imaging reports through the EMR as part of routine activities. The wide spectrum of clinical specialties mean there are widely varied needs for diagnostic image interpretation, and for clinical image and video image consumption. There is a similarly wide spectrum of images and video that must be accessed, reviewed, and manipulated. This spectrum includes DICOM (digital imaging and communications in medicine) diagnostic images common to cardiology, obstetrics, radiology, and other specialties. Additionally, health organizations frequently make some forms of scanned paper documentation available throughout the EMR via image viewers. To meet the enterprise viewing needs of many clinical users to review many content types within an organization, enterprises are looking to a single multi-purpose application: an enterprise image viewer (Roth et al., 2016). A traditional full version PACS typically includes local storage of images, tailored to specialty specific diagnostic tools with a higher degree of operational specialty workflow support, but more limited features for viewing from within the EMR context.

Even within a single specialty, the current state of the art involves a variety of systems that doctors need to access to order diagnostic tests for patients, track the status, review and interpret results, clarify treatment options and suggestions, and communicate with the patient. PACS systems are isolated islands of data that often do not communicate with each other, and they each present data differently, appropriate to each specialty's workflow (MicroMarket Monitor, 2015). Specialists, such as cardiologists, often access several separate systems daily to do their work, with no ability to engage directly with patients. Access from outside the health network often does not exist. The current situation leads to wasted time by specialist physicians who can otherwise focus on their patients. See Figure 1.

Figure 1. Current market state of the art

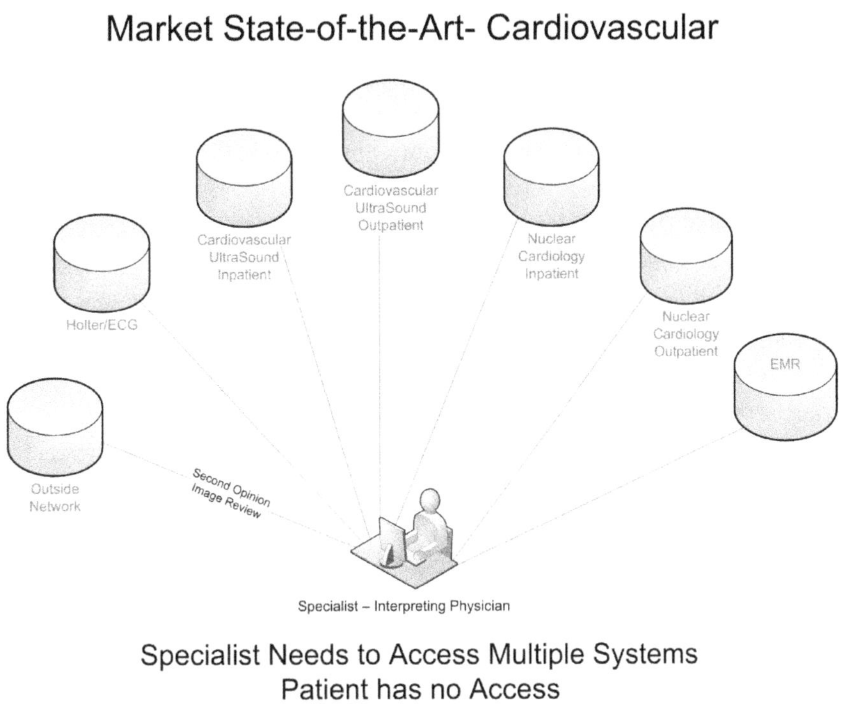

In larger health care institutions, it is increasingly obvious that separate image archives for every department are not cost effective or scalable. The solution is to have each department's PACS assigned only to a local cache, and archive to an enterprise archive that drives a universal clinical viewer. It sounds simple, but unfortunately not many PACS can truly work with third-party Integration of the Health Care Enterprise Compliant Image Archive (Langer, 2009).

PACS have been in existence for several years and have become an integral part of the infrastructure of radiology and imaging departments across the world. However, although the core technology continues to evolve and improve, key practical issues involved in the implementation of a PACS, with associated maintenance, troubleshooting, training, and integration issues still remain and, if anything, continue to increase in complexity as dependence on PACS grows. To make matters more complex, the closely associated field of teleradiology involves seamlessly integrating a varied PACS across locations, as well as across continents (Kalyanpur et al., 2010).

Since the adoption of PACS in the late nineties and early 2000s, imaging exams have been stored digitally, and film has effectively been eliminated. There is a misconception that the shift to digital imaging helped medical image exchange eliminate any potential image loss that was happening with printed image films. Unfortunately, this is not the case: despite the most recent advances in digital imaging, most hospitals still keep losing their imaging data, with these losses going completely unnoticed. As a result, not only does image loss affect the faith in digital imaging but it also affects patient diagnosis and daily quality of clinical work (Oglevee et al., 2014).

Furthermore, when patients travel from provider to provider, healthcare is still wrestling with image availability at the point of care. Patients receive digital copies of their imaging studies on CDs with the risk that this fragile media could be damaged and become unreadable. CDs also can be easily misplaced or lost by the patient, and some patients simply forget to bring their CDs to the appointment. Each CD burner manufacturer created their own approach to storing the images, reports, and image viewer on the CD—no two are exactly alike. At the receiving end, the images are sometimes viewed using the viewer on the CD, but more commonly copied from the CD, updated with local patient and order information, and loaded into the local PACS. This requires a significant manual effort in order to get the outside images into the radiologists' familiar local environment and tools.

If the CD was bad or damaged in some way, it may not be not possible to view or retrieve all images. And rarely are the reports available with the images. Despite significant progress, image-sharing practices need to be modernized to take advantage of the electronic exchange of images with related reports.

Electronic exchange provides opportunities for improved operational workflows that can positively impact patient care, reduce cost, improve patient and clinician satisfaction, and can even increase revenue opportunities in key service lines. CD-based image exchange has laid an important foundation to support the emerging next generation of interoperable, standards-based image exchange (Vreeland et al. 2016).

NEW PARADIGM: SOCIAL NETWORKING TECHNOLOGY

Social networking may be the answer. It is a proven communication and coordination model that we applied to facilitate outpatient-imaging interpretation and expert consults both in-house as well as outsourced. Social networking can be implemented via a web-based interface portal to link doctors, diagnostic imaging techs, experts and patients for remote diagnosis; and to speed access to images, data, and history; which ultimately cuts the time to the correct treatment plan.

Social networking technologies are tools that allow users to create connections, communicate, and share interests online (Gunawardena et al., 2009) and are being used in medicine in a variety of ways. A systematic review found that technology-based interventions for people living with HIV show promise for encouraging medication adherence, sexual risk reduction, decreased drug use, increase health literacy, and improvements in depressive symptoms (Noar & Willoughby, 2012). Recruiting children for research provides another example of how the use of social networking may improve access to difficult-to-reach pediatric research participants (Close et al., 2013).

The social networking communication and information sharing medium has the power to revolutionize the way physicians interact with their patients and fellow health care workers. When managed correctly, it can provide a great way for doctors to communicate and educate others. For example, a surgeon used Twitter during a robotically assisted partial nephrectomy to let other surgeons know that a total nephrectomy was not necessary, despite the large tumor size (Prasana et al., 2011).

A social networking solution can facilitate single point access to images, data and patient history with secure messaging and reporting so that doctors and caregivers can communicate effectively and access the information they need to make informed decisions about patients.

The Secure Portal

A patient portal that creates a secure social network of primary care physicians with their patients and with specialty interpreting physicians is a clinical tool that can uniquely improve treatment outcomes and maximize incentive bonuses in a capitated payment environment. A software system that allows a primary care physician to: order diagnostic studies (i.e., echocardiograms, vascular studies, nuclear stress tests, etc.); review results with the interpreting physician (i.e., cardiologist, radiologist, etc.); get detailed explanations about the patient's specific condition and the recommended treatment plan; access an information library with details about the patient's specific condition; and, be able to share this information directly with the patient. This allows a primary care physician to retain interaction with the patient and only incur a specialty consult with a specialist when they jointly determine the need together. This empowers patients to take a more active role in determining their treatment plans and saves the health network money.

The new technology paradigm uses social networking concepts, an implementation of which is called the Diagnostic Modality Interface Portal1™. This interface layer and portal technology model could help care providers improve patient outcomes by facilitating initial risk stratification and remote consults with experts, thereby reducing admissions and readmissions. This is a pioneering digital health technology model that utilizes concepts from social networking to make treatment recommendations timelier and to make patient care more effective. Additionally, an interface portal addresses the lack of specialists in underserved areas, and ease accessibility for ageing populations.

Specialists and other caregivers are dedicated professionals who will manage to get their jobs done no matter what. When there is a need to confer on difficult diagnostic image interpretations and no formal tool is available, they will resort to using whatever technologies are available, including non-secure smartphone apps. The author has heard from several practicing cardiologists in the USA, Europe and Israel that getting information from the source to an interpreting physician even within the same medical or hospital network is often such a challenge under their professional time constraints that they resort to sending medical images to each other via WhatsApp in order to confer on difficult interpretations. Instead, a secure portal application would facilitate consults and provide tracking and reporting of the various opinions that can be integrated into the EMR for access by all the patient's caregivers.

Implementation of the Social Networking Model

The technology paradigm presented in this chapter proposes facilitating integrated care for patients using a social networking model. This has been implemented as a pioneering Diagnostic Modality Interface Portal that facilitates single point access to images, data and patient history with doctor messaging so that telemedicine services will accelerate faster. The implementation is a web accessible outpatient interpretation and reporting layer that interfaces with PACS systems for messaging and reporting. This technology links doctors, diagnostic devices, imaging technicians, and patients for remote diagnosis and to reach consensus on the best treatment plan. The portal also provides infrastructure for data from patient monitoring devices and smartphone apps, as well as future tools such as Artificial Intelligence Image Analysis.

The Diagnostic Modality Interface Portal creates a single access layer to all diagnostic and history event information and facilitates a platform for remote interpretation and reporting for cardiologists, radiologists, and other interpreting physicians via a single online log in. Using an interface layer, diagnostic tests can be administered locally by a sonographer or nuclear technologist, and then be interpreted by a specialist who may be sitting at a remote clinic or who may be working at home. A pre-screening evaluation can determine if the patient needs to travel for a physical exam or procedure, and thus reduces patient referrals and hospital admissions. See Figure 2.

Figure 2. Diagnostic modality interface portal to achieve care coordination vision

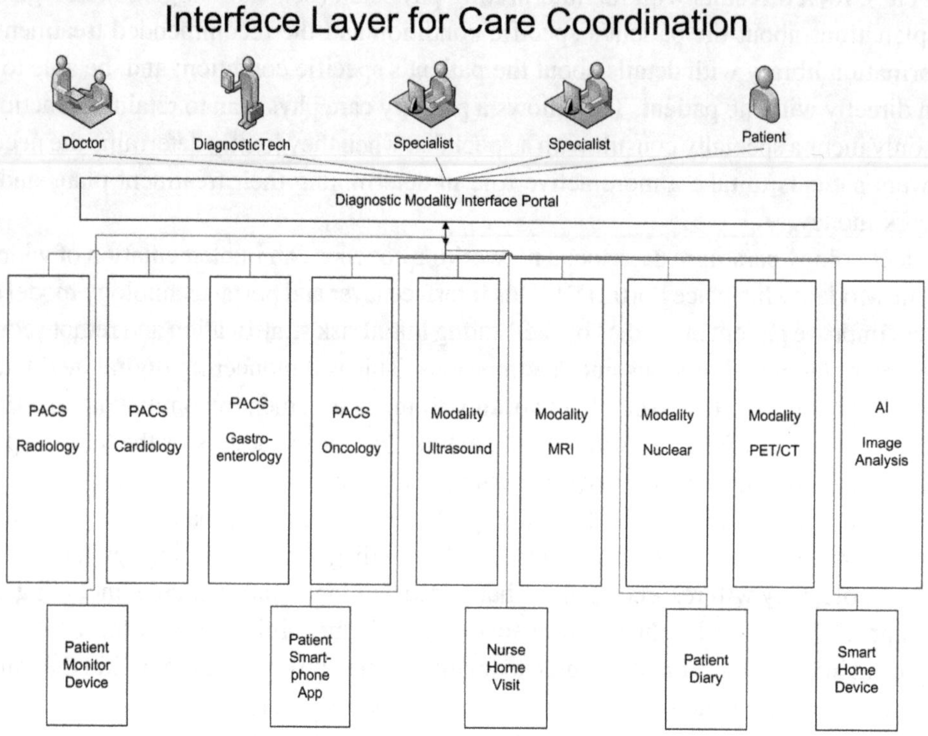

The implementation is complete with an algorithm that enables data visualization of patient events and diagnostic tests and images in a timeline, and with private messaging between the doctors, and diagnostic techs about each study. This algorithm improves the doctor-expert workflow by merging social networking concepts with legacy web-based medical diagnostic models. Caregiver coordination functionality facilitates joint decision-making, while patient access empowers them to seek specialty consultation and expert advice.

Online shared access to critical data is secured by pre-authorized user restrictions and permissions. As the rise in outsource telemedicine providers around the world attests, patient data and image sharing across medical institutions can be accomplished when there is a strong enough motivator for regulatory bodies to allow it. Using industry standard DICOM file exports from all modalities such as electrocardiogram (ECG/EKG), echocardiogram (ECHO), ultrasound, CT scan (CT), PET scan (PET), MRI, and nuclear imaging, it is possible to interface directly to the diagnostic machine or to the PACS for the diagnostic data, and to the EMR system to import daily worklists and export reports with interpretation results.

The modality interface layer also has the capability to accept data from Holter monitors, mobile telemetry apps, home patient follow-up visit reports for monitoring and evaluation, and pre-operative risk assessment that the doctors, nurses, and technicians can upload to the system directly by themselves, and into the patient folder. The portal also provides infrastructure for data from patient monitoring devices, and smartphone apps as well as future tools such as Artificial Intelligence Image Analysis.

In the Diagnostic Modality Interface Portal implementation of the social networking model, the portal automatically converts files (e.g. images, clips, and data from DICOM or other modality specific formats) into jpeg, mp4, and PDF formats as appropriate, so they can be easily and quickly accessed by doctors from any computer without installation of any special client software like a DICOM reader or modality specific application software.

Access at Point of Care

The new social networking model presented in this chapter consolidates data, measurements, history, and images thus enabling secure sharing among caregivers and patients at any point of care no matter how remote. In an area that lacks a local specialist, this solution extends specialty care to underserved populations where a mobile diagnostic tech can perform an exam. In an area where specialists are available, this solution expedites second and third opinions.

Single point access to images and patient history and doctor messaging sounds like it would be a software application that is already in use by every doctor in every serious medical facility. However, it is not in use, nor is it trivial to achieve.

The new paradigm is unique in that it provides a single layer that interfaces to the PACS and/or to all diagnostic modalities together with a patient portal. Besides providing access, the implementation of this model provides a private messaging platform for secure communication among doctors, experts, technicians and patients. Its reporting, scheduling and tracking capabilities, and standards-based connectivity to PACS, EMR, and any diagnostic device in hospital as well as patient managed apps and devices, lets users bypass layers of legacy systems. Table 1 shows the main advantages of the new social networking paradigm implemented as a Diagnostic Modality Interface Portal compared with the limitations of the current state of the art.

Why Now

The widespread adoption of smartphones and social networking applications has created an environment where geographic distance is no longer viewed as a handicap that must be tolerated. In addition, as diagnostic devices become more and more prevalent, to meet growing demand for diagnostic tests, there is more formalization of roles, training and certification requirements of sonographers and other diagnostic imaging technicians that varies by country.

Table 1. Advantages of the diagnostic modality interface portal implementation

Diagnostic Modality Interface Portal	Pitfall that it Addresses	What it Provides
Social Networking Model with a Patient Event Timeline	Communication Access Population Coverage	Improves care coordination among doctors and other experts to cut decision time and drives engagement with patients via access to history and recommendations at point of care
Customizable Structured Reporting	Workflow	Speeds the workflow for the Interpreting Physician
Single Access Point for data and images	Interoperability	Physicians have access at office or home to review studies
Patient Portal	Patient Engagement	Encourage consults and access in emergencies
Private Messaging platform among caregivers that patients cannot access	Coordination	Secure communication by and between doctors, specialists, and technicians for clarifications

The growing availability of outsource specialists encourages patients to demand specialty and sub-specialty expertise from their medical providers, which will put more pressure on the systemic workflow problems. In the USA, the Bureau of Labor Statistics expects that job growth from 2016-2026 for diagnostic medical sonographers and cardiovascular technologists and technicians is 17% (U.S. Department of Labor, 2018).

In an article published by Healthcare in Europe.com, Angelo La Leggia, a clinical scientist, specialized in Echocardiography explains "The use of sonographers has potential in promoting screening programs within the medical specialties, reduce waiting lists for patients to have access to an ultrasound service, reduce the number of more advanced and expensive imaging modalities (reducing patient's radiation exposure) and reduce hospital lengths of stay and related costs. Employing sonographers would enable doctors to dedicate and commit more time towards the patients' care thus optimizing the competences of different healthcare professionals and share responsibilities" (D'Abate & La Leggia, 2017). Similarly, the European Association of Nuclear Medicine has published clear guidelines for requisite "Competencies for the European Nuclear Medicine Technologist." They contend that defining the tasks that may be performed, may also contribute to the standardization and quality assurance of nuclear medicine practice in Europe (EANM Technologists Committee, 2018).

A Model that Keeps the Patient in Center Focus

The social networking model uniquely fills the void of the capabilities that are lacking in the current state of the art by consolidating information data, measurement, history, and images; and facilitating sharing of that information among caregivers and patients at the point of care as well as remotely. The social networking model places the patient squarely in control of their condition history with access to medical summaries and PDF reports, and their individual timeline of medical events. The model enables a cross platform application designed for speed and high volume that can be accessed by any web capable device and gives interpreting physicians needed access to study images to independently verify measurements. This also facilitates expert consults with patients' interpreting physicians.

Simplifies the Workflow Despite Many Moving Parts

Figure 3 shows the streamlined basic workflow enabled by the interface layer.

The simplified workflow supported by the Diagnostic Modality Interface Portal implementation of the social networking model, keeps all caregivers connected on the current issue for which the patient presented. Together with the patient's medical history, and integration of ongoing data from devices and nurse visits, interpreting physicians can see the entire picture about the patient and recommend the most appropriate treatment accordingly. Additionally, with this technology, doctors can improve their productivity and see more patients.

Patient Access

The patient portal functionality is intended to make sure that patients have access to their history and reports so that they can seek other expert advice as well as never be caught short in an emergency. The level of information that the patient can upload by themselves or access by themselves can be limited by their primary care provider or other entity that manages their data. As far as the patient's caregivers

Figure 3. Simplified workflow

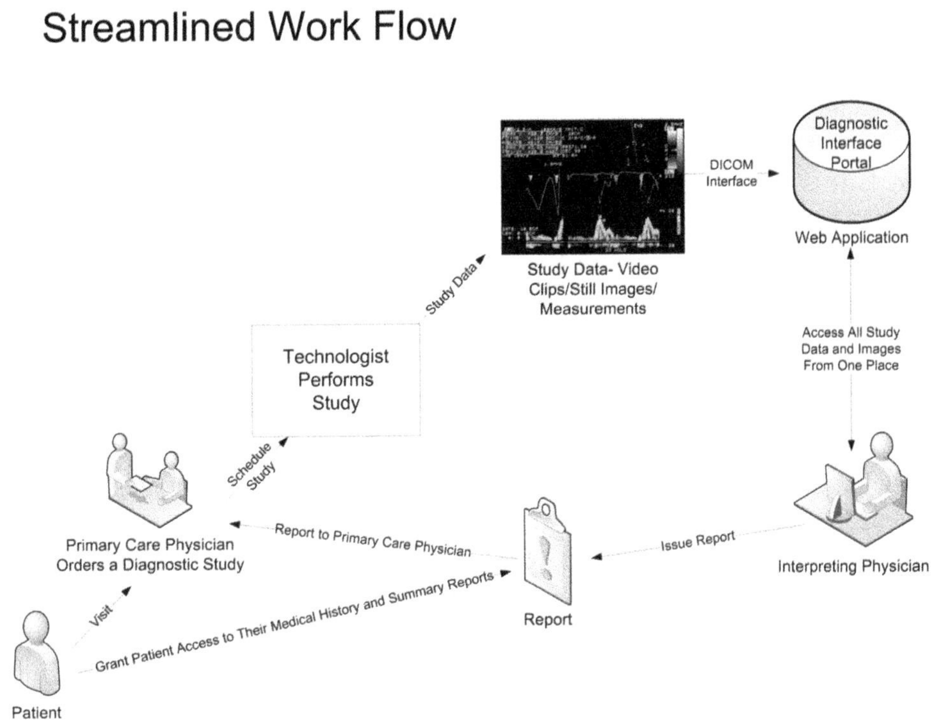

are concerned, questions and answers between the doctors and specialists can remain private and not available to the patient. In cases where a primary care physician is advised to have a psychologist present when presenting an interpreting physician's or other expert's findings and opinions, they can limit access by the patient so that they cannot access these reports and opinions until after the primary care physician discusses them directly with the patient.

In addition, with the right permission settings, an interface portal can potentially fill the role of a UHR (universal health record), as it is patient-centered, and the information available to patients also can be fully controlled by them. Similarly, as the portal interfaces to diagnostic modalities like ultrasound, nuclear imaging, and PACS systems; technically the portal can just as effectively interface with other portals of the patient's various health care providers. If there is an operational or regulatory mandate available that allows the sharing of PHI (private health information) by and between healthcare organizations– as per a patient's permission and instruction – then all of the patient's data and history can be available through one log-in on the portal.

This could eliminate the major shortcoming of most patient portals today, namely, access to data across multiple organizations and institutions. With an interface portal implementation, patients and caregivers will no longer have a fragmented view of individual patient data.

Similarly, the interface portal model can also facilitate a patient's PHR (personal health record), by allowing the patient to maintain all of their care information as well as upload data from personal monitoring devices, health smartphone apps, and smart home devices like medical toilets, and daily diaries of their wellbeing.

PHRs can be set with certain thresholds so that if any of the patient generated data or home device generated data exceeds a certain pre-defined threshold, the patient's primary care physicians can be automatically notified. This would make it easier for caregivers to maintain continuous communication with patients, not just episodic, and to track chronic conditions and illnesses and post-discharge follow-up so that they could enact early interventions.

Raising the Bar

Technology takes time to be deployed in hospitals and healthcare networks, and introducing a new technology will require clearly defined and demonstrable added value. An interface portal offers such added value. PACS system vendors continually expand the features and use cases of their systems, but their software applications were built to meet the needs of specific specialties and departments, and as such they are restricted by their current architectures. By design, the interface portal model introduces a new single interface layer that sits atop of and connects all PACS, EMR, and native diagnostic modalities for requisite access and sharing.

Organizing patient information around a single access point enables specialists to remain focused on analyzing the data and translating it into an appropriate plan of care. This is a vast improvement over current inefficiencies whereby doctors log in to multiple systems to interpret various test results, which could lead to frustration and possible distraction from their primary focus on the patient's plan of care. This is an excellent opportunity to dramatically improve not only the method of work, but the diagnosis itself, which can rely on a whole set of findings, analyses and perspectives to interpret the information and diagnose the problem. Driving a core strategy to become the leading care coordination technology for all medical specialties, this model can achieve an ambitious vision of becoming the social network for medicine.

Pros and Cons of the Portal Model

The pros can be summarized as follows:

1. Doctors and Specialists can consult with colleagues internal to their institutions as well as provide consults on an outsource basis to colleagues outside their institution and access patient data and image files from any web capable device. This will improve workflow and quality of interpretations.
2. Diagnostic Imaging Technologists can automate data entry and image upload to multiple systems used by their client doctors. They can enter patient demographic information and study measurements only once and have access to structured reports as consulting doctors may require as well as provide timely quality assurance review. With the Diagnostic Modality Interface Portal, technologists can do away with handing CDs to patients.
3. Hospitals can easily expand the specialties and subspecialties they offer to patients via outsourcing on a pay-per-use basis, conduct more pre-operative assessments, and reduce admissions and referrals.
4. Patients can access their medical history and reports. They will never be stranded in an emergency, and they can obtain other expert consults.

The cons can be summarized as follows:

1. Deploying an interface portal will involve integration with existing systems for a healthcare provider. From their perspective, this translates into scheduling and allocation of resources and commensurate management decisions involved.
2. The factors involved in determining the return on investment (ROI) need to be identified and the ROI needs to be calculated.
3. There needs to be a champion within the healthcare provider to push for initial use of an interface portal. In each hospital or healthcare network, this may be a different specialist or department depending on the individual hospital's needs.

CASE STUDIES

The social networking model serves all medical specialties and remote medical act services using telemedicine systems. For illustrative purposes, three use cases are presented to help illustrate the applicability of the steps required to accomplish all of the functionality of this model.

Outpatient Scenario

A 57-year-old female presents to her primary care physician with complaints of shortness of breath, lower extremity swelling and decreased exercise tolerance. She denies any chest discomfort but does attest to 3 pillow orthopnea and paroxysmal nocturnal dyspnea worsening over the last 6 weeks. The primary care physician appropriately suggests an immediate cardiac consultation. However, the nearest cardiology practice is approximately 90 minutes' drive away and the next available appointment is in 4 weeks.

Patient Care Decision Point: What would be the most efficient way to do an echocardiogram (ECHO) to evaluate the heart murmur? Is there a way to arrange for a cardiology consultation sooner than waiting four weeks?

With the new model presented in this chapter, the following would occur: Diagnostic cardiac echo test (ECHO) would be performed by a sonographer at the primary care physician's office with local or mobile ultrasound imaging equipment, and a cardiologist specialist would interpret the results remotely. The interpreting cardiologist will have access to the patient's relevant medical history for comparison. Additionally, questions and answers with the primary care physician would clarify what to discuss with the patient. This would allow for risk stratification of the cardiac patient without requiring her to travel and without the delay required to see a traditional cardiologist or visit to an emergency room.

Inpatient Scenario: Emergency Consult

A 45-year-old male presents to the emergency room with complaints of substernal chest pain and shortness of breath. His symptoms started about 15 minutes prior to arrival in the emergency department. He rates the pain an 8 out of 10 on a scale of 1 to 10. He states that the pain radiates to his jaw and left arm. There is associated nausea and diaphoresis. After initial triage was performed a 12-lead EKG was obtained. The emergency room physician on call reviewed the electrocardiogram and was uncertain regarding the implications. There was no cardiologist on call available for further consultation.

Decision point: Is it appropriate to administer TPA to this patient? Should he be transferred to a tertiary center for primary PCI? What is appropriate management at this time?

At this time, consultation with the cardiologist able to review the EKG and decide regarding acute management of this patient's chest discomfort would seem to be the most appropriate and desirable situation. If an interface portal would be available, the following would/could occur:

The emergency room staff would contact the telemedicine service and the interpreting physician on call would immediately be in touch with the emergency room doctor. A video consultation would be set up with the assistance of the nursing staff or via smartphone or computer app. After obtaining a history by interviewing the patient via video conferencing, examining the patient via video conferencing and reviewing the EKG data, the cardiologist would dictate a full consultation and the emergency room physician and staff would have access to the consultation. An appropriate decision regarding the patient's care would be made. On the remote end, the interpreting physician on-call, would log into the interface portal. A full consultation followed by a verbal sign out would not be necessary. The full consultation report would be generated by the interpreting physician on the portal. The hospital would subsequently, by direct electronic data interface (EDI), enter the report into their EMR system.

Women's Health Organization: Fetal Echocardiogram

A Women's Health Organization that provides counseling, referrals and support, to all those seeking professional help in overcoming difficulties starting a family is finding this social networking model to be a good fit for the needs of their patients. This organization's discreet and caring counselors possess a unique synthesis of pastoral wisdom and specialized training in modern reproductive medicine. Professional supervisors on their staff certify the genetic integrity of fertility treatments worldwide. In the course of its work consulting and advising on critical issues that may arise during pregnancy, this organization refers patients for potential multiple medical and religious/conscience consults on fetal echocardiograms and general fetal ultrasounds and other medical diagnostic studies. The organization needs an easily accessible way to consolidate patient diagnostic information with images and expert opinions so that they can facilitate consults quickly when emergencies arise.

Interface portal technology is a good fit for this women's health organization to meet its specialized needs by:

1. Introducing information sharing technology that will speed up the time it takes couples to get results from their diagnostic imaging tests and identify the correct treatment plan within the guidelines of the patient's religious or spiritual background.
2. Greatly shortening the time to reach a decision on a pregnancy and recommendations for abortion or alternate courses of treatment.
3. Enabling access to a wider pool of experts who may be medical and spiritual or religious as per the patient's life choices.
4. Improving the quality of the decisions via faster and more-timely sharing of information among the experts on difficult pregnancies.

Figure 4 presents a high-level view of the fetal echocardiogram use case within the general streamlined workflow that is facilitated by the Diagnostic Modality Interface Portal.

Figure 4. Fetal echocardiogram use case

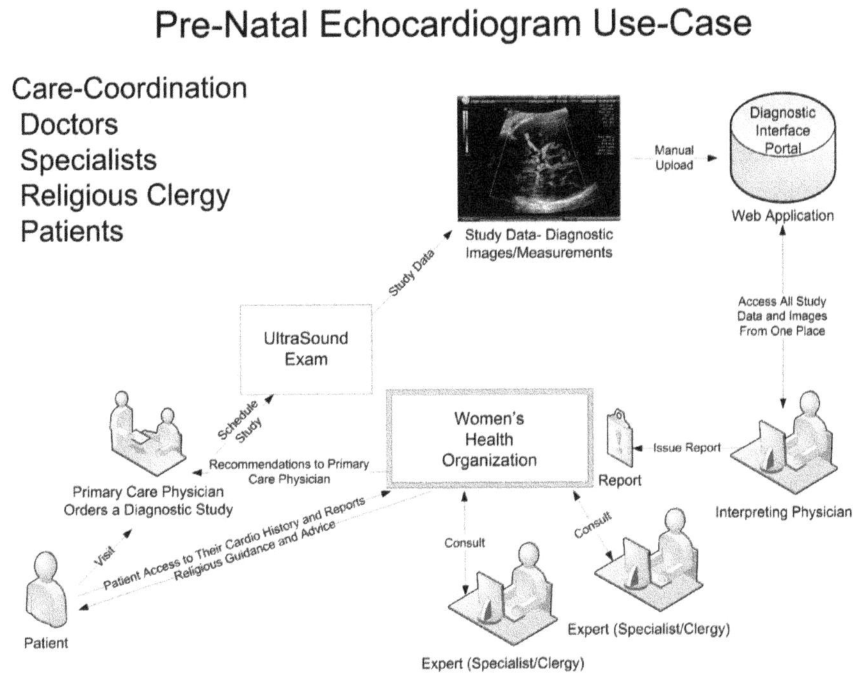

DEPLOYMENT CONFIGURATIONS

An interface portal can be deployed either as an in-house software application or on the public cloud as a secure and scalable software as a service (SaaS) application. It can be accessed by any web device with a standard login that can support multi-factor authentication. All areas of medicine that require expert care coordination are supported, so the user base can grow fast. Key to portal implementation is that it provides a web accessible software platform for all medical clinicians to interpret medical diagnostic studies with structured reporting and empower patients to seek other expert opinions. Patient history can include data and images from all diagnostic modalities such as clinical data, diagnostic imaging studies such as echocardiograms, electrocardiograms, CT scans, PET scans, MRI, ultrasound, nuclear imaging testing, Holter monitors, mobile telemetry applications, home patient follow-up visits for monitoring and evaluation, and pre-operative risk assessment.

Early Adopters

The recent expanding availability of telemedicine services indicates that there is a business case for specialists, doctors, payers, hospital networks and patients. Building a platform for remote interpretation and reporting that follows the interface portal model outlined in this chapter has potential for immediate use in the USA and elsewhere. Initial users of this type of an interface portal could be doctors in under-served areas, at regional medical centers, and primary care medical practices; and in diagnostic imaging services. Using this new model, diagnostic tests such as Nuclear Stress, Echocardiograms, EKGs, and general ultrasound can be administered locally by a sonographer or nuclear imaging tech. The data and images will be reviewed and interpreted remotely by a specialist sitting elsewhere. The remote specialist will do an initial evaluation of the patient and determine if the patient needs to travel for a physical exam with a specialist or for a procedure. This pre-screening decreases unnecessary, costly patient referrals and reduces hospital admissions.

In addition, other users of this type of interface portal would be specialists who consult with colleagues. In conversations that the author has had with doctors in Colorado, New York, Zurich, Copenhagen and Israel, they said that technology that implements this model will enable them to stop using WhatsApp to share images and consult with each other. They recognize the Diagnostic Modality Interface Portal as an information sharing consult and reporting solution that they and their colleagues can use to communicate with each other on difficult interpretations across their hospital departments and institutions. They stated that they recognize its added value as an add-on interface layer to their existing PACS systems, interfacing with DICOM and HL7 industry standards. Beyond hospital departments for in-house coordination among specialties and specialists, the user base can quickly expand to outsource consult providers and diagnostic imaging services.

COMMERCIAL OPPORTUNITY

In the USA, the general rule is that a doctor can provide medical care to a patient remotely as long as the physician is licensed in the state where the patient presents him/herself for treatment. Some states go so far as to allow telemedicine services by a physician who is not even licensed their state as long as he or she is licensed in another state.

Reimbursement rates for services rendered by telemedicine may involve some differences from "physically in-person" for certain services, but on the whole, they are same. In fact, Medicare does not make a distinction in their reimbursement rates. According to the American Telemedicine Association (ATA) "Many "telehealth" services, such as remote radiology, pathology and some cardiology, are covered simply as "physician services." For traditional fee-for-service beneficiaries living in rural areas, Medicare covers physician services using videoconferencing. The approximately 14 million beneficiaries in Medicare Advantage (managed care) plans have complete flexibility in using telehealth, if their provider offers the service. ATA is pushing the Centers for Medicare and Medicaid, and Congress to remove the arbitrary restrictions that limit telehealth coverage, so that all beneficiaries can get this great benefit. "

The compelling urgency for telemedicine is that specialists are in short supply, and a shortage of cardiologists is projected to get even worse. For example, as reported in the Journal of the American College of Cardiology (JACC), there are currently at least 4,000 too-few cardiologists to fill open private-practice and academic positions, and this shortfall is predicted to rise to 16,000 by 2050 (Cullen et al., 2016).

The good news is that using the right technology model like the Diagnostic Modality Interface Portal, interpreting physicians can provide specialty diagnostic services to a much wider catchment area and patient base. These services can be provided off-line for outpatient consults as well as in real-time for inpatient support and emergency room care. Examination data is collected from the patient by a technician using a diagnostic device like an ultrasound machine, and then uploaded to a server. An interpreting physician can then read the study and issue a report and recommendations some time later. He/she does not need to physically touch the patient. These services can be very profitable. Individual reimbursement rates vary by payer and by country. In the USA, the Centers for Medicare & Medicaid Services (CMS) generally set a baseline reference. CMS Reimbursement rates for imaging and diagnostic services are set by procedure and are composed of professional reimbursement as well as technical reimbursement.

Professional Component means the amount the physician gets paid for providing the diagnosis and putting his/her license and reputation on the line. Technical Component is the amount to cover the overhead needed to enable the physician to examine the patient and provide the diagnosis. This includes facilities, diagnostic equipment, nurses, technicians, etc. A single patient for a single cardio related event can have several studies ordered that are separate billable events. Expanding a specialist's patient base using a Diagnostic Modality Interface Portal would enable them to interpret more studies and issue billable and reimbursable diagnoses via the web.

Revenue Models

Following the popular revenue model for web based PACS offerings; a Diagnostic Modality Interface Portal can be priced fee-per-study on a software as a service (SaaS) basis. However, considering that interface portal technology also fits within a hospital or other medical institution, an on-premise license would be appropriate. As a result, there appear to be two basic revenue models for this application:

1. Software as a service for individual specialists and small specialty outsource groups- Fee per Study
2. Enterprise Software for hospital and/or regional medical groups- License Fee

With respect to on-premise licensing or enterprise license, base pricing of the portal could be a combination of how much the enterprise can earn by using a system such as this through billing procedures and how much they would save in having a specialist on staff as well as volume of studies. The author recommends that a detailed business case be developed.

TRANSLATING SPECIALIST CARE COORDINATION INTO FUNCTIONALITY

The social networking model improves patient care by connecting the principal people involved with the necessary and relevant information. It consolidates patient medical diagnostic tests, ongoing monitoring, and event data from multiple sources and then enabling a consolidated visualization in a timeline shared with patient and caregivers. The interface portal described herein, thus creates social networking interactions between patients and physicians (interpreting and ordering) and nurses and diagnostic technicians for communication; questions and answers; and information sharing about a patient's specific medical condition and history; as well as to trigger and facilitate a tele-consult. Using an interface portal, caregivers can read and interpret native diagnostic images, and encourage patients to securely access and update their medical histories when they experience health related events.

By presenting patient's medical history and visualizing test data and images as a timeline of events, this model creates a secure social network for medical care that patients can access and share with trusted experts and caregivers as they see fit. This allows and encourages patients to maintain a secure health diary by posting symptoms in their timelines like: "went to visit the emergency room, they told me x" and "I had difficulty walking up the hill today". This effectively establishes a patient portal combined with a clinical interpretation and reporting platform for physicians that not only allows access to their medical records but also enables patients to add to their personal medical record and share it with their medical caregivers who can respond to it. Use of a patient timeline to create an interoperable social network information exchange for medical diagnostic information empowers patients to take control of their health and keeps them engaged in the ongoing treatment of their conditions.

The interface portal can be built to support study interpretations in batch mode, scheduled as per interpreting physician's schedule. The portal can also enable remote guidance of diagnostic technologists by a consulting physician as well as interpretation for remote emergency support for medical services such as cardiology, pre-natal and general radiology.

Future Steps

An interface portal could be the base on which to deploy additional diagnostic care coordination features. Future integration of Artificial Intelligence (AI) image analysis capability into the portal will bring yet another high value tool to the interpreting specialists and further improve their accuracy and workflow. Ultimately, this type of technology is a solution to universal access, by enabling health networks to meet currently unmet needs for medical care due to cost, travel distance and wait time; reducing unnecessary use of expensive hospital care and stabilizing health workforce imbalances and shortages to cover aging populations.

Considering that the Health IT market was $134Bn worldwide in 2016 and will exceed $280Bn by 2021 as quoted by the US government Global Healthcare Technologies Team (2017), an expert care coordination platform that meets the needs of the market today and for the future is high value. For the sub-segments of PACS technology the UK, Germany and France form the biggest markets within Europe, presently valued at $4.4bn, $4.0bn and $3.3bn per annum respectively, and account for 46% of all European revenues see IPACSO Innovation Framework for CT Security PACS Market and Spending Trends Overview (Seldeslachts, 2019).

Each type of user: doctor, technician, patient and so forth has specific permissions for what they are able to access, view and download within each patient's study and event timeline, as well as what they can upload or create such as images, reports, or events. The author together with a team of other professionals has implemented this social networking model as the Diagnostic Modality Interface Portal.

CONCLUSION

Social networking technology has the potential to facilitate care coordination among medical specialists and improve patient care. An implementation of the social networking model for this purpose is the Diagnostic Modality Interface Portal. This interface portal presents patient medical events, diagnostic data and images for each of the involved care givers and the patient, and thereby creates social networking interaction between patients and physicians (interpreting and ordering) for communication, questions and answers, and information sharing about a patient's specific cardiac history. In addition, primary care physicians and patients alike can use the interface portal alike to trigger and facilitate a tele-consult with specialists.

For example, cardiovascular diseases (CVDs) are the number one cause of death worldwide. Improving patient outcomes and financial pressures have forced a shift from invasive and costly procedures to enhanced workflow and integrated approaches to diagnosing and treating heart disease using innovations in high-precision imaging technology. Clinicians have tools to improve patient care, and reduce healthcare costs, but these technologies are often slow and difficult to access when needed most.

Using an interface portal, patient diagnostic studies can be accessed seamlessly and accurately so that clinicians can conveniently read and interpret them locally or remotely, coordinate treatment with patients and other caregivers, and encourage patients to securely access their cardiac histories and update them when they experience events so that they can share information with care-givers when needed.

The interface portal merges social networking concepts with web based medical diagnostic access to allow interpreting physicians, specialists who may be located remotely to access all relevant medical material including patient history, data and images and have these data before their eyes in an integrative and systemic manner; while engaging patients with controlled but direct access. This improves joint decision-making by physicians and encourages patients to seek specialty consultation.

Additionally, the expert coordination functionality described in this chapter can accelerate the adoption of telemedicine services around the world, through the improvements it brings to specialist workflow together with the patient portal. This new social networking model uniquely enables access and sharing by and among those authorized users who need the information when they need it and where they need it. The author believes that by implementing this innovative model correctly, it can become the leading expert coordination technology for all medical specialties and that it can become a leading social network for medicine.

REFERENCES

Aller, M. B., Vargas, I., Coderch, J., & Vázquez, M. L. (2017). Doctors' opinion on the contribution of coordination mechanisms to improving clinical coordination between primary and outpatient secondary care in the Catalan national health system. *BMC Health Services Research*, *17*(1), 842. doi:10.1186/s12913-017-2690-5 PubMed

Andriole, K., Badano, A., Crawford, J., Chang, P., Flynn, M., Reiner, B., ... Seibert, J. (2004). AAPM/RSNA Tutorial on Equipment Selection: PACS Equipment Overview. *Radiographics*, *24*(1), 313–334. doi:10.1148/rg.241035137 PubMed

Bandon, D., Lovis, C., Geissbühler, A., & Vallée, J. P. (2005). Enterprise-wide PACS: Beyond Radiology, an Architecture to Manage All Medical Images. *Academic Radiology*, *12*(8), 1000–1009. doi:10.1016/j.acra.2005.03.075 PubMed

Bodenheimer, T. (2008). Coordinating care—A perilous journey through the health care system. *The New England Journal of Medicine*, *358*(10), 1064–1071. doi:10.1056/NEJMhpr0706165 PubMed

Bureau of Labor Statistics, U.S. Department of Labor. (2018). Occupational Outlook Handbook: Diagnostic Medical Sonographers and Cardiovascular Technologists and Technicians, Including Vascular Technologists. Retrieved from https://www.bls.gov/ooh/Healthcare/Diagnostic-medical-sonographers.htm

Callen, J., Paoloni, R., Li, J., Stewart, M., Gibson, K., Georgiou, A., ... Westbrook, J. (2013). Perceptions of the effect of information and communication technology on the quality of care delivered in emergency departments: A cross-site qualitative study. *Annals of Emergency Medicine*, *61*(2), 131–144. doi:10.1016/j.annemergmed.2012.08.032 PubMed

Carrasqueiro, S., Esteves, A., Marques, L., Martins, D., Pereira, C., & Ramalho, A. (2017). EU state of play on telemedicine services and uptake recommendations (Report No. D7.1.2). Retrieved from https://ec.europa.eu/health/sites/health/files/ehealth/docs/ev_20171128_co09_en.pdf

Close, S., Smaldone, A., Fennoy, I., Reame, N., & Grey, M. (2013). Using information technology and social networking for recruitment of research participants: Experience from an exploratory study of pediatric Klinefelter syndrome. *Journal of Medical Internet Research*, *15*(3), e48. doi:10.2196/jmir.2286 PubMed

Codari, M., Pesapane, F., & Sardanelli, F. (2018). Artificial intelligence in medical imaging: Threat or opportunity? Radiologists again at the forefront of innovation in medicine. *European Radiology Experimental*, *2*(1), 35.

Cullen, M. W., Ijioma, N. N., Jayaram, N., Kithcart, A. P., Narang, A., Rajagopalan, B., ... Sinha, S. S. (2016). The supply and demand of the cardiovascular workforce: Striking the right balance. *Journal of the American College of Cardiology*, *68*(15), 1680–1689.

D'Abate, F., & La Leggia, A. (2017, June 16). The role of sonographers: future professionals across Europe? Retrieved from https://healthcare-in-europe.com/en/news/the-role-of-sonographers-future-professionals-across-europe.html

Data Bridge Market Research. (2016). Europe Departmental PACS Market – Industry Trends and Forecast to 2024 (Report No. DBMR-1215). Retrieved from https://databridgemarketresearch.com/reports/europe-departmental-pacs-market/

EANM Technologists Committee. (2018). *Competencies for the European Nuclear Medicine technologists*. Staffordshire, U.K: BNMS Technology Group.

Elhauge, E. (2010). *The fragmentation of U.S. health care: Causes and solutions*. New York, NY: Oxford University Press; doi:10.1093/acprof:oso/9780195390131.001.0001.

EU eHealth Stakeholder Group. (2014). Widespread Deployment of Telemedicine Services in Europe. (Report No. DAE KA 13/2). Retrieved from http://www.vitlab-resater.eu/sites/default/files/TelemedicinedeploymentreportEHSG.pdf

euro.who.int. (2019). Data and statistics. Retrieved from http://www.euro.who.int/en/health-topics/Health-systems/health-workforce/data-and-statistics

European Commission. eHealth. (2012). Communication from the Commission To the European Parliament, the Council, The European Economic and Social Committee and The Committee of the Regions (Report No. COM 736). Retrieved from https://eur-lex.europa.eu/legal-content/EN/TXT/PDF/?uri=CELEX:52012DC0736&from=EN

Finucane, M. L., Slovic, P., Hibbard, J. H., Peters, E., Mertz, C. K., & MacGregor, D. G. (2002). Aging and decision-making competence: An analysis of comprehension and consistency skills in older versus younger adults considering health-plan options. *Journal of Behavioral Decision Making*, *15*(2), 141–164. doi:10.1002/bdm.407

Forrest, C. B., Glade, G. B., Baker, A. E., Bocian, A., von Schrader, S., & Starfield, B. (2000). Coordination of specialty referrals and physician satisfaction with referral care. *Archives of Pediatrics & Adolescent Medicine*, *154*(5), 499–506. doi:10.1001/archpedi.154.5.499 PubMed

Gandhi, T. K., Sittig, D. F., Franklin, M., Sussman, A. J., Fairchild, D. G., & Bates, D. W. (2000). Communication breakdown in the outpatient referral process. *Journal of General Internal Medicine*, *15*(9), 626–631. doi:10.1046/j.1525-1497.2000.91119.x PubMed

Gunawardena, C. N., Hermans, M. B., Sanchez, D., Richmond, C., Bohley, M., & Tuttle, R. (2009). A theoretical framework for building online communities of practice with social networking tools. *Educational Media International*, *46*(1), 3–16. doi:10.1080/09523980802588626

Hsiao, C. J., Hing, E., Socey, T. C., & Cai, B. (2010). Electronic medical record/electronic health record systems of office-based physicians: United States, 2009 and preliminary 2010 state estimates. National Center for Health Statistics, 2001-2011. Available from http://www.cdc.gov/nchs/data/hestat/emr_ehr_09/emr_ehr_09.htm

Kalyanpur, A., Singh, J., & Bedi, R. (2010). Practical issues in picture archiving and communication system and networking. *The Indian Journal of Radiology & Imaging*, *20*(1), 2. doi:10.4103/0971-3026.59743 PubMed

Kripalani, S., LeFevre, F., Phillips, C. O., Williams, M. V., Basaviah, P., & Baker, D. W. (2007). Deficits in communication and information transfer between hospital-based and primary care physicians: Implications for patient safety and continuity of care. *Journal of the American Medical Association*, *297*(8), 831–841. doi:10.1001/jama.297.8.831 PubMed

Kutner, M., Greenburg, E., Jin, Y., & Paulsen, C. (2006). The Health Literacy of America's Adults: Results from the 2003 National Assessment of Adult Literacy. NCES 2006-483. National Center for Education Statistics. Available from https://files.eric.ed.gov/fulltext/ED493284.pdf

Langer, S. (2009). Issues surrounding PACS archiving to external, third-party DICOM archives. *Journal of Digital Imaging*, *22*(1), 48–52. doi:10.1007/s10278-008-9125-0 PubMed

Medpac. (2012, June). Report to the Congress: Medicare and the Health Care Delivery System. Retrieved from http://www.medpac.gov/docs/default-source/reports/jun12_entirereport.pdf

MicroMarket Monitor. (2015). Europe Departmental Picture Archiving and Communication System (PACS) Market by Product (Radiology PACS, Cardiology PACS, Others), by Deployment), by End User (Hospitals, Laboratories, Physicians), by Component - Analysis and Forecast to 2019 (Report No. DE 1001). Retrieved from http://www.micromarketmonitor.com/market/europe-departmental-pacs-5624333279.html

Morton, S., Shih, S. C., Winther, C. H., Tinoco, A., Kessler, R. S., & Scholle, S. H. (2015). Health IT–enabled care coordination: A national survey of patient-centered medical home clinicians. *Annals of Family Medicine*, *13*(3), 250–256. doi:10.1370/afm.1797 PubMed

Noar, S. M., & Willoughby, J. F. (2012). eHealth interventions for HIV prevention. *AIDS Care*, *24*(8), 945–952. doi:10.1080/09540121.2012.668167 PubMed

O'Malley, A. S., & Reschovsky, J. D. (2011). Referral and consultation communication between primary care and specialist physicians: Finding common ground. *Archives of Internal Medicine*, *171*(1), 56–65. PubMed

OECD/EU. (2018). *Health at a Glance: Europe 2018: State of Health in the EU Cycle. Paris/EU*. Brussels, Belgium: OECD Publishing.

Oglevee, C., & Pianykh, O. (2015). Losing Images in Digital Radiology: More than You Think. *Journal of Digital Imaging*, *28*(3), 264–271. doi:10.1007/s10278-014-9748-2 PubMed

Ontario, H. Q. (2013). Electronic tools for health information exchange: An evidence-based analysis. *Ontario Health Technology Assessment Series*, *13*(11), 1–76. Available from http://www.hqontario.ca/en/documents/eds/2013/full-report-OCDM-etools.pdf PubMed

Picture archiving and communication system. (2019, Jan. 22). Retrieved from https://en.wikipedia.org/w/index.php?title=Picture_archiving_and_communication_system&action=info

Practical-patient-care.com. (2019). TeleConsult Europe - Maximise radiology efficiency with expertise on demand - Practical Patient Care. Retrieved from http://www.practical-patient-care.com/contractors/imaging-diagnostics-and-analysis/teleconsult-europe/

Prasanna, P. M., Seagull, F. J., & Nagy, P. (2011). Online social networking: A primer for radiology. *Journal of Digital Imaging*, *24*(5), 908–912. doi:10.1007/s10278-011-9371-4 PubMed

Roth, C. J., Lannum, L. M., Dennison, D. K., & Towbin, A. J. (2016). The current state and path forward for enterprise image viewing: HIMSS-SIIM collaborative white paper. *Journal of Digital Imaging*, *29*(5), 567–573. doi:10.1007/s10278-016-9887-8 PubMed

Schoen, C., Osborn, R., Huynh, P. T., Doty, M., Zapert, K., Peugh, J., & Davis, K. (2005). Taking The Pulse Of Health Care Systems: Experiences Of Patients With Health Problems In Six Countries: Patients' voices can provide policy leaders with a window onto what is happening at the front lines of care. *Health Affairs*, *24*(Suppl1), W5-509–W5-525. doi:10.1377/hlthaff.W5.509

Seldeslachts, U. (2019). PACS Market and Spending Trends Overview. Retrieved from https://ipacso.eu/11-uncategorized/157-pacs-market-and-spending-trends-overview.html

Social networking service. (2019, Feb. 18). Retrieved from https://en.wikipedia.org/w/index.php?title=Social_networking_service&oldid=884010054

U. S. Department of Commerce. (2017). Health Information Technology Industry Snapshot. Retrieved from https://build.export.gov/build/groups/public/@eg_main/@byind/@healthtech/documents/webcontent/eg_main_114799.pdf

Vreeland, A., Persons, K. R., Primo, H. R., Bishop, M., Garriott, K. M., Doyle, M. K., ... Bashall, C. (2016). Considerations for exchanging and sharing medical images for improved collaboration and patient care: HIMSS-SIIM collaborative white paper. *Journal of Digital Imaging*, *29*(5), 547–558. doi:10.1007/s10278-016-9885-x PubMed

World Health Organization. (2016). Health Services Delivery Programme Division of Health Systems and Public Health. Integrated care models: An overview. Retrieved from http://www.euro.who.int/__data/assets/pdf_file/0005/322475/Integrated-care-models-overview.pdf

KEY TERMS AND DEFINITIONS

Artificial Intelligence in Medical Imaging: In an article titled, "Artificial intelligence in medical imaging: threat or opportunity? Radiologists again at the forefront of innovation in medicine" published in 2018 by European Radiology Experimental reports: "one of the most promising areas of health innovation is the application of artificial intelligence (AI), primarily in medical imaging. With an irreversible increase in the amount of data and the possibility to use AI to identify findings either detectable or not by the human eye, radiology is now moving from a subjective perceptual skill to a more objective science… The higher efficiency provided by AI will allow radiologists to perform more value-added tasks, becoming more visible to patients and playing a vital role in multidisciplinary clinical teams" (Coder, Pesapane & Sardanelli, 2018).

DICOM: Digital imaging and communications in medicine which includes diagnostic images common to cardiology, obstetrics, radiology, and other specialties.

Holter Monitor: This is a battery powered device, made to be portable. It measures heart activity (ECG) continuously and records the data for analysis.

Integrated Care: eHealth systems and services with strong user involvement, focusing on interoperability and the integration of emerging patient-centric technologies for cost-effective healthcare" (WHO, 2016, p. 4).

PHR (Personal Health Record): Allows patient to maintain all their care information as well as uploaded data from personal monitoring devices, health smartphone apps, and smart home devices like medical toilets, and daily diaries of their wellbeing.

Telemedicine: Technology-enabled practice of medicine that focuses on remote diagnosis, treatment, and follow-up of patients. In the modern era this means use of computer, Internet and often mobile technologies.

UHR (Universal Health Record): Patient-centered information available to and often controlled by patients. Contains all health care information and history.

ENDNOTE

1 ™ Diagnostic Modality Interface Portal is a trademark of CardioLync, Inc.

Section 4
Underserved Populations

Chapter 15
Use of a Mobile App by Older People in an Integrated Care Setting

Bella Azaria
Assuta Medical Centers, Israel

Rachelle Kaye
Assuta Medical Centers, Israel

Reut Ron
Assuta Health Services Research Institute, Israel

Ofer Chen
Samson Assuta Ashdod University Hospital, Israel

Michal Bar-Ilan
Samson Assuta Ashdod Hospital, Israel

Alona Sigalov Zlatkin
Samson Assuta Ashdod Hospital, Israel

Erela Rotlevi
Maccabi Healthcare Services, Israel

Michal Yeshayahu
Maccabi Healthcare Services, Israel

Josep Roca
University of Barcelona, Spain

Isaac Cano
Hospital Clinic de Barcelona, Spain

Erik Baltaxe
https://orcid.org/0000-0003-2353-3822
Hospital Clinic de Barcelona, Spain

Jordi de Batlle
Institut de Recerca Biomedica de Lleida, Spain

Gerard Torres
Institut de Recerca Biomedica, Spain

Maarten Lahr
University Medical Center Groningen, The Netherlands

DOI: 10.4018/978-1-7998-0047-7.ch015

ABSTRACT

The current study analyzes the information collected and the lessons learned during the first six months of the CONNECARE project in Israel, in order to assess the use of the mobile technology by patients, their motivations and obstacles; as well as their satisfaction. As of the middle of February 2019, 59 patients were recruited and 18 discharged from the project and completed the feedback questionnaires. Based on preliminary data presented in this chapter, as measured against the McGaughey et al. Research Framework, it can be concluded that the usage of the CONNECARE mobile platform can be rated as moderate. The analysis together with insights from the literature, suggest that usage of the CONNECARE app could be improved by introducing additional features that would increase patients' motivation to use the system as well as its full integration into usual healthcare processes.

INTRODUCTION

The use of mobile apps by the elderly is receiving increasing attention and there are an increasing number of apps on the market targeting this populations, particularly in the area of health care. These include apps for monitoring such as *iBP Blood Pressure and Instant Heart Rate: Heart Rate and Pulse Monitor*; provision of medical health care advice such as *My Medical, WebMD* and *AskMD*; and medication reminders such as *Pill Reminder Pro, Pillboxie, MedCoach,* and *MediSafe* (Hurst, 2018; iYogi, 2018). These apps are intended to be used by the patient for self-care at home. Several studies have investigated motivation as well as design issues. Among these, there is a growing conviction and preliminary evidence that mobile apps can support chronic disease management (Quinn et al., 2011; Bexelius et al., 2010; Carrasco et al., 2008; Lester et al., 2010). However, chronic disease management (CDM) apps have not lived up to their potential because relatively few patients are willing to pay for the digital tools. Huckman and Stern maintain that the more likely customers are health care organizations (Huckman & Stern, 2018). Despite this, there have been relatively fewer studies done specifically on the use of mobile apps by complex chronically ill older adults within an organizational based -integrated health care setting as an aid to treatment adherence, self-management and interaction with healthcare professionals. CONNECARE, a project funded by the European Commission's HORIZON 2020 program, is currently being conducted in Ashdod, Israel by Samson Assuta Ashdod Hospital and Maccabi Healthcare Services. The project focuses on digitally enabled integrated care for complex, chronically ill older adults. The digital platform being comprises a mobile app accompanied by a wearable device for the patients that is interfaced with a computerized case management platform operated by the health professionals.

The purpose of this chapter is to analyze the information collected and the lessons learned during the course of the CONNECARE project to date, in order to: assess the use of the mobile technology by the patients in the project in Israel including their motivations and obstacles as well as satisfaction; its effects on patient – healthcare professional interaction; and, the extent to which the use of the mobile technology contributed to patient empowerment and self-management, patient quality of life and care integration. The McGaughey, Zeltman, and McMurtey (2013) research framework was used to guide analysis in this study. It delineates the relationships between motivation, obstacles, ease of use, adoption and actual usage. The objective was to better understand the best use of mobile technology for the elderly in a healthcare setting, address all factors in our research model, and investigate implications related to appropriate technology design for this population.

BACKGROUND

Digitally Enabled Integrated Care

The digital transformation of health care is high on the agenda in all developed countries and is receiving especially high visibility in the European Union with its publication on 25th April 2018 by the European Commission of the Communication on Digital Transformation of Health and Care in the Digital Single Market that identifies three priorities:

- Citizens' secure access to their health data, also across borders;
- Personalized medicine through shared European data infrastructures;
- Citizen empowerment with digital tools for user feedback and person-centered care using digital tools to empower people to look after their health, stimulate prevention and enable feedback and interaction between users and healthcare providers.

Side by side with the movement toward digitalization of healthcare, is the growing conviction regarding the necessity of integrated care to meet the needs of an aging population with an increasing chronic disease burden. While the notion of integrated care was discussed in the late 1990s, a first attempt to define integrated care was offered by Kodner and Spreeuwenberg in 2002 (Kodner & Spreeuwenberg, 2002). Many subsequent definitions were put forth including one proposed by the World Health Organization (WHO Europe, 2016).

The notion of digitally enabled integrated care began to gain significant traction in Europe during the last decade. An indication of its importance has been the willingness of the European Commission to fund projects supporting the development of telehealth and telecare in the 7th European Research Framework (FP7) as well as the AAL (Ambient Assisted Living) Program, jointly funded by the European Commission and member and associated States (including Israel). This emphasis intensified in the European HORIZON 2020 program (2013-2020). On July 30, 2014, the EC published a call for proposals entitled "PHC-25 -2015: Advanced ICT systems and services for integrated care" with a deadline for submission of April 2015. Assuta Medical Centers was invited to be a member of a consortium that successfully submitted the CONNECARE Proposal, which was funded at the end of 2015 and launched in April 2016. Assuta's motivation for joining the project was its ambition for its new hospital being built in Ashdod which was strongly focused on its vision to be a "hospital with a community" and a hub for an integrated care system in the Ashdod area, coordinating the care between the new hospital, community healthcare services and social services.

Israel has been a pioneer in Health IT and its second largest Health Plan, Macccabi Healthcare Services, was one of the first healthcare organizations, internationally, to implement Electronic Medical Records on an organization-wide basis. Israel was an early adopter of telemedicine and was among the earliest to provide its citizens with access to their medical information via web-based patient portals. This was followed by the development and implementation of mobile apps giving both patients and clinicians access to the EMR via smartphone and tablet. Thus, the journey toward digitally supported integrated care in Israel has been part of an ongoing process of digital innovation.

The CONNECARE Project

CONNECARE is a multi-country project funded by the European HORIZON 2020 program to develop and implement a digitally enabled integrated care service. It is being implemented in two areas of Catalonia, Spain (Lleida and Barcelona), in Groningen, Netherlands and in Ashdod, Israel by Assuta Ashdod Hospital and Maccabi Healthcare Services.

Integrated Care for purposes of the CONNECARE project and this chapter is defined according to the definition set out in the report of the HSPA Expert Group on Integrated Care called *BLOCKS: Tools and methodologies to assess integrated care in Europe* (European Commission, 2017a). The definition for "[i]ntegrated care includes initiatives seeking to improve outcomes of care by overcoming issues of fragmentation through linkage or coordination of services of providers along the continuum of care." (European Commission, 2017, p. 2).

The CONNECARE Project is first and foremost an integrated care service based on a patient-centered integrated care model. From an organizational perspective, the integrated care model implemented in Ashdod is a case management model focused on integration and continuity of care between the hospital and primary and secondary healthcare in the community. The CONNECARE project aims to overcome the fragmentation of care by coordinating hospital and community healthcare services using digital technology, specifically mobile technology, for community dwelling, chronically ill patients that have been admitted to the hospital and will be discharged back to the community.

The primary digital tools being used by the patients are a mobile app accompanied by a wearable device (Fitbit watch) that tracks steps and motion, heart rate and sleep quality. The app collects the information from the wearable on a continuous basis, and in addition. includes tasks, reminders, alerts, questions and questionnaires and a chat feature for messaging. The app interacts with a digital case management platform operated by health professionals, in the Israeli program, primarily by nurse case managers and physical therapists. The Israeli project focuses on two groups of patients: complex chronic patients 60+ who are Maccabi members with an unplanned admission to Assuta Ashdod hospital via the Emergency department (Case 1) and Maccabi complex chronic patients 55+ scheduled for major elective surgery in Assuta Ashdod Hospital (Case 2).

The patients scheduled for elective surgery enter the program 3-4 weeks prior to surgery. A hospital- based Care Manager assesses the patient and refers the patient to a pre-surgery habilitation program coordinated by the Assuta Ashdod Physical Therapy Department to strengthen the patient both physically and emotionally prior to surgery, including a supervised and non-supervised physical exercise training program. Patients receive the wearable (a Fitbit watch and the Fitbit app) together with the CONNECARE app, along with instructions and training in their use. The pre-habilitation program is a combination of supervised activity in the physical therapy department, supplemented by nutritional consultation where needed and emotional support; as well as a program of activities and exercises to be performed at home. The patient's activity and adherence to the program at home is monitored by the professional staff with ongoing feedback – both through the chat feature of the app and by phone.

Both groups of patients (post-surgery and those with an unplanned hospitalization) are picked up by the Maccabi Nurse Case managers during their hospital stay and are then followed by them post-discharge for 3 months, using a combination of the app and Fitbit, phone calls and occasional face-to-face visits, either in the Maccabi Integrated Care Unit in the hospital or at the patient's home. The Maccabi Nurse Case managers develop a care plan based on the hospital medical and nursing discharge plans under the guidance of the patient's primary care physician. Post discharge services in the community are arranged for and coordinated, usually prior to discharge or immediately following discharge. The post discharge plan is translated by the nurse case managers into tasks and entered into the health professional's case management platform. These tasks are automatically transmitted to the patient's app, where he receives notifications of his tasks, reminders, alerts, and questions regarding task performance as well as tracking how he feels and his overall status. The information from the Fitbit as well as everything entered by the patient into the app is transmitted in near real time back to the dashboard so that the case managers can monitor the patient's adherence and progress. In addition to monitoring and ongoing interaction with the health professional, patients are also supported in making appointments and dealing with bureaucratic hurdles in receiving coordinated care in the community.

From a research perspective, recruitment of patients into the project began in July 2018 and will continue until August 2019. The study uses implementation research methodology based on the Standards for Reporting Implementation Studies (StaRI) framework and checklist (Pinnock et al., 2017). A matched control group for both intervention groups will be created using the Maccabi database and compared using propensity scoring. The study measures selected clinical status outcomes as well as healthcare utilization outcomes but focuses predominantly on the evaluation of the implementation and the use of the mobile technology by the patients in the intervention groups.

The digital platform, both the mobile app for patients and the case management platform for clinicians, have been designed and developed using a co-design methodology. The use of the platform by the healthcare professionals has had its ups and downs, but by and large has been successfully implemented with ongoing modifications and refinements to meet their needs.

However, the adoption and actual use of the mobile app and Fitbit watch by the patients in the CONNECARE project has been fraught with challenges, many of which have been addressed in the past by previously published studies. These challenges include: motivation; the unique user characteristics of the older adult; designing the app geared to the special needs of the older users; and, the training/learning process for using the app.

The CONNECARE Mobile Solution

The CONNECARE mobile app for chronic patients is not a stand-alone app, but the patient component of an interactive digital system between the patient and healthcare professionals, and a platform for coordination among health professionals. Because of the interactive nature of the digital platform, the app can only be properly presented and understood within the context of its interaction with the healthcare professional via the CONNECARE case management platform.

In this section, the authors present the app as it transacts with the clinician platform. The screen shots are in English, but the platform used by the clinicians in Israel is in Hebrew and the app for the patients is in English, Hebrew and Russian. The patient can only access the app once he has been registered by the healthcare professional as a patient in the case management platform.

The first steps of the process are the creation of the patient in the clinician dashboard and the medical and functional evaluation of the patient (See Figure 1).

The clinician then creates a care plan, which is translated into tasks for the patient. The healthcare professional defines the task in terms of start and end date, frequency, quantity, and times of day (determines when a reminder will pop up). See Figure 2. The task then appears as a notification in the patient's app. In the following example, the physical therapist has prescribed physical activity, specifi-

Figure 1. Screen from the clinician dashboard - a patient's care plan

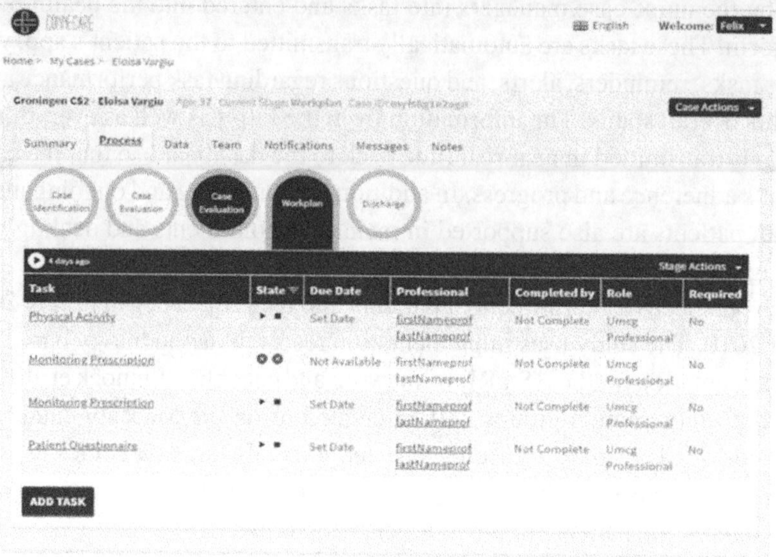

cally walking. The patient receives the instruction in the app – he synchronizes his Fitbit with the app and when he sees that the app is active (See Figure 3 and Figure 4), he puts the Fitbit watch on his wrist.

The Fitbit transmits the patient's steps and heart rate to the app, and the patients can monitor their own activity and see their walking trend over time. See Figure 5. The app transmits the information to the clinician platform so that the healthcare professionals can monitor his progress and provide feedback. See Figure 6.

Figure 2. Screen from the clinician dashboard - physical activity task form

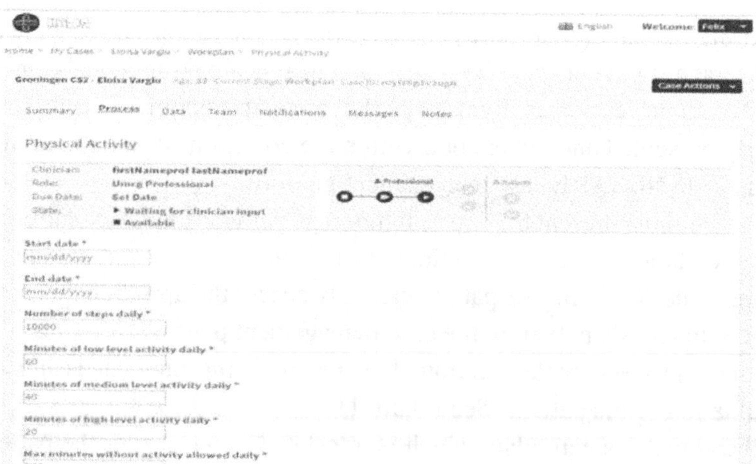

Figure 3. The patient's app - physical activity task pop-up remainder

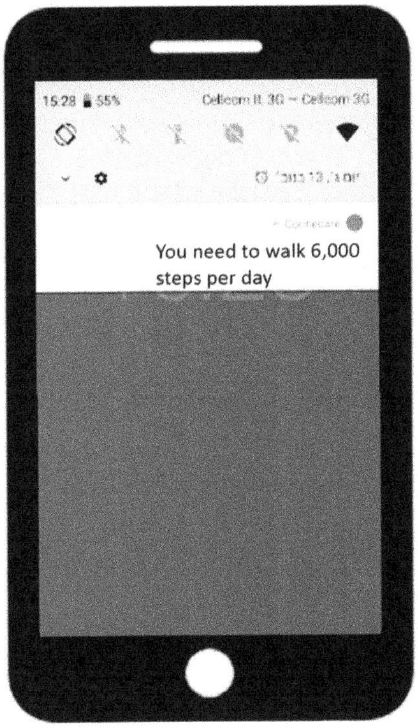

Figure 4. The patient's app - measurements home page

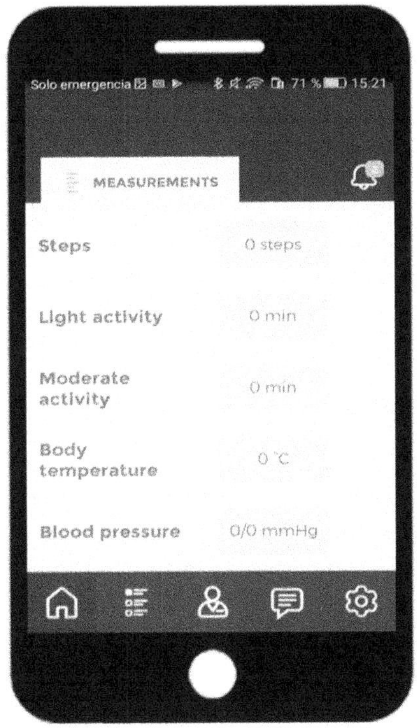

Figure 5. The patient's app - trend of daily steps over time

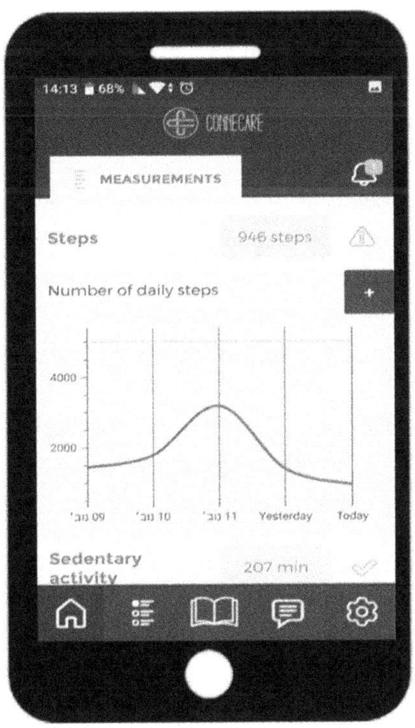

Figure 6. Screen from the clinician dashboard - monitoring the trend of patient's daily steps over time

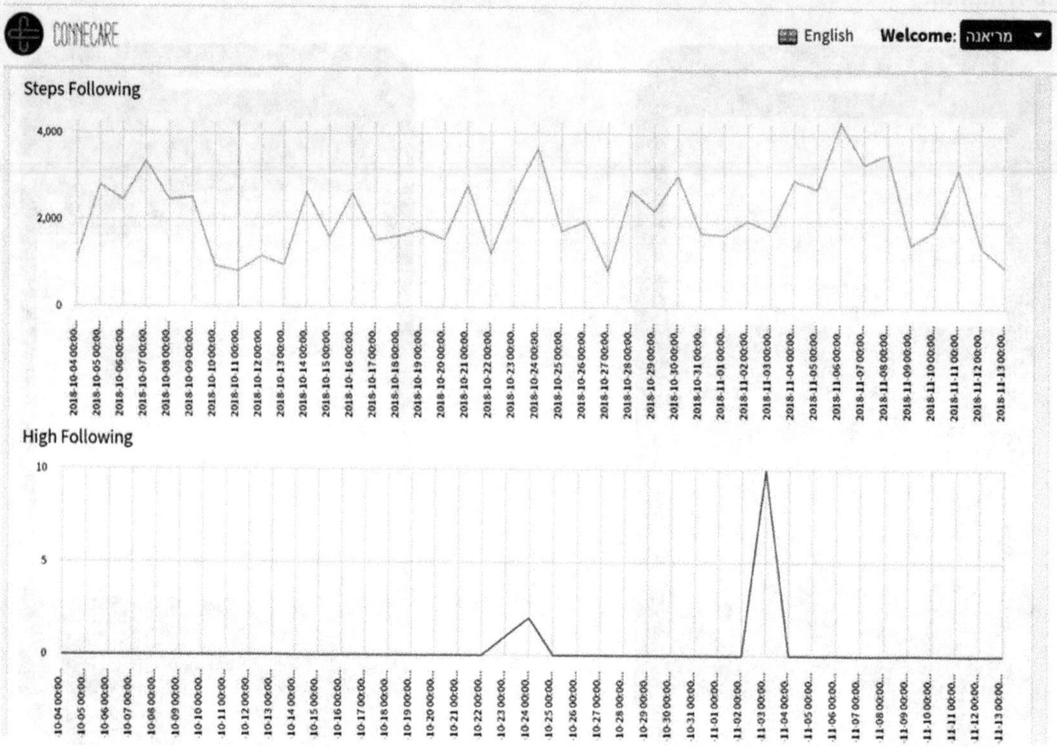

The clinician can also prescribe additional types of physical activity as part of the care plan, and the patient will get notifications and reminders about these as well, and be asked to report whether he has performed them. See Figure 7. The clinician can also prescribe additional tasks, such as blood pressure monitoring. The patient can use a blood pressure cuff with Bluetooth that transmits to the app. See Figure 8.

The patient can see his current blood pressure levels in the app, and he can also see his blood pressure trends over time. See Figure 9 and Figure 10. The clinician can also monitor the patient's blood pressure on the clinician platform. See Figure 11. Other features include nutrition reminders, medication monitoring, glucose level monitoring and other biometric measures.

One of the most important features of the app is the messaging function that enables asynchronous interaction between the patient and the healthcare professional. In the following example, the nurse case manager sends a message to the patient giving him positive feedback on his walking and asking about his appointment with the orthopedic surgeon. See Figure 12. The patient is notified on the app that he has a message, reads the message and responds with a question relative to the prescription he received from the doctor and takes a picture of the prescription and sends it to the nurse. The nurse receives the prescription and the question in the clinician dashboard and can then respond to the patient. See Figure 13.

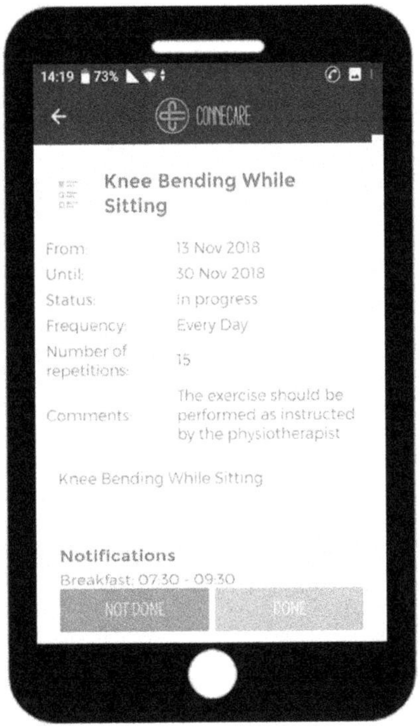
14:19 73%
CONNECARE
Knee Bending While Sitting
From 13 Nov 2018
Until 30 Nov 2018
Status In progress
Frequency Every Day
Number of repetitions 15
Comments The exercise should be performed as instructed by the physiotherapist
Knee Bending While Sitting
Notifications
Breakfast: 07:30 - 09:30
NOT DONE
DONE

Figure 7. The patient's app - notifications of prescribed physical exercise

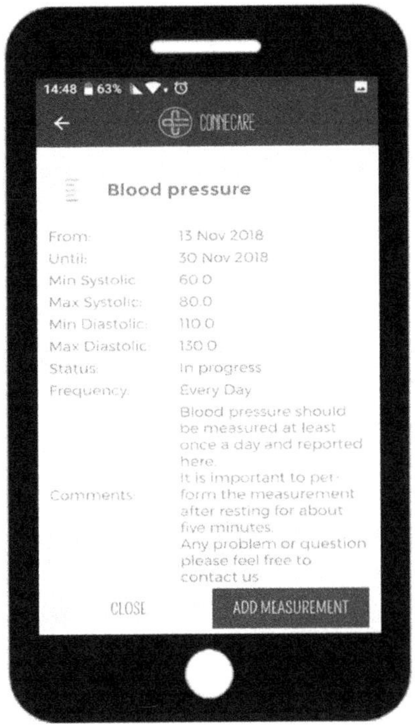

Figure 8. The patient's app - notifications to measure blood pressure

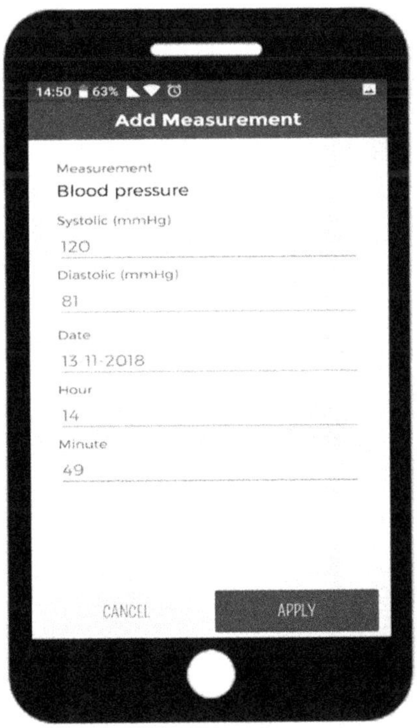

Figure 9. The patient's app - blood pressure values input screen

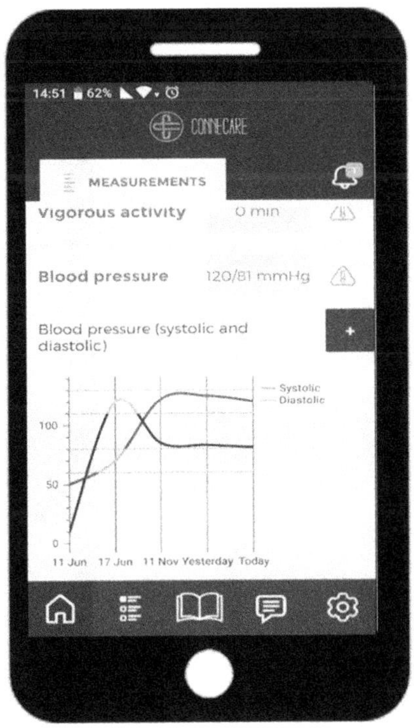

Figure 10. The patient's app - blood pressure trends over time

Figure 11. Screen from the clinician dashboard - patient blood pressure trends over time

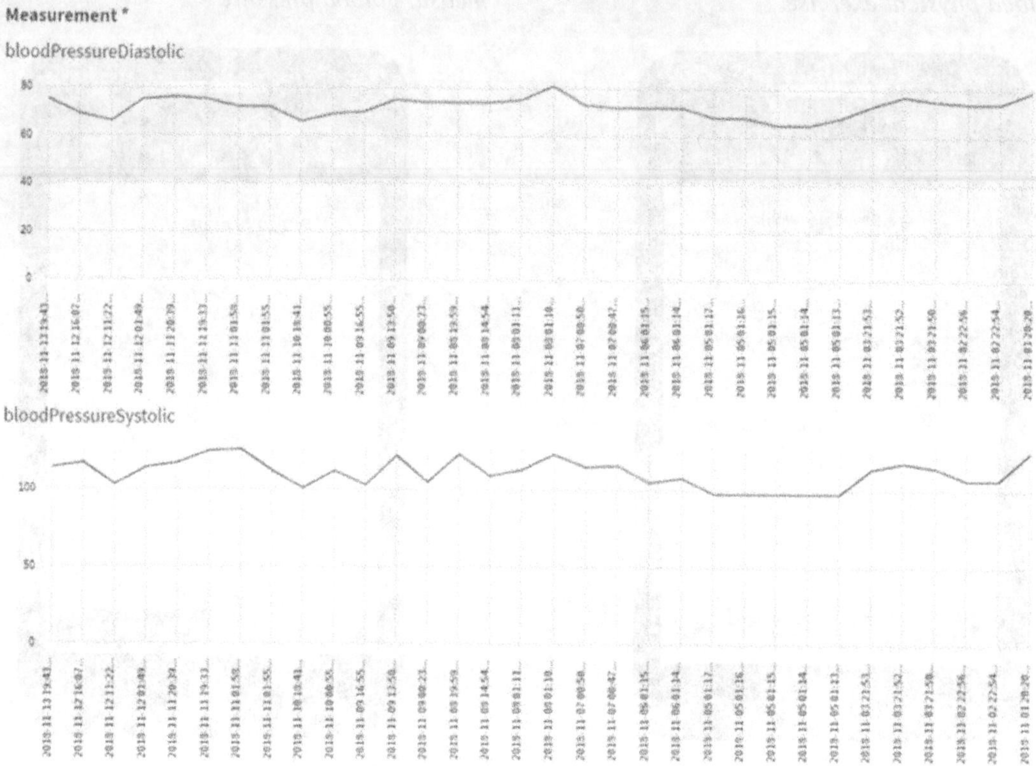

Figure 12. The patient's app - messaging

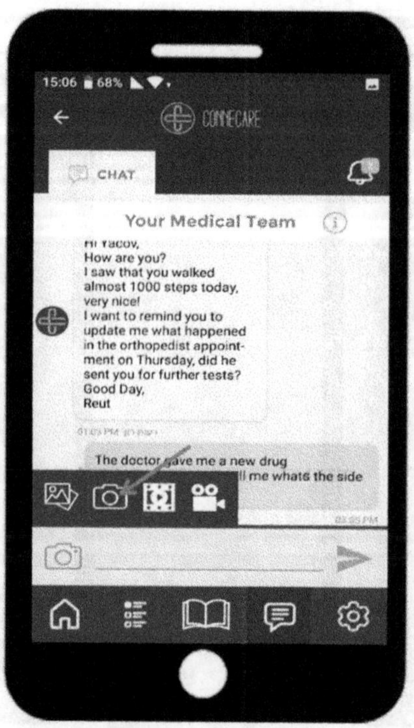

Figure 13. Screen from the clinician dashboard – messaging

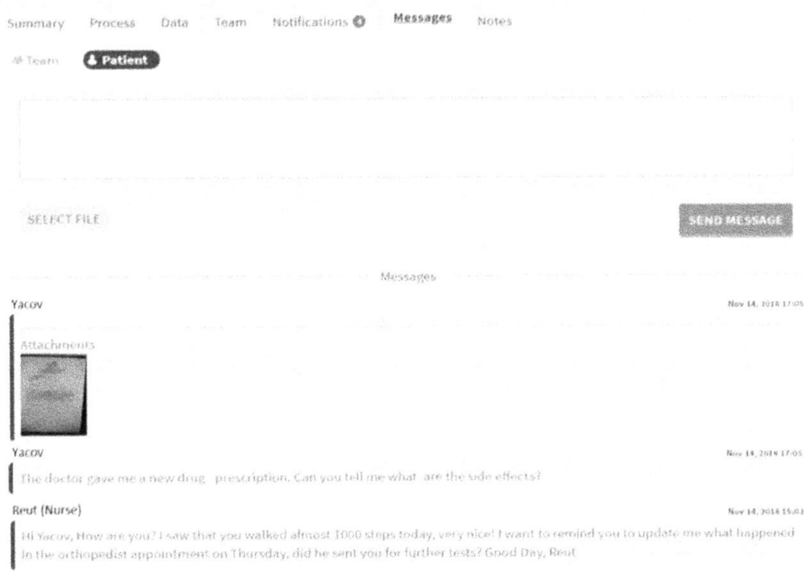

MOBILE TECHNOLOGY USE ASSESSMENT FOR CHRONICALLY ILL, OLDER ADULTS

Assessment Framework and Methodology

The research framework proposed by McGaughey, Zeltmann, and McMurtrey (2013) was used in this chapter for assessing the use of the CONNECARE mobile technology by the patients in this project. The sources of information for the assessment were data documented on an ongoing basis by the staff regarding patient usage of the mobile system and its various features. Additionally, patient feedback was collected from those who were discharged from the study using the following instruments: *Satisfaction with the Technology Measures, EQ-5D, The Person Centered Coordinated Care Experiences Questionnaire (P3CEQ)*, items G1-G4 adapted from the *Nijmegen Continuity Questionnaire (NCQ)*, and *System Usability Scale (SUS)*. This was supplemented by observations by the clinical staff as well as the research staff documented in a structured implementation log and in the minutes of regular staff meetings as well as anecdotal information from both patients and clinical staff. There are additional data regarding health status (before and after) as well as other outcomes that will be measured for comparison with the control group that will be analyzed at the end of the project. The analysis addresses the following major issues:

- Motivation
- Obstacles: human factor (user characteristics), service-related, device-related
- Ease of use
- Training
- Support
- Usage (high, medium, low)

Results

The patient recruitment period for the project in Israel was ongoing at the time of this chapter's development and was expected to cover the time period from July 2018 to August 2019. As of the middle of February 2019, 59 patients had been recruited (28 males and 31 females ranging from ages 58-79 with an average age of 66.8). Most of the patients were married (76%), defined themselves as having middle socioeconomic status (86%), and had university education (58%). Twenty-one patients were recruited prior to major elective surgery and underwent or are currently undergoing the pre-habilitation program with the Fitbit and the app as well as post-discharge follow-up, and 38 have been recruited in the hospital during their inpatient stay after an unplanned admission via the emergency room and received or are receiving post-discharge follow up for three months with the Fitbit and app. 14 patients (24% - 9 from Case 1 and 5 from Case 2) dropped out of the project prior to completing the entire course and 18 patients have been discharged from the project and have completed the feedback questionnaires. Of the 14 patients who dropped out of the project ahead of schedule, eight (57%) were single (divorced or widowed). It should be noted that the feedback results reported here are on the first 18 patients recruited who had to cope with problems with the mobile technology that have since been resolved, so that these results reflect this limitation.

The following sections summarize the overall results. Detailed results can be found in the Appendix.

Usage (n = 59 Patients)

Devices Used

71% of the patients used or are using their smartphone while the remaining 29% are using a tablet. The main reason for tablet use is that the patients owned an old smartphone that cannot support the app. Of the patients using tablets, the majority are using a tablet provided by the project with a SIM card due to difficulties with WIFI in the home. All patients received a Fitbit watch, provided by the project.

Actual Use (n = 45, Excluding Patients Who Left the Study Ahead of Schedule)

82% of the patients measured steps with the Fitbit, with or without the app. 42% of the patients reported performance of tasks other than the walking assigned to them in the care plan via the app. 55% of the patients who were required to monitor their blood pressure used this feature of the app. 32% of the patients used the messaging function

Use by Case (Case 1 -Unplanned Admission; Case 2 – Elective Surgery)

Case 1: 76% counted steps, 41% reported performing assigned tasks, 24% used the messaging.
Case 2: 90% counted steps, 43% reported performing assigned tasks, 44% used the messaging.

Demographic Variables Affecting Usage

Age was not a strong factor in use, although those above 74 years old tended to use both the Fitbit and the app less, with the exception of the oldest patient in the study (age 79) who used all features regularly. Gender was not a strong factor in use, except for the use of the messaging feature, which was used significantly more by female patients. The patient's marital status had a significant impact on their participation in the project and usage. Although the vast majority of patients were married (76%) there is clearly a significantly lower usage pattern for the unmarried patients. This was true even in Fitbit use (93% for married patients compared to 60% for single patients). Education level was not a significant factor influencing usage, although the messaging feature was used less by patients with higher education levels (university degrees). This may be a random finding, and it will be interesting to see whether this finding persists in the final sample. The impact of the patient's socio-economic level on their use of mobile technology was inconclusive as only eight (14%) patients defined themselves as having low or high (not middle) socioeconomic status.

Change in Frequency of Usage over Project Course: As co-design is a major feature of the CONNECARE project, the app is being continuously improved and refined with new features added. The improvement of the app did not affect Fitbit usage which has been relatively high throughout the project. It did, however, affect performance of tasks in the app to some extent. Messaging was not available at the start of the project and there was increased use since the feature became available but not as rapidly as expected.

Satisfaction With the Technology (n=18 Patients Completed and Discharged)

The satisfaction questionnaire contained four question with a scale of 1-10 (1=Low, 10=high, NA= didn't use the technology). The questionnaire was completed separately for the Fitbit watch and the app. The results were significantly higher for the Fitbit watch than the app. The average scores for the Fitbit and app are in Table 1.

Table 1. Satisfaction with the technology average scores for the Fitbit and app (n=18)

Question	Fitbit watch	Connecare App
Overall impression	9	6.77
User friendliness	8.63	7.17
Ability to use	8.81	6.83
Would you recommend this to someone else?	9.54	7.40

System Usability Scale (SUS) (n=17)

The system usability scale questionnaire comprised 10 statements with five possible ratings from strongly disagree (1) to strongly agree (5). The percent of patients who rated each statement 4 or above (agree-strongly agree) for each question was:

- I think that I would like to use this system frequently = 35%
- I found the system unnecessarily complex = 18%
- I thought the system was easy to use = 53%
- I would need the support of a technical person to be able to use this system = 24%
- I found the various functions in this system were well integrated = 59%
- I thought there was too much inconsistency in this system = 12%
- I would imagine that most people would learn to use this system very quickly = 53%
- I found the system very cumbersome to use =12%
- I felt very confident using the system = 41%
- I needed to learn a lot of things before I could get going with this system = 29%

Overall, the proportion of patients who agreed with positive statements about the app were relatively low, but surprisingly, the percent of patients who agreed with the negative statements were even lower.

Patient Comments

Patients added an explanatory comment to their ratings. Some patients felt that the app helped them, was well integrated and felt that most people could learn to use it, but others cited various problems with using the app and cited that they needed repeated training and were helped in its use by their spouse or children. The comments also strongly support the finding that the patients were much more satisfied with the Fitbit than the app and felt that it was more useful for them. The specific comments shed light on some of the obstacles as well as positive aspects of the mobile technology. They also indicate that the context of integrated care service was important. Sample comments included:

Critical Comments

- Some of the data on the Fitbit and the app was in English so I could not understand them
- The watch is simple to use but I got in trouble with the app – synchronizing them is difficult
- Using the app would have been easier if it had been integrated with the Maccabi app which I know and use
- It would help if the app had a reminder to charge the watch
- If the app supported making appointments with my doctor it would have been more efficient for me
- Having to remove the watch to shower is a nuisance
- I only used the watch – I gave up on the app

Positive Comments

- The project is fantastic, provides reminders to drink water, feedback on sleep quality, all of the features
- The app should be accessible to all patients as it is really helpful
- This project helps me organize my day reminding me to take medication, drink water, walk
- The project gave me a sense of safety and security, attention, caring and support
- The app and watch encouraged self-discipline
- I wanted to do more fitness, especially after my last hospitalization, but couldn't bring myself to do it … using the Fitbit really encouraged me to walk more

Rating the Integrated Care Service, Continuity of Care and Perception of Health State (n=18)

While not directly related to the subject of this chapter, which focuses on the use of the mobile technology in the project, it is important to note that most patients felt they were more often than not involved in decisions about their care, received moderate support from the team, always received enough information and felt that they were treated as a "whole person" rather than a disease or condition. Interestingly enough, while they were satisfied with their relationship with the clinical staff, most did not perceive continuity of care among the clinical team. At the end of the three-month post discharge follow-up, they perceived their health state as very good as measured by EQ-5D. In response to the request to rate their health status from 100 (the best health state you can imagine) to 0 (the worst health state you can imagine) the median was 77.5 with highest being 100 and the lowest being 50.

Observations of the Staff as Recorded in the Implementation Log

The implementation log is a record of obstacles encountered from the start of the pilot in July 2018. As there is a strong element of co-design in the project, many of the problems with the mobile technology were addressed and features were added or solutions found. For example, initially there were problems with patients remembering their user name and password, which became an issue as the password would expire if the patients were not using the app on a regular basis. This problem was addressed and resolved. There were also equipment problems. The preferred option was for patients to use their own smartphones but many had old phones that could not support the app. The solution was to provide them with tablets. This led to another issue, which was that, even though they claimed they had WIFI at home, they couldn't remember the password to their WIFI. This was solved by giving them tablets with a SIM card so that they were not dependent on WIFI.

In the early part of the project, patients had to open the app to see notifications and reminders. This was changed so that the patients received pop-ups on their phone or tablet even when the app was closed (just like the pop-ups from text messages and WhatsApp). The staff reported that for many patients, despite the fact that they were trained on Fitbit and app use, and received a simply stated very explicit user manual with lots of pictures of screen shots showing how to use each feature, they forgot or couldn't "get it''.

A recurring phenomenon among many patients was embarrassment at not understanding how to work with the application and / or the Fitbit. Many patients were ashamed to say that they did not understand or did not remember. The staff was very respectful and empathetic, and conducted repeated training sessions both on the telephone and in face-to-face meetings. A number of attempts were made to involve patients' children or other family member to assist in the use of the app at home. This experience was successful in a small number of cases. Either the children did not have the time or patience to help their parents with the app, or the patient did not want the help of his children (mostly because of embarrassment at needing help).

DISCUSSION

The preliminary results on the use of the CONNECARE mobile device, show a clear preference and greater comfort level with the Fitbit watch than the app. This was supported by the structured feedback from the first 18 patients to complete the CONNECARE program and staff observation that seemed to indicate that patients viewed the overall program as supportive, were happy to use the Fitbit, but were not highly motivated to use the app. Not only because it required significantly more effort than the Fitbit, but because they apparently did not perceive enough "added value" to warrant the extra effort.

Motivation

The purpose of the CONNECARE mobile technology was explicitly to improve the health status of the patient, prior to surgery and post-discharge from the hospital. The functions were designed to help improve adherence to the treatment plan, to provide emotional support and a sense of security, and to empower the patient by giving him feedback, both in terms of self-monitoring as well as feedback from the clinicians. In this respect, the CONNECARE mobile platform only met several key needs identified in the literature. Gao and Koronios (2010) identify the key needs of senior citizens in their daily life, as health monitoring needs, personal information needs, social needs, leisure and sale needs, and safety and privacy needs. Older adults are motivated to use mobile technology if they perceive that it contributes to their *Quality of Life* (Qol). Martína, Martinb, and Medranoa (2011) compared Qol components identified by older people, needs found in their review of the research and the AAL (Ambient Assisted Living Program) model, and found a high degree of consistency. Qol components were:

- *Family and other relationships/contact with others* (maintain social contact with mobile phone as communication device);
- *Emotional well-being* (feeling safe and secure, safety, security and privacy, peace of mind);
- *Independence/mobility/autonomy* (freedom of movement, enjoyment, self-actualization);
- *Social/leisure activities/enjoyment* (self-actualization, hobbies, learning and education);
- *Finances/standard of living* (working life);
- *Own health/health of others* (healthier independent life, health and wellness, home care, chores and supply with goods.

In addition to intrinsic life-related motivations, a significant factor in the use of mobile technology by older adults is user satisfaction. Young Seok Lee (2007) found that user satisfaction was affected by three attributes of mobile phones: usefulness, ease of use, and pleasure of use. Another relevant insight from the literature is that for older adults to accept mobile health technology, it must represent a clear benefit to them and fit with their goals, expectations, and lifestyles (Jorunn et al., 2017).

While it is important to distinguish between patient motivation to adhere to medical treatment recommendations and the motivation to use an app as a tool to support adherence to treatment, both raise the question of key motivating factors and factors that impede or deter. Studies on medication adherence have identified the following key deterrents:

- Lack of family/social support;
- Economic factors such as unemployment, poverty, issues of affordability;
- Perceived benefit – asymptomatic patients are less motivated to adhere to a treatment regimen;
- Patient unfriendliness.

While lack of family/ social support was a factor in recruitment of patients to the study, once recruited it did not appear to be a major factor affecting use. Likewise, economic factors were not perceived to be an issue as patients received the mobile technology free of charge. However, perceived benefit and user friendliness were key issues. Lack of doctor- patient relationship (or more broadly – professional-patient relationships) is also cited as an important factor. There was a close and ongoing relationship between health professionals and the patient in CONNECARE. However, while the patient's doctors were supportive, they were not actively involved. An additional factor for lack of adherence to treatment cited in studies on adherence to treatment – not only medication, but other forms of treatment such as physical therapy, is low self- efficacy - the patient's beliefs about their capabilities to produce designated levels of performance required by the treatment regimen (Kagolianni, 2011). While the rationale for using a health related mobile app is to empower the patient and increase the patient's sense of self efficacy, it may be counterbalanced by a sense of anxiety and helplessness in the technical mastery of the use of the app, which then acts to discourage its use.

The CONNECARE app addressed only some of the Qol components listed identified as important to older adults. The CONNECARE app did not address the patients' social needs – in terms of contact with family and friends or leisure activities. It also did not address finances or standard of living. The level of actual usage, as well as the feedback from the first 18 patients recruited, seem to indicate insufficient motivation for using the app. The perception of the staff and the researchers is that because they could use the Fitbit without using the app, they had less motivation to use the app. They could see the number of steps they walked, as well as their heart rate from the Fitbit, and the Fitbit is by far simpler and easier to use, requiring little effort from the patient except to remember to charge it and to take it off before bathing and then put it back on. Another observation of the staff was that CONNECARE patients do not always perceive the benefit as they still have recourse to face-to-face care with their doctor and other health professionals, and communication with their nurse case manager by phone. Thus, the use of the app, even for messaging, was not sufficiently compelling. Patients from Case 2, admitted for major elective surgery, would appear to have exhibited a higher level of adherence to their care plan and the use of both the Fitbit and the app. This may be related to the fact that the benefit was perceived as more immediate and compelling as part of their preparation for their upcoming surgery. Patients noted that the pre-habilitation program, supported by the app, increased their sense of independence and improved their mobility, giving them greater confidence that they could cope with the challenge of surgery.

Obstacles

Human Factors

User characteristics of older adults is a key factor. Young Sook Lee (2007) found that older adults are generally conservative mobile phone users, who use a few functions of mobile phones and perceive their phone to be difficult to use. Sri Kurniawan noted that older people are passive users of mobile phones, that they experience fear of consequences of using unfamiliar technology, and that most preferred design features that are aids for declining functional abilities (Kurniawan, 2008). Another study showed that older people require more time to complete tasks on mobile devices and describes problems such as the size of the screen to read information, the size of menus and interfaces issues (Lin, Hsieh, & Shiang, 2009). These elements are being experienced in the CONNECARE patient's use of the CONNECARE app. While not true of all patients, many do tend to be passive users, and there has been the challenge of overcoming the fear of using unfamiliar technology. A more common experience of CONNECARE patients has been embarrassment due to their inability to use all of the features resulting in a sense of low self-efficacy. As the co-design of the app is an ongoing process throughout the lifetime of the project, these issues are being addressed with app refinements.

Service Related

The feedback from the 18 patients who have completed the project did not indicate a lack of satisfaction with the service for the devices, although there were times when the app suddenly stopped working and patients needed help getting it back on-line. Some patients had difficulty accessing the WIFI in their homes (particularly those with tablets) but this was perceived more as a user problem than a service problem. Cost was not an issue as the Fitbits and tablets were provided by the project.

Device Related

This was an issue for more than a quarter of the patients who either did not have smartphones or had older smartphones that could not support the app. Providing tablets did not fully resolve the problem until the project started to provide tablets with SIM cards. Even using the Fitbit has its challenges: it requires activation of Bluetooth on the phone or tablet; remembering to charge the Fitbit once a week; and, remembering to remove it before showering and putting it back on after.

Ease of Use

Ease of use is often referred to as usability, that includes characteristics such as: (1) learnability, how easily users can accomplish basic tasks the first time they use the system; (2) efficiency, how fast users can perform a task after they have learned the design; (3) memorability, how easily users can re-establish good use of the system; (4) low error rate; (5) satisfaction, how pleasant users find the system; and (6) utility, the functionality of the system (Nielsen, 2012). Usability has been a major factor and challenge for the implementation of the CONNECARE app as indicated by the lower satisfaction rating of the app compared with the Fitbit which is perceived as easy to learn and easy to use, error free, and satisfying to use. The usability of the app improved over the course of the project and was reflected in increasing use of additional features beyond counting steps as the project progressed.

Training and Support

Training and Support have been crucial in the CONNECARE project. Training consisted of face-to-face on hands training supplemented by a very detailed users' manual with many visual aids and screen shots of all of the app's screens with arrows and detailed instructions illustrating all of the functions. Nonetheless, repeated training has been necessary frequently and staff reports repeated phone conversations sometimes as long as a half an hour re-explaining and walking the patient through the use of the app and the Fitbit. In addition to the ongoing support of the nurse case managers, technical support has been provided where necessary. This is consistent with Leung et al. (2012) results regarding how older adults learn to use mobile technology. Leung et al. showed that the preference for trial-and-error decreases with age, and while over half of older respondents and participants preferred using the instruction manual, many reported difficulties using it. A useful approach was found to be an example help system, Help Kiosk, designed to support older adults' learning to use mobile devices.

Usage Rating

The McGaughey et al. (2013) model categorized usage as being high, medium or low. In the words of the authors: "Use can be low, as in the case when a senior owns a smartphone and uses it only for making calls, or perhaps not at all. High use as we define it, is not just using a lot of minutes for phone calls, it is getting the full benefit of the device's functionality, like taking pictures, sending text messages, using the calendar, alarms, or reminders, etc. Moderate use lies somewhere between the two extremes" (p. 190). Based on the preliminary data presented in this chapter on the results of the first 6 months of the CONNECARE pilot, as measured against the McGaughey et al. (2013) research framework, it can be concluded that on average, usage of the CONNECARE mobile platform for patients at this stage in the project can be rated as medium/moderate, with the app having a relatively low usage, both in terms of frequency of use and the number of functions used and the Fitbit having a relatively high usage. The analysis that has been done here together with insights from the literature, suggest that the usage of the CONNECARE app could be improved by introducing additional features that would increase the patients' motivation to use more of the system's functions with greater frequency. This could include additional quality of life components such as a feature that would enable messaging and easy communication with family and friends in addition to communication with the Nurse Case Managers and additional memory aids like appointments and a broader spectrum of reminders (Kurniawan, 2008). Motivation might also be increased if the app could be more flexible with regards to the type of activity it automatically tracks and not be limited to automatic tracking of steps alone (Coughlin et al., 2016). Other aspects that may increase motivation are rewards/positive feedback for the performance of assigned tasks and gamifications (West et al., 2017).

CONCLUSION

An important limitation of the lessons learned is that the CONNECARE mobile technology was developed as part of a research and development project and is constantly being upgraded in response to patient and staff feedback. Thus, at this point in time, the CONNECARE mobile app is not a finished product ready to go to market and will continue to be improved over the next 6 months. Nonetheless, important lessons have been learned that may be applicable in general to the use of mobile technology by older adults in the healthcare setting:

1. In 2019, as opposed to a decade ago, it is increasingly difficult to make generalizations about the needs and skills of "older adults". Most older adults have mobile phones. Many older adults use basic apps. While only 72% of the patients are using their smartphones in this project, this is not because they don't have a smartphone, but because they have a model not capable of supporting the CONNECARE app, which may, in fact, be a limitation of the app. Likewise, as seen from patient comments, responses to the app vary greatly: some patients don't like it and some patients love it.
2. Older adults, in general, still do not use mobile technology with the same ease as people under the age of 40, for whom smartphones are second nature and are rapidly replacing all other IT devices. WhatsApp is rapidly replacing email. Older adults (particularly above the age of 70) are using fewer functionalities than younger people, are using those functionalities that are easy to learn and easy to use, and that provide them with significant added value.
3. The CONNECARE experience so far raises the question as to how much benefit older adults see in health monitoring. The Fitbit watch is a simple, easy to use technology and yet only 82% of the study participants were willing to use it on a regular basis.
4. The fairly overwhelming preference for the Fitbit over the app suggests the most successful mobile technology for older adults (and perhaps the younger population as well) may be wearables, but would prefer wearables that are waterproof and have overcome the limitation of needing to be recharged.
5. Andrew Sixsmith in his chapter on Technology and the Challenge of Aging (2013) makes a point of emphasizing that mobile technologies in healthcare *cannot work in isolation, and should be seen as part of an integrated care solution that enhances the formal and informal networks of care that already exist.* The CONNECARE experience supports this. Many patients were able to overcome the obstacles and use both the Fitbit and the app because it was a part of their relationship with the clinical staff and because the clinical staff urged them to use it and supported them in their use. In assessing the technology and the project using the various questionnaires, patients tended to comment on the project as a whole, not only the mobile technology, confirming that they recognized it was part of a larger program.

It would appear to be a foregone conclusion that smartphones are becoming ubiquitous even among older adults and that they use an increasing number of apps that they perceive as enabling them to do things that are important to them. However, medical and healthcare apps are not among the most used. A recently published AARP research report on a representative sample of 1520 Americans 50+ found that 73% of the 50-69 age group and 55% of the 70+ group owned a smartphone. Yet, only 33% of the 60-69 group and 21% of the 70+ group used apps to manage or receive medical care (Anderson, 2017). There is a consensus in the literature that health and medical care management apps have great potential and at the same time are facing hurdles in adoption. The area in which research has thus far not been sufficient is in the implementation of healthcare management apps by healthcare organizations such as HMOs, Health Plans, or Regional and National Health systems. All of the Health Plans in Israel have apps that enable their members to access their patient portals on their mobile phones, that enable them to see their medical information and even to perform functions such as renewing prescriptions and making appointments, but the development of organization-wide apps for tracking vital signs and managing care are still in their infancy. This adds an additional dimension of importance to the CONNECARE project, which aims to implement a multi-functional healthcare management app within a hospital and community healthcare organization setting in order to support patient empowerment and integrated care. The lessons learned thus far can be useful in informing healthcare organizations and systems as they move forward acting as a catalyst for further research in this area.

REFERENCES

Anderson, G. O. (2017). Technology Use and Attitudes among Mid-Life and Older Americans, AARP research. Retrieved from https://www.aarp.org/content/dam/aarp/research/surveys_statistics/technology/info-2018/atom-nov-2017-tech-module.doi.10.26419%252Fres.00210.001.pdf

Bexelius, C., Löf, M., Sandin, S., Trolle Lagerros, Y., Forsum, E., & Litton, J. E. (2010). Measures of physical activity using cell phones: Validation using criterion methods. *Journal of Medical Internet Research*, *12*(1), e2. doi:10.2196/jmir.1298 PMID:20118036

Carrasco, M. P., Salvador, C. H., Sagredo, P. G., Márquez-Montes, J., González de Mingo, M. A., Fragua, J. A., ... Monteagudo, J. L. (2008). Impact of patient-general practitioner short-messages-based interaction on the control of hypertension in a follow-up service for low-to-medium risk hypertensive patients: A randomized controlled trial. *IEEE Transactions on Information Technology in Biomedicine*, *12*(6), 780–791. doi:10.1109/TITB.2008.926429 PMID:19000959

Coughlin, S.S., Whitehead, M., Sheats, J.Q., Mastromonico, J., & Smith, S. (2016). A Review of Smartphone Applications for Promoting Physical Activity. Jacobs J. Community Med, 2, 021.

Europe, W. H. O. (2016). Strengthening people-centred health systems in the WHO European Region: framework for action on integrated health services delivery. Retrieved from http://www.euro.who.int/__data/assets/pdf_file/0004/315787/66wd15e_FFA_IHSD_160535.pdf?ua=1

European Commission. (2017). Expert Group on Health Systems Performance Assessment, BLOCKS. Tools and methodologies to assess integrated care in Europe. Retrieved from http://ec.europa.eu/health/sites/health/files/systems_performance_assessment/docs/2017_blocks_en_0.pdf

Gao, J., & Koronios A. (2010). Mobile Application Development for Senior Citizens. PACIS 2010 Proceedings, 65.

Huckman, R. S., & Stern, A. D. (2018). Why Apps for Managing Chronic Disease Haven't Been Widely Used, and How to Fix It. *Harvard business Review*. Retrieved from https://hbr.org/2018/04/why-apps-for-managing-chronic-disease-havent-been-widely-used-and-how-to-fix-it

Hurst, J. (2018). The Best Apps and Tools for Older People. Retrieved from https://www.lifehack.org/278271/the-best-apps-and-tools-for-older-people

iYogi. (2018). 10 Best Medical Apps for Seniors. Retrieved from www.iyogi.com/editors-pick/10-best-medical-apps-for-seniors.html

Jorunn, L. H., Beatrix, V., Clemens, B., Chris, T., Taraldsen, K., Pijnappels, M., ... Mellone, S. (2017). Mobile Health Applications to Promote Active and Healthy Ageing. *Sensors (Basel)*, *17*(3), 622. doi:10.339017030622 PMID:28335475

Kagolianni, A. (2011). Factors affect in patient adherence to medication regimen. *Health Science Journal*, *5*(3), 157–158.

Kodner, L. D., & Spreeuwenberg, C. (2002). Integrated care: Meaning, logic, applications, and implications – a discussion paper. *International Journal of Integrated Care*, *2*(4), e12. doi:10.5334/ijic.67 PMID:16896389

Kurniawan, S. (2008). Older people and mobile phones: A multi-method investigation. *International Journal of Human-Computer Studies*, *66*(12), 889–901. doi:10.1016/j.ijhcs.2008.03.002

Lester, R. T., Ritvo, P., Mills, E. J., Kariri, A., Karanja, S., Chung, M. H., ... Plummer, F. A. (2010). Effects of a mobile phone short message service on antiretroviral treatment adherence in Kenya (WelTel Kenya1): A randomised trial. *Lancet*, *376*(9755), 1838–1845. doi:10.1016/S0140-6736(10)61997-6 PMID:21071074

Leung, R., Tang, C., Haddad, S., McGrenere, J., Graf, P., & Ingriany, V. (2012). How older adults learn to use mobile devices: Survey and field investigations. ACM Trans, 3, Article 11.

Lin, C. J., Hsieh, T. L., & Shiang, W. J. (2009). Exploring the Interface Design of Mobile Phone for the Elderly. *Human Centered Design*, *5619*, 476–481. doi:10.1007/978-3-642-02806-9_55

Martína, L., Martinb, S., & Medranoa, C. (2011). Mobile applications in an aging society: Status and trends Inmaculada Plazaa. *Journal of Systems and Software*, *84*(11), 1977–1988. doi:10.1016/j.jss.2011.05.035

McGaughey, R., Zeltmann, S. M., & McMurtrey, M. (2013). Motivations and obstacles to smartphone use by the elderly: Developing a research framework. *International. Journal of Electronic Finance*, *7*(3/4), 177–195. doi:10.1504/IJEF.2013.058601

Nielsen, J. (2012). Usability 101: Introduction to Usability. Retrieved from https://www.nngroup.com/articles/usability-101-introduction-to-usability

Pinnock, H., Barwick, M., Carpenter, C. R., Eldridge, S., Grandes, G., Griffiths, C. J., ... Taylor, S. J. C. (2017). Standards for Reporting Implementation Studies (StaRI): Explanation and elaboration document. *BMJ Open*, *7*(4). doi:10.1136/bmjopen-2016-013318 PMID:28373250

Quinn, C. C., Shardell, M. D., Terrin, M. L., Barr, E. A., Ballew, S. H., & Gruber-Baldini, A. L. (2011). Cluster-randomized trial of a mobile phone personalized behavioral intervention for blood glucose control. *Diabetes Care*, *34*(9), 1934–1942. doi:10.2337/dc11-0366 PMID:21788632

Sixsmith, A. (2013). Chapter 2 Technology and the Challenge of Aging. In A. Sixsmith, & G. Gutman (Eds.), Technologies for Active Aging, 7 International Perspectives on Aging, Springer Science+Business Media, New York, NY. p. 10-11.

West, J. H., Belvedere, L. M., Andreasen, R., Frandsen, C., Hall, P. C., & Crookston, B. T. (2017). Controlling Your "App"etite: How Diet and Nutrition-Related Mobile Apps Lead to Behavior Change. *JMIR mHealth and uHealth*, *5*(7), e95. doi:10.2196/mhealth.7410 PMID:28694241

Young, S. L. (2007). Older adults' user experiences with mobile phones: identification of user clusters and user requirements. (*Dissertation submitted to the Faculty of the Virginia Polytechnic Institute and State University in partial fulfillment of the requirements for the degree of Doctor of Philosophy in Industrial and Systems Engineering*).

KEY TERMS AND DEFINITIONS

AAL (Ambient Assisted Living Program): A funding program that works towards creating market-ready products and services for older people, co-financed by the European Commission (through HORIZON 2020) and 17 countries.

Case Management: A collaborative process of assessment, planning and care coordination to meet an individual's comprehensive healthcare needs coordinated by a designated case manager – in the case of CONNECARE in Israel, by nurse case managers.

CONNECARE: Acronym for "Personalised Connected Care for Complex Chronic Patients" the formal name of the project funded by a grant from the European Commission.

Digitally Enabled Integrated Care: Integrated health and social care that coordinate the care for a patient among the various sectors – hospital, primary care, specialist care and social services supported by digital technologies such as electronic medical/health records, case management platforms, patient portals, mobile technology, etc.

Digital Single Market: A policy belonging to the European Single market that covers digital marketing, e-commerce and telecommunications. It is a part of the Digital Agenda for Europe 2020 as defined in the document *A Digital Single Market for Europe* by the European Commission published in May 2015.

Elective Surgery: Surgery that is scheduled in advance because it does not involve a medical emergency.

Electronic Medical Records (EMRs): Digital versions of patient charts in clinician offices, clinics, health plans and hospitals, mostly used for diagnosis and treatment in this chapter. Used interchangeably with electronic health records that contain information from most or all clinicians involved in the patient's care, at least within a given sector such as a community network or a hospital.

HORIZON 2020 Program: The HORIZON 2020 program is the 8th iteration of the European Framework Program for Research and Innovation that is financed and operated by the European Commission and provides grants to proposals responding to published calls from 2014-2020.

Implementation Research: An integrated concept that links research and practice in order to improve the implementation of health policies, programs and practices. It is multidisciplinary and focuses on practical approaches to improve implementation and to enhance equity, efficiency, scale-up, sustainability and ultimately, to improve people's health.

Maccabi Healthcare Services: The second largest Health Fund in Israel covering 25% of the population (more than 2 million people) responsible for covering and providing all of the services in the public basket of services under the Israel National Health Insurance Law.

Maccabi Integrated Care Unit: This unit is operated by Maccabi and physically situated in Samson Assuta Ashdod Hospital. Its purpose is to do joint discharge planning with hospital staff for Maccabi patients and to assure a seamless transition back to the community by coordinating the services required by the patient in the community post discharge.

Samson Assuta Ashdod Hospital: The newest public general hospital to be built in Israel – the first after 40 years – in the city of Ashdod, Israel's fifth largest city. The hospital opened its doors in 2017 and aims to be a hub for integrated care, working cooperatively with Israel's four Health Funds and Social Services.

APPENDIX

Table 2. Demographic variables of 59 patients recruited July 2018 - February 2019

Patient number	Recruitment date	Age	Gender	Marital status	Education level	Socio-economic	Status 02/2019
1001	01/08/2018	61	female	Married	Tertiary	Medium	Released at the end
1002	31/07/2018	70	female	Married	BA	High	Released at the end
1003	01/08/2018	65	male	Married	Tertiary	Medium	Released at the end
1004	06/08/2018	65	female	Married	MA	Medium	Left ahead of schedule
1005	15/08/2018	65	male	Married	BA	Medium	Released at the end
1006	27/08/2018	68	female	Married	BA	Medium	Released at the end
1007	17/09/2018	79	male	Married	Tertiary	Medium	Released at the end
1008	25/09/2018	70	male	Married	High school	Medium	Released at the end
1009	25/09/2018	65	female	Married	BA	Medium	Released at the end
1010	11/10/2018	61	female	Married	High school	Medium	Left ahead of schedule
1011	15/10/2018	74	male	Divorcee	High school	Medium	Left ahead of schedule
1012	16/10/2018	69	male	Married	Tertiary	Medium	Released at the end
1013	17/10/2018	68	male	Married	Tertiary	Medium	Released at the end
1014	23/10/2018	75	female	Married	High school	Medium	Released at the end
1015	23/10/2018	59	female	Divorcee	Tertiary	Low	Left ahead of schedule
1016	13/11/2018	78	male	Married	Tertiary	Low	Released at the end
1017	11/11/2018	68	female	Married	MA	Medium	Released at the end
1018	06/11/2018	64	female	Divorcee	Tertiary	Medium	Left ahead of schedule
1019	07/11/2018	70	male	Married	BA	Medium	Released at the end
1020	23/11/2018	69	male	Married	MA	Medium	Active followup
1021	29/11/2018	71	male	Married	MA	Medium	Active followup
1022	02/12/2018	72	female	Married	MA	Medium	Active followup
1023	03/12/2018	66	male	Widower	High school	Medium	Left ahead of schedule
1024	04/12/2018	71	male	Divorcee	Tertiary	Medium	Active followup
1025	05/12/2018	61	female	Divorcee	Tertiary	Medium	Left ahead of schedule
1026	18/12/2018	69	female	Married	BA	Low	Active followup
1027	16/12/2018	66	female	Married	High school	Medium	Active followup
1028	23/12/2018	69	male	Married	Tertiary	Medium	Active followup
1029	26/12/2018	72	female	Widow	MA	Medium	Active followup
1030	01/01/2019	63	male	Divorcee	Tertiary	Medium	Active followup
1031	01/01/2019	72	female	Married	High school	High	Active followup
1032	08/01/2019	75	female	Divorcee	MA	Low	Left ahead of schedule
1033	15/01/2019	69	male	Married	Tertiary	Medium	Active followup
1034	20/01/2019	71	female	Widow	MA	Medium	Left ahead of schedule

continues on following page

Table 2. Continued

Patient number	Recruitment date	Age	Gender	Marital status	Education level	Socio-economic	Status 02/2019
1035	11/02/2019	71	male	Married	MA	Medium	Active followup
1036	06/02/2019	68	male	Married	Tertiary	Medium	Active followup
1037	06/02/2019	64	female	Married	Tertiary	Medium	Active followup
1038	13/02/2019	71	male	Married	BA	High	Active followup
2001	12/07/2018	60	female	Married	High school	Medium	Released at the end
2002	16/07/2018	71	male	Married	MA	Medium	Released at the end
2003	20/08/2018	78	female	Married	Tertiary	Medium	Left ahead of schedule
2004	13/09/2018	60	female	Married	High school	Medium	Released at the end
2005	25/09/2018	62	male	Married	Tertiary	Medium	Left ahead of schedule
2006	07/10/2018	60	female	Divorcee	Tertiary	Medium	Left ahead of schedule
2007	10/10/2018	60	female	Divorcee	Tertiary	Medium	Released at the end
2008	25/10/2018	66	male	Married	High school	Medium	Left ahead of schedule
2010	20/11/2018	72	female	Married	MD / PHD	Medium	Active followup
2011	22/11/2018	61	male	Married	BA	Medium	Active followup
2012	03/12/2018	69	male	Married	Tertiary	Medium	Active followup
2013	04/12/2018	70	female	Divorcee	High school	Medium	Active followup
2014	12/12/2018	61	male	Married	BA	Medium	Active followup
2015	26/12/2018	68	male	Divorcee	MD / PHD	High	Active followup
2016	31/12/2018	60	female	Married	MD / PHD	Medium	Left ahead of schedule
2017	13/01/2019	62	female	Married	High school	Medium	Active followup
2018	14/01/2019	58	female	Married	Tertiary	Medium	Active followup
2019	28/01/2019	58	female	Married	High school	Medium	Active followup
2020	31/01/2019	62	male	Married	BA	Medium	Active followup
2021	11/02/2019	58	male	Married	Tertiary	Medium	Active followup
2022	11/02/2019	60	female	Married	High school	Medium	Active followup

Table 3. Actual use of mobile technologies (N=59)

Patient number	Equipment	Steps monitoring	Tasks	Blood pressure	Messages
1001	Personal mobile phone	V	partial	V	NR
1002	Personal mobile phone	V	V	V	NR
1003	Tablet	V	X	NR	NR
1004	Personal mobile phone	NR	NR	NR	NR
1005	Tablet	partial	X	NR	NR
1006	Personal mobile phone	X	X	NR	NR
1007	Tablet	V	partial	X	V

continues on following page

Table 3. Continued

Patient number	Equipment	Steps monitoring	Tasks	Blood pressure	Messages
1008	Personal mobile phone	V	partial	NR	X
1009	Personal mobile phone	partial	X	X	X
1010	Personal mobile phone	NR	NR	NR	NR
1011	Personal mobile phone	X	X	NR	X
1012	Personal mobile phone	V	X	NR	X
1013	Personal mobile phone	V	X	V	X
1014	Personal mobile phone	X	X	NR	X
1015	Personal mobile phone	NR	NR	NR	NR
1016	Tablet	X	X	X	X
1017	Tablet	V	V	V	V
1018	Personal mobile phone	X	X	X	X
1019	Personal mobile phone	V	V	NR	X
1020	Tablet	V	X	V	X
1021	Tablet	partial	X	NR	X
1022	Personal mobile phone	V	V	V	X
1023	Personal mobile phone	NR	NR	NR	NR
1024	Personal mobile phone	X	X	NR	X
1025	Personal mobile phone	partial	X	NR	X
1026	Personal mobile phone	partial	X	partial	X
1027	Personal mobile phone	V	V	V	V
1028	Personal mobile phone	V	V	V	V
1029	Tablet	partial	X	X	X
1030	Tablet	V	partial	V	V
1031	Personal mobile phone	V	X	NR	X
1032	Personal mobile phone	X	X	X	X
1033	Personal mobile phone	V	partial	NR	X
1034	Personal mobile phone	X	X	NR	X
1035	Tablet	V	V	NR	V
1036	Tablet	V	X	NR	X
1037	Tablet	V	V	NR	V
1038	Personal mobile phone	V	V	NR	X
2001	Personal mobile phone	partial	partial	NR	NR
2002	Tablet	V	V	NR	NR
2003	Personal mobile phone	partial	X	NR	NR
2004	Personal mobile phone	V	V	V	V
2005	Personal mobile phone	partial	X	X	X

continues on following page

Table 3. Continued

Patient number	Equipment	Steps monitoring	Tasks	Blood pressure	Messages
2006	Personal mobile phone	partial	X	X	X
2007	Personal mobile phone	V	V	V	V
2008	Personal mobile phone	X	X	NR	X
2010	Tablet	partial	X	NR	X
2011	Personal mobile phone	V	X	NR	X
2012	Personal mobile phone	partial	X	NR	X
2013	Personal mobile phone	V	partial	X	partial
2014	Personal mobile phone	V	V	NR	X
2015	Tablet	X	X	X	X
2016	Personal mobile phone	partial	X	NR	V
2017	Personal mobile phone	V	V	NR	V
2018	Tablet	V	V	NR	X
2019	Personal mobile phone	V	X	NR	X
2020	Tablet	V	V	NR	V
2021	Personal mobile phone	V	X	NR	V
2022	Personal mobile phone	V	X	NR	V

Table 4. Technology satisfaction questionnaire (N=18)

Patient number	Fitbit watch				Connecare App			
	Overall impression	User friendliness	Ability to use	Would you recommend this to someone else?	Overall impression	User friendliness	Ability to use	Would you recommend this to someone else?
1001	10	10	10	10	NA	NA	NA	NA
1002	10	10	5	9	9	9	5	NA
1003	7	8	6	10	5	7	4	10
1005	9	9	10	8	7	5	8	6
1006	5	3	3	NA	1	NA	NA	NA
1007	10	10	10	10	8	8	8	8
1008	10	10	10	10	NA	NA	NA	NA
1012	5	3	9	NA	6	6	7	NA
1013	10	8	10	10	4	5	2	2
1014	10	8	10	9	3	3	3	3
1017	10	10	10	10	10	10	10	10
1018	NA	NA	NA	NA	NA	NA	NA	NA
1019	10	10	10	NA	NA	NA	NA	NA

continues on following page

Table 4. Continued

Patient number	Fitbit watch				Connecare App			
	Overall impression	User friendliness	Ability to use	Would you recommend this to someone else?	Overall impression	User friendliness	Ability to use	Would you recommend this to someone else?
1020	10	10	10	10	10	7	7	10
2002	10	10	10	10	7	7	10	7
2004	10	10	10	10	10	10	10	10
2009	NA	NA	NA	NA	NA	NA	NA	NA
2011	8	9	8	8	8	9	8	8
Average	**9.00**	**8.63**	**8.81**	**9.54**	**6.77**	**7.17**	**6.83**	**7.40**

Table 5. System usability scale questionnaire (N=18)

Q1	I think that I would like to use this system frequently
Q2	I found the system unnecessarily complex
Q3	I thought the system was easy to use
Q4	I would need the support of a technical person to be able to use this system
Q5	I found the various functions in this system were well integrated
Q6	I thought there was too much inconsistency in this system
Q7	I would imagine that most people would learn to use this system very quickly
Q8	I found the system very cumbersome to use
Q9	I felt very confident using the system
Q10	I needed to learn a lot of things before I could get going with this system

Table 6. Patient responses

Patient number	Q1	Q2	Q3	Q4	Q5	Q6	Q7	Q8	Q9	Q10
1001	2	3	3	3	3	NA	NA	NA	NA	NA
1002	1	2	4	1	3	3	4	2	4	4
1003	5	2	4	5	5	2	5	2	5	4
1005	2	3	3	2	2	3	3	3	3	3
1006	1	5	1	5	1	1	1	5	1	5
1007	5	2	4	4	4	1	4	2	4	2
1008	5	1	5	1	5	1	3	1	3	3
1012	1	2	4	2	4	2	4	2	4	2
1013	1	5	2	2	2	3	2	4	2	4
1014	2	3	3	2	3	3	4	2	3	4

continues on following page

Table 6. Continued

Patient number	Q1	Q2	Q3	Q4	Q5	Q6	Q7	Q8	Q9	Q10
1017	2	2	5	1	4	2	5	1	5	2
1018	3	3	3	5	3	2	2	2	3	3
1019	2	5	3	3	4	4	3	2	3	2
1020	5	2	2	2	4	2	4	2	2	3
2002	3	2	4	2	4	4	2	3	3	1
2004	5	2	5	2	4	2	4	1	5	1
2009	NA	NA	NA	NA	NA	NA	NA	NA	NA	NA
2011	4	2	4	2	4	2	4	2	4	2
Average	2.88	2.71	3.47	2.59	3.47	2.31	3.38	2.25	3.38	2.81
% of respondents over 3	35%	18%	53%	24%	59%	12%	53%	12%	41%	29%

Table 7. Person-centered coordinated care experiences questionnaire (N=18)

Q1	F1. Did you discuss what was most important for YOU in managing your own health and wellbeing?
Q2	F2. Were you involved as much as you wanted to be in decisions about your care?
Q3	F3. Were you considered as a 'whole person' rather than just a disease/condition in relation to your care?
Q4	F4. Did your care-team involve your family/friends/carers as much as you wanted?
Q5	F5. Did you have enough support from your care team to help YOU to manage your own health and wellbeing?
Q6	F6. Did you receive useful information at the time you need it to help you manage your health and wellbeing?

Table 8. Responses

Patient #	Q1	Q2	Q3	Q4	Q5	Q6
1001	3	4	4	2	2	4
1002	1	2	4	4	4	4
1003	2	4	1	1	4	4
1005	1	1	1	1	1	1
1006	4	4	4	1	4	4
1007	2	4	4	NA	4	4
1008	4	4	4	4	4	4
1012	1	1	2	1	1	1
1013	4	4	4	4	4	4
1014	4	3	4	3	4	4
1017	4	4	4	4	4	4
1018	4	3	3	1	3	3
1019	1	1	4	4	1	1
1020	2	2	2	NA	4	4

continues on following page

Table 8. Continued

Patient #	Q1	Q2	Q3	Q4	Q5	Q6
2002	2	2	4	1	2	3
2004	1	2	1	1	2	1
2009	2	4	4	2	4	4
2011	4	4	1	NA	4	4
Average	2.56	2.94	3.06	2.27	3.11	3.22
% of respondents over 3	39%	50%	61%	28%	61%	67%

Table 9. Items G1-G4 adapted from the Nijmegen continuity questionnaire (N=18)

Q1	G1. My care providers transfer information very well to one-another
Q2	G2. My care providers work together very well
Q3	G3. My care providers are very well connected
Q4	G4. My care providers always know what one-another is doing
Q5	G5. I have to wait too long to obtain a service or appointment

Table 10. Responses to items G1-G4 adapted from the Nijmegen continuity questionnaire

Patient number	Q1	Q2	Q3	Q4	Q5
1001	1	1	1	1	4
1002	1	1	1	NA	5
1003	1	1	1	1	2
1005	1	1	NA	3	4
1006	3	1	2	2	3
1007	NA	2	2	NA	NA
1008	NA	NA	1	NA	NA
1012	2	4	NA	4	NA
1013	1	1	1	1	NA
1014	1	1	1	1	4
1017	NA	1	1	1	1
1018	2	2	3	2	1
1019	NA	NA	NA	1	5
1020	2	2	2	2	4
2002	2	3	3	NA	NA
2004	1	2	NA	1	NA
2009	1	1	1	1	1
2011	1	1	1	1	5
Average	1.43	1.56	1.50	1.57	3.25
% of respondents less than 3	72%	78%	67%	67%	22%

Chapter 16
mHealth Collaboration for Social Good:
Lessons on Adaptability

Hope Koch
Baylor University, USA

Shelby L. Garner
Baylor University, USA

Gina Green
Baylor University, USA

Julia Hitchcock
Baylor University, USA

Zonayed Mahid
Washington State University, USA

Carolin Elizabeth George
Bangalore Baptist Hospital, India

Philip Young
Baylor University, USA

ABSTRACT

The World Health Organization lauds mobile health (mHealth) technology as a means of creating stronger healthcare systems and improving health-related outcomes. This chapter reports on an action research study examining the development of a mHealth technology hypertension app to help people living in India's urban slums and rural villages take better care of their health. The collaboration involved a multidisciplinary team of U.S.-based academic researchers, and India-based healthcare and technology professionals. This study suggests that traditional Western-based project management approaches alone are insufficient when developing technology for social good. Specifically, the study finds that team, process, and technology adaptability are key to successfully developing healthcare technology to serve at-risk populations in resource-constrained areas. Implications of these findings to systems development research are discussed.

DOI: 10.4018/978-1-7998-0047-7.ch016

INTRODUCTION

Mobile Health (hereinafter mHealth) technologies have the potential to improve the accessibility to and personalization of medical care, particularly in limited resource settings (WHO Global Observatory for eHealth, 2011). The World Health Organization (WHO) describes mHealth as using mobile technologies to support public health practice, and advocates for its use to improve health care delivery systems around the world (2011). Mobile technologies may be particularly useful in India given the country's large percentage of people lacking basic health care and the country's technical prowess (Garner, Sudia, & Rachaprolu, 2018). In recent years smart phone and Internet access has surpassed roadway and other infrastructure in India (Garner et al., 2018). In one study, many physicians and nurses report using smart phones to support their everyday health care practice in India. Unfortunately, these healthcare providers struggle to find credible and culturally appropriate mHealth applications to teach the population about the growing rate of non-communicable diseases like hypertension. Most mobile resources currently available in India were created in the western world with many concepts that may not translate to the Indian population where diet and lifestyle are different (Garner et al., 2018).

This chapter reports on an action research project aimed at developing a mHealth application to help people living in India's urban slums and rural villages understand how to prevent and manage hypertension. Hypertension is a major contributor to cardiovascular disease, and is the leading cause of death in India and around the globe (World Health Organization, 2016; Zhou et al., 2017). This chapter describes the creation of a hypertension mHealth application that overcame the shortcomings of other health applications used in India's urban slums and rural villages.

The development team included a cross-cultural, multi-disciplinary group of medical, technology and creative professionals who donated resources to the project. The development team's belief systems, values and realities often starkly contrasted with the daily realities of the people it aimed to help with the mHealth application. This divide made conducting analysis with the people difficult and pushed the boundaries of traditional systems development theories (Walls, Widmeyer, & El Sawy, 1992). In fact, the team found that many traditional project management and control techniques were ineffective (Tiwana & Keil, 2009) and bringing this project to successful completion required adaptability. The objective of this research is to highlight the role of adaptability, not project management control techniques, in developing mHealth systems to help people with limited resources, education and access to health care take better care of their health.

BACKGROUND

This section highlights insights from the research streams that informed the study. These streams include: mHealth, systems development project management, social innovation collaboration and adaptability.

Implications and Benefits of mHealth

The rapid global advancement of wireless mobile technologies and recent proliferation of cellular networks in growing economies such as India, creates an optimal milieu for mHealth use (WHO Global Observatory for eHealth, 2011). Ninety percent of people living in a low and middle income countries have access to a mobile phone with mobile-cellular subscriptions (Sondaal et al., 2016). The United Nations and World Health Organization report that mHealth application are effective in improving health outcomes world-wide and reducing disease burdens such as HIV/AIDS, tuberculosis and malaria. In health care, a variety of disciplines are testing the effectiveness of mHealth including general, specialized, emergency, and disaster health services (WHO Global Observatory for eHealth, 2011).

Several health care studies highlight the promise of mHealth. A systematic review designed to assess the effect of mHealth interventions for women, before during and after pregnancy, finds that mHealth interventions increase women's use of health services, health facilities, and vaccination rates (Sondaal et al., 2016). In India, mHealth studies find that unidirectional text messaging is an effective way to remind patients about follow-up care (Sondaal et al., 2016). Given the encouraging results of mHealth, researchers need to design and test mHealth applications for vulnerable populations such as people who cannot read and do not have the financial resources to pay for cellular service (Walsham, 2017). A review of the mHealth literature and practice indicates that India's most vulnerable populations do not have access to culturally appropriate apps to teach them how to improve their health outcomes.

Managing Systems Development

Developing a culturally appropriate app requires systems development and project management processes. The former refers to the broad set of activities performed to ensure the accurate and efficient definition, design and implementation of software artifacts. Project management refers to the broad set of activities required to plan, coordinate and track the work of individuals involved in the systems development effort to ensure stated objectives are met. Without these processes, mistakes can occur. Four common categories of project mistakes include people, process, product, and technology (Nelson, 2007). Given that 88% of reported IS project mistakes are people or process related (Nelson, 2007), effective project management is essential.

One of the definitive sources of project management best practices comes from the Project Management Institute (PMI). The PMI (2017) developed the "Project Management Body of Knowledge" which defines project management as "the application of knowledge, skills, tools, and techniques to project activities to meet project requirements. The PMI decomposes project management into initiation, planning, executing, monitoring and controlling, and closing. Monitoring, often discussed as an antecedent to or part of control, involves obtaining information about a controlee's behavior, as opposed to control, which is acting on that information to change a controlee's behavior (Eisenhardt, 1985).

Control is important in outsourced IS development projects, where the controller (i.e., the client) and the controlee (i.e., the vendor) may have different priorities given that they work for different organizations often in different countries (Dibbern, Goles, Hirschheim, & Jayatilaka, 2004). A comprehensive review of research on IS project control finds that communicational and evaluational congruence are critical in outsourced systems development projects (Wiener et al., 2016). Organizations often outsource routine projects with clear, measurable objectives such as updating legacy systems, building programs to execute core functions like billing and accounting, and routine website maintenance (Dibbern et al., 2004). In these cases, contracts and compensation define the controllers' and the controlees' roles and align their objectives. IS research on outsourced systems that require elements of creativity and entertainment is limited (Dibbern et al., 2004). Additionally, little is known about what controller-controlee relationships look like when building technology for social good, and when IS success depends on voluntarily use of the system.

Social Innovation Collaborations

When building systems to empower vulnerable populations to take better care of their health, a social innovation collaboration approach, rather than the traditional control relationships discussed above, may be more effective. Social innovation collaborations bring together stakeholders from a variety of disciplines as partners, rather than as controllers and controlees, to develop social goods (Phills, Deiglmeier, & Miller, 2008). A social good is "a novel solution to a social problem that is more effective, efficient, sustainable, or just than the existing solutions and for which the value created accrues primarily to society as a whole rather than private individuals (Phills et al., 2008, p. 36)."

Insights from social innovation collaboration studies suggest integrating adaptability and flexibility with control techniques that are typically used in systems development. A study of a social innovation collaboration between nonprofit organizations finds that stakeholder flexibility is necessary to sustain initiatives to successful conclusions; yet too much variation in the development process may cause initiatives to deviate from the original purpose (Dufour, Lessard, & Chamberland, 2014, p. 69). Similarly, when developing systems, research finds that adaptive leadership and the ability to adapt to change is vital to complex collaborations, but too little control can result in chaos (Augustine et al., 2005). These lessons suggest the need to supplement traditional control-based systems development processes with adaptability when developing technology in social innovation collaborations. However, little is known about what adaptability looks like in this context.

Adaptability

Adaptability is critical to innovation (Vorhies, Harker, & Rao, 1999). Adaptability recognizes that, at times, success depends on reconfiguring resources and goals in response to challenges and opportunities (Chakravarthy, 1982; Tuominen, Rajala, & Möller, 2004). Three types of adaptability inform this study: team adaptability, process adaptability and technology adaptability.

Team Adaptability. Teams that adapt to change perform better than those that do not (Salas, Sims, & Burke, 2005). Team adaptability is defined as "a change in team performance, in response to a salient cue or cue stream, that leads to a functional outcome for the entire team (Burke, Stagl, Salas, Pierce, & Kendall, 2006, p. 1190)." Adaptive teams can properly evaluate a situation, achieve a coherent understanding of the new situation, change their plans according to the new situation, coordinate their work in response to a change, and learn from their experience (Schmidt, Kude, Tripp, Heinzl, & Spohrer, 2013).

Adaptability is critical for social innovation collaboration teams because of the complexities these collaborations address and the limited resources. Many social innovation collaborations bring diverse stakeholders together to tackle serious problems such as the environment, poverty and health (Head & Alford, 2013). The magnitude of these problems, the uncertain environment, and the goal of creating a social good, rather than a profit, often involves limited financial resources to create the social good (Aarons, Hurlburt, & Horwitz, 2011). Given this, teams may have to adapt to new strategies, take on additional responsibilities or change processes (Richardson, Kettinger, Banks, & Quintana, 2014a).

Process adaptability. Process adaptability is the degree of discretion over work activities and decisions during a project (Tatikonda & Montoya-Weiss, 2001, p. 156). Process adaptability is critical when developing systems because system development is a complex process (Conboy, 2009). For example, the required functionality of a newly developed system is often ill-defined at the outset (Lee & Xia, 2005).

Changes in user requirements, priorities and external environments increase the complexity (Benbya & McKelvey, 2006). If not properly addressed, these changes could lead to project failure (Kappelman, McKeeman, & Zhang, 2006). A project teams' process adaptability impacts project performance (Lee & Xia, 2005) by speeding up the development process, reducing project time delays, and helping teams meet their development objectives (Susman & Dean Jr, 1992). Process adaptability is especially important when developing social good information technologies for marginalized populations (Oreglia & Srinivasan, 2016).

Technology adaptability: Technology adaptability refers to the extent that the developed system can support various technological needs (Tallon & Pinsonneault, 2011). Adaptable technology has several features that can accommodate environmental changes. These include the ability to adjust to changing requirements, easily modify the system and its components, and support different strategies (Patten, Whitworth, Fjermestad, & Mahindra, 2005). Adaptive technology may be especially important to address complex social problems because the environment is uncertain (Weber, Reichert, & Rinderle-Ma, 2008).

Summary

In summary, developing technology through a social innovation collaboration may require introducing elements of adaptability into the traditional systems development process. These elements might impact how the team functions, the process they use to develop the technology, and the technology itself. This chapter describes an action research project to develop and implement a mHealth application that helps people in India's urban slums and rural villages learn about hypertension and its effects on health. The following sections describe the research method and case background, followed by recommendations, and implications for future collaborations focused on developing technology for social good.

METHOD: ACTION RESEARCH

Research Setting: The Problem Situation

This chapter reports on a social innovation collaboration between U.S. based researchers, a hospital in India (hereinafter HospitalCo) and two India-based technology vendors (hereinafter AnimationCo and AppCo) to develop and implement mobile technology that helps marginalized and illiterate populations in India better understand hypertension. The social innovation collaboration was part of a university's initiative to bring researchers together to address serious problems facing society. This collaboration brought together researchers from nursing, art, statistics and information systems. These researchers partnered with practitioners from India including a leading hospital, an animation development company and an application development company. All names are pseudonyms.

Our initial theory was that the researchers could outsource building the mHealth app to vendors from India because these vendors could build a culturally tailored mHealth hypertension app at a reasonable cost. The researchers would apply traditional project management techniques to ensure the vendors developed a quality product, on-time. This report chronicles how this theory played out in this action research project. The project offers insight into the interactions between two socially and culturally different groups that collaborated to build the mHealth application. The researchers found that adaptability on the part of all stakeholders, especially the U.S. researchers, was critical in bringing the mHealth application to completion. This was critical in this social innovation collaboration where the environment was uncertain, resources were limited and most stakeholders donated resources to the project.

Why Action Research

Action research assumes that "the best way to study a complex social process is by introducing changes into that process and observing the effects. The theory underlying the intervention is validated by the extent to which these changes successfully solve problems in the setting" (Baskerville & Stage, 1996, p. 492). Involving "practical problem solving with theoretical relevance" (Mumford, 2001, p. 12), action research consists of the action and the reaction. The action is the intervention that attempts to remedy the real-world problem and the reaction is the stakeholder's response to the intervention. This study's intervention follows the five phases of the action research cycle: diagnosing, action planning, action taking, evaluating and specifying learning (Baskerville & Wood-Harper, 1996).

Data Collection

To understand the project context, the researchers used multiple data sources to triangulate findings including direct observation, group meetings, semi-structured interviews and e-mail communications. Data collection spanned February 2017-March 2018. The data collection efforts involved building a case study database with all data sources including transcribed interviews and 53 pages of field notes detailing all meetings, personal interactions and reflections on the project. Since the team was located in India and the U.S., most stakeholder communication occurred via email or Skype. The researchers collected 352 emails and observed ten Skype meetings, each approximately 60 minutes long. During the course of the study, the researchers interviewed every stakeholder involved in the project.

To analyze the data, the researchers used NVIVO, a qualitative analysis software package. This involved open and focused coding. This coding process allowed reviewing the projects' overall process and gaining greater insight into the interactions and collaboration between the U.S. and India stakeholders. As the researchers analyzed the data, the researchers wrote memos, had weekly discussions and read literature. The literature review spanned the fields of population health, social innovation collaboration and project management. The researchers initially relied upon control theory in IS project management to plan the project (Wiener et al., 2016). As the project unfolded, adaptability emerged as a key theme. As a result, the researchers reviewed the adaptability literature and reanalyzed the data identifying instances of adaptability. This analysis helped devise lessons for others engaged in cross-cultural, social innovation collaborations, to build technology for marginalized populations.

CASE: ADAPTABILITY IN DEVELOPING THE MHEALTH APP

This case describes how the researchers designed and built the mHealth hypertension application. This case illustrates how the researchers modified their initial theories of project management control with adaptability in order to develop a quality mHealth application on time.

Diagnosing: The Need to Scale Hypertension Education

The first step in the action research cycle is diagnosing, which involves defining the problem (Baskerville & Wood-Harper, 1996). The directors of HospitalCo's community health department were struggling to provide low-cost health services to the growing population of residents living in India's slums and rural areas. HospitalCo had approximately 20 community health workers tasked with serving more than 800,000 residents. In the quote below the assistant director of community health explains the challenges they faced reaching people who spoke different languages and had limited understanding of anatomy:

In our area, people speak 5-6 different languages with multiple dialects. People without education, were not able to understand the complexity of the disease. The fact that hypertension can affect many organs like the heart and kidney was tough for them to imagine when they do not know what heart and kidney means. Animation could make them understand all these concepts.

As the director of community health explains above, mobile technology could alleviate some of the current challenges and it promised more scalability and consistency than the current process of oral teaching with paper counseling cards. Moreover, the counseling cards portrayed Western characters and were not tailored to the target population's reality including living conditions, culture, language or educational levels. Developing a mHealth app to teach people about hypertension would allow HospitalCo's community health workers to reach more people and provide a consistent message. The app required several adaptability features including the ability to: (1) overcome language barriers with animation and translation into three languages; (2) divide the health message into short segments customized to the recipients' needs; and (3) collect data on knowledge, learning and social demographics.

Action Planning: Using Project Management to Plan the App's Development

HospitalCo needed a partner to fund and oversee the development of the mHealth app, launching the second stage of action research--action planning. In this stage, HospitalCo's community health directors shared their vision with their long-term partner—a nursing professor and researcher. The nursing researcher applied for a university funded social innovation grant to develop the mHealth app.

This grant required that the nursing professor (1) bring a cross-discipline group of researchers together to address some of the world's toughest problems and (2) develop innovative technology. The cross-discipline group of researchers brought creativity, project management, technology development and statistical expertise to address healthcare problems. The team envisioned developing a virtual reality simulation. Virtual reality involves "using computer graphics systems in combination with display and interface devices to create an interactive three-dimensional computer-generated environment that provides an immersion effect (Pan, Cheok, Yang, Zhu, & Shi, 2006)." Initially the team envisioned developing a character that participants could manipulate and see the health impacts. For example, having the character take a walk and lose weight.

In March 2017, AcademicU provided a $56,000 grant and the AcademicU-HospitalCo team began searching for external partners to build the technology. HospitalCo's community health directors recommended that AppCo build the application, which included a pre and post test to assess the app's effectiveness in teaching people about hypertension. This educational assessment had several *adaptability* features including: (1) the tests were in three different languages; (2) the app, health workers or participants could read the questions as well as listen to the questions; (3) when people missed a question the app gave the correct answer and allowed participants to replay and review animation segments; and (4) participants could skip questions. AppCo recommended that AnimationCo, a leading animation and entertainment provider in India, build the virtual reality portion of the mHealth app. After meeting with

Each stakeholder brought a unique, complementary resource. As Indian nationals, the stakeholders (i.e., AnimationCo, AppCo, and HospitalCo) understood India's norms including its culture, medical system and people. The community health directors offered medical and cultural consultation on the project and opportunities to test and implement the app with hundreds of people living in India's slums. The nursing professor managed the project and envisioned this as the beginning of many projects to address health issues in India. The researchers involved with this project coined themselves the "Healthy India Team."

In the action planning stage, the research team drew upon their combined field expertise to build their working theory about how to build the mHealth application. This involved meeting with the vendors, specifying the business requirements and holding scheduled meetings to ensure the vendors met deadlines. To ensure vendor compliance, the team developed contracts with project milestones, deliverables and payment schedules. While the researchers were aware of differences between U.S. and India business practices, the researchers weren't fully prepared for the degree or scope of adaptability needed and the residual effect it would have on the project from start to finish.

Action Taking: Building the mHealth App Required Adaptability

In the action taking stage, the team built the mHealth app. This involved writing the script, creating the animation, developing the app and incorporating virtual reality components. The paragraphs that follow show how this process unfolded including the critical role that adaptability played in turning the vision of the mHealth app into reality.

Creating the Script and Storyboard

Based on their understanding of India's health care system and the community's needs, the nursing professor in consultation with HospitalCo's community health physicians developed a script, which the creative director turned into a storyboard. The script and storyboard addressed how to: define hypertension, prevent hypertension, identify hypertension symptoms, and seek professional care. HospitalCo's physicians consulted medically on the script's accuracy and translation into three languages commonly spoken in the communities HospitalCo served.

Animation Building

In the quote below, the creative director explains AnimationCo's motivation for joining the project.

When we met with AnimationCo's CEO we learned AnimationCo was not signing up for any financial reason. Our resources to pay them are limited. AnimationCo wants their name associated with the project and they want to help the people of India.

After receiving an initial payment, AnimationCo assigned their development team in India to make the animation and the university researchers scheduled the first of many Skype meetings with AnimationCo. Recognizing the time difference, the nursing professor scheduled the meeting for 6:00 am in the United States, which was still within normal working hours in India. While the Healthy India Team had developed a script and storyboard, they gave AnimationCo creative leeway to develop the virtual reality simulation component of the project. During the first Skype meeting, the nursing professor explained, "We need to brand this as a virtual reality simulation, balance the fun vs. the education. If we want more grant money the virtual reality must be there." In response to this request, AnimationCo's U.S.-based liaison responded:

We'll play around with what we can do within the budget, maybe a character that you can do different things to, like lay on the couch and watch TV or eat bad foods and [how] that impacts how the character looks

After the initial meeting, the India delivery office took over the project. The India office was unclear about the virtual reality simulation component, what they were supposed to do and how much virtual reality simulation they could do for the money. After one Skype meeting AnimationCo's creative manager responded, "I need to check with my boss on whether we can deliver the virtual reality." Once the U.S. based researchers referred the Chief Executive Officer to the signed contract, he committed to support the virtual reality simulation, even though this was not AnimationCo's core competency. AnimationCo proceeded with the project with the efficiency of a factory production line. It created the 2-dimensional characters, animatics, 3-dimensional characters, the audio script translated into three languages, and finally the fully textured animation.

The process of making the animation proceeded as follows. AnimationCo provided the first draft of the characters which the nursing professor shared via email with the team. The India-based physicians and the U.S.-based research team conveyed their feedback to the nursing professor in a variety of formats. Everyone used email, but at times the U.S.-based research team used text messages and the India-based physicians used What's App, a social media platform. The nursing professor sent the compiled feedback to AnimationCo's creative manager to modify the deliverables. The team repeated this cycle regularly between September 2017-November 2017. Once AnimationCo completed the black and white 2D line animatics in late October 2017, AnimationCo suspended the regularly scheduled Skype meetings which the Healthy India Team was using to maintain creative input, ensure script adherence and ensure AnimationCo delivered a quality project on time. When the Healthy India Team tried to schedule the next Skype meeting, AnimationCo's creative manager responded:

We'd prefer to provide deliverables over email and schedule Skype meetings only if necessary. Indian holidays are approaching, and we'll have irregular work schedules.

The Healthy India Team agreed because AnimationCo was hitting its targets and the time had changed in America. The now 12.5-hour time difference made Skype meetings more challenging. AnimationCo was unwilling to extend its workday forcing the U.S. based Healthy India Team to conduct 5:00 am Skype meetings.

During these meetings the U.S. based creative director, whose role was to oversee the creative vision of the project, would ask repeatedly for information regarding AnimationCo's decisions made during the development of the animation and software development tools used. AnimationCo's production manager and creative manager responded in ways that indicated they didn't understand what the U.S.-

based creative director wanted, didn't want to share their development process, or didn't want to disrupt their factory-like production process. During these awkward moments, the U.S. based Healthy India Team, would gloss over AnimationCo's unwillingness to share the interim work products, tools and processes. This situation highlights the U.S.-based creative director's role adaptability. Her role was reduced to charting the creative direction of the animation and overseeing the animation making process. This somewhat reduced oversight was an important decision made in an effort to ensure AnimationCo met the animation completion deadline for field implementation. As a result of the loss of U.S. creative director's oversight, the animation suffered in several key ways discussed next.

The first deliverable was the 2D character designs. The team was pleased yet provided some feedback:

Can we have the lady in saree? Indians don't look too trim and fit in their middle age. I stand for a cuter and plumpy version of the characters. Can they make the monkey a little more cute? After visiting our target group, I believe they are too perfect, I would like to see the attendant wearing sandals, darken his skin considerably.

The nursing professor sent the combined feedback to AnimationCo. AnimationCo then revised the 2D designs and shared the English audio track. More animation character development available for consideration and critique required another feedback cycle. While the feedback slowed the project's delivery, it increased the animation's medical accuracy, cultural understanding and creative entertainment value. In the following quote, the nursing professor highlighted the team's sensitivity to culture and socioeconomic status:

One thing that we want to be sensitive about is that we are not being too stereotypical to one socioeconomic group because that could come off as offensive to others - particularly when funded by Americans.

In this quote, the nursing professor expressed concern about Americans, with little knowledge of Indian culture, developing content. She worried about offending the viewers who might perceive that Americans are looking down on India as a low to middle income nation.

Even though the animation's purpose was to teach about hypertension, the U.S.-based creative director directed AnimationCo to ensure the animation was entertaining and interesting to a wide range of people. The quote below highlights the conversations she had with AnimationCo:

As for the monkey he is generic, is there some feature the animators could exploit to give him a unique look. I don't feel he needs to be cuter per say. But I would like to see a selected "monkey" feature individualized to make his presence cuter. The monkey's sweeping gestures are effective, adding interest and just enough entertainment for the viewership to grow fond of him.

Because of their heavy patient workloads, the physicians, at times, offered feedback past the deadline, which caused all stakeholders to adapt their processes and expectations. The U.S.-based researchers wanted to gather all the feedback, especially the physicians' feedback, and send it to AnimationCo. When the physicians' feedback was late, the U.S.-based researchers had to decide if it was worth sending the feedback to AnimationCo. On one hand, the physicians' feedback was most critical because they were the project champions---if AnimationCo didn't include their feedback it could have resulted in an animation the physicians did not approve of and would not use. On the other hand, sending AnimationCo late feedback disrupted their product process and could cause rework, resulting in increased costs that might harm the quality of the animation and AnimationCo's willingness to do future work. In the end, this process resulted in all parties adapting. Sometimes the U.S.-based researchers decided it was not worth disrupting AnimationCo's production process with additional feedback that may result in rework. At other times, AnimationCo had to rework the animation based on late feedback.

AnimationCo completed their work in early January 2018 and the quality was better than the team imagined. Given the time and cost it took to build the animation with all the feedback cycles, and AnimationCo's willingness to take on additional development for the app, the U.S.-based researchers abandoned the virtual reality simulation component. AnimationCo thought they fulfilled their virtual reality simulation obligation by delivering moving icons of characters swimming, biking and running, but the U.S.-based researchers could not use these icons at this late stage of development. In an effort to deliver the project and build goodwill with AnimationCo for future collaborations, the nursing professor did not enforce the virtual reality simulation component of AnimationCo's contract.

App Building

AppCo built the mobile application, which included AnimationCo's animation and a platform to collect demographic information about the people that viewed the animation, what they had learned and their geographic location. Building the app involved some unexpected tedious work developing icons and audio files, in three languages, for the pre and post test. The U.S.-based researchers assumed AppCo would develop everything related to the app, but AppCo would not agree to develop the icons, audio or text files because it was not specified in their contract. As a small company looking to expand its technology in India's health care sector and make a profit, AppCo was unwilling to adapt and assume this extra burden. Given their language barrier and limited Indian cultural knowledge, the Healthy India Team turned to AnimationCo to develop the icons, audio files and text files. AnimationCo agreed to complete the additional work even though it was beyond the scope of their contract and expertise. This created project bottlenecks when AnimationCo outsourced the sound bites to an external vendor, leaving AppCo waiting on icons and sound from AnimationCo.

Communication with AppCo was problematic. Initially, the U.S.-based researchers conducted a Skype meeting with AppCo to specify the requirements. This was followed by a second meeting which was largely unproductive. AppCo's Internet connection was poor and the project managers AppCo assigned to the project were facing issues external to this project, leaving us with an AppCo customer liaison on the call who was unfamiliar with our team and our project. The liaison didn't understand the creative director's questions or requests for background products. As a result, the researchers resorted to managing AppCo over email. Unfortunately, the researchers encountered several difficulties evaluating AppCo's work products: the file sizes were too large; AppCo developed and tested the app on Androids, which the U.S. -based researchers did not have easy access to; and the U.S. researchers did not understand Hindi or Kannada languages.

Both the U.S. researchers and AppCo adapted their expectations and accepted a reduction in quality to work through this process. The U.S.-based researchers adjusted their app completion deadline to the date they needed the app for pilot testing. As soon as they arrived in India, the U.S. researchers visited AppCo to view the work products. As promised, AppCo completed everything and was only waiting on a few icons and audio files from AnimationCo. Getting AnimationCo to deliver the missing files required the U.S.-based nursing professor act as a liaison between AppCo and AnimationCo. This involved the U.S. nursing professor physically visiting AnimationCo's corporate offices and explaining what audio files were needed to complete the App. AnimationCo immediately assigned someone to the issue and within hours delivered the missing audio files to the nursing professor's hotel, demonstrating their adaptability and responsiveness.

Before pilot testing the app with human subjects the team had to secure the Institutional Review Board's approval, from both the U.S. university and HospitalCo in India, to protect human subjects and patient privacy. This process required adaptability. Researchers had to ensure research procedures and laws were adhered to in both countries, requiring several drafts and rewrites of the Institutional Review Board protocol. To protect patient privacy and security of international data transfer, the app did not collect identifying or sensitive information. The team worked with AppCo to ensure all features of the app used pictorial icons with audio overlay (in 3 languages) so that people who could not read could easily understand all aspects of the app including informed consent. Adapting the app to be user friendly to individuals who were illiterate was crucial to ensuring the app's success reaching and empowering marginalized populations.

To ensure the app reached marginalized populations, the researchers worked with HospitalCo's community health workers, who took the app on an Android tablet to standing health clinics in the urban slums and rural villages and went door to door visiting people in the community. The community health workers sat with each participant, gave them the option of not participating and guided them through the app. The app contained a built-in consent process, which the researchers adapted for use in places where Internet connectivity was unavailable. At the end of each workday, when the community health worker returned to HospitalCo, the data collected on the Android was uploaded to a secure server. This data was shared with the U.S.-based researchers who performed statistical analysis on the data. Data collection and transfer also required adaptability. The team experimented with several iterations of an Excel spreadsheet that used non-identifiable coded data and met Internal Review Board requirements, international data privacy laws and security protocols.

Evaluating

Completing the action research cycle involved the researchers and practitioners assessing whether the theory the team used to guide the intervention actually worked—was it effective, and did it relieve the problem (Baskerville & Wood-Harper, 1996)? This research evaluated the effectiveness of the project management techniques the researchers believed would lead to a quality mHealth hypertension app, delivered on time. In the action planning stage, the researchers envisioned that project management control techniques such as contracts specifying deliverables, milestones and meetings would ensure the vendors built the virtual reality simulation on time. However, when the researchers tried to implement these techniques in the action taking stage, adaptability on the part of all stakeholders, surpassed project management controls in terms of helping build a quality mHealth application on-time.

Because geographic distance, time zone differences and device compatibility issues kept the project from meeting the artificial project deadline, the researchers adapted the deadline to the date they actually needed the application for pilot testing. When the researchers arrived in India in February 2018, they met with the vendors and addressed the issues with immediate face-to-face meetings. The vendors prioritized the project and delivered the completed mHealth app within 48 hours, just in time to share it with the India stakeholders and begin field testing.

The second method of evaluating the project was quality. Did the project champions like the mHealth app? Did they believe it would help them teach marginalized, at risk populations in India about hypertension? The interviews with and observations of the directors of HospitalCo's community health program, the physicians and community health workers indicated they believed the mHealth app was a high-quality product. Several aspects of the mHealth app pleased them including its: interactivity, cultural appropriateness and ability to educate in an entertaining way. With regard to interactivity, the app allowed viewers to select different video segments appropriate for their health learning outcomes. This superseded the previous process where health workers carried paper counseling cards into underserved communities with Western characters and society. As shown in Figure 1, the app has culturally appropriate figures speaking the same language and residing in a similar community setting as the intended audience.

The community health physicians' actions indicated that the mHealth app passed their quality standards. These included showing the app to peer departments at the hospital, training the community health workers how to use the app, allowing us to demonstrate the app at a rural clinic and arranging a community viewing of the full-length animation. This range of venues gave the researchers an opportunity to assess the users' acceptance of the app. Unfortunately, at times the users struggled to see and hear the animation. The users preferred watching the animation in small groups, sometimes with as many as 15 people. In these groups, the 5*7 screen size of the Androids was too small, and the volume was too low. This was exacerbated because most viewing occurred outside on the streets and created issues with the sun on the Androids and street noise. The researchers dealt with this partially by purchasing external speakers that connected to the Androids. Despite the challenges, the users' actions including gathering around in small groups to watch the animation, smiling, asking questions and coming up with suggestions for future apps, lead us to believe that users' acceptance of the app was very positive. To-date, over 500 people have participated in the pre and post test survey and the results indicate that the participants learned about hypertension from using the app (Garner et al., 2019).

Figure 1. A frame from the hypertension mHealth app

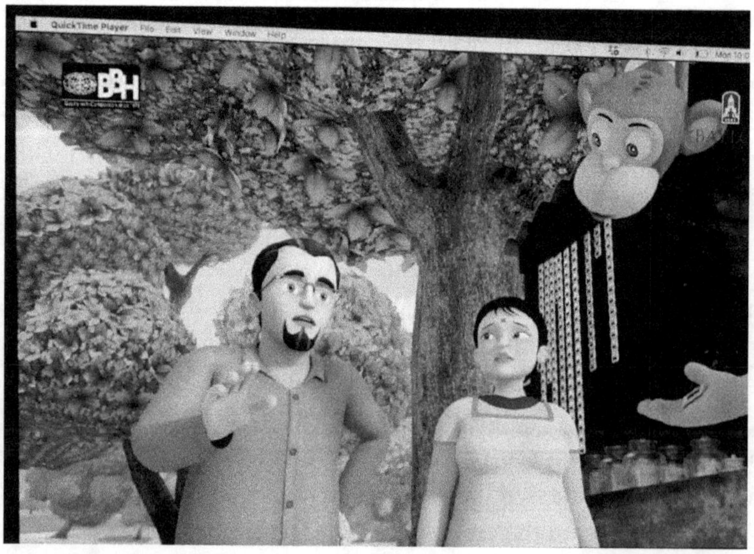

SOLUTIONS AND RECOMMENDATIONS

The purpose of this action research project was to provide insight into building a mHealth app in situations where: (1) the app is a social good addressing a serious problem (2) most of the stakeholders are donating project resources and (3) the project leaders, who are controlling the project, have limited knowledge of the daily realities of the people who will build and be helped by the app. Based on what the researchers learned in this process, this study offers three recommendations for others working under these circumstances.

Recommendation 1: Adaptability May Outweigh Traditional Control in Project Management

In the action planning stage, the researchers believed that effective project management techniques were critical to building the app. However, as the researchers started building the app, they realized that adaptability on the part of all the stakeholders, especially the U.S. researchers initiating the project, was key.

Table 1 shows that adaptability cuts across teams, processes and technology. Team adaptability involves an interplay of vision and team members' role adaptability. The U.S. researchers and the India technology vendors ultimately achieved a shared vision of success for the project, which involved trade-offs and role adaptability. Trade-offs involved the U.S. researchers settling for less (i.e., foregoing the virtual reality simulation component) and AnimationCo doing more (i.e., creating icons and sound bites). Role adaptability involved the U.S. researchers assuming additional roles as liaisons between the vendors and surrendering some creative license and process control to AnimationCo.

Process adaptability deals with how the project was accomplished. Most of the process adaptability occurred as the U.S. team adapted their project management techniques to meet the reality of working with vendors in another country who were donating resources to the project. Process adaptability included time, communication method, feedback and deadlines/milestones. Given that the vendors were working on the project at reduced costs, the vendors, rather than the client, often dictated time and communication methods. This meant the U.S. team accepted meetings during normal sleeping hours and gave up the control technique of periodic Skype meetings in favor of the vendor's preference for email communication. This impacted feedback, deadlines and milestones. The U.S. team emailed feedback to AnimationCo so they could rework the characters and animation. Not having the back and forth common in conversations left the U.S. team ill-informed about the impact this feedback had on AnimationCo's process. At times, the U.S. team didn't send late feedback out of concern that it would cause more delays and cost overruns. Given that communication between the U.S. team and AnimationCo was now mostly occurring over email, AnimationCo was having trouble understanding the importance of supplying the correct audio and sound files to AppCo. These communication struggles had two results. First the U.S. team adjusted their artificial project deadlines and set deadlines based on when they needed the app for pilot testing during their India trip. Second, the U.S. team scheduled physical meetings to address the outstanding sound and icon development issues that they couldn't resolve over email.

Recommendation 2: Let the Recipients Adapt Technology to Their Needs

In some cases, the recipients (HospitalCo) used the technology in ways the researchers did not intend with the initial research project; however, having adaptable technology and being adaptable about how

Table 1. Adaptability examples

PROJECT INITIATORS **US-based Researchers and India-based Hospital**	**TECHNOLOGY DEVELOPERS** **India-based—AppCo & AnimationCo**
TEAM ADAPTABILITY	
Project Vision: Settling for less: U.S. research team accepts AnimationCo's delivery of an animated video and some gif files of character exercising instead of the virtual reality simulation specified in the contract	Project Vision: Doing more: AnimationCo builds animations of characters exercising to fulfill the virtual reality component of the contract even though this is beyond their core competency
Role Adaptability: U.S.-based creative director gives more control over creative license and process to AnimationCo when AnimationCo is unwilling to respond to her requests for information on their development process. U.S.-based nursing professor takes on a liaison role to get AnimationCo to deliver the necessary audio files and icons to AppCo	Role Adaptability: AnimationCo assumes the role of developing icons and sound bites for the pre and post test when AppCo would not take on this responsibility. AppCo puts different people into roles when circumstances such as traffic or family issues prevents a person from fulfilling their role
PROCESS ADAPTABILITY	
Time: Accepts meetings outside normal U.S. work and sleep hours	
Communication Method: Had to communicate over email when: (1) AnimationCo's suspended periodic Skype meetings; and (2) Skype meeting with AppCo proved unproductive	Communication Method: Met with U.S.-based researchers face-to-face to resolve outstanding issues
Feedback: Team provided feedback on the vendor's progress via text messaging, email or What's App. Sometimes U.S.-based team didn't send feedback to AnimationCo if it was late and would disrupt AnimationCo's production process.	Feedback: AnimationCo reworked animation and characters based on feedback even when this caused rework to AnimationCo's factory-like production process
Deadline and milestones: Adjusted artificial deadlines when the project fell behind. Adjusted process of evaluating work products from email to face-to-face meetings due to technology compatibility and translation issues associated with email.	Deadline and milestones: AppCo and AnimationCo went the extra mile to meet real deadlines. Prioritized rework while the U.S. team was in India. Delivered revised deliverables to the researchers' work site.
TECHNOLOGY ADAPTABILITY	
Translation: Application available in three languages. Animation transcends language and literacy barriers.	
Segmentation: Ability to segment the health application into short messages customized to the recipients' needs.	
Assessment: (1) the health workers or participants could read or play assessment and demographic questions; (2) the app gave the correct answer to missed questions and directed participants to the segment of the animation that covered the missed information; (3) participants could skip assessment and demographic questions.	
Use: HospitalCo uses Android technology in a variety of ways beyond the app including health screenings. Once the assessment research was complete, HospitalCo incorporates the full animation into its daily work practices. The animation reaches beyond its target audience of adults living in India's urban slums and rural villages to a variety of demographics including children and medical workers. People adapt the animation, which the researchers envisioned as an individual learning tool, into a group learning tool. The power of the group reinforces the message. AppCo uses the Animation to support new business. HospitalCo and AcademicU use the app for research.	

the recipients use the technology were key to meeting the overall objective of helping the people of India take better care of their health. Table 1 shows how the recipients adapted the technology's features to their needs. These included translation, segmentation, assessment and use. Since the mHealth application translated into three languages, it allowed health care workers to work with people they normally could not communicate with. Segmentation allowed health workers to only play parts that recipients needed and not overwhelm the recipients with too much information. Users could customize the assessment to their objectives. For instance, health care workers used the score on the assessment to determine what additional hypertension education to provide and users could skip the assessment all together. Most importantly, HospitalCo could use the Android technology that delivered the mHealth hypertension app to serve many different purposes including screenings and electronic medical records.

Recommendation 3: Human Values Should Form the Basis of Adaptability Decisions

Human values, which are integral to ethical, compassionate and safe relationship-centered healthcare (Rider et al., 2014), formed the basis of the adaptability decisions. Human values include human welfare, universal usability, and autonomy (Friedman & Kahn Jr, 2007). Human welfare is the good fortune, health, happiness and prosperity of individuals, communities and societies (Friedman & Kahn Jr, 2007). Improving human welfare was the overall vision for the project which led to the stakeholders' willingness to adapt. Effective, caring, and skilled communication are essential to maintaining human value which is manifested through the interaction process (Rider et al., 2014). Understanding that the U.S. researchers needed to be physically on the ground in India to enhance team communication when implementing the app, led to all stakeholders adapting their processes to make this happen. The U.S. researchers sacrificed some quality and functionality to get the app in the hands of the people that needed it most. The technology vendors prioritized rework and delivered products at the field site. And, HospitalCo adjusted work processes to implement the app during the researchers India visit.

Universal usability refers to the notion that all people who want to use a technology could be successful users (Friedman & Kahn Jr, 2007). The app addressed universal usability by designing for populations that many technology designers may forget. This includes illiterate people, with low education levels and few resources. The app's design fostered a dialogue between learners and the content rather than focusing on the physical interaction at the interface.

Autonomy is achieved when users have control over the technology and can use it for different goals (Friedman & Kahn Jr, 2007). This project achieved autonomy by giving HospitalCo, its health workers and the people discretion over how they used the technology. For example, HospitalCo could use the Androids to deliver the animation or in other ways that helped the people. The health care workers had considerable discretion to teach individuals or communities, to show segments and to supplement the health message.

RESEARCH IMPLICATIONS

Traditional project management approaches, characterized by rigid, linear actions, have difficulty accommodating the changes that are inherent in cross-cultural, social innovation collaborations (Augustine et al., 2005). The traditional approaches tend to emphasize early, lengthy planning, then ongoing governance including monitoring, controlling, change and risk management, and the like, to ensure agreed-upon plans are adhered to (Project Management Institute, Inc., 2017). In the context of a cross-cultural collaboration between the U.S. and India for social good, this study affirms the importance of using agile management techniques that emphasize control adaptability, in the management processes of these complex, less-defined systems (Augustine et al., 2005).

The research shows how cross-cultural and cross-discipline collaborations that create mHealth innovations can evolve from one technology vision to another based on project context, creating the need to exhibit adaptability in both the collaboration process and the end-product. In the present study, the initial technology requirement was to build a mHealth virtual reality simulation-based app for hypertension education. In the end, a 3-D animation-based mHealth education app was developed instead and proved to be the more appropriate technology. This act of adjustment in technology vision both affirms and adds to existing knowledge in adaptive management of systems development efforts.

Second, the study also adds to systems development knowledge that often assumes that technology requirements are established early on and should be implemented as requested. When this is not done it is often interpreted as failure. The present research demonstrates that not implementing some technology requirements as initially specified may result in a successful project. When tackling complex, less-defined problems in a social innovation context, initial technology requests based on Western values may require adjustment to the cultural context, to ensure intended recipients can effectively use the technology

FUTURE RESEARCH DIRECTIONS

As the nature of societal problems become more complex, there is a growing need for scholars and practitioners to work together toward developing sustainable solutions that resolve societal issues (Deng, Joshi, & Galliers, 2016; Richardson, Kettinger, Banks, & Quintana, 2014b). This need is particularly important for fields like information systems, that have historically focused on organizational and managerial problems rather than societal problems (Trauth, Joshi, & Yarger, 2018). Globalization allows large diversity among groups developing solutions, which may introduce cultural division and misunderstanding of user needs. The research provides guidance on the advantages of adaptability over traditional control throughout the management of a project. Future research may further this project's contributions by extending the role of adaptability in the management process to larger or different projects as well as other cultural settings. Future research could additionally extend the insights into the use and impacts of adaptability in the implementation and diffusion processes of mHealth innovations.

CONCLUSION

Academics and practitioners need to work together to "create better and more valuable knowledge for both camps (Lanamäki, Stendal, & Thapa, 2011, p. 130)" and solve the world's toughest problems. The chapter reports on a collaboration between academics and practitioners spanning a variety of fields including academia, medicine, entertainment and technology development. In examining the social innovation collaboration that created mHealth technology for social good, the researchers found that adaptability at the team member, process and technology levels is essential to developing mHealth technology for marginalized populations. In the end, the collaboration resulted in a culturally appropriate app for patient empowerment. The app empowered vulnerable populations with high rates of illiteracy and limited financial resources to take better care of this health. The process of designing and developing this app answers calls by the World Health Organization (2011) and researchers of information and communication technology for development (Zheng & Walsham, 2008) to empower vulnerable populations with mHealth. Hopefully, this research will encourage more multi-discipline, multi-cultural social good collaborations, to assist people developing healthcare-related technologies for forgotten populations.

ACKNOWLEDGMENT

This research was supported by a Baylor University Social Innovation Collaboration grant and Bangalore Baptist Hospital.

REFERENCES

Aarons, G., Hurlburt, M., & Horwitz, S. (2011). Advancing a conceptual model of evidence-based practice implementation in public service sectors. *Administration and Policy in Mental Health*, *38*(1), 4–23. doi:10.100710488-010-0327-7 PMID:21197565

Baskerville, R. L., & Stage, J. (1996). Controlling prototype development through risk analysis. *Management Information Systems Quarterly*, *20*(4), 482–504. doi:10.2307/249565

Baskerville, R. L., & Wood-Harper, A. T. (1996). A critical perspective on information systems action research. *Journal of Information Technology*, *11*, 235–246. doi:10.1177/026839629601100305

Benbya, H., & McKelvey, B. (2006). Toward a complexity theory of information systems development. *Information Technology & People*, *19*(1), 12–34. doi:10.1108/09593840610649952

Burke, C. S., Stagl, K. C., Salas, E., Pierce, L., & Kendall, D. (2006). Understanding team adaptation: A conceptual analysis and model. *The Journal of Applied Psychology*, *91*(6), 1189–1207. doi:10.1037/0021-9010.91.6.1189 PMID:17100478

Chakravarthy, B. S. (1982). Adaptation: A promising metaphor for strategic management. *Academy of Management Review*, *7*(1), 35–44. doi:10.5465/amr.1982.4285438

Conboy, K. (2009). Agility from first principles: Reconstructing the concept of agility in information systems development. *Information Systems Research*, *20*(3), 329–354. doi:10.1287/isre.1090.0236

Deng, X., Joshi, K. D., & Galliers, R. D. (2016). The duality of empowerment and marginalization in microtask crowdsourcing: Giving voice to the less powerful through value sensitive design. *Management Information Systems Quarterly*, *40*(2), 279–A19. doi:10.25300/MISQ/2016/40.2.01

Dibbern, J., Goles, T., Hirschheim, R., & Jayatilaka, B. (2004). Information systems outsourcing: A survey and analysis of the literature. *SIGMIS Database*, *35*(4), 6–102. doi:10.1145/1035233.1035236

Dufour, S., Lessard, D., & Chamberland, C. (2014). Facilitators and barriers to implementation of the AIDES initiative, a social innovation for participative assessment of children in need and for coordination of services. *Evaluation and Program Planning*, *47*, 64–70. doi:10.1016/j.evalprogplan.2014.07.006 PMID:25150926

Eisenhardt, K. M. (1985). Control: Organizational and Economic approaches. *Management Science. Linthicum, 31*(2), 134.

Friedman, B., & Kahn, P. H. Jr. (2007). Human values, ethics, and design. In *The human-computer interaction handbook* (pp. 1223–1248). Boca Raton, FL: CRC Press.

Garner, S. L., George, C. E., Young, P., Hitchcock, J., Koch, H., & Green, G. … Gift, N. (2019). Effectiveness of an mhealth application to improve hypertension health literacy in India. *WHO-South East Asia Journal of Public Health, Under Review*. Retrieved from https://www.journals.elsevier.com/public-health

Garner, S. L., Sudia, T., & Rachaprolu, S. (2018). Smart phone accessibility and mHealth use in a limited resource setting. *International Journal of Nursing Practice, 24*(1), e12609. doi:10.1111/ijn.12609 PMID:29159919

Head, B., & Alford, J. (2013). Wicked problems: Implications for public policy and management. *Administration & Society, 47*(6), 711–739. doi:10.1177/0095399713481601

Kappelman, L. A., McKeeman, R., & Zhang, L. (2006). Early warning signs of IT project failure: The dominant dozen. *Information Systems Management, 23*(4), 31–36. doi:10.1201/1078.10580530/46352.23.4.20060901/95110.4

Lanamäki, A., Stendal, K., & Thapa, D. (2011). Mutual informing between IS academia and practice: Insights from KIWISR-5. *Communications of the Association for Information Systems*, 123–132.

Lee, G., & Xia, W. (2005). The ability of information systems development project teams to respond to business and technology changes: A study of flexibility measures. *European Journal of Information Systems, 14*(1), 75–92. doi:10.1057/palgrave.ejis.3000523

Martensson, P., & Lee, A. S. (2004). Dialogical action research at Omega Corporation. *Management Information Systems Quarterly, 28*(3), 507–536. doi:10.2307/25148648

Mumford, E. (2001). Advice for action researchers. *Information Technology & People, 14*(1), 12–27. doi:10.1108/09593840110384753

Nelson, R. R. (2007). IT project management: Infamous failures, classic mistakes, and best practices. *MIS Quarterly Executive, 6*(2).

Oreglia, E., & Srinivasan, J. (2016). ICT, Intermediaries, and the transformation of gendered power structures. *Management Information Systems Quarterly, 40*(2), 501–510. doi:10.25300/MISQ/2016/40.2.13

Pan, Z., Cheok, A. D., Yang, H., Zhu, J., & Shi, J. (2006). Virtual reality and mixed reality for virtual learning environments. *Computers & Graphics, 30*(1), 20–28. doi:10.1016/j.cag.2005.10.004

Patten, K., Whitworth, B., Fjermestad, J., & Mahindra, E. (2005). Leading IT flexibility: anticipation, agility and adaptability. In *Americas Conference on Information Systems Proceedings*, Omaha, NE: Association for Information Systems.

Phills, J. A., Deiglmeier, K., & Miller, D. T. (2008, Fall). Rediscovering social innovation. Stanford Social Innovation Review; Stanford, 6(4), 34–43.

Project Management Institute, Inc. (2017). *Guide to the Project Management Body of Knowledge* (6th ed.). Newton Square, PA: Project Management Institute. Retrieved from https://www.pmi.org/pmbok-guide-standards/foundational/pmbok

Richardson, S., Kettinger, W., Banks, M., & Quintana, Y. (2014a). IT and Agility in the social enterprise: A case study of St Jude children's Research Hospital's "Cure4Kids" it-platform for international outreach. *Journal of the Association for Information Systems, 15*(1), 1–32. doi:10.17705/1jais.00351

Rider, E. A., Kurtz, S., Slade, D., Longmaid, H. E. III, Ho, M.-J., Pun, J. K., ... Branch, W. T. Jr. (2014). The International charter for human values in healthcare: An interprofessional global collaboration to enhance values and communication in healthcare. *Patient Education and Counseling, 96*(3), 273–280. doi:10.1016/j.pec.2014.06.017 PMID:25103181

Salas, E., Sims, D. E., & Burke, C. S. (2005). Is there a "big five" in teamwork? *Small Group Research, 36*(5), 555–599. doi:10.1177/1046496405277134

Schmidt, C., Kude, T., Tripp, J., Heinzl, A., & Spohrer, K. (2013). *Team adaptability in agile information systems development.* In P*roceedings of the 34*[th] *International Conference on Information Systems,* Milan, Italy: Association of Information Systems.

Sondaal, S. F. V., Browne, J. L., Amoakoh-Coleman, M., Borgstein, A., Miltenburg, A. S., Verwijs, M., & Klipstein-Grobusch, K. (2016). Assessing the Effect of mhealth interventions in improving maternal and neonatal care in low- and middle-income countries: A systematic review. *PLoS One, 11*(5). doi:10.1371/journal.pone.0154664 PMID:27144393

Susman, G. I., & Dean, J. W., Jr. (1992). Development of a model for predicting design for manufacturability effectiveness. Integrating Design and Manufacturing for Competitive Advantage, 207–227.

Tallon, P. P., & Pinsonneault, A. (2011). Competing perspectives on the link between strategic information technology alignment and organizational agility: Insights from a mediation model. *Management Information Systems Quarterly, 35*(2), 463.

Tatikonda, M. V., & Montoya-Weiss, M. M. (2001). Integrating operations and marketing perspectives of product innovation: The influence of organizational process factors and capabilities on development performance. *Management Science, 47*(1), 151–172. doi:10.1287/mnsc.47.1.151.10669

Tiwana, A., & Keil, M. (2009). Control in internal and outsourced software projects. *Journal of Management Information Systems, 26*(3), 9–44. doi:10.2753/MIS0742-1222260301

Trauth, E., Joshi, K. D., & Yarger, L. K. (2018). ISJ Editorial. *Information Systems Journal, 28*(6), 989–994. doi:10.1111/isj.12201

Tuominen, M., Rajala, A., & Möller, K. (2004). How does adaptability drive firm innovativeness? *Journal of Business Research, 57*(5), 495–506. doi:10.1016/S0148-2963(02)00316-8

Vorhies, D. W., Harker, M., & Rao, C. (1999). The capabilities and performance advantages of market-driven firms. *European Journal of Marketing, 33*(11/12), 1171–1202. doi:10.1108/03090569910292339

Walls, J. G., Widmeyer, G. R., & El Sawy, O. A. (1992). Building an information system design theory for vigilant EIS. *Information Systems Research, 3*(1), 36–59. doi:10.1287/isre.3.1.36

Walsham, G. (2017). ICT4D research: Reflections on history and future agenda. *Information Technology for Development, 23*(1), 18–41. doi:10.1080/02681102.2016.1246406

Weber, B., Reichert, M., & Rinderle-Ma, S. (2008). Change patterns and change support features–enhancing flexibility in process-aware information systems. *Data & Knowledge Engineering, 66*(3), 438–466. doi:10.1016/j.datak.2008.05.001

WHO Global Observatory for eHealth. (2011). *mHealth: New horizons for health through mobile technologies.* (No. 3). Retrieved from http://www.who.int/goe/publications/goe_mhealth_web.pdf

Wiener, M., Mahring, M., Saunders, C., & Remus, U. (2016). Control configuration and control enactment in information systems projects: Review and expanded theoretical framework. *Management Information Systems Quarterly, 40*(3), 741–774. doi:10.25300/MISQ/2016/40.3.11

World Health Organization. (2016). *WHO | World Health Statistics 2016: Monitoring health for the SDGs.* Retrieved from http://www.who.int/gho/publications/world_health_statistics/2016/en/

Zheng, Y., & Walsham, G. (2008). Inequality of what? Social exclusion in the e-society as capability deprivation. *Information Technology & People, 21*(3), 222–243. doi:10.1108/09593840810896000

Zhou, B., Bentham, J., Cesare, M. D., Bixby, H., Danaei, G., Cowan, M. J., & Cisneros, J. Z. (2017). Worldwide trends in blood pressure from 1975 to 2015: A pooled analysis of 1479 population-based measurement studies with 19·1 million participants. *Lancet, 389*(10064), 37–55. doi:10.1016/S0140-6736(16)31919-5 PMID:27863813

KEY TERMS AND DEFINITIONS

Adaptability: Incorporating flexibility into the technology, process and team dynamics of a project.

Community Health: Hospital divisions that provide free and low-cost healthcare services to marginalized populations in India.

Community Health Worker: People tasked with providing basic healthcare education to marginalized populations in India; usually understand the community's social structure and values.

Control: Management practices used to understand and influence the agreed-upon outcomes of a project.

mHealth Hypertension App: A software application designed to teach people in India how to prevent and manage hypertension. Consists of an entertaining animation and a questionnaire to collect demographic information and assess learning.

Rural Village: Geographic regions in India where distance and socioeconomics conditions hinder access to mainstream education and healthcare.

Social Innovation Collaboration: Diverse stakeholders donating time and resources to address a social problem.

Urban Slum: Geographic regions in India with high population density, limited resources and limited understanding of how to prevent non-communicable diseases.

Chapter 17
Common-Sense Epidemiology in the Age of Electronic Patient Records (EPR)

Shirly Bar-Lev
Ruppin Academic Center, Israel

Dizza Beimel
Ruppin Academic Center, Israel

ABSTRACT

Encouraging patients to play a more active role in their health care is crucial for healthcare planning and for the design of services. This chapter shifts the scholarly focus from practitioners' decision making to that of laypersons' trying to make sense of the lab results available on their EPRs. The authors developed a methodology to capture the relationship between information formats (graph, numeric, or verbal), laypersons' assessment of the conditions' gravity, and their preferred course of action. Focusing on the effect of "not knowing" on laypersons' preferred courses of action, our findings show that formats that left respondents less able to understand the results—namely, the numeric and verbal formats—produced a lower sense of urgency, and correspondingly, less inclination to actively seek professional help. The chapter takes a step toward deriving practical recommendations as to how personal clinical information should be communicated, to improve laypersons' interpretation of the information's significance.

INTRODUCTION

The accessibility of personalized medical information via Electronic Patient Records (EPRs) has significantly changed the way laypersons self-assess their health, consult physicians, and engage with medical advice (Bylund, Gueguen, Sabee, Imes, Li, & Sanford, 2007; Levin-Zamir, Baron-Epel, Cohen, & Elhayany, 2016). The EPR is commonly defined as a data repository containing patients' health information accumulated throughout the course of the patient's life. Through its retrieval functions it is expected to allow authorized persons (health professionals, patients, or administrators) easy access to stored patient information (Berg, 2004). Giving patients access to their own records can support pa-

DOI: 10.4018/978-1-7998-0047-7.ch017

tients in shared decision making and in managing their own care. It can also improve communication with health care professionals. However, laypersons who use EPRs can and often do view the results of medical tests and procedures before interacting with their health care providers, and the meaning they attach to such information can significantly affect their decision making and subsequent follow-up care. Despite growing use of EPRs, little is known about their effect on patients' decision-making capabilities and engagement. It therefore behooves us to learn how the exposure of people with no medical training to complex medical terminology and to raw medical data affects the risk of harm from self-diagnosis and self-treatment (Bhavnani 2002; Beck, Richard, Nguyen-Thanh, Montagni, Parizot, & Renahy, 2014; Levin-Zamir et al. 2016).

This chapter aims to narrow this gap in the literature by appraising how the formatting of personalized health information (specifically, test results) in EPRs affects how well individuals understand the information, how they assess its gravity, and their chosen course of action in response. We hypothesize a relationship between the information format (graphic, numeric or verbal), laypersons' assessment of the situation, and preferred courses of action. We tested our hypotheses using an online survey with a sample of healthy Israeli volunteers. Finally, we offer a nuanced account of ways in which the online presentation of personalized health information can empower and constrain patients in the management of their health and that of their families (Iyawa, Herselman, & Botha, 2016; Lupton & Maslen, 2019).

This chapter proceeds as follows. We first describe the state of Health Information Technologies (HIT) in the Israeli healthcare system. The next section reviews current discussions on lay epidemiology and its possible implications for the design of the EPR. In the third and fourth sections we describe the methodology and design of the study, then present our findings. We conclude by discussing the study's limitations, and its implications for improving the communication of personalized health information.

BACKGROUND

Like many health care systems around the world, Israel's system is facing enormous and unprecedented financial and capacity pressures, leading to what Koh et al. (2012) called a "cycle of costly 'crisis care'" (see also Koh, Berwick, Clancy, Baur, Brach, Harris, & Zerhusen, 2012); Simmons, Wolever, Bechard, & Snyderman, 2014; Paz-Fuchs, Mandelkern, & Galnoor, 2018; Baim-Lance, Tietz, Lever, Swart, & Agins, 2019). In response to such challenges, governments are keen to support plans that serve to simultaneously re-organize and coordinate care while engaging the patient in the process of care delivery and self-management of health (Lupton & Maslen, 2019). The implementation of EPR systems is part of what has been called the "digital health ecosystem" – a complex network of digital platforms (including mobile applications, wearable self-tracking devices, medical imaging, genomics, and personalized medicine) designed, in part, to facilitate patients' participation in the healthcare delivery process (see Iyawa, Herselman, & Botha, 2016). In this context, access to relevant and personalized information is believed to increase laypersons' control over their health and its determinants, and thereby improve their health (Lupton & Maslen, 2019).

The digital health promise is founded on the expectation that patients can, should, and will assume greater responsibility for understanding and managing their health, including chronic health conditions. But what do we know about the relationship between information and patients' engagement?

Scholars describe patient engagement in terms of a continuum characterized by how much information flows between patient and provider, how active is patients' role in care decisions, and how involved patients or patient organizations become in policy making (Carman, Dardess, Maurer, Sofaer, Adams, Bechtel, & Sweeney, 2013). At the full partnership end of the continuum, patients have direct access to their records, can see notes from clinicians, and can add or edit information. The record, in these cases, reflects the entire experience of care from the perspectives of both the patient and clinicians. To date, the EPR system implemented in the four Israeli Health Maintenance Organizations (HMOs) gives patients direct access to their lab results and allows them to perform several administrative procedures. Patients can use their electronic records to receive individual medical feedback, access prescriptions, and conduct e-consultations with their family doctor. But they cannot see a diagnosis list, nor contribute or correct information. These restricted capacities position the current interface at the midpoint of the engagement continuum. Despite its limitations, to date, the EPR constitutes the most comprehensive source of personalized health information accessible to Israeli patients.

Israel has a high rate of EPR adoption in community health delivery systems. Indeed, as early as 2003, more than 4.6 million patient records were entered by nearly 5000 primary care physicians (i.e., family medicine, internal medicine, pediatrics, and OB/GYN) in Israel's four major HMOs, leading Margalit, Roter, Dunevant, Larson, & Reis (2006) to describe electronic records in Israeli primary care as an almost fully immersed environment. In March 2018, the Israeli government launched an ambitious plan to invest NIS 1 billion ($287 million) to create a digital database containing the medical files of some 9 million residents, and make them available to patients, researchers and enterprises.[1] The program mandates the establishment of a specialized medical database which will include information provided voluntarily by patients. Thus, while the program is primarily designed to speed up commercialization of products and help companies penetrate the market, it will surely revolutionize the way patients manage and relate to their personal health information.

THEORETICAL FOCUS

Over the last three decades, taking account of subjective and lay viewpoints on health has become a "sine qua non of adequate health assessments" (Prior, 2003, p. 42), and forms the basis of collaborative models of care delivery. In light of this trend, scholars interested in lay epidemiology have focused mainly on subjective ways of knowing (Prior, 2003; Knight and Mattick, 2006; Copelton & Valle, 2009), often conceived as key to a democratized and customer-sensitive system of health care (Prior, 2003). In their seminal 1991 paper, Davison, Davey-Smith, and Frankel coined the term "lay epidemiology" to designate how lay beliefs about the causes, course and management of illness affect people's attitudes and behaviors. Lay epidemiology fits within what Lovatt et al. (2015, p. 1913) call a "social constructivist ontology" which emphasizes how people interpret and make sense of health and illness, and how these interpretations relate to actions, practices and behaviors. While standard epidemiology focuses largely on health outcomes at a population level, lay epidemiology is concerned with patients' decision making and behaviors in relation to their own individual lives.

Another stream of researchers shifted attention from subjective ways of knowing to examining the different ways in which laypeople and experts interpret medical facts to assess the severity of illness (Prior, 2003; Keselman & Smith, 2012). Jemmott, Croyle, and Ditto (1988) introduced the term "common sense epidemiology" to distinguish the ways in which laypersons gather information and interpret it to make sense of health and disease (p. 56). These scholars have shown that laypersons construe the symptoms, causes, course, and consequences of disease in relation to the circumstances of their own lives (Jemmott, Croyle, & Ditto, 1988; Levy, Weinstein, Kidney, Scheld, & Guarnaccia, 2008; Copelton & Valle, 2009; Pilnick & Zayts, 2014). Prior (2003) points out that while laypeople may be "experts" in their own experiences, they are "rarely skilled in matters of (medical) fact gathering, or in the business of diagnosis…[and] they can often be plain wrong about the causes, course and management of common forms of disease and illness." It has also been established that when presented with the same information, laypeople and experts draw different conclusions about risk (Levy et al., 2008; Jauho, 2017). However, one aspect of lay epidemiology that has received scant attention is the interpretation of personalized medical information viewed via EPRs (Pyper, Amery, Watson, & Crook, 2004; Keselman & Smith, 2012).

Growing efforts to make health care more patient-centered have sensitized both practitioners and scholars to the ways laypersons respond to uncertainty (Han, Klein, and Arora, 2011). There are of course multiple varieties of uncertainty, each causing distinct psychological effects and warranting different courses of action. In this chapter, we focus on uncertainty with regard to the meaning of lab results obtained through EPRs. We here follow Pichler & Hesson (2016, p. 4), who point out that "IDK [i.e., the statement "I don't know"] functions as a cognitive claim of insufficient knowledge." That is, the concept of uncertainty used here implies a "subjective perception of ignorance" (Han, Klein, & Arora, 2011, p. 829) regarding the meaning of information presented. We ask how this subjective awareness of insufficient knowledge or incomprehension motivates laypersons' actions.

In our study, we operationalized uncertainty as "I don't know" responses to questions about the meaning of anonymized lab results presented in one of three formats: numeric expressions, graphs, or verbal expressions. "I don't know" responses were taken to reflect perceived incoherence (i.e., poor understanding) of the presented information. We pose two research questions: 1) Does the way medical information is presented (verbally, numerically, or graphically) affect laypersons' level of uncertainty, above and beyond the effect of control variables? 2) Does the level of uncertainty affect laypersons' preferred course of action above and beyond the effect of control variables? We examine a number of social and demographic factors as control variables, including gender, age, education, attitudes towards health and illness, and familiarity with the EPR system. Formally, we propose three hypotheses:

Hypothesis One: The three information formats (verbal, numeric, and graphic) will yield different levels of accuracy in assessing the gravity of the healthcare condition.

Hypothesis Two: The three information formats (verbal, numeric, and graphic) will yield different levels of uncertainty regarding the health condition.

Hypothesis Three: The lower the perceived coherence (understandability) of the information provided, the more proactive people are likely to be in seeking help or information.

METHODS

Sample and Procedure

We presented 298 respondents with authentic (anonymized) patient lab results relating to 10 important but non-life-threatening health conditions using either numeric expressions, graphs, or verbal expressions (see under "Information formats" below). Participants were then asked to assess the gravity of the hypothetical patient's condition and the course of action they would follow if they were that patient. Participants were randomly assigned to receive one of two versions of the questionnaire. Both versions contained the same scenarios and questions, differing only in the presentation of the test results. Each of the three formats was randomly distributed between the two versions of the questionnaire, such that for each scenario we were able to juxtapose two of the three possible formats.

Perceived illness level has been found to affect both underuse and overuse of healthcare services (Prior, Evans, & Prout, 2011; Hajek, Bock, & König, 2017). We were therefore interested in how laypeople in ordinary, everyday, non-clinical settings interpret health information they can routinely retrieve from the EPR. For this purpose, we used an online survey with a sample of healthy volunteers. An initial sample of participants was recruited through the researchers' networks of contacts. We then employed the snowball sampling method, asking potential respondents to virally distribute the link to the questionnaire to others in their own networks. The two versions of the questionnaire were randomly distributed to individuals who clicked on the link. The link was operative for a period of two weeks. By the end of the data collection period the link had been distributed to over 350 individuals, of whom 298 completed the questionnaire and were found eligible to participate in the study. The exclusion criteria were handing in an incomplete form, or being a physician, a nurse, or an alternative practitioner.

Design

We designed two versions of an online questionnaire based on 10 hypothetical medical decision-making scenarios extracted from authentic EPRs. In each scenario, a series of symptoms had led the family doctor to request a lab test or series of tests. We presented our participants with the scenarios and associated lab results. The lab results were presented in one of three formats: numeric expressions, graphs, or verbal expressions (see below). After reading the scenarios and viewing the results, participants were asked to assess the gravity of the hypothetical condition, and what course of action they would follow if they were the patient.

The lab tests (blood work or cultures) were ordered to investigate or test for one of the following: menstrual arrest; hemoglobin deficiency; infection; hepatitis B; streptococcus (a throat infection); or a routine cholesterol check. We chose these conditions and tests because they are relatively common, likely to be only moderately serious, and in most cases potentially applicable to both men and women. Each scenario contained a short description of the hypothetical patient's symptoms and the possible consequences of poor treatment.

Two physicians and a nurse served as an expert panel. Each one independently reviewed the scenarios and confirmed the accuracy and reliability of the information provided. The two physicians were family doctors who ran their own community clinics. The nurse was employed in an emergency department in a medical center located in northern Israel.

An example follows: *For several weeks, Ayala had been feeling more tired than usual. She is pale and experiences a general feeling of laxity. During a visit to her family doctor, he recommended checking her hemoglobin level. Hemoglobin is a molecule found in red blood cells that carries the oxygen from the lungs to the tissues of the body. Ayala took the test and received the following result:*

Figure 1. An example of one scenario with graphic (version A) and numeric (version B) presentations of information

Version A Version B

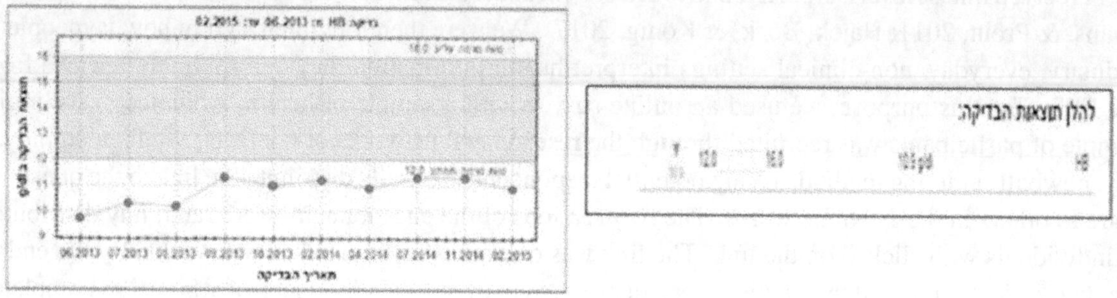

Tools and Measures

Information Formats

We extracted lab results in three different formats from authentic electronic patient records. Results presented in the verbal format included the name of the diagnosis, test, or condition, with a short explanation and/or recommendation from the physician. The numeric format comprised a single measure or a series of measures presented in table form, sometimes with an indication of the norm. The graphic format comprised a graph containing the current measurement, previous measurements, and an indication of the norm. Four scenarios juxtaposed numeric and graphic presentations, two juxtaposed graphic and verbal presentations, and three juxtaposed numeric and verbal presentations. One scenario was identical in both versions of the questionnaire and presented verbal information.

Perceived Gravity of Condition

After reading each scenario, participants were asked to assess the gravity of the hypothetical health condition. Perceived gravity ranged from 1=very low to 5=very high, with 6= don't know. For the sake of comparison, we asked our expert panel (the two physicians and nurse described above) to assess the actual gravity of each of the scenarios.

Uncertainty

The sixth option in the gravity scale, namely "don't know," was used to measure how participants assessed the coherence, or understandability, of the information presented. A choice of the "don't know" response indicated that the participant acknowledged having difficulty interpreting the lab results. We measured the proportion of "don't know" responses for each scenario. The higher the number, the greater the uncertainty.

To test whether difficulty understanding the results reflected incoherence of the presented information or something else, we asked six assessors (three researchers, and the three medical professionals on our expert panel) to independently rate the coherence of the information supplied for each version of the ten scenarios. The independent assessors measured coherence as a combination of four indicators: determinacy (i.e., exactness) of the information presented (yes/no); perspective (i.e., are the results shown as a snapshot in time or in relation to previous measurements); presence of a norm (showing whether the present results are normal or abnormal); and presence of a general explanation. Each indicator was assessed on a scale of 1=very low to 5=very high or 6 = not relevant. For each version of each scenario we measured the number of respondents who chose option 6 ("don't know") in the gravity scale and correlated these responses with those of our expert assessors. We found a strong correlation between our participants' assessments and those of our experts, indicating that our expert assessors and laypersons perceived the coherence of the information supplied in similar terms ($r[20] = 0.640$, $P<0.05$).

Accuracy

We measured the accuracy (i.e., correctness) of participants' assessments of the gravity of the health condition against those of the physicians and nurses by subtracting the former from the latter. Positive values meant that the participant underestimated the gravity of the condition, a value of zero meant that the participant correctly assessed the gravity of the condition, and negative values meant that the participant overestimated the gravity of the condition. This variable ranged from -0.35 to 3.75. We then turned this into a categorical variable named accuracy (>0=1; 0=2; <0=3).

Courses of Action

After providing their assessment of the condition's gravity, participants were asked which of four courses of action they would likely follow if they were the patient: call a doctor; search the Internet; do nothing and wait for the doctor to call them; and do nothing and wait for their next visit to the doctor. We identified the first two options (call a doctor or search the Internet) as more proactive, and the second two (wait for the doctor's call or for a scheduled visit) as less proactive.

Demographics and Control Variables

Before responding to the scenarios, respondents were asked demographic questions and questions about the main control variables. The demographic characteristics of the sample are shown in Table 1.

With respect to the control variables, one set of questions addressed how often respondents used their own EPR to perform various tasks, such as viewing lab results, scheduling appointments, or downloading forms (8 items; $\alpha = 0.88$). These items were measured on a six-point scale where 1= I have never used this function, 2= rarely, 5= frequently, and 6= I am not aware that this function exists. Another set covered participants' health status, attitudes towards self-care, and responsiveness to medical or health recommendations (7 items; $\alpha = 0.620$). These items were measured on a 5-point scale where 1=rarely and 5= frequently. Reliability for all these variables was acceptable, and all items appeared to be worthy of retention, resulting in a decrease in the alpha if deleted. A third set of questions elicited participants' information-seeking behaviors (whether participants tend to seek medical information and help mainly from a doctor, family or friends, online health forums, or websites). Participants' information-seeking behaviors are shown in Table 2.

Table 1. Descriptive statistics: Demographics (N=298, full questionnaire)

Criterion	No of respondents	% of respondents
Age	N=255 M=36.12, SD=13.734	Missing values 43
18-39	127	49.8
40-59	75	29.4
60 and older	53	20.8
Gender	N= 269	Missing values 29
Male	112	41.6
Female	157	58.4
Religious self-definition	N=270	Missing values 28
Secular	237	88%
Traditional	24	9.8%
Religious (orthodox)	9	3.3%
Marital status	N=267	Missing values 31
Single	138	51.7
Married	124	46.4
Divorced	5	1.9
Parents to children under 18 years	N=268	Missing values 30
Yes	79	29.5
No	189	70.5
Health status	N=270	Missing values 28
Poor	7	6.2
Good	46	17
Very Good	136	50.4
Excellent	81	30
Income	N=269	Missing values 29
Below average	132	49.1
Around average	22	8.2
Above average	82	30.5
Far above average	33	12.3
Education	N=269	Missing values 29
High school	80	29.7
Academic	172	63.9
other	17	6.3
HMO	N=268	Missing values 39
Clalit	126	47
Maccabi	95	35.4
Leumit	20	7.5
Meuhedet	27	10.1

Table 2. Prevalent sources of information

Variables	Doctor	Family/Friends	Forums	Websites
Information about treatment	55.6 (N=144)	5.4 (N=14)	7.3 (N=19)	31.7 (82)
Recommendation for a doctor/clinic/hospital	29.2 (N=76)	40.8 (N=106)	15.4 (N=40)	14.6 (N=38)
Emotional support in coping with emotional state	12.5 (N=32)	78.6 (N=202)	5.4 (N=14)	3.5 (N=9)

RESULTS

The descriptive statistics of the sample can be found in Table 1. Here we highlight some findings from the questions on health status, health behaviors or attitudes, and use of EPRs. Based on the full sample (N=298), seven respondents (2%) claimed to be in poor health, while 263 (88%) reported being in good or very good health. Fifty-five respondents (18%) reported suffering from a chronic illness, and 21 respondents (7%) reported suffering from some type of physical limitation. Age was positively correlated with feeling responsible for one's health (r[213]=0.139, P<0.001), and negatively correlated with postponing regular checkups (r[213]=-0.162, P<0.001). Forty-six out of 268 respondents (17.2%) reported that they regularly visit alternative healers. Our respondents reported visiting the doctor only after attempting to self-care (M=4.8, std=0.437), and agreed that maintaining a healthy lifestyle was important (M=4.69, std=0.57). They also reported generally complying with their doctor's recommended regime (M=4.36, std=0.844). Half the respondents (N=130) said they turn to their doctor for a consultation, while 25% (N=65) turn to a family member, 22.7% (N=59) consult medical websites for information, and only 2.3% (N=6) consult online health forums.

Seventy-one percent of our participants (N=173) reported that they frequently read their lab results via the EPR, while 7.7% (N=23) were not aware of being able to view their lab results via the EPR, and another 10% (N=30) claimed to have never viewed lab results via the ERP. Women tend to consult the EPR significantly more than men (t[216]=-3.6, P<0.001). However, these differences disappear when looking at use of the EPR solely for the purposes of viewing lab results and viewing personal recommendations. Results of the multiple linear regression to predict the level of EPR use indicate that there was a collective significant effect of gender, age, education, health status, and income on EPR use (F(5,240) = 4.187, p = .000, R2 = .080). The individual predictors were examined further and indicated that only income (Beta = .258; t = 2.660, p = .008), health status (Beta = -.129; t = -1.980, p < .046) were significant predictors in the model. Gender, age, and education were not predictive of EPR use.

Hypothesis Testing

H1 predicted that the three information formats (verbal, numeric, and graphic) would yield different levels of accuracy in assessing the gravity of the healthcare condition.

To fully understand the behavioral implications of uncertainty or "not knowing," we looked at another measure of lay comprehension, namely accuracy in the interpretation of the gravity of the health condition (Keselman & Smith, 2012). Figure 2 displays the proportion of "don't know" answers for each scenario, and Figure 3 displays the disparities between our participants and the experts in the assessment of gravity for each scenario. Together, the two capture two aspects of comprehension: acknowledged failure to understand; and an assumption of understanding while misinterpreting the results.

Figure 2. The proportion of "do not" know answers of each version of the scenarios

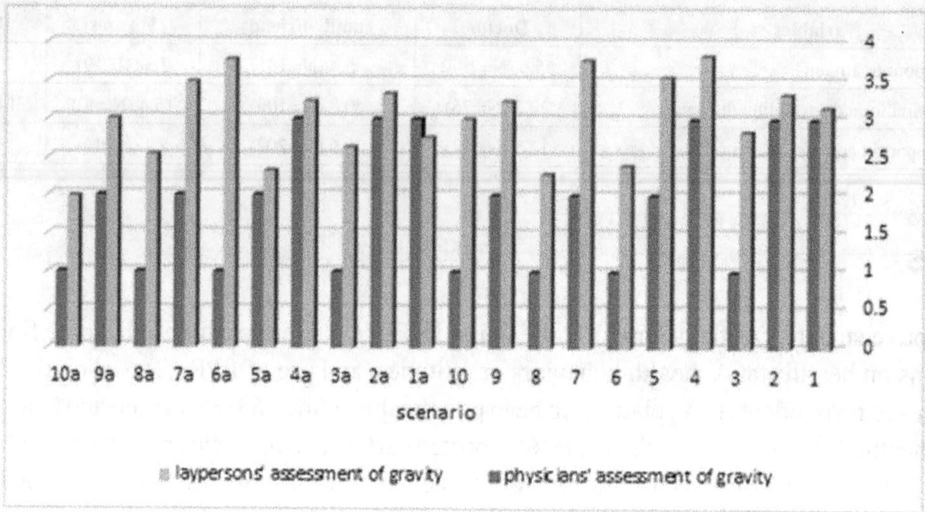

Figure 3. Participants' and Experts' assessments of gravity, for each scenario

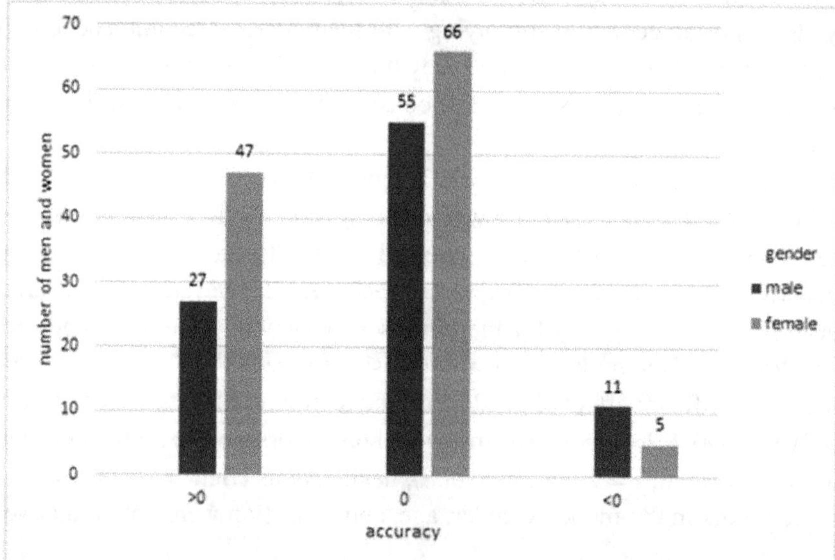

A paired-samples t-test was conducted to compare the participants' assessments of gravity and the experts'. In general, there was a significant difference between the participants' (M=3.02, SD=1.14) and experts' (M=1.9, SD=0.85) assessments of gravity, t(18)=-6.624, p = 0.000. These results suggest that the medical professionals tended to interpret the gravity of the health conditions as less severe than the participants. However, both the participants and the professionals interpreted the gravity of most conditions as low, or moderately low. Figure 3 displays both experts' and participants' assessments of gravity for each scenario.

Table 3. A paired-samples t-test to compare participants' and the experts' assessments of gravity based on information formats

Information format			Mean	N	Std. Deviation	t Mean
Numeric	Pair 1	Expert assessment	2.1667	6	.98319	-.87350
		Participants assessment	3.0402	6	.38946	
Verbal	Pair 1	Expert assessment	1.7778	9	.83333	-1.18900
		Participants assessment	2.9668	9	.56317	
Graph	Pair 1	Expert assessment	1.8000	5	.83666	-1.29280
		Participants assessment	3.0928	5	.74946	

P< 0.05

A second paired-samples t-test was conducted to compare the participants' and experts' assessments of gravity based on the three information formats. Table 3 clearly suggests that the participants were fairly accurate in the general trend, but tended to overestimate the conditions' gravity in all three formats. Looking specifically at the three formats, compared to the professionals' assessments, participants displayed a relatively high level of inaccuracy (measured as the difference between the laypeople's assessments and the experts') when information was displayed in the graphic format, less so in the verbal, and the least in the numeric format. In other words, for those respondents who hazarded a gravity assessment (as opposed to those who chose the "don't know" option), information was most difficult to interpret correctly when presented graphically, and easiest to interpret correctly when presented numerically. These findings confirm H1, showing that over and above the control variables, the format in which information is presented affects how people interpret it. Figure 4 displays the comparison of experts' and laypersons' assessments of gravity according to the information format.

Figure 4. A comparison of experts' and laypersons' assessments of gravity according to information formats

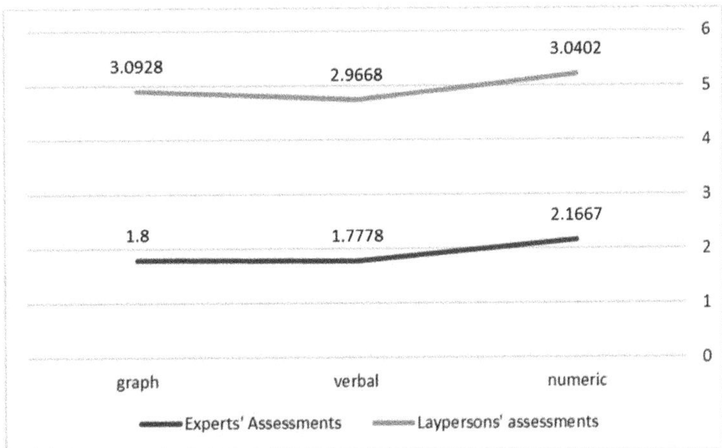

A two-way ANOVA was performed to examine the effect of gender and age on accuracy. There was a significant interaction between the effects of gender and age on accuracy, F(2, 204) =8.118, p < .0000. However, simple main effects analysis showed that there were no significant main effects between gender and accuracy, nor between age and accuracy. An independent t-test to test the effect of gender on accuracy confirmed there were no significant differences between men and women in level of accuracy. However, a one-way between-subjects ANOVA to compare the effect of age on accuracy showed a significant effect of age at the p<.00 level for all three age groups, F(2, 210) = 4.94, p = 37.233. Post hoc comparisons using the Tukey HSD test indicated that the mean score for participants aged 18–39 (M = 1.98, SD = 0.54) was significantly different from the scores for those aged 40–59 (M = 1.28, SD = 0.79) and those aged 60 or over (M=1.3, SD=0.6). The findings show no differences between those aged 40–59 and those aged 60 or above. Taken together, these results suggest that with greater age (at least up to a certain point), people tend to be more accurate in interpreting the gravity of health conditions based on the information presented to them.

To further probe the data, we conducted a multiple linear regression to predict level of accuracy. These results point to a significant association between accuracy and gender, age, education, health status, income, and EPR use (F(1,244) = 15.409, p < .001, R2 = .059). Examining the individual predictors, only age (Beta = .186; t = -3.063, p = .002) was a significant predictor of accuracy in the model. Gender, education, health status, income, and EPR use were not predictive of accuracy.

H2 posited that the three information formats (verbal, numeric, and graphic) would differ in their coherence levels (understandability).

Results of the multiple linear regression to predict uncertainty (i.e., "don't know" answers) point to a significant collective association between uncertainty and gender, age, health status, EPR use, perceived gravity of the condition, and accuracy (F(6,203) = 5.804, p < .001, R2 = .146). Looking at the individual predictors independently, only gender (Beta = .155; t = 2.352, p = .002), gravity (Beta = -.247; t=-3.043, p = .003), and accuracy (Beta = -446; t=-5.431, P<0.000) were significant predictors, while age, health status and EPR use were not predictive of uncertainty. Women tended to choose the "don't know" option (M=14.312; sd=3.8) significantly more than men (M=13.16; sd=3.6), t (267) =1.799, P=0.014. It is noteworthy that these differences disappeared when age was factored in. As Figure 5 shows, a two-way ANOVA was conducted to examine the effect of gender and age on uncertainty. There was a statistically insignificant interaction between the effects of age and gender on uncertainty, F (2, 246) =2.231, p = .11). Participants aged 18–39 were significantly more inclined to choose the "don't know" option than those aged 40–59 (P<0.000), while those aged 40–59 were less likely to choose "don't know" than those aged 60 or over (P<0.000), creating a U-shaped pattern. While the interaction of gender and age on level of accuracy was statistically insignificant, it indicates an interesting trend that should be explored further.

To test the effect of the three information formats (verbal, numeric, and graphic) on coherence levels (understandability), we performed a linear regression to predict uncertainty based on the information format (Beta = -.706, t(17) =-3.921, p < .001, (F(2,17) = 8.181, p < .001, R2 = .492). Next, we performed a one-way ANOVA to test the differences between the three information formats in responses indicating uncertainty. The ANOVA yielded a statistically significant difference between the three groups (F(2,17) =9.789, p = .001). A Tukey post-hoc test revealed that uncertainty was lowest when information was presented in the graphic format (M=5.35, min=1.30-max= 7.4) and highest when it was presented in the numeric format (M=15.9, min=10.70, Max=21), with a significant difference between them (P<0.000). There was an insignificant difference between the graphic and verbal formats (P=0.405), with uncertainty slightly higher in the latter than in the former (M=8.18, min=3; Max=15.8). In general, the findings

Figure 5. Two-way ANOVA to test the effects of gender and age on level of uncertainty

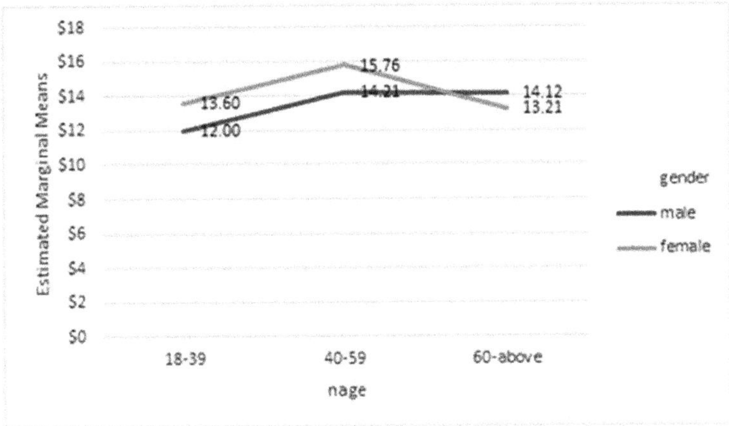

indicate that respondents found the numeric format most difficult to understand and the graphic format the easiest, thus confirming H2. However, as will be recalled, participants displayed a relatively high level of inaccuracy (measured as the difference between the laypeople's and experts' assessments) when information was displayed in the graphic format, less so in the verbal, and the least in the numeric format. Figure 6 displays the distribution of "don't know" responses by information format.

H3 predicted that the greater the uncertainty, the more proactive people are likely to be in seeking help or information.

We expected that respondents who realized they did not understand the information (and who therefore chose the "don't know" response to the gravity question) would favor more proactive measures, defined as contacting a doctor immediately or searching for information on the Internet. A Pearson correlation revealed an inverse relationship between "don't know" responses and participants' tendency to report they would call a doctor ($r=-0.184$, $p<001$), and a positive relationship between "don't know" and the

Figure 6. Levels of uncertainty ("do not know") according to information format

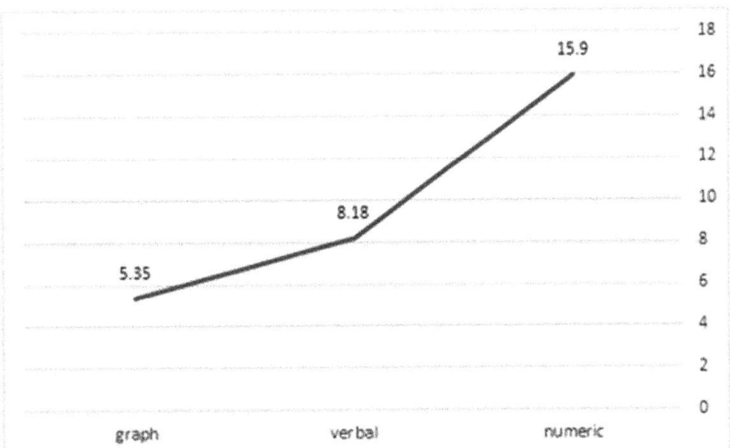

Table 4. Correlations between incoherence and preferred action (N=298)

Measure	1	2	3	4
1. Call doctor Sig. (2-tailed)		-.097 .094	-.260*** .000	-.061 .296
2. Internet use Sig. (2-tailed)	-.097 .094		.482*** .000	.467*** .000
3. Wait for doctor to call Sig. (2-tailed)	-.260*** .000	.482*** .000		.779*** .000
4. Wait for visit to doctor Sig. (2-tailed)	-.061 .296	.467*** .000	.779*** .000	
5. Don't know Sig. (2-tailed)	-.184*** .001	-.438*** .000	.442*** .000	.448*** .000

***p<0.01

other three courses of action: searching the Internet (r=0.438, P<001), waiting for the doctor to call them (r=0.442, P<.005), or waiting for their next visit to the doctor (r=0.488, P<.005) (see Table 4). Thus, the greater the perceived incoherence of the information presented, the less likely participants were to say they would immediately call their family doctors. Rather, they were more likely to say they would search the Internet for information, wait for their next doctor's appointment, or wait for their doctor to contact them. Consulting the Internet for information was positively correlated with waiting for the doctor to call and waiting for one's next visit to the doctor (r[298]=0.482, P<0.001; r[298]=0.467, P<0.001, respectively).

A linear regression to test participants' preferred course of action under conditions of uncertainty confirmed our previous findings (F(4,293) = 33.433, p < .001, R2 = .313). The analysis revealed that immediately calling the doctor (Beta = -.135; t = -2.623, p = .009), searching the Internet (Beta = .256; t = 4.572, p < .000) and waiting for the next visit to the doctor (Beta = .354; t=4.393, P<0.000) were significant predictors in the model. Waiting for the doctor to call was found insignificant in this model. These findings suggest that people who fail to understand information presented in an EPR are likely to react by searching the Internet for information, or postponing discussion of the results until their next visit to the doctor. Our hypothesis that the greater the uncertainty, the more proactive people are likely to be in seeking help or information was rejected.

DISCUSSION

Using hypothetical scenarios taken from authentic EPRs, we showed that the format in which medical information is presented plays a central role in how well individuals understand the information, their assessment of the associated health condition, and subsequently their likely choice of action. In general, those participants who assessed the gravity of the health condition on a 5-point scale rather than choosing "don't know" (and who, therefore, presumably felt they understood the information sufficiently to make an assessment) tended to slightly overestimate the gravity of the condition, compared with assessments by medical professionals. The consistency of this finding suggests that clinicians and laypeople often understand medical information differently (see also Han, Klein, & Arora, 2011; Keselman & Smith, 2012; Rosenfeld & Weinberg, 2012; Lupton, 2013; Pilnick & Zayts, 2014). We found that high perceived gravity was the only predictor of immediately calling the doctor as the likely course of action, suggesting that overestimating the import of test results seen on EPRs may result in unnecessary visits to the physician. Equally, underestimating the gravity of a condition may lead to underuse of health care facilities. In this regard, those formats that left respondents less able to understand the results – particularly the numeric format – produced a lower sense of urgency, and correspondingly, less inclination to actively seek professional help. Thus, uncertainty regarding the meaning of the lab results drove participants to shift the burden of responsibility to their doctors, as well as to delay actively seeking medical services. These findings are especially striking since participants' assessments were generally unrelated to EPR use, nor to gender, income, education, or health status. Age was the only demographic variable found to predict assessments of the health condition, with younger age associated with greater perceptions that a given condition was a serious cause for concern. We attribute this finding to younger participants' relative paucity of experience with the health system generally, and with changes in their own health more particularly.

Our study focused on how laypersons interpret results of routine check-ups and lab tests provided directly to patients via electronic patient records. One of the central features of digital medicine is the individualization of detailed data. The underlying assumption of the digital project is that the better laypersons' access to detailed physiological data, the more likely they will be to take an active, engaged role in their own health care (Lupton, 2013). Alas, online access to personal medical information (especially when it is not properly explained or put into context) can be harmful. It can cause short-term distress (e.g., depression, anxiety, poorer perceptions of health, and psychological distress) and in the worst cases, lead people to avoid future screenings (Dubey, Mathew, Iglar, Moineddin, & Glazier, 2006; Armon & Taker, 2013; Lupton, 2013).

Research into the implications of personalized health information on laypersons' use of healthcare services is still in its early stages, with few demonstrations of measurable clinical impact (Skolbekken, 2019). The two factors most often cited as contributing to excessive rehospitalization and overcrowding in primary care are poor communication and poor coordination during care transitions (Durand, Palazzolo, Tanti-Hardouin, Gerbeaux, Sambuc, & Gentile, 2012; Gouge, 2018). Laypersons use information to build representations of health and illness, and the results of this process influence their decisions to act. A study on laypersons' interpretation of personalized risk statistics with regard to the risk of getting cancer showed that people often reject their personal risk numbers as invalid (Scherer, Ubel, McClure, Greene, Alford, Holtzman, & Fagerlin, 2013). However, findings on the effects of information formats are mixed and nuanced. In the case of antenatal screening tests, for instance, it has been shown that laypersons display a better understanding of the information when a verbal or narrative format is used (Michie, Lester, Pinto, & Marteau, 2005), yet are more likely to take up genetic testing when presented with numeric risk information (Wilson, Ferguson, & Thorn, 2011; Pilnick & Zayts, 2014). Moreover, when the probability of an outcome is expressed in verbal terms, the framing of the problem (whether negative or positive) has an influence on parents' decisions regarding antenatal testing, whereas when presented with the same information in numeric terms, the framing of the problem has almost no effect on the parents' decision (Welkenhuysen, Evers-Kiebooms, & d'Ydewalle, 2001). Looking further, a variety of studies in the health domain demonstrate that presenting information via graphs increases perceptions of risk as well as readiness to choose safer alternatives than when risk is communicated numerically (Dambacher, Haffke, Groß, & Hübner; 2016). Dambacher et al. explain that information conveyed in graphic form tends to be interpreted more intuitively than numeric information, thus lending an impression of understandability. Hence, under certain conditions, graphical components can have a stronger influence on decisions than information in another format (Bodemer & Gaissmaier, 2012; Dambacher, Haffke, Groß, & Hübner, 2016). Similarly, we found that our participants tended to perceive information presented via graphs to indicate higher levels of severity than when presented in verbal or numeric terms. Participants thus were most inaccurate in interpreting results presented in graphic form.

With laypeople now being expected and encouraged to regularly assess their own physiological markers and monitor their own health – responsibilities that were once the preserve of health care providers – it is paramount that personal health information be communicated in a format that ensures precision and minimizes uncertainty.

LIMITATIONS

Like all studies, ours is subject to limitations. First, even though the health information we supplied was drawn from authentic records, it was presented in the context of hypothetical scenarios. As such, our results may not accurately reflect how people respond to their own personalized health information. Future inquiries should consider ways of delving deeper into how people might interpret their own health information, using a combination of quantitative and qualitative methods. Second, despite our sample's diversity in terms of demographics, experience with the EPR system and health beliefs, our research design prevented us from reaching relatively isolated minority groups within the Israeli population, such as Arabs, ultraorthodox Jews, and immigrants of Ethiopian or French descent. Future studies should study the role of cultural diversity in the interpretation of personalized health information. This may require specific methodologies that control for language proficiencies while maintaining the authenticity of the information formats, something that was beyond the scope of our study. However, we can assume that if native Israelis, highly proficient in Hebrew, demonstrated significant deficiencies in comprehension, members of these populations will as well.

Finally, our sample is predominantly young and fairly well educated. Future research should examine uncertainty and comprehension of the three information formats with a broader, more representative sample of the population.

PRACTICAL IMPLICATIONS

Our findings show that technical aspects of EPRs – specifically, the format in which information is presented – may influence how people interpret the information, and their subsequent engagement with their health and with any health conditions. In addition, our findings point to a difference between simply understanding medical information (a function of the coherence of the information provided) and an ability to interpret the information's significance. We found that "don't know" responses were highest for the numeric format and lowest for the graphic format, suggesting that the numeric format is most difficult to understand and the graphic format the easiest. But in scenarios where respondents hazarded a guess as to the gravity of a given condition, they were more often wrong when information was presented graphically compared with numerically. In other words, people were more likely to admit they did not understand information presented in a numeric format; but when they believed they understood the information, they were more likely to misinterpret the gravity of the condition when the information was presented in the graphic format. These findings, if replicated over additional studies with representative samples, have implications for the design of EPRs at the practical level.

Policymakers increasingly believe that encouraging patients to play a more active role in their health care can improve quality, efficiency, and health outcomes (Coulter & Ellins, 2007; Koh, Brach, Harris, & Parchman, 2013). However, engaging patients in their own personal health care fundamentally relies on their ability to obtain, process, communicate, and understand basic health information. To date, there is no consensus as to what an EPR should contain (Keselman & Smith, 2012), and personalized medical information is typically presented in a way that is biased toward expert knowledge. So long as system designers and policy makers keep envisioning the medical expert as the customer/provider of the information, and the patient or layperson as merely a user of the information, relatively few people will become proficient enough to properly understand and act on available health information.

Clearly, if patients are to become effectively involved in their own care, careful design of EPRs is warranted, based on an understanding of patients' information needs and decision-making processes. Future research should continue to identify technical aspects of information presentation that lead laypeople astray, so that policy makers and software designers can make appropriate design decisions and develop needed comprehension support tools.

CONCLUSION

Our study offers new insights into how patients respond to medical records authored by health professionals. Our findings suggest that high levels of uncertainty can result in shifting more of the burden of patient care back to the clinician. This can offset current expectations for greater levels of patient self-care. Our study thus suggests that a paradigmatic shift in the way we think about information as a catalyst of self-care is in order. Toward this end, we need to recognize the layperson and not the clinician as the target of information. Presenting laypersons with discrete pieces of information devoid of context and a sense of progress or meaning does little to engage them in their own care. We call for further research to investigate how EPRs can best be designed so that patients are not just given information, but as Goetz (2010) put it, given an opportunity to act on it.

REFERENCES

Armon, G., & Toker, S. (2013). The role of personality in predicting repeat participation in periodic health screening. *Journal of Personality*, *81*(5), 452–464. doi:10.1111/jopy.12021 PMID:23126563

Asmundson, G. J., Abramowitz, J. S., Richter, A. A., & Whedon, M. (2010). Health anxiety: Current perspectives and future directions. *Current Psychiatry Reports*, *12*(4), 306–312. doi:10.100711920-010-0123-9 PMID:20549396

Baim-Lance, A., Tietz, D., Lever, H., Swart, M., & Agins, B. (2019). Everyday and unavoidable coproduction: Exploring patient participation in the delivery of healthcare services. *Sociology of Health & Illness*, *41*(1), 128–142. doi:10.1111/1467-9566.12801 PMID:30084113

Beck, F., Richard, J. B., Nguyen-Thanh, V., Montagni, I., Parizot, I., & Renahy, E. (2014). Use of the internet as a health information resource among French young adults: Results from a nationally representative survey. *Journal of Medical Internet Research, 16*(5), e128. doi:10.2196/jmir.2934 PMID:24824164

Berg, M. (2003). *Health information management: Integrating information and communication technology in health care work.* Abingdon, UK: Routledge. doi:10.4324/9780203563298

Bhavnani, S. K. (2002, April). Domain-specific search strategies for the effective retrieval of healthcare and shopping information. In CHI'02 Extended Abstracts on Human Factors in Computing Systems (pp. 610-611). ACM. doi:10.1145/506443.506508

Bodemer, N., & Gaissmaier, W. (2012). Risk communication in health (pp. 621–660). New York, NY: Springer Netherlands.

Bylund, C. L., Gueguen, J. A., Sabee, C. M., Imes, R. S., Li, Y., & Sanford, A. A. (2007). Provider–patient dialogue about Internet health information: An exploration of strategies to improve the provider–patient relationship. *Patient Education and Counseling, 66*(3), 346–352. doi:10.1016/j.pec.2007.01.009 PMID:17329062

Carman, K. L., Dardess, P., Maurer, M., Sofaer, S., Adams, K., Bechtel, C., & Sweeney, J. (2013). Patient and family engagement: A framework for understanding the elements and developing interventions and policies. *Health Affairs, 32*(2), 223–231. doi:10.1377/hlthaff.2012.1133 PMID:23381514

Copelton, D. A., & Valle, G. (2009). "You don't need a prescription to go gluten-free": The scientific self-diagnosis of celiac disease. *Social Science & Medicine, 69*(4), 623–631. doi:10.1016/j.socscimed.2009.05.012 PMID:19559513

Coulter, A., & Ellins, J. (2007). Effectiveness of strategies for informing, educating, and involving patients. *British Medical Journal, 335*(7609), 24–27. doi:10.1136/bmj.39246.581169.80 PMID:17615222

Dambacher, M., Haffke, P., Groß, D., & Hübner, R. (2016). Graphs versus numbers: How information format affects risk aversion in gambling. *Judgment and Decision Making, 11*(3), 223–242.

Davison, C., Smith, G. D., & Frankel, S. (1991). Lay epidemiology and the prevention paradox: The implications of coronary candidacy for health education. *Sociology of Health & Illness, 13*(1), 1–19. doi:10.1111/1467-9566.ep11340301

Dubey, V., Mathew, R., Iglar, K., Moineddin, R., & Glazier, R. (2006). Improving preventive service delivery at adult complete health check-ups: The Preventive health Evidence-based Recommendation Form (PERFORM) cluster randomized controlled trial. *BMC Family Practice, 7*(1), 44. doi:10.1186/1471-2296-7-44 PMID:16836761

Durand, A. C., Palazzolo, S., Tanti-Hardouin, N., Gerbeaux, P., Sambuc, R., & Gentile, S. (2012). Non-urgent patients in emergency departments: Rational or irresponsible consumers? Perceptions of professionals and patients. *BMC Research Notes, 5*(1), 525. doi:10.1186/1756-0500-5-525 PMID:23006316

Eng, T. R. (2002). eHealth research and evaluation: Challenges and opportunities. *Journal of Health Communication, 7*(4), 267–272. doi:10.1080/10810730290001747 PMID:12356287

Fetterolf, D. E. (1999). A Framework for Evaluating Underutilization of Health Care Services. *American Journal of Medical Quality, 14*(2), 89–97. doi:10.1177/106286069901400204 PMID:10446670

Goetz, T. (2010). *The decision tree: Taking control of your health in the new era of personalized medicine*. Emmaus, PA: Rodale.

Gouge, C. (2018). "Getting the knowledge right": Patient communication, agency, and knowledge. *The Journal of Medical Humanities, 39*(4), 535–551. doi:10.100710912-016-9389-1 PMID:27017829

Hajek, A., Bock, J. O., & König, H. H. (2017). Association of general psychological factors with frequent attendance in primary care: A population-based cross-sectional observational study. *BMC Family Practice, 18*(1), 48. doi:10.118612875-017-0621-5 PMID:28340559

Han, P. K., Klein, W. M., & Arora, N. K. (2011). Varieties of uncertainty in health care: A conceptual taxonomy. *Medical Decision Making, 31*(6), 828–838. doi:10.1177/0272989X10393976 PMID:22067431

Iyawa, G. E., Herselman, M., & Botha, A. (2016). Digital health innovation ecosystems: From systematic literature review to conceptual framework. *Procedia Computer Science, 100*, 244–252. doi:10.1016/j.procs.2016.09.149

Jauho, M. (2017). Contesting lifestyle risk and gendering coronary candidacy: Lay epidemiology of heart disease in Finland in the 1970s. *Sociology of Health & Illness, 39*(7), 1005–1018. doi:10.1111/1467-9566.12542 PMID:28236330

Jemmott, J. B., Croyle, R. T., & Ditto, P. H. (1988). Commonsense epidemiology: Self-based judgments from laypersons and physicians. *Health Psychology, 7*(1), 55–73. doi:10.1037/0278-6133.7.1.55 PMID:3257734

Keselman, A., & Smith, C. A. (2012). A classification of errors in lay comprehension of medical documents. *Journal of Biomedical Informatics, 45*(6), 1151–1163. doi:10.1016/j.jbi.2012.07.012 PMID:22925723

Knight, L. V., & Mattick, K. (2006). "When I first came here, I thought medicine was black and white": Making sense of medical students' ways of knowing. *Social Science & Medicine, 63*(4), 1084–1096. doi:10.1016/j.socscimed.2006.01.017 PMID:16519978

Koh, H. K., Berwick, D. M., Clancy, C. M., Baur, C., Brach, C., Harris, L. M., & Zerhusen, E. G. (2012). New federal policy initiatives to boost health literacy can help the nation move beyond the cycle of costly "crisis care.". *Health Affairs, 31*(2), 434–443. doi:10.1377/hlthaff.2011.1169 PMID:22262723

Koh, H. K., Brach, C., Harris, L. M., & Parchman, M. L. (2013). A proposed "health literate care model" would constitute a systems approach to improving patients' engagement in care. *Health Affairs, 32*(2), 357–367. doi:10.1377/hlthaff.2012.1205 PMID:23381529

Levin-Zamir, D., Baron-Epel, O. B., Cohen, V., & Elhayany, A. (2016). The association of health literacy with health behavior, socioeconomic indicators, and self-assessed health from a national adult survey in Israel. Journal of Health Communication, 21(sup2), 61-68.

Levy, A. G., Weinstein, N., Kidney, E., Scheld, S., & Guarnaccia, P. (2008). Lay and expert interpretations of cancer cluster evidence. *Risk Analysis: An International Journal, 28*(6), 1531–1538. doi:10.1111/j.1539-6924.2008.01110.x PMID:18795998

Lovatt, M., Eadie, D., Meier, P. S., Li, J., Bauld, L., Hastings, G., & Holmes, J. (2015). Lay epidemiology and the interpretation of low-risk drinking guidelines by adults in the United Kingdom. *Addiction (Abingdon, England)*, *110*(12), 1912–1919. doi:10.1111/add.13072 PMID:26212155

Lupton, D. (2013). Quantifying the body: Monitoring and measuring health in the age of mHealth technologies. *Critical Public Health*, *23*(4), 393–403. doi:10.1080/09581596.2013.794931

Lupton, D., & Maslen, S. (2019). How women use digital technologies for health: Qualitative interview and focus group study. *Journal of Medical Internet Research*, *21*(1), e11481. doi:10.2196/11481 PMID:30681963

Mantwill, S., & Schulz, P. J. (2017). Low health literacy and healthcare utilization among immigrants and non-immigrants in Switzerland. *Patient Education and Counseling*, *100*(11), 2020–2027. doi:10.1016/j.pec.2017.05.023 PMID:28559092

Margalit, R. S., Roter, D., Dunevant, M. A., Larson, S., & Reis, S. (2006). Electronic medical record use and physician–patient communication: An observational study of Israeli primary care encounters. *Patient Education and Counseling*, *61*(1), 134–141. doi:10.1016/j.pec.2005.03.004 PMID:16533682

Michie, S., Lester, K., Pinto, J., & Marteau, T. M. (2005). Communicating risk information in genetic counseling: An observational study. *Health Education & Behavior*, *32*(5), 589–598. doi:10.1177/1090198105278562 PMID:16148206

Neter, E., & Brainin, E. (2019). Association Between Health Literacy, eHealth Literacy, and Health Outcomes Among Patients With Long-Term Conditions. *European Psychologist*, *24*(1), 68–81. doi:10.1027/1016-9040/a000350

Paz-Fuchs, A., Mandelkern, R., & Galnoor, I. (Eds.). (2018). The privatization of Israel: the withdrawal of state responsibility. Berlin, Germany: Springer. doi:10.1057/978-1-137-58261-4

Pichler, H., & Hesson, A. (2016). Discourse-pragmatic variation across situations, varieties, ages: I don't know in sociolinguistic and medical interviews. *Language & Communication*, *49*, 1–18. doi:10.1016/j.langcom.2016.04.002

Pilnick, A., & Zayts, O. (2014). "It's just a likelihood": Uncertainty as topic and resource in conveying "positive" results in an antenatal screening clinic. *Symbolic Interaction*, *37*(2), 187–208. doi:10.1002ymb.99

Prior, L. (2003). Belief, knowledge and expertise: The emergence of the lay expert in medical sociology. *Sociology of Health & Illness*, *25*(3), 41–57. doi:10.1111/1467-9566.00339 PMID:14498929

Prior, L., Evans, M. R., & Prout, H. (2011). Talking about colds and flu: The lay diagnosis of two common illnesses among older British people. *Social Science & Medicine*, *73*(6), 922–928. doi:10.1016/j.socscimed.2010.09.054 PMID:21186076

Pyper, C., Amery, J., Watson, M., & Crook, C. (2004). Patients' experiences when accessing their online electronic patient records in primary care. *The British Journal of General Practice*, *54*(498), 38–43. PMID:14965405

Rosenfeld, D., & Weinberg, D. (2012). Domestic practice, situated contingency and adherence to medical directives: A call for research. *Social Theory & Health*, *10*(1), 42–60. doi:10.1057th.2011.9

Scherer, L. D., Ubel, P. A., McClure, J., Greene, S. M., Alford, S. H., Holtzman, L., ... Fagerlin, A. (2013). Belief in numbers: When and why women disbelieve tailored breast cancer risk statistics. *Patient Education and Counseling*, *92*(2), 253–259. doi:10.1016/j.pec.2013.03.016 PMID:23623330

Simmons, L. A., Wolever, R. Q., Bechard, E. M., & Snyderman, R. (2014). Patient engagement as a risk factor in personalized health care: A systematic review of the literature on chronic disease. *Genome Medicine*, *6*(2), 16. doi:10.1186/gm533 PMID:24571651

Skolbekken, J. A. (2019). Online risk numbers–helpful, meaningless or simply wrong? Reflections on online risk calculators. *Health*. PMID:30678517

Welkenhuysen, M., Evers-Kiebooms, G., & d'Ydewalle, G. (2001). The language of uncertainty in genetic risk communication: Framing and verbal versus numerical information. *Patient Education and Counseling*, *43*(2), 179–187. doi:10.1016/S0738-3991(00)00161-0 PMID:11369151

Wilson, J. L., Ferguson, G. M., & Thorn, J. M. (2011). Genetic testing likelihood: The impact of abortion views and quality of life information on women's decisions. *Journal of Genetic Counseling*, *20*(2), 143–156. doi:10.100710897-010-9335-8 PMID:21057975

ADDITIONAL READING

Berg, M. (2003). *Health information management: Integrating information and communication technology in health care work*. Routledge. doi:10.4324/9780203563298

Berg, M., & Timmermans, S. (2000). Orders and their others: On the constitution of universalities in medical work. *Configurations*, *8*(1), 31–61. doi:10.1353/con.2000.0001

Bowker, G., Star, S. L., Gasser, L., & Turner, W. (2014). *Social science, technical systems, and cooperative work: Beyond the great divide*. Psychology Press. doi:10.4324/9781315805849

Lupton, D. (2014). *Digital sociology*. Routledge. doi:10.4324/9781315776880

KEY TERMS AND DEFINITIONS

Common-Sense Epidemiology: A concept concerned with how laypersons interpret medical information to make sense of the symptoms, causes, course, and consequences of disease. The layperson-as-epidemiologist metaphor implies an agent (layperson) who actively gathers information and interprets it to make sense of his or her health condition. Scholars in the field of e-literacy also look at the personal resources that laypersons mobilize in this process of sense-making.

E-Health Literacy: E-health literacy is commonly defined as Health as the use of emerging information and communication technology, especially the Internet, to improve or enable health and health care (Eng,, 2001).

Electronic Patient Records (EPRs): Electronic Patient Records are also referred to as Electronic Medical Records or Electronic Health Records. All refer to a computerized system that systematically collects and electronically stores patient- and population-level health information in a digital format. They are primarily used by health care professionals to perform administrative and clinical functions. Patients are allowed varying levels of online access to their records.

Health Information Technology (HIT): Covers the research, design, and application of information technologies in healthcare settings, including the design, development, creation, use and maintenance of information systems to support clinical and administrative processes. In the past two decades, the implementation of HIT in primary and tertiary care settings has revolutionized healthcare policy and care management.

Health Literacy: The World Health Organization defines health literacy as "the cognitive and social skills which determine the motivation and ability of individuals to access, understand, and use information to promote and maintain good health" (World Health Organization, 1998, p.20). Since then, the Institute of Medicine has expanded the definition to include the skills necessary to making "appropriate health decisions" (Neter and Brainin, 2019).

Overutilization of Health Services: Overutilization of services refers to excessive use of medical services. Overutilization related to patient choice is often related to disease conviction - the belief that bodily sensations and changes are due to disease processes. This can motivate maladaptive coping behaviors such as: reassurance seeking, recurrent checking, and information searching (Asmundson, Abramowitz, Richter, Whedon, 2010; Mantwill & Schulz, 2017).

Patients' Engagement in Health Care: Patient engagement refers to the relationship between patients and health care providers as they work together to "promote and support active patient and public involvement in health and healthcare, and to strengthen their influence on healthcare decisions, at both the individual and collective levels (Coulter & Ellins, 2007).

Uncertainty: Here uncertainty refers to a person's doubt about the meaning of information. This type of uncertainty means that the person is aware of not knowing how to make sense of the information provided to him.

Underutilization of Health Services: Underutilization of services refers to a state where patients do not receive the full range of necessary services due to inadvertent problems with access to services, under prescription of services, or due to patients' choice to avoid care (Fetterolf, 1999).

ENDNOTE

[1] https://www.timesofisrael.com/despite-privacy-concerns-israel-to-put-nations-medical-database-online/

Chapter 18
Impact of Information Technology on Patient Confidentiality Rights:
A Perspective

Abba Amsami Elgujja
https://orcid.org/0000-0003-0476-8810
University of Salford, UK

ABSTRACT

Advances in information technology, be it by way of social media or use of the electronic medical information systems, has changed the way we deal with patient confidential information. The hitherto clear professional relationship with the patient has been blurred using social media, just like the unprecedented rate at which electronic health information is used to access and share patient's confidential information among healthcare professionals. However, given the special professional relationship of confidence which traditionally bonds the healthcare practitioner with the patient, use of these technologies by the healthcare professionals portends the risk of breach of that duty of confidentiality. Although the patient's right to demand confidentiality of his information is not absolute, an unlawful breach could result in a crime, actionable tort, or become a subject of disciplinary action. This chapter undertakes a general review of the benefits and dangers of embracing these new information technologies and their impact on the confidentiality of sensitive health data.

INTRODUCTION

Advances in information technology have led to diverse impact on patient experience in healthcare (Rauv, 2017). Information technology, be it by way of social media, use of the electronic medical information systems or web-based other smart applications/tools is, therefore, a welcome idea. Its use heralds numerous far-reaching benefits for health communication between and among the public, patients, and health professionals. However, it also has changed the way we deal with confidential patient informa-

DOI: 10.4018/978-1-7998-0047-7.ch018

tion. The impact of technology on non-financial outcomes such as patient satisfaction and quality is gaining interest (Wallwiener, Wallwiener, Kansy, Seeger, & Rajab, 2009). Information is the lifeblood of modern medicine, while the health information technology (HIT) infrastructure could be considered as its circulatory system. Without that system, neither individual physicians nor health care institutions can perform at their best or deliver the highest-quality care (Wallwiener et al., 2009).

Health information technology (IT) has the potential to improve the health of individuals and the performance of providers, yielding improved quality, cost savings, and greater engagement by patients in their own health care (Buntin, Burke, Hoaglin, & Blumenthal, 2011). As the transition of healthcare from paper to an increasingly electronic world ensues, a new debate over privacy of individually identifiable health information has emerged. The concept of privacy and confidentiality ensures a win-win situation for both the patient and the healthcare professional. Healthcare professionals need the confident patient to divulge all pertinent information necessary for diagnosing and treating the patient, while the patients need to feel confident that they can receive needed health care without the risk that their private information will be inappropriately disclosed. Any such concerns might result in withholding of information and lead to potentially negative clinical consequences (Kuhn, 2011).

Major sources of disagreement over privacy issues can sometimes be traced back to the use of different definitions for key terms. Therefore, it would be proper to define the terms with a view avoiding confusion during the discussion in the subsequent sections. Many at times, we feel tempted to use the terms "privacy" and "confidentiality" interchangeably as if they bear one and the same meaning or connotation. The terms privacy and confidentiality are sometimes distinguished on the basis that privacy refers to physical matters, while confidentiality refers to informational material (Goodman, Miller, & Informatics, 2006). In other words, the right to privacy is the limitation placed on the right of others to have access to information about, or the physical space, of an individual (James, 1975). It should be noted that the privacy limitation placed on information is regarding unlawful access rather than its unlawful sharing with (or disclosure to) third parties, which comes within the ambit of confidentiality.

Conversely, confidentiality is simply, the duty to maintain patient's private information revealed during a professional relationship (Folkman, 2000). The information sought to be protected must be unique to that particular patient (as opposed to information that could be attributable to any person qua person) (Everstine et al., 1980). The lawful access to patient's private data or other similar information of this kind, therefore, creates an obligation in, or a commitment by the healthcare professionals to keep that data in confidence (Parent, 1983).

Privacy is the right of patients for their personal information not to be accessed and divulged (disclosed) to others, while confidentiality is the obligation of all holders of Individually Identifiable Health Information (IIHI) to protect the information according to the privacy interests of the patients to whom the information relates (US Department of Health and Human Services, 2001). A patient expects (trusts) that data that have been shared with a provider will not be further shared inappropriately. On the other hand, individually identifiable health information is any health data or record that could be correlated with a particular individual (Kuhn, 2011).

Patient privacy must be a major consideration in the development of information systems. Systems have to be designed not only to meet current legal requirements, but to anticipate future requirements. The system has to put into consideration, the multiple conflicting interests, to wit, the patient's interest to ensure that no one has unnecessary access to his data, the hospital administrator's interest to ensure an unimpeded access to data needed for management, and the physicians' interest to avoid time-consuming limitation on medical practice. (Brannigan, 1992). In addition to the electronic health information systems, other information technologies that have impact on healthcare and the patient, is the advent of Internet communication, and especially the social media. These technologies have the potential of "inadvertently blurring the interface between work and personal time (Thompson et al., 2008) as well as their professional relationship (Nelson & Staggers, 2014). Patients, too, mostly unknowingly, do leave behind a trail of personal information during their online explorations for answers to their health issues. (Denecke et al., 2015a).

Many hospitals have introduced electronic health information systems (also called, E-health) to replace the traditional paper-based medical records (Bah et al., 2011) and implement electronic systems (Alsulame, Khalifa, & Househ, 2016 p. 204). The advantage of enhanced convenience of accessibility and distribution of health information attributable to electronic health information system also creates the dangers related to privacy and confidentiality of patients' data (Barrows, Jr. & Clayton, 1996). Because they contain large amounts of highly detailed clinical information about patients in an extremely compact form that can be easily stored and rapidly transmitted between healthcare professionals and institutions.(Sade, 2010) In Saudi Arabia, the use of electronic health record system is a new experience for many of the health care professionals that could create a new ethical-legal dilemma about their duty of confidentiality.

This risk is further compounded by the ubiquitous nature of those technologies all over the world. The world continues to embrace them even the more on every evolving day. For instance, in Saudi Arabia, as part of its popularly coined Vision 2030, the Kingdom has an ambitious technological growth plan in the healthcare sector to ensure a smooth integration of medical records among their health care institutions. The plan includes the integration of electronic health information records of the primary healthcare clinics with that of the specialist tertiary health institutions to enable healthcare professionals to, securely and seamlessly, share patient data as they deal with millions patients annually (Chikhaoui, Sarabdeen, & Parveen, 2017, p. 7). In view of the increasing and rapid demand for healthcare services, and a blossoming ICT community, this ambitious government's plan could help it achieve its vision of becoming a regional and global leader in IT healthcare systems development and adoption (Chikhaoui et al., 2017, p.7). Several indicators seem to suggest that the healthcare industry could maintain the momentum of its rapid growth, at least, in the near future. The most prominent indicator of this direction is the growing desire among the current population to improve their wellbeing (Chikhaoui et al., 2017, p.7). In addition to the immensely growing Saudi healthcare workforce (Health, 2013), the Kingdom of Saudi Arabia has been welcoming hundreds of thousands of healthcare practitioners from all over the globe (The Saudi Commission for Health Specialties, 2014). This could have a significant implication on the clinicians' perceptions related to patient confidentiality given the diversity of their training and practice backgrounds.

However, integration or interlace of electronic health records between entities or among clusters of hospitals could present a huge challenge and a serious concern related to unauthorized access, security violation, and difficulties in securing a safe and seamless transfer from one hospital to another (Chikhaoui et al., 2017, p.8). Consequently, the increasing electronic health information systems would require a suitable legal and ethical environment that safeguards data privacy, security and confidentiality. In particular, there must be respect, and taking responsibility, for fundamental human rights and, especially, the right to privacy and confidentiality of sensitive patient's data by the healthcare professionals and health institutions (Chikhaoui et al., 2017, p. 8).

In addition to the dangers attributable to the adoption of electronic health information systems by healthcare institutions in most of the countries all over the world, another factor that could affect the patient's confidentiality rights is the use of social media for healthcare communication. Therefore, given to the special professional relationship of confidence which traditionally bonds the healthcare practitioner with the patient, use of these technologies by the healthcare professionals portends a new risk of breach of that duty of confidentiality. Although the patient's right to demand confidentiality of his information is not absolute, an unlawful breach could result in a crime, actionable tort or become a subject of disciplinary action.

The focal point is the impact of these information technologies on the confidentiality of patients' personal data, and the possible gap, if any, between technology and the law, has been adequately bridged. It also explores the adequacy of the legal safeguard of patient confidentiality in view of the new challenges brought about by the use of information technologies. On the other hand, it also attempts to proffer practical ways of ensuring that, in spite of the technologies, practitioners maintain their solemn duty of securing and maintaining the confidentiality of the patients' sensitive health information.

Although the approach would be a holistic review of the prevailing challenges all over the world, the author's approach is heavily influenced by his experience in the Saudi Arabian healthcare system, and in many instances, the expositions might apply globally, but only to the Saudi Arabian jurisdictions. It would not be surprising, therefore, to find several references made to the Saudi Arabian jurisdictions in this chapter. Another point worthy of note is that, this review is made from the legal purview.

As much as technologies have brought about numerous benefits to humanity, patients and healthcare delivery, its limitations and dangers associated with its use cannot easily be discounted. In particular, the easy accessibility and the ease of distribution of information through the advances in information technologies have also made personal individually identifiable health information vulnerable to unjustifiable disclosure to third parties. It would seem necessary to examine the impact of information technology on patient confidentiality with a view to identifying ways to curtail possible unlawful breaches.

THE IMPACT OF INFORMATION TECHNOLOGY ON PATIENT CONFIDENTIALITY

E-Privacy remains a challenge, as highly advanced privacy invasive technologies continue to emerge and evolve, exposing more private data than previously envisaged (Alharbi & Zyngier, 2012). Increasingly, personal data ends up in a *bucket* of data that can be used and re-used for all kinds of known and unknown purposes. This poses critical questions on the requirements for gathering, storing, analyzing and ultimately erasing data. Little is known about these systems, how they impact privacy and civil liberties, and how they address accuracy problems (Cannataci, 2017).

In many countries, laws have lagged behind the advances in technology, leaving significant lacunae in the adequacy of data protections (Campaign, 2001). The recent advances in the information technologies and social media networking seem to be a new challenge to managing the patient's confidential information. Saudi Arabia has witnessed a spectacular progress in health care, arguably the best among its peers, and is investing heavily in electronic health information systems and aiming to build a single electronic health system by 2020 (MOH, 2017). Consequently, the use of electronic medical information systems is on the rise in Saudi Arabia, perhaps because, during the preceding decade, the implementation of an electronic health information system for hospitals has been among the top priorities of Saudi Arabia. On the other hand, Internet use is becoming ubiquitous among the Saudi public and health care professional. For instance, statistics show that, as of the first quarter of the year 2012, about half (47.5%) of the Saudi populations use the Internet of which 82% of these utilize Facebook, while the number of

Twitter users has risen exponentially. The trend is expected to steadily rise even higher recently (Al-Khalifa & Garcia, 2013).

However, recently, concerns related to patient confidentiality breaches have been increasing as healthcare information management is increasingly becoming more digitized, disseminated and portable without a commensurate knowledge of the root cause of breaches in confidentiality. This creates a new and complex challenge to the healthcare professionals and organizations in their bid to establish proper controls and security (Kamoun & Nicho, 2014).

To emphasize this further, stories surrounding the UK's experience with mass surveillance through bulk acquisition of patients' data could be quite disturbing. In mid-2015, a public hospital contracted with Google DeepMind Technologies Limited, an information technology company that had no prior experience in healthcare services, to develop software using patients' health information from the Trust's database (Powles & Hodson, 2017). The data package involved patient identifiable information including demographic details, the results of every blood tests recorded at the hospital in the previous five years before the transfer, and the electronic records of patients' diagnoses, procedures and treatment courses while at the hospital (Powles & Hodson, 2017). The dilemma was in the choice of the right approach to deploy data-driven innovations to improve patient care and at the same time maintaining public trust in the use and security of their sensitive health information (King et al., 2018).

The Special Rapporteur on Privacy Cannataci (2017) stressed this, when he stated thus:

There is also growing evidence that the information held by states, including that collected through bulk acquisition or "mass surveillance" is increasingly vulnerable to being hacked by hostile governments or organised crime. The risk created by the collection of such data has nowhere been demonstrated to be proportional to the reduction of risk achieved by bulk acquisition. (Cannataci, 2017)

It is evident that some of the data protection principles were not followed in the contract. The Data Protection Act (DPA), 1998 (and the recently created General Data Protection Regulation (GDPR), 2016 which became applicable in May, 2018) require that the purpose for which personal data is processed must be clearly stated by the data controller, at a time no later than when the information is collected (purpose specification principle). Under section 22 of the DPA (and Article 5 (1) (b) of the recently created GDPR), where an information is processed for an alternative purpose, there must be a corresponding legal basis since the data controller cannot rely on the initial legal basis. The Trust initially claimed that the identifiable patient data was being processed for the purpose of direct patient care, however, investigation had found out, the purpose was actually for the clinical safety testing of *Streams* app developed by Google. The Trust had already shared the patient's data long before a privacy impact assessment agreement formalized (Powles & Hodson, 2017).

Presently, under Clause 40 of the GDPR (2016), the data controllers that did not fulfil the data protection principle requiring that the data controllers must, unless exempted by some other legitimate basis (as laid down by law), obtain consent of the data subject before lawfully sharing their personal data with third parties. The change in the initial purpose of processing the patient records for patient care to another one for testing an app rules out the assumption of implicit consent. Where processing is based on the data subject's consent, the controller should be able to show evidence that the data subject has freely given an informed consent in writing to the processing operation (a separate consent for any subsequent processing under Clause 42, GDPR). The evidence should demonstrate that the data subject is aware of, among other particulars, the identity of the controller and the purposes of the processing for his data, and that he/she was given the option to refuse or withdraw consent without detriment. Therefore, because the patients have not been properly informed, they were unable to exercise their right to opt out from the program which would have effectively prevented the processing of their personal data (Powles & Hodson, 2017).

Furthermore, Clause 49 of the GDPR requires that the personal data should be processed to the extent strictly necessary and proportionate for the purposes of ensuring network and information security. The Trust was unable to justify that sharing such a huge bulk of patient health records was necessary and proportionate for testing of the application. The impression left in the mind of the data subject, would seem to be that although they did not expect that the Trust would share their data with a third party company for testing a mobile application, they were not informed of the fact that it would occur. The Information Commissioner's Office conclusion was that this sharing of patients' data was in violation of the 1998 Data Protection Act (Powles & Hodson, 2017).

From the foregoing, we could deduce that despite the great advantages of adopting the electronic health information technologies, that enhances convenience of accessibility and distribution of health information, it also creates the risk related to privacy and confidentiality of patients' data. As can be seen from the Google case, his risk is real, and the impact it could cause to patients could be huge. Unfortunately, other information technologies, including social media use, eHealth concepts etc., too, portend similar risks to patient confidentiality.

ELECTRONIC MEDICAL RECORDS/E-HEALTH INFORMATION RISKS

The increasing demand for advanced information technology in the health sector is seemingly outpacing the law and regulations governing confidentiality rights. The health care settings, too, are embracing the fluidity of the changes happening in the society where they operate as they strive to meet the challenges of increased demand for higher quality medical services for less money in an increasingly competitive business environment. Therefore, healthcare providers and research institutions are searching for solutions that would maximize efficiency at a reduced cost (Chikhaoui et al., 2017, p.6).

Developing countries face several challenges associated with maintaining the confidentiality of health-related information, which include the data subjects' "diminished autonomy, language barriers, limited health literacy, and cultural barriers resulting from paternalism and social diversity" (Nair & Ibrahim, 2015, p. 211). Unfortunately, one of the limitations of the Saudi Arabian policy considerations for privacy and confidentiality is that, the Arabic culture gives priority to family values over individual autonomy and encourages conformity to family norms. Although this may have helped in protecting physical and proprietary privacy, data privacy of the data subjects could face significant challenges in such environment (Edwards, 2016).

It is apparent that the modern health institutions of both the developed and developing countries have continued to embrace and adopt the electronic health information systems in an unprecedentedly massive rate. There has been a varying rate of growth in the use of electronic health information systems or electronic medical record system in Saudi Arabia. Despite the exponential growth of electronic medical record system in a particular region Saudi Arabia reported (Bah et al., 2011), it is still generally lagging behind as reported in others (Hasanain, Vallmuur, & Clark, 2015; Jabali & Jarrar, 2018). However, many hospitals are in varying stages of introducing electronic health information systems to replace the traditional paper-based medical records and implement electronic systems (Alsulame et al., 2016).

The use of electronic health record systems is a new experience for many of health care institutions and professionals that could create a new ethical-legal dilemma about their duty of confidentiality.

Recently, there has been a noticeable shift in our understanding of health information systems and technologies, which raises concerns about their safe use by health professionals (Fernandez-Luque, Elahi, Grajales, & Iii, 2009). It is understandable that the proliferative use of electronic health information systems for health care delivery presents significant benefits for the patients and the health care providers in terms of enhancing patient autonomy, improving patient treatment outcomes, advances in health research and public health surveillance, etc. However, it also presents new legal challenges including that of privacy and confidentiality of identifiable health information (Hodge, Gostin, & Jacobson, 1999). For instance, Alhammad's (2017, p. 3) assessment of "outpatients' attitudes and expectations towards electronic personal health records (ePHR) systems in secondary and tertiary hospitals in Riyadh, Saudi Arabia" buttresses just that. The study noted that three-quarters of respondents believed that the security and confidentiality of their private health information are important (75%). The author, however, lamented that more research is required to further explore the ePHR privacy concerns of patients and the key factors in improving the use of ePHRs among specific populations (Alhammad, 2017).

Despite the varying degrees of awareness to their right to privacy, most patients do understand that the issue of confidentiality is important but are, nevertheless, in favor of permitting their healthcare providers and some family members to have access to healthcare or research related data. For instance, Alahmad and others studied a cross-section of patients for their attitude towards medical and genetic confidentiality in the Saudi research bio bank. Most respondents agreed to some specifically justifiable disclosures, however, they emphasized the importance of maintaining patient/donor confidentiality (Alahmad, Hifnawy, Abbasi, & Dierickx, 2016).

Similarly, other studies have shown patients' qualified acceptance of medical students in their care for confidentiality breach concerns (Al Ghobain et al., 2016) or show a preference for a physical examination by a lone physician (Al-Harbi & Al-Harbi, 2010). Some patients, who were studied on their attitude towards shared medical appointments, have shown a preference for an individual appointment approach because of concerns about possible unwarranted disclosure of confidential information to strangers (Alhowimel, 2013). The author, therefore, argues that patient confidentiality could be a decisive factor to patients in their willingness to freely disclose pertinent information to their healthcare professionals (Alkabba, Hussein, Albar, Bahnassy, & Qadi, 2012). Confidentiality could be a decisive factor to patients in their willingness to freely disclose pertinent.

IMPACT OF SOCIAL MEDIA ON PATIENT CONFIDENTIALITY

Apart from the increasing use of electronic health information systems, the social media that is now becoming part of daily life experience for a majority of people with access to the Internet, too, pose similar risks of breaches of confidentiality (Ahmed et al., 2013; Farnan et al., 2013). Social media use has, apparently, become ubiquitous in all facets of society, including and especially, among healthcare professionals. This might relate to the availability and accessibility to the Internet and other information technologies across the globe. Unlike before the proliferation of Internet and social media when people interacted on face-to-face basis, by mail or telephones, individuals have suddenly found themselves interacting with strangers who might be far across the borders. This sudden emergence of blurred boundaries of relationships has the potential to affect the confidential professional relationship between the healthcare professionals and the patients (Casella, Mills, & Usher, 2014). This development could potentially raise the temptation for Internet users to, unknowingly, carelessly, or negligently, share even sensitive data with completely unknown, or partially known third parties on the Internet.

Social media are a user-created content and communications tool hosted on a web-based application which may be in a form of networking sites e.g. Facebook or Twitter; media sharing sites e.g., Instagram; or blogs. Their popularity is rapidly rising from 'obscurity to ubiquity' (Bosslet, 2011) over the recent years. Social media is now used in almost all sectors of human endeavours, be it social, professional, academic, business or even in the healthcare sector. Just like in the other sectors, its use is even accelerating more quickly than envisaged (George, Rovniak, & Kraschnewski, 2013 p. 4). Social media is now increasingly being used for, among others, disseminating information among patients and professional colleagues (George et al., 2013), and recently, as source of data for surveillance and research (McKee, 2013). In the same vein, the use of social media among healthcare professionals is on the rise reaching about 90% among doctors and much higher among medical students as of 2011 (Prasanna, Seagull, & Nagy, 2011).

The professional relationship between the patient and healthcare professionals may be under a threat with the advent of the Internet, and more specifically, the large-scale use of social media platforms by individuals in society, health care professionals inclusive. For, instance, in the U.S., the scale of Facebook's online network is immense, with an estimated number of 149 million Americans using it every month, with each one connected to an average of 214 people (Collingwood, 2013). The growth of the number of people with Internet access continues to rise and a consequence of this is that it is becoming the norm for people to conduct significant parts of their lives through online social networks. Similarly, just like elsewhere, the daily use of Internet among adults has increased tremendously in the UK from about 60% in 2010 (White & Selwyn, 2013) to nearly 90% in 2015 (Meeker, 2015), and this figure might continue to increase.

Social media platforms generally enable users to form an online profile, to share personal information, to learn and keep up to date with knowledge, to facilitate virtual attendance at medical conferences, and to measure impact within a field (Roupret et al., 2014, p. 629). In addition, in this respect, Facebook offers something unprecedented, i.e., a direct real time access to an individual's social network, and without the need for tedious network registration by participants (Cobb & Graham, 2012, p. 571). Facebook provides such tools as *pages* and *groups* that allow self-enrolment and sharing of information via groups, and *applications* that provide direct access to all the aforementioned tools (Cobb & Graham, 2012). These facilities offered by the social media seem to create a virtual communication environment that could potentially affect how and what we communicate to whom, more especially within the context of the professional relationship between the patient and the health professionals.

This is even more so social media use amongst health care professionals continue to increase. For instance, recent estimates of the use of social media by doctors has escalated dramatically from 41% in 2010 to 90% in 2011, whereas the rates of use have been found to be above 90% for medical students (George et al., 2013, p. 454). Among pharmacy students in the UK, for example, a study showed that most of the respondents (91.8%) reported using social networking web sites, with 98.6% using Facebook and 33.7% using Twitter (Hall, Hanna, & Huey, 2013 p. 9). A growing minority of physicians also uses social media to communicate directly with patients to augment clinical care (Ventola, 2014, p. 491).

Conversely, patients join and use social media for increasing their knowledge about their health conditions, for social support, for exchanging advice among themselves (Antheunis, Tates, & Nieboer, 2013) and for self-help (Hamm et al., 2000). A majority of modern patients, more especially those with chronic conditions, seek social media and other online sources to obtain information on health issues, to link up with others with similar conditions, and to participate more actively in decisions affecting their health care. This ubiquitous use of social media by both health care professionals and patients over the last several years shows that these technologies will soon be part of modern medicine (George et al., 2013, p. 454).

However, by their nature, medical practice and social media use are contradictory. Medicine, by its nature involves private communications, privacy, confidentiality, and formal conduct, whereas social media entails values sharing and openness, connection and transparency, and informality. Therefore, any attempt to converge the two could create some concern in the professional practice (George et al., 2013, p. 454). Hence, social media fora, like Facebook, Twitter, WhatsApp as well as the ubiquitous search engines like Google, are raising an unprecedented level of medical legal/ethical dilemmas as health care professionals around the world struggle to responsibly incorporate these new technologies into their professional lives (Devi, 2011, p. 1141).

Undoubtedly, these concerns might have stemmed from the issues of privacy/confidentiality, consent, and other ethical issues of consequence to health professionals (George et al., 2013, p. 454). In addition, emerging evidence abound showing that medical professionals have discovered a new means of safely and productively navigating through social media for use in health care. These moves could illustrate that social media has been accepted as a tool to complement modern medical practice as it could provide unprecedented opportunities for cost-effective 2-way communication between health professionals and patients (George et al., 2013, p. 454). In spite of the currently available privacy safeguards, and the ability of users to navigate safely, there still exists the potential risks of blurring the boundaries to professional confidential relationships.

The use of social media through smart phones or computer has become a common outlet where patient's confidential information could be leaked because practitioners are mostly likely to use it for exchanging information about patient care (including sensitive patient information). Although patient's privacy is among the top dilemmas for public and private healthcare practitioners in Saudi Arabia (Ebad, Jaha, & Al-Qadhi, 2014), it is instructive to note that Saudi literature on medical/clinical ethics remains limited in terms of volume and scope (Alkabba et al., 2012). A study by Al Qaryan et al. (2016) has noted that a significant proportion of medical interns used personal mobiles to keep in contact with team members regarding the patient, while some 16% of participants did not have any security features on their smartphones. Although this study relates to medical interns and final year students, in the absence of similar Saudi study on qualified professionals, its findings could serve as a tip of an iceberg in this respect.

This discussion is undertaken within the context of the larger society in which social media is considered a useful tool for sharing personal information with friends and family members in their social circle, within which health providers may find themselves involved just like any other member of the society. The public, the patient as well as healthcare professionals use it frequently because of its distinctive features e.g., encouraging greater interactions with others, it is free, available, shared, and has personalized information; and it is readily accessible with wider coverage (Moorhead et al., 2013, p. 8). It can also be used to provide peer/social/emotional support or to support public health surveillance, and therefore, has the potential to influence health policy.

The main challenge that healthcare professionals face on social media is how to keep appropriate professional relationships boundaries safe when interacting with patients online and, how to ensure that patient privacy/confidentiality is maintained (Alsughayr, 2015, p. 108). Therefore, the health care professionals' online behaviour and content of their posts can adversely affect their professional reputation, which may ultimately have far-reaching consequences on their careers as well. Unsurprisingly, the UK's General Medical Council advises doctors to "make sure that (their) conduct at all times justifies their patients' trust in them and the public's trust in the profession" (General Medical Council, 2018).

Social media, whether used by individual healthcare professionals, by healthcare institutions or by the patients has a lot to offer in terms of creating new approach to networking, seeking and sharing information about health needs, or communicating with others. Social media has created opportunities for communications between healthcare professionals and institutions on the one hand, and the patients on the other, as well as communication among patient populations. However, the hitherto clear confidential relationship and boundary becomes blurred with individually identifiable health information.

Benefits of Social Media in Healthcare Communication

Without doubt, social media heralds numerous all-encompassing benefits for health communication between and among the public, patients, and health professionals. Social media users can control the dynamics of interaction and therefore, increase the frequency and number of interactions. So, social media provides readily available, shared, and customized health information to deal with health issues (Adams, 2010, p. e89), with a potential to improving health outcomes (Moorhead et al., 2013).

Social media has largely affected the practice of healthcare professions, perhaps most publicly by facilitating improved communication with and among patients (von Muhlen, Ohno-Machado, 2012, p.777). One of the main benefits of social media for health care communication is the availability and broadened access to health information for all, irrespective of gender, age, socio-economic status, race, or geographic locality, as compared to conventional communication approaches (Moorhead et al., 2013, p. 11/36). Social media also can provide for easier and wider access than the traditional methods where some people, such as youth and those in lower socioeconomic groups would not have easy access to health information (Moorhead et al., 2013). Interestingly, Facebook offers something unprecedented, i.e., a direct access to someone's social network, without the necessity of enrollment by participants (Cobb & Graham, 2012).

In addition, health related social media sites have changed traditional patient–physician relationships. They provide an accessible platform for discussing sensitive and complex issues / information with health professionals. In some social networking sites, patients form groups, share experiences and assist each other (Colineau & Paris, 2010). It is quite interesting to note that social media has, in many ways, broadly affected medical practice, perhaps, by enabling increased communication with and among patients. Instances include the use of social media, e.g., Twitter or Facebook, to conduct emergency broadcasts during natural disasters. (von Muhlen et al., 2012 p. 777).

Not only patients alone form communities on social media. Social media provide health care professionals with the wherewithal to share professional information, to debate health care issues related to policies and/or practices, and post beneficial comments for both patients and fellow colleagues (Nyongesa, Munguti, Omondi, & Mokua, 2014, p. 3). Health care professionals also can use social media to potentially improve patient's health outcomes, develop a professional network, keep up to date with news and discoveries, motivate patients on their illnesses and treatment options, as well as provide reliable health information to the community (Ventola, 2014 p. 491). For instance, the *Google Hangout* platform provides a forum where health care providers can communicate or interact with his or her patients, follow up on their conditions and proffer appropriate measures before complications set in (Nyongesa, Munguti, Omondi, & Mokua, 2014, p. 3).

The era of communicating disease information through leaflets and pamphlets is running toward extinction giving in to the easy, available and low-cost use of social media fora. Therefore, many health care professionals and institutions take advantage of these benefits that become available by merely joining the social media platform (Nyongesa et al., 2014, p. 2). An example of such experience is the one shared by the European Association of Urologists where the association used the social media to keep its members updated with urologic literature and news, followed live reportage of academic conferences, participated in discourse on a barrage of ideas, and networked with colleagues from around the world (Roupret et al., 2014, p. 628); and engaged with academic medical content (Roupret et al., 2014, p. 629). Conversely, health care institutions are increasingly involved in the social media both as a marketing avenue and a platform for providing information about their available services (Nyongesa et al., 2014, p. 3).

Social media not only supports healthcare processes through gathering and sharing information among communities and groups but, also supports patient empowerment, by getting patients into the position to take control of their healthcare needs (Denecke et al., 2015, p. 137). The communities of networking and data sharing platforms encourage and support sharing experiences about their sickness conditions, and treatment options/outcomes, as well as enabling members to track personal health and be actively involved in their own care (Denecke et al., 2015b).

Another health communication use of social media is in the field of public health surveillance. Social media are recently being seen as a source of data for surveillance and research by providing an opportunity for real time and, at relatively low cost, communication tool to track public concerns or capture discourses undertaken outside traditional media channels (McKee, 2013 p. 298). These may include monitoring public response to health issues, tracking and monitoring disease outbreak, identifying target areas for intervention efforts, and for disseminating pertinent health information to targeted communities (Moorhead et al., 2013, p. 8/36). Moreover, social media also is used to recruit patients for clinical trials based on social-media profiles or the mining of such data for epidemiological studies, or to crowdsource answers to individual clinical questions, e.g., use of posted tweets data to detect and monitor disease activity such cholera outbreaks (Denecke et al., 2015, p. 137).

While social media are primarily used for social interactions and keeping in touch with friends and family, we have realized from the foregoing that they are increasingly being used for health-related purposes (Ahmed et al., 2013, p. 328). Social media can also contribute to medicine by improving communication with patients, enhancing professional development, and contributing to public health research and service (Winkelstein, 2013, p. 454), thereby enhancing outcomes (Fisher & Clayton, 2012, p. 100). However, discourse on the limitations and dangers of social media use health care has overshadowed consideration of its potential benefits (Winkelstein, 2013).

Social media has obviously come to stay in our society. It has become ubiquitous in our lives, and it seems to transcend to every nook and crannies of our lives. Furthermore, social media offers society many benefits as individuals, professionals or healthcare organizations. It allows unhinged communications between and among individuals, groups, and between individuals and organizations. These communications include healthcare communications. However, the question remains: is there any limitation(s) or inherent to, or associated with, risks caused by social media used for healthcare communications? The next section attempts to answer this question.

Limitations and Dangers of Social Media for Healthcare Communication

There is no doubt that social media use in health care is a welcome idea. However, it has its own limitations and dangers. The quality of information derived from social media interactions is usually variable and inconsistent, as social media tools are largely an informal and unregulated tool used for data collection, sharing, and dissemination (Moorhead et al., 2013, p. 11/36). Both patients (and the public at large) as well as health care professionals may encounter certain barriers to social media use. For patients and other users of social media, their main concern is the risk of privacy infringement, and the unreliability of the information obtained therein. Whereas the professionals' main barriers were inefficiency and lack of skills (Antheunis et al., 2013).

Apart from the limitations alluded to previously and the enormous benefits already considered, all users of social media should be cautious of the inherent risks associated with the unaccredited nature of its informational content (Nyongesa et al., 2014, p. 3). Moreover, social media use also has the potential to create dual (professional versus private) relationships between health care professionals and patients, or blur the boundaries of the patient/professional relationship (Aylott, 2011; Casella et al., 2014). The potential risk associated with breaching patient confidentiality or posting unprofessional content (M. von Muhlen et al., 2012, p. 779) can be brought about by the "immediate and extensive visibility of online postings, and their permanence on the sites" (Marnocha et al., 2015, p. 119).

It is no wonder, therefore, that the press is awash with headlines of reports implicating health care professionals in unprofessional conduct on social media. ''Medical students' cadaver photos get scrutiny after images show up online'' (Heyboer, 2010), ''Nursing students expelled from university after posting pictures of themselves posing with a human placenta on "Facebook'' (Daily Mail, 2011), "Five nurses were fired for Facebook postings", etc., (Fink, 2011). Similarly, twenty-three incidents of patient information postings on social networking sites by NHS staff were reported to the Information Commissioner's Office in 2011 alone. These incidents involved 13 medical personnel from 11 trusts across the UK including a doctor who was dismissed for posting a picture of a patient on Facebook (Caldicott, 2013, p. 52).

In addition, in the year 2012, severe data losses in England were reported to the Department of Health mostly involving the loss or theft of data. Almost one-third were related to unauthorized disclosures (Caldicott, 2013, p. 49). Another report released to Guardian Healthcare showed that 16 trusts had brought 72 separate actions against their staff for inappropriately using social media at various times between 2008 and October 2011. The 'inappropriate use" included inappropriate conversations/comments on/about patient/patient-care or, posting pictures of the workplace on social media platforms (Laja, 2011). More often, social media users are unaware of the risks of wrongful disclosure of personal information online, (Adams, 2010) or of sharing harmful or incorrect advice on social media (Adams, 2010, p. 391-400). Just like other members of the public, it is clear that some clinicians use social media in their professional lives, but the respect for privacy remains a concern to everyone (Ventola, 2014). Therefore, discussion of the dangers of these technologies in medicine has overwhelmed consideration of positive applications (George et al., 2013).

As much as social media offers us benefits, there are attendant risks of the breach of confidentiality associated with its use in healthcare communications. It would, therefore, require all healthcare professionals and organizations to use it with caution, lest, professional boundaries become blurred, and individually identifiable health information becomes at risk of being unlawfully shared with third parties.

eHEALTH AND mHEALTH IMPACTS ON PATIENT'S CONFIDENTIALITY RIGHTS

Another evolving new technology that is used for collecting and managing patients' health information is the eHealth concept. E-health is a rather new healthcare practice supported by information technology that evolved within the preceding decade (Della Mea, 2001). This concept is referred to as *eHealth* for any kind online or offline computer-based application or electronic device, or *mHealth* for any (mobile) monitoring system that healthcare professionals use in healthcare practices to monitor or improve the patient's health status (Kampmeijer, Pavlova, Tambor, Golinowska, & Groot, 2016). Other similar concepts with like impact on patient confidentiality include *ePrescribing* (access to prescribing options, printing prescriptions to patients and sometimes electronic transmission of prescriptions from doctors to pharmacists), *telemedicine* (physical and psychological diagnosis and treatments at a distance, including telemonitoring patients' functions), wearables, fitness trackers, and others still evolving.

E-Health or similar applications offer healthcare professionals an access to medical knowledge and patient data at the point of care but studies have emphasized that they could be potentially dangerous (Lewis & Wyatt, 2014). These new applications potentially empower patients to get healthier or possibly enhance clinicians to become more effective and efficient (Musiat, Goldstone, & Tarrier, 2014). Physicians now have new ways to conduct professional communication, have easier access to decision support and expedited, efficient specialist consultation (Bromwich & Bromwich, 2016). However, these advantages of eHealth are not without some corresponding disadvantages. There are a number of concerns related to treatment credibility, user privacy and confidentiality. The potential risks to recording, storing and sharing patient information or images on such devices is further heightened if electronic mobile devices are hacked, lost or stolen (Bromwich & Bromwich, 2016). Basically, mobile security risks are high because *eHealth* tools give hackers an "easier direct access to more valuable organizational assets than any other intrusion point" (Gruessner, n.d.). Reports of data protection violations seem to even outweigh magnitude of real damage to health caused by health apps (Albrecht, 2016).

The key to successful data protection related to eHealth is the consistent implementation of existing laws along with obtaining valid informed consent, freely given, to enable data users to make their own decisions with regards to sharing their data (Albrecht, 2016, p. 26). The modern Internet-enabled smartphones with health technologies are easy to use and portable, but they are an easy prey for hackers. This is because a smartphone is like a micro-computer that has a microphone, a camera, a GPS and an antenna to connect from, and share all information including telephone numbers, address, emails, photos, contacts and, bank accounts and credit cards anywhere. Therefore, a smartphone could be a dangerous treasure of sensitive information that arguably is part of lives, but at a very high risk (Alvarez, McGlaughlin, & Wirth, 2017).

Apart from the e-Health tools discussed supra, there are several technologies in the hospitals, malls, public places and the street that collect, analyze and store our personal data on daily basis. Consequently, by merely walking out of one's home to work or school, multiple cameras track movement making it possible to reconstruct one's tracks with great precision, although the subject did not know about it nor give his consent. More often, signposts in public places alert people of the presence of CCTV cameras, whereupon, the only option open for non-consent is to avoid going to such places. However, that would mean that one could only avoid these cameras in modern cities by staying indoors, at home without going out to work. This would not only be impracticable but would have serious ramifications on society. Therefore, it could be argued that these serious privacy concerns create new challenges to the privacy laws. As a result, it is appropriate to assess whether adequate legal protections exist as safeguards for information privacy and confidentiality exist under current laws, or whether substantial gaps in the legal regime need to be filled with new laws or regulations.

E-Health technologies, no doubt, offer patients and doctors, the ability to remotely interact and communicate regarding diagnosing and managing patient ailments without the necessity for a face-to-face encounter. However, use of these tools, along with cloud services, allow for collection and processing of huge amount of health information which may, ultimately come to the possession of third parties without the knowledge and consent of the data subjects.

HAS THE LAW ADEQUATELY PROTECTED PATIENT CONFIDENTIALITY RIGHTS?

More often than not, laws lag behind modern developments which could include technological advancement (Dror, 1958). Novel technological innovation often raises gray areas in prevailing laws (Herz, 2009). It is not unexpected, therefore, that conventional law is unable to apply precisely on innovations and advancements in technology over time. It would have been sufficient that key principles are available to support adequate and extensive protection of human rights in a digital age (Electronic Frontier Foundation, 2014). Unfortunately, gaps exist between regulations provided by laws and the technological revolution, which grows even wider proportionately to the speed of technology advancement. Consequently, gaps in privacy laws, too, are widening rapidly (Wadhwa, 2014).

There is no doubt that novel technological advancements have potentially positively impacted humans' lives, although, using these technologies could portend potential security risks and challenges (Chikhaoui, Sarabdeen, & Parveen, 2016, p. 3): "[l]aw is always going to be playing catch up to technology," Bridget Treacy, leader of UK Privacy and Information Management practice at law firm Hunton & Williams in UK, had once asserted (Burn-Murdoch, 2013). It has been argued that the main problem with information security in health care is not technology, but a lack of cohesive security rules and policy. Relevant policy must shape technology and guide its use, and not the other way around. Security policy defines what is to be protected, to what reasonable degree protections will be afforded, and who is privileged to access protected items. (Randolph, 1996). Although, in every country, there are an array of privacy and data protection laws and regulations, they are not without a number of significant flaws. Often, in response to fast and often unforeseen dynamics in the technological landscape of privacy, surveillance, and data sharing, the law reactively and irregularly develops in a sporadic manner, thereby giving rise to gray areas in the protection of individuals' rights of privacy and confidentiality.

Major barriers to adopting cloud computing includes the lack of practical knowledge among users, and weak laws dealing with privacy. Privacy issues have almost always delayed the adoption of cloud computing (Chikhaoui et al., 2017, p. 10). Many countries do not yet have comprehensive data protection laws though they have devised strategic plans for privacy protection (Chikhaoui et al., 2017, p. 8). In countries, like Saudi Arabia and Nigeria, to mention two, have scattered pieces of legislation on patient confidentiality spread across several laws. They are lacking in both structure and substance. For instance, there is no available definition of "personal data", data processor, or safeguards against abuse in any of the existing Saudi Arabian legislation (Chikhaoui et al., 2017, p. 8).

Another explanation for lapses in the law is that, except for some recent regulations e.g., the European General Data Protection Regulation (GDPR) (European Union, 2016), most existing laws on information privacy and confidentiality are not based on standardized data protection principles. This means each piece of law, be it legislation, case law, or professional code must be contextualized to understand and interpret its impact. As a result, determining each case regarding data collection, processing and storage becomes burdensome. The ripple effect includes increased risks of privacy and confidentiality breaches and abuses by unlawful disclosure to unknown third parties. Modern data protection law should provide adequate safeguards from potential risks of arbitrary misuse of patients' personal data. In respect to Saudi Arabian settings, the assessment by triple test has shown that such safeguards are defective and inadequate.

CONCLUSION

There is no doubt that advances in information technology are fast-evolving, and transforming our lives in many ways. The transformation includes healthcare delivery. Health professionals can now use technology to easily and efficiently diagnose, treat and rapidly follow up on their patients. Patients can seek health information, tips and advice on the Internet or through social media. Social media can be used in crowdsourcing for research, contact tracing during disaster, epidemics and outbreaks. It is no longer in dispute that information benefits society in many ways.

However, technology, especially and particularly information technology, be it social media or electronic health information systems, or eHealth concepts, have made our social interaction easier, and improved the way patients and the healthcare professionals interact within the purview of confidential professional relationships. For these relationships to thrive, and nurture required mutual trust between patient and healthcare professionals, the latter commits to their duty to maintain the confidentiality of any personal information the patient divulges to enable them to identify and treat his ailment smoothly and successfully. However, advances in modern information technology have created a potential risk to this right of confidentiality which the patient has always enjoyed, as protected by the laws.

It has been argued that the laws are not able to keep up with the technology revolution. This ensuing gap potentially gives way to unresolved gray areas. Of course, some regional bodies are making efforts to reduce, if not eliminate such risks. A good example of such effort is the European Union's General Data Protection Regulation, 2016 which came into effect on May 26th, 2018. It not only laid down basic data protection principles, but also gave rights and powers to data subjects, in this case, the patients, to control how, who and for how long his/her personal data may be processed and shared. While the GDPR may be considered a wakeup call to all countries to optimize their laws to deal with the impact of technologies on the patient's confidentiality rights, professional bodies and regulators should also tailor their professional ethics and code to be contemporaneous with the advances in technology, as well as ensure compliance with same, and the law.

Technology is good for the patient, the healthcare professional and society at large, but it must be used with caution against the attendant risk to the closely guarded trust created by the professional relationships between them. Trust is difficult to gain and easy to lose (Pattinson, 2017).

ACKNOWLEDGMENT

I genuinely acknowledge and highly appreciate the review and contribution of my PhD research supervisor, Dr. Nicolas Kang-Riou of Salford Business School, University of Salford, Greater Manchester. My appreciation also goes for Dr. Augustine Edobor Arimoro, of University of Cape Town, for his review and invaluable input that immensely helped shaped the chapter.

REFERENCES

Adams, S. A. (2010). Blog-based applications and health information: Two case studies that illustrate important questions for Consumer Health Informatics (CHI) research. *International Journal of Medical Informatics*, *79*(6), e89–e96. doi:10.1016/j.ijmedinf.2008.06.009

Ahmed, O. H., Sullivan, S. J., Schneiders, A. G., Anderson, L., Paton, C., & McCrory, P. R. (2013). Ethical Considerations in Using Facebook for Health Care Support: A Case Study Using Concussion Management. *PM & R*, *5*(4), 328–334. doi:10.1016/j.pmrj.2013.03.007

Al Ghobain, M., Alghamdi, A., Arab, A., Alaem, N., Aldress, T., & Ruhyiem, M. (2016). Patients' perceptions towards the participation of medical students in their care. *Sultan Qaboos University Medical Journal*, *16*(2), 224–229. doi:10.18295qumj.2016.16.02.014

Al-Harbi, M., & Al-Harbi, K. (2010). Patient attitudes towards interns and medical students rotating in dermatology clinics in Almadinah Almunawwarah Region, Saudi Arabia. *Sultan Qaboos University Medical Journal*, *10*(3), 377–381.

Al-Khalifa, H. S., & Garcia, R. A. (2013). The state of social media in Saudi Arabia's higher education. *International Journal of Technology and Educational Marketing*, *3*(1), 65–76. doi:10.4018/ijtem.2013010105

Alahmad, G., Hifnawy, T., Abbasi, B., & Dierickx, K. (2016). Attitudes toward medical and genetic confidentiality in the Saudi research biobank: An exploratory survey. *International Journal of Medical Informatics*, *87*, 84–90. doi:10.1016/j.ijmedinf.2015.12.015

Albrecht, U.-V. (2016). Rationale. *Chances and Risks of Mobile Health Apps (CHARISMHA)*, 2–5.

Alhammad, O. S. (2017). Assessing Outpatients' Attitudes And Expectations Towards Electronic Personal Health Records (ePHR) Systems. In *Secondary and Tertiary Hospitals In Riyadh*. Saudi Arabia: McMaster University.

Alharbi, I. M., & Zyngier, S. (2012). A holistic view on the opportunities and risks faced by Saudi Arabia government in their adoption of the new law regulating electronic privacy. *WIAR 2012; National Workshop on Information Assurance Research*, 1–7.

Alhowimel, M. H. (2013). Attitudes of physicians toward implementing shared medical appointments at national guard family medicine centers in Riyadh. *Value in Health*, *16*(7), A538. doi:10.1016/j.jval.2013.08.1354

Alkabba, A. F., Hussein, G. M. A., Albar, A. A., Bahnassy, A. A., & Qadi, M. (2012). The major medical ethical challenges facing the public and healthcare providers in Saudi Arabia. *Journal of Family & Community Medicine*, *19*(1), 1–6. doi:10.4103/2230-8229.94003

Alqaryan, S., Alkhalifa, M., Alharbi, M., Alabaishi, S., & Aldrees, T. (2016). Smartphones and professionalism : A cross-sectional study on interns and final-year medical students. *International Journal of Medical Research & Health Sciences*, *5*(9), 198–202.

Alsughayr, A. (2015). Social media in healthcare: Uses, risks, and barriers. *Saudi Journal of Medicine and Medical Sciences*, *3*(2), 105. doi:10.4103/1658-631X.156405

Alsulame, K., Khalifa, M., & Househ, M. (2016). E-Health status in Saudi Arabia: A review of current literature. *Health Policy and Technology*, *5*(2), 204–210. doi:10.1016/j.hlpt.2016.02.005

Alvarez, B., McGlaughlin, C., & Wirth, A. (2017). The benefits and risks of health technology in the digital era – HIMSS Privacy and Security. Retrieved from https://staysafeonline.org/blog/health-technology-digital-era-benefits-risks/

Antheunis, M. L., Tates, K., & Nieboer, T. E. (2013). Patients' and health professionals' use of social media in health care: Motives, barriers and expectations. *Patient Education and Counseling*, *92*(3), 426–431. doi:10.1016/j.pec.2013.06.020

Aylott, M. (2011). Blurring the boundaries: Technology and the nurse-patient relationship. *British Journal of Nursing (Mark Allen Publishing)*, *20*(13), 810–812, 814–816. doi:10.12968/bjon.2011.20.13.810

Bah, S., Alharthi, H., El Mahalli, A. A., Jabali, A., Al-Qahtani, M., & Al-kahtani, N. (2011). Annual survey on the level and extent of usage of electronic health records in government-related hospitals in Eastern Province, Saudi Arabia. Perspectives in Health Information Management / AHIMA, American Health Information Management Association.

Barrows, R. C. Jr, & Clayton, P. D. (1996). Privacy, confidentiality : And electronic medical records. *Journal of the American Medical Informatics Association*, *3*(2), 139–148. doi:10.1136/jamia.1996.96236282

Bosslet, G. T. (2011). Commentary: The good, the bad, and the ugly of social media. *Academic Emergency Medicine*, *18*(11), 1221–1222. doi:10.1111/j.1553-2712.2011.01197.x

Brannigan, V. M. (1992). Protecting the privacy of patient information in clinical networks: Regulatory effectiveness analysis. *Annals of the New York Academy of Sciences*, *670*(1 Extended Clin), 190–201. doi:10.1111/j.1749-6632.1992.tb26090.x

Bromwich, M., & Bromwich, R. (2016). Privacy risks when using mobile devices in health care. CMAJ : Canadian Medical Association Journal = Journal de l'Association Medicale Canadienne, 188(12), 855–856. doi:10.1503/cmaj.160026

Buntin, M. B., Burke, M. F., Hoaglin, M. C., & Blumenthal, D. (2011). The benefits of health information technology: A review of the recent literature shows predominantly positive results. *Profiles of Innovation in Healthcare Delivery*, *30*(3). doi:10.1377/hlthaff.2011.0178

Burn-Murdoch, J. (2013, April 12). Data protection law is in danger of lagging behind technological change. *The Guardian*.

Caldicott, F. (2013). Information: To share or not to share. Information Governance Review. Information: To Share or Not to Share.

Campaign, G. I. L. (2001). *Privacy and Human Rights: An International Survey of Privacy Laws and Practice*. Global Internet Liberty Campaign.

Cannataci, J. A. (2017). Report of the Special Rapporteur on the right to privacy A/HRC/34/60.

Casella, E., Mills, J., & Usher, K. (2014). Social media and nursing practice: Changing the balance between the social and technical aspects of work. *Collegian (Royal College of Nursing, Australia), 21*(2), 121–126. doi:10.1016/j.colegn.2014.03.005

Chikhaoui, E., Sarabdeen, J., & Parveen, R. (2016). Privacy and security issues in the use of clouds in E-Health in the Kingdom Of Saudi Arabia. In Communications of the IBIMA (pp. 1–18). doi:10.5171/2017.369309

Chikhaoui, E., Sarabdeen, J., & Parveen, R. (2017). Privacy and security issues in the use of clouds in e-Health in the Kingdom of Saudi Arabia. Communications of the IBIMA, 1–18. doi:10.5171/2017.369309

Cobb, N. K., & Graham, A. L. (2012). Health behavior interventions in the age of facebook. *American Journal of Preventive Medicine, 43*(5), 571–572. doi:10.1016/j.amepre.2012.08.001

Colineau, N., & Paris, C. (2010). Talking about your health to strangers: Understanding the use of online social networks by patients. *New Review of Hypermedia and Multimedia, 16*(1-2), 141–160. doi:10.1080/13614568.2010.496131

Collingwood, L. H. (2013). Privacy protection under the English legal system: is it adequate given the challenges raised by online communicating between individuals? (Doctoral dissertation, Kingston University).

Della Mea, V. (2001). What is e-health?: The death of telemedicine? *Journal of Medical Internet Research, 3*(2), E22. doi:10.2196/jmir.3.2.e22

Denecke, K., Bamidis, P., Bond, C., Gabarron, E., Househ, M., Lau, A. Y., ... Hansen, M. (2015a). Ethical issues of social media usage in healthcare. *Yearbook of Medical Informatics, 10*(1), 137–147. doi:10.15265/IY-2015-001

Denecke, K., Bamidis, P., Bond, C., Gabarron, E., Househ, M., Lau, A. Y. S., ... Hansen, M. (2015b). Ethical issues of social media usage in healthcare. *Yearbook of Medical Informatics, 10*(1), 137–147. doi:10.15265/IY-2015-001

Devi, S. (2011). Facebook friend request from a patient? *Lancet, 377*(9772), 1141–1142. doi:10.1016/S0140-6736(11)60449-2

Dror, Y. (1958). Law and Social Change. *Tulane Law Review*, 33.

Ebad, S. A., Jaha, E. S., & Al-Qadhi, M. A. (2014). Analyzing privacy requirements: A case study of healthcare in Saudi Arabia. *Informatics for Health & Social Care, 41*(1), 47–63. doi:10.3109/17538157.2014.965301

Edwards, L. (2016). Privacy, Security and data protection in smart cities: A critical EU law perspective. *European Data Protection Law Review*, *2*(1), 28–58. doi:10.21552/EDPL/2016/1/6

Electronic Frontier Foundation. (2014). *NECESSARY & PROPORTIONATE: International Principles on the Application of Human Rights Law to Communications Surveillance*. Retrieved from http://www.ohchr.org/Documents/Issues/Privacy/ElectronicFrontierFoundation.pdf

European Union. (2016). Regulation 2016/679 of the European Parliament and the Council of the European Union. *Official Journal of the European Communities, 2014*(April), 1–88.

Everstine, L., Everstine, D. S., Heymann, G. M., True, R. H., Frey, D. H., Johnson, H. G., & Seiden, R. H. (1980). Privacy and confidentiality in psychotherapy. *The American Psychologist*, *35*(9), 828–840. doi:10.1037/0003-066X.35.9.828

Farnan, J. M., Sulmasy, L. S., Worster, B. K., Chaudhry, H. J., Rhyne, J. A., & Arora, V. M. (2013). Online medical professionalism: Patient and public relationships: Policy Statement From the American College of Physicians and the Federation of State Medical Boards. *Annals of Internal Medicine*, *158*(8), 620. doi:10.7326/0003-4819-158-8-201304160-00100

Fernandez-Luque, L., Elahi, N., Grajales, F. J., & Iii, F. J. G. (2009). An analysis of personal medical information disclosed in youtube videos created by patients with multiple sclerosis. In Studies in Health Technology and Informatics (pp. 292–296). doi:10.3233/978-1-60750-044-5-292

Fink, J. (2011, Nov. 19). Five nurses fired for Facebook postings. Scrubs.

Fisher, J., & Clayton, M. (2012). Who gives a Tweet: Assessing patients' interest in the use of social media for health care. *Worldviews on Evidence-Based Nursing*, *9*(2), 100–108. doi:10.1111/j.1741-6787.2012.00243.x

Folkman, S. (2000). Privacy and Confidentiality. In B. D. Sales, & S. Folkman (Eds.), *Ethics in research with human participants* (1st ed., p. 215). American Psychological Association.

General Medical Council. (2018). Confidentiality - GMC good medical practice. Retrieved from https://www.gmc-uk.org/ethical-guidance/ethical-guidance-for-doctors/confidentiality

George, D. R., Rovniak, L. S., & Kraschnewski, J. L. (2013). Dangers and opportunities for social media in medicine. *Clinical Obstetrics and Gynecology*, *56*(3), 453–462. doi:10.1097/GRF.0b013e318297dc38

Goodman, K. W., Miller, R. A., & Informatics, H. (2006). Ethics and health informatics : Users, standards, and outcomes. In E. H. Shortliffe, & J. J. Cimino (Eds.), *Biomedical Informatics Computer Applications in Health Care and Biomedicine* (3rd ed., pp. 379–402). New York, NY: Springer. doi:10.1007/0-387-36278-9_10

Gruessner, V. (n.d.). Why mobile security risks are healthcare's biggest liability. Retrieved from https://mhealthintelligence.com/news/why-mobile-security-risks-are-healthcares-biggest-liability

Hall, M., Hanna, L.-A., & Huey, G. (2013). Use and views on social networking sites of pharmacy students in the United Kingdom. *American Journal of Pharmaceutical Education*, *77*(1), 9. doi:10.5688/ajpe7719

Hamm, M. P., Chisholm, A., Shulhan, J., Milne, A., Scott, S. D., Given, L. M., & Hartling, L. (2000). Social media use among patients and caregivers: a scoping review. doi:10.1136/bmjopen-2013

Hasanain, R. A., Vallmuur, K., & Clark, M. (2015). Electronic medical record systems in Saudi Arabia: Knowledge and preferences of healthcare professionals. *Journal of Health Informatics in Developing Countries*, *9*(1), 23–31.

Health, M. (2013). Saudi Arabia Ministry of Health Achievements 2013.

Herz, M. (2009). Law lags behind: FOIA and affirmative disclosure of information. *Cardozo Public Law, Policy, and Ethics Journal*, *7*(3).

Heyboer, K. (2010, March 26). Medical students' cadaver photos gets scrutiny after images show up online. New Jersey Real-Time News.

Hodge, J. G. Jr, Gostin, L. O., & Jacobson, P. D. (1999). Legal issues concerning electronic health information: Privacy, quality, and liability. *Journal of the American Medical Association*, *182*(15), 1466–1471. doi:10.1001/jama.282.15.1466

Jabali, A. K., & Jarrar, M. (2018). Electronic health records functionalities in Saudi Arabia: Obstacles and major challenges. *Global Journal of Health Science*, *10*(4), 50. doi:10.5539/gjhs.v10n4p50

James, R. (1975). Why privacy is important. *Philosophy & Public Affairs*, *4*(4), 323–333.

Kamoun, F., & Nicho, M. (2014). Human and organizational factors of healthcare data breaches: The Swiss cheese model of data breach causation and prevention. [IJHISI]. *International Journal of Healthcare Information Systems and Informatics*, *9*(1), 42–60. doi:10.4018/ijhisi.2014010103

Kampmeijer, R., Pavlova, M., Tambor, M., Golinowska, S., & Groot, W. (2016). The use of e-health and m-health tools in health promotion and primary prevention among older adults: A systematic literature review. *BMC Health Services Research*, *16*(S5), 290. doi:10.118612913-016-1522-3

King, D., Karthikesalingam, A., Hughes, C., Montgomery, H., Raine, R., Rees, G., & Team, O. (2018). Letter in response to Google DeepMind and healthcare in an age of algorithms. *Health and Technology*, *8*(1–2), 11–13. doi:10.100712553-018-0228-4

Kuhn, T. (2011). Health Information Technology and Privacy- American College of Physicians A Position Paper July 2011.

Laja, S. (2011, Nov. 9). Trusts reveal staff abuse of social media | Healthcare Professionals Network | The Guardian. *The Guardian*.

Lewis, T. L., & Wyatt, J. C. (2014). mHealth and mobile medical Apps: A framework to assess risk and promote safer use. *Journal of Medical Internet Research*, *16*(9), e210. doi:10.2196/jmir.3133

Mail, D. (2011, Jan. 3). Four nursing students expelled from university after posting pictures of themselves posing with a human placenta on Facebook. *Daily Mail*.

Marnocha, S., Marnocha, M. R., & Pilliow, T. (2015). Unprofessional content posted online among nursing students. *Nurse Educator*, *40*(3), 119–123. doi:10.1097/NNE.0000000000000123

McKee, R. (2013). Ethical issues in using social media for health and health care research. *Health Policy (Amsterdam), 110*(2–3), 298–301. doi:10.1016/j.healthpol.2013.02.006

Meeker, M. (2015). 2015 Internet Trends. Retrieved from https://www.kleinerperkins.com/perspectives/2015-Internet-trends

Moh, S. (2017). National E- Health Strategy - MOH Initiatives 2030. Retrieved from https://www.moh.gov.sa/en/Ministry/nehs/Pages/vision2030.aspx

Moorhead, S. A., Hazlett, D. E., Harrison, L., Carroll, J. K., Irwin, A., & Hoving, C. (2013). A new dimension of health care: Systematic review of the uses, benefits, and limitations of social media for health communication. *Journal of Medical Internet Research, 15*(4), e85. doi:10.2196/jmir.1933

Musiat, P., Goldstone, P., & Tarrier, N. (2014). Understanding the acceptability of e-mental health-attitudes and expectations towards computerised self-help treatments for mental health problems. *BMC Psychiatry, 14*(1), 109. doi:10.1186/1471-244X-14-109

Nair, S. C., & Ibrahim, H. (2015). Assessing subject privacy and data confidentiality in an emerging region for clinical trials: United Arab Emirates. *Accountability in Research, 22*(4), 205–220. doi:10.1080/08989621.2014.942452

Nelson, R., & Staggers, N. (2014). *Health Informatics : An Interprofessional Approach*. Elsevier Health Sciences.

Nyongesa, H., Munguti, C., Omondi, C., & Mokua, W. (2014). Harnessing the power of social media in optimizing health outcomes. *The Pan African Medical Journal, 18*, 1–5. doi:10.11604/pamj.2014.18.290.4634

Parent, W. A. (1983). A new definition of privacy for the law. *Law and Philosophy, 2*(3), 305–338. doi:10.1007/BF00144949

Pattinson, S. D. (2017). Medical Law and Ethics (5th ed.). London, UK: Sweet and Maxwell.

Powles, J., & Hodson, H. (2017). Google DeepMind and healthcare in an age of algorithms. *Health and Technology, 7*(4), 351–367. doi:10.100712553-017-0179-1

Prasanna, P. M., Seagull, F. J., & Nagy, P. (2011). Online social networking: A primer for radiology. *Journal of Digital Imaging, 24*(5), 908–912. doi:10.100710278-011-9371-4

Rauv, S. (2017, June 14). The impact of technology in healthcare. Retrieved from https://www.elcomcms.com/resources/blog/the-impact-of-technology-in-healthcare-trends-benefits-examples

Roupret, M., Morgan, T. M., Bostrom, P. J., Cooperberg, M. R., Kutikov, A., Linton, K. D., ... Catto, J. W. F. F. (2014). European Association of Urology (@Uroweb) recommendations on the appropriate use of social media. *European Urology, 66*(4), 628–632. doi:10.1016/j.eururo.2014.06.046

Sade, R. M. (2010). Breaches of health information: Are electronic records different from paper records? *The Journal of Clinical Ethics, 21*(1), 39–41.

The Saudi Commission for Health Specialties. (2014). *Code of Ethics for Healthcare Practitioners*. Saudi Commission for Health Specialties.

Thompson, L. A., Dawson, K., Ferdig, R., Black, E. W., Boyer, J., Coutts, J., & Paradise Black, N. (2008). The intersection of online social networking with medical professionalism. *Journal of General Internal Medicine, 23*(7), 954–961. doi:10.100711606-008-0538-8

US Department of Health and Human Services. (2001, Sept. 5). Protecting the privacy of patients health information. Retrieved from https://aspe.hhs.gov/basic-report/protecting-privacy-patients-health-information

Ventola, C. L. (2014). Social media and health care professionals: Benefits, risks, and best practices. *P&T, 39*(7), 491.

von Muhlen, M., & Ohno-Machado, L. (2012). Reviewing social media use by clinicians. *Journal of the American Medical Informatics Association, 19*(5), 777–781. doi:10.1136/amiajnl-2012-000990

Wadhwa, V. (2014). Laws and ethics can't keep pace with technology. Retrieved from https://www.technologyreview.com/s/526401/laws-and-ethics-cant-keep-pace-with-technology/

Wallwiener, M., Wallwiener, C. W., Kansy, J. K., Seeger, H., & Rajab, T. K. (2009). Impact of electronic messaging on the patient-physician interaction. *Journal of Telemedicine and Telecare, 15*(5), 243–250. doi:10.1258/jtt.2009.090111

White, P., & Selwyn, N. (2013). Moving on-line? An analysis of patterns of adult Internet use in the UK. *Information Communication and Society, 16*(1), 1–27. doi:10.1080/1369118X.2011.611816

Winkelstein, P. (2013). Medicine 2.0: Ethical challenges of social media for the health profession. In C. George, D. Whitehouse, & P. Duquenoy (Eds.), *eHealth: Legal, Ethical and Governance Challenges* (pp. 227–243). Berlin, Germany: Springer Berlin Heidelberg; doi:10.1007/978-3-642-22474-4_10

KEY TERMS AND DEFINITIONS

Confidentiality: Literally, it is the state of keeping or being kept secret or private. In medical practice, confidentiality is the duty to keep and/or maintain (not to unlawfully disclose to third person) the patient's private information (secrets) revealed during a professional relationship.

Data Controller: A person, or an organization that determines the purpose and means of collecting and processing a person's personal data. For example, in the case of health information systems, the person responsible for deciding what data are collected, the purpose for its use, and the way and manner it may be processed.

eHealth: A novel technological concept that enables an electronic delivery of healthcare services online via the Internet.

Electronic Health Information System: An electronic system used by healthcare facilities to collect, store, manage and share a patient's electronic health or medical records for the purpose of patient care, research and quality management.

Electronic Health Records: An electronic form of the patient's paper-based medical or health record that can be instantaneously made securely and promptly available to authorized persons.

General Data Protection Regulation (GDPR): A legal framework that sets guidelines for the collection and processing of personal information from individuals who live in the European Union.

Health Information Technology (IT): Information technology applied to health and health care.

Individually Identifiable Health Information (IIHI): Information, including demographic data, that relates to: the individual's physical or mental health or condition (past, present or future), the provision of health care (including the payment therefor) to the individual that identifies (or for which there is a reasonable basis to believe it can be used to identify) the individual (See 45 C.F.R. § 160.103 HIPAA).

mHealth (mobile health): The use of mobile phones or other wireless (mobile) technology in healthcare, medical practice or public health.

Personal Data: Any information or different pieces of information that relates to a particular identified or identifiable living individual.

Privacy: The right of individuals, in the exercise of their autonomy, to control access to their private personal information by others.

Social Media: Websites and applications that enable users to create and share content or to participate in social networking.

Compilation of References

Aarons, G., Hurlburt, M., & Horwitz, S. (2011). Advancing a conceptual model of evidence-based practice implementation in public service sectors. *Administration and Policy in Mental Health*, *38*(1), 4–23. doi:10.100710488-010-0327-7 PMID:21197565

Aas, E. (2017). Prepare providers for telemedicine: 3 critical training areas. Retrieved from http://managedhealthcareexecutive.modernmedicine.com/managed-healthcare-executive/news/prepare-providers-telemedicine-3-critical-training-areas

Abbas, R. M., Carroll, N., & Richardson, I. (2018). in technology we trust: Extending TAM from a healthcare technology perspective. Paper presented at the *2018 IEEE International Conference on Healthcare Informatics (ICHI)*. 10.1109/ICHI.2018.00051

Abbott, A. (2004). Icelandic database shelved as court judges' privacy in peril. London, UK: Nature Publishing Group. doi:10.1038/429118b

Abouelmehdi, K., Beni-Hessane, A., & Khaloufi, H. (2018). Big healthcare data: Preserving security and privacy. *Journal of Big Data*, *5*(1), 1. doi:10.118640537-017-0110-7

Abraham, C., & Michie, S. (2008). A taxonomy of behavior change techniques used in interventions. *Health Psychology*, *27*(3), 379–387. doi:10.1037/0278-6133.27.3.379 PMID:18624603

Abràmoff, M. D., Lavin, P. T., Birch, M., Shah, N., & Folk, J. C. (2018). Pivotal trial of an autonomous AI-based diagnostic system for detection of diabetic retinopathy in primary care offices. *npj Digital Medicine*, *1*(39), 1-8.

Adams, S. A. (2010). Blog-based applications and health information: Two case studies that illustrate important questions for Consumer Health Informatics (CHI) research. *International Journal of Medical Informatics*, *79*(6), e89–e96. doi:10.1016/j.ijmedinf.2008.06.009

Addady, M. (2016). A new study of telemedicine services finds bad diagnoses. Retrieved from http://fortune.com/2016/05/16/telemedicine-services/

Adjerid, I., Adler-Milstein, J., & Angst, C. (2018). Reducing Medicare spending through electronic health information exchange: The role of incentives and exchange maturity. *Information Systems Research*, *29*(2), 341–361. doi:10.1287/isre.2017.0745

Adler, N. E., Boyce, T., Chesney, M. A., Cohen, S., Folkman, S., Kahn, R. L., & Syme, S. L. (1994). Socioeconomic status and health: The challenge of the gradient. *The American Psychologist*, *49*(1), 15–24. doi:10.1037/0003-066X.49.1.15 PMID:8122813

Afolayan, T., Aiterebhe, E. F., & Mejabi, V. (2015). Mobile phone usage in rural communities in Kwara state, Nigeria. *Inform Technolt*, *12*(2), 1–15.

Agar, M. H. (1996). *The professional stranger: An informal introduction to ethnography*. New York, NY: Academic Press.

Agboola, S. O., Ju, W., Elfiky, A., Kvedar, J. C., & Jethwani, K. (2015). The effect of technology-based interventions on pain, depression, and quality of life in patients with cancer: A systematic review of randomized controlled trials. *Journal of Medical Internet Research, 17*(3), e65. doi:10.2196/jmir.4009 PMID:25793945

Agency for Integrated Care. (2016). *Introduction to Home Care*. Singapore. Retrieved from https://www.aic.sg/sites/aicassets/AssetGallery/HCIK_BOOKLET 02_FA-5(Online).pdf

Ahmed, O. H., Sullivan, S. J., Schneiders, A. G., Anderson, L., Paton, C., & McCrory, P. R. (2013). Ethical Considerations in Using Facebook for Health Care Support: A Case Study Using Concussion Management. *PM & R, 5*(4), 328–334. doi:10.1016/j.pmrj.2013.03.007

Ajzen, I. (1991). The theory of planned behavior. *Organizational Behavior and Human Decision Processes, 50*(2), 179–211. doi:10.1016/0749-5978(91)90020-T

Akerkar, S. M., & Bichile, L. S. (2004). Health information on the internet: Patient empowerment or patient deceit? *Indian Journal of Medical Sciences, 58*(8), 321–326. PMID:15345885

Akiyama, M., & Byung-Kwang, Y. (2016). A systematic review of the economic evaluation of telemedicine in Japan. *Journal of Preventive Medicine and Public Health, 49*(4), 183–196. doi:10.3961/jpmph.16.043 PMID:27499161

Al Ghobain, M., Alghamdi, A., Arab, A., Alaem, N., Aldress, T., & Ruhyiem, M. (2016). Patients' perceptions towards the participation of medical students in their care. *Sultan Qaboos University Medical Journal, 16*(2), 224–229. doi:10.18295qumj.2016.16.02.014

Alaeddini, A., Yang, K., Reddy, C., & Yu, S. (2011). A probabilistic model for predicting the probability of no-show in hospital appointments. *Health Care Management Science, 14*(2), 146–157. doi:10.100710729-011-9148-9 PMID:21286819

Alahmad, G., Hifnawy, T., Abbasi, B., & Dierickx, K. (2016). Attitudes toward medical and genetic confidentiality in the Saudi research biobank: An exploratory survey. *International Journal of Medical Informatics, 87*, 84–90. doi:10.1016/j.ijmedinf.2015.12.015

Alam, M., D'Este, C., Banwell, C., & Lokuge, K. (2017). The impact of mobile phone based messages on maternal and child healthcare behaviour: A retrospective cross-sectional survey in Bangladesh. *BMC Health Services Research, 17*(1), 434. doi:10.118612913-017-2361-6 PMID:28645278

Albrecht, U.-V. (2016). Rationale. *Chances and Risks of Mobile Health Apps (CHARISMHA)*, 2–5.

Alepis, E., & Lambrinidis, C. (2013). M-health: Supporting automated diagnosis and electonic health records. *SpringerPlus, 2*(1), 103. doi:10.1186/2193-1801-2-103 PMID:23556144

Alhammad, O. S. (2017). Assessing Outpatients' Attitudes And Expectations Towards Electronic Personal Health Records (ePHR) Systems. In *Secondary and Tertiary Hospitals In Riyadh*. Saudi Arabia: McMaster University.

Alharbi, I. M., & Zyngier, S. (2012). A holistic view on the opportunities and risks faced by Saudi Arabia government in their adoption of the new law regulating electronic privacy. *WIAR 2012; National Workshop on Information Assurance Research*, 1–7.

Al-Harbi, M., & Al-Harbi, K. (2010). Patient attitudes towards interns and medical students rotating in dermatology clinics in Almadinah Almunawwarah Region, Saudi Arabia. *Sultan Qaboos University Medical Journal, 10*(3), 377–381.

Alhowimel, M. H. (2013). Attitudes of physicians toward implementing shared medical appointments at national guard family medicine centers in Riyadh. *Value in Health, 16*(7), A538. doi:10.1016/j.jval.2013.08.1354

Alkabba, A. F., Hussein, G. M. A., Albar, A. A., Bahnassy, A. A., & Qadi, M. (2012). The major medical ethical challenges facing the public and healthcare providers in Saudi Arabia. *Journal of Family & Community Medicine, 19*(1), 1–6. doi:10.4103/2230-8229.94003

Al-Khalifa, H. S., & Garcia, R. A. (2013). The state of social media in Saudi Arabia's higher education. *International Journal of Technology and Educational Marketing, 3*(1), 65–76. doi:10.4018/ijtem.2013010105

Allam, A., Kostova, Z., Nakamoto, K., & Schulz, P. J. (2015). The Effect of Social Support Features and Gamification on a Web-Based Intervention for Rheumatoid Arthritis Patients: Randomized Controlled Trial. *Journal of Medical Internet Research, 17*(1), e14. doi:10.2196/jmir.3510 PMID:25574939

Allam, A., Schulz, P. J., & Krauthammer, M. (2017). Toward automated assessment of health Web page quality using the DISCERN instrument. *Journal of the American Medical Informatics Association, 24*(3), 481–487. doi:10.1093/jamia/ocw140 PMID:27707819

Aller, M. B., Vargas, I., Coderch, J., & Vázquez, M. L. (2017). Doctors' opinion on the contribution of coordination mechanisms to improving clinical coordination between primary and outpatient secondary care in the Catalan national health system. *BMC Health Services Research, 17*(1), 842. doi:10.1186/s12913-017-2690-5 PubMed

Almodovar, A. S., Surve, S., Axon, D. R., Cooper, D., & Nahata, M. C. (2018). Self-directed engagement with a mobile app (Sinasprite) and its effects on confidence in coping skills, depression, and anxiety: Retrospective longitudinal study. *JMIR mHealth and uHealth, 6*(3), e64. doi:10.2196/mhealth.9612 PMID:29549066

Alpay, L., Van Der Boog, P., & Dumaij, A. (2011). An empowerment-based approach to developing innovative e-health tools for self-management. *Health Informatics Journal, 17*(4), 247–255. doi:10.1177/1460458211420089 PMID:22193825

Alqaryan, S., Alkhalifa, M., Alharbi, M., Alabaishi, S., & Aldrees, T. (2016). Smartphones and professionalism : A cross-sectional study on interns and final-year medical students. *International Journal of Medical Research & Health Sciences, 5*(9), 198–202.

Alsughayr, A. (2015). Social media in healthcare: Uses, risks, and barriers. *Saudi Journal of Medicine and Medical Sciences, 3*(2), 105. doi:10.4103/1658-631X.156405

Alsulame, K., Khalifa, M., & Househ, M. (2016). E-Health status in Saudi Arabia: A review of current literature. *Health Policy and Technology, 5*(2), 204–210. doi:10.1016/j.hlpt.2016.02.005

Alvarez, B., McGlaughlin, C., & Wirth, A. (2017). The benefits and risks of health technology in the digital era – HIMSS Privacy and Security. Retrieved from https://staysafeonline.org/blog/health-technology-digital-era-benefits-risks/

American Academy of Ophthalmology. (2019). About the IRIS@ registry. Retrieved from https://www.aao.org/iris-registry/about

Ammenwerth, E., Schnell-Inderst, P., & Hoerbst, A. (2012). The impact of electronic patient portals on patient care: A systematic review of controlled trials. *Journal of Medical Internet Research, 14*(6), e162. doi:10.2196/jmir.2238 PMID:23183044

Ancker, J. S., Barrón, Y., Rockoff, M. L., Hauser, D., Pichardo, M., Szerencsy, A., & Calman, N. (2011). Use of an electronic patient portal among disadvantaged populations. *Journal of General Internal Medicine, 26*(10), 1117–1123. doi:10.100711606-011-1749-y PMID:21647748

Anders, C., & Cassidy, A. (2014). Effective organizational change in healthcare: Exploring the contribution of empowered users and workers. *International Journal of Healthcare Management, 7*(2), 132–151. doi:10.1179/2047971913Y.0000000061

Anderson, G. O. (2017). Technology Use and Attitudes among Mid-Life and Older Americans, AARP research. Retrieved from https://www.aarp.org/content/dam/aarp/research/surveys_statistics/technology/info-2018/atom-nov-2017-tech-module.doi.10.26419%252Fres.00210.001.pdf

Anderson, E. S., Hsieh, D. M., & Alter, H. J. (2016). Social emergency medicine: Embracing the dual role of the emergency department in acute care and population health. *Annals of Emergency Medicine*, *68*(1), 21–25. doi:10.1016/j.annemergmed.2016.01.005 PMID:26921967

Anderson, E. S., Lippert, S., Newberry, J., Bernstein, E., Alter, H. J., & Wang, N. E. (2016). Addressing social determinants of health from the emergency department through social emergency medicine. *The Western Journal of Emergency Medicine*, *17*(4), 487–489. doi:10.5811/westjem.2016.5.30240 PMID:27429706

Anderson, R. M., & Funnell, M. M. (2010). Patient empowerment: Myths and misconceptions. *Patient Education and Counseling*, *79*(3), 277–282. doi:10.1016/j.pec.2009.07.025 PMID:19682830

Andreu-Perez, J., Poon, C. C. Y., Merrifield, R. D., Wong, S. T. C., & Yang, G.-Z. (2015). Big data for health. *IEEE Journal of Biomedical and Health Informatics*, *19*(4), 1193–1208. doi:10.1109/JBHI.2015.2450362 PMID:26173222

Andriole, K., Badano, A., Crawford, J., Chang, P., Flynn, M., Reiner, B., ... Seibert, J. (2004). AAPM/RSNA Tutorial on Equipment Selection: PACS Equipment Overview. *Radiographics*, *24*(1), 313–334. doi:10.1148/rg.241035137 PubMed

Anguera, J. A., Boccanfuso, J., Rintoul, J. L., Al-Hashimi, O., Faraji, F., Janowich, J., ... Gazzaley, A. (2013). Video game training enhances cognitive control in older adults. *Nature*, *501*(7465), 97–101. doi:10.1038/nature12486 PMID:24005416

Anonymous. (2018). Screen Time. *Physician Leadership Journal*, *5*(1), 80.

Antheunis, M. L., Tates, K., & Nieboer, T. E. (2013). Patients' and health professionals' use of social media in health care: Motives, barriers and expectations. *Patient Education and Counseling*, *92*(3), 426–431. doi:10.1016/j.pec.2013.06.020

Apple Inc. (2017). Apple Heart Study launches to identify irregular heart rhythms. Retrieved from https://www.apple.com/newsroom/2017/11/apple-heart-study-launches-to-identify-irregular-heart-rhythms/

Archer. (2019). The importance of healthcare data analytics in an EMR. Retrieved from https://www.archer-soft.com/en/blog/importance-healthcare-data-analytics-emr

Armon, G., & Toker, S. (2013). The role of personality in predicting repeat participation in periodic health screening. *Journal of Personality*, *81*(5), 452–464. doi:10.1111/jopy.12021 PMID:23126563

Asmundson, G. J., Abramowitz, J. S., Richter, A. A., & Whedon, M. (2010). Health anxiety: Current perspectives and future directions. *Current Psychiatry Reports*, *12*(4), 306–312. doi:10.100711920-010-0123-9 PMID:20549396

Association of British Neurologists. (2017). Acute Neurology Services Survey. Retrieved from http://www.theabn.org/media/docs/ABN%20publications/ABN%20acute%20neurology%20survey%20final%2013%20March%202017.pdf

Atallah, N., Khalifa, M., El Metwally, A., & Househ, M. (2018). The prevalence and usage of mobile health applications among mental health patients in Saudi Arabia. *Computer Methods and Programs in Biomedicine*, *156*, 163–168. doi:10.1016/j.cmpb.2017.12.002 PMID:29428068

Atasoy, H., Greenwood, B. N., & McCullough, J. S. (2018). The digitization of patient care: A review of the effects of electronic health records on health care quality and utilization. *Annual Review of Public Health*, *40*(1), 487–500. doi:10.1146/annurev-publhealth-040218-044206 PMID:30566385

Aujoulat, I., D'hoore, W., & Deccache, A. (2007). Patient empowerment in theory and practice: Polysemy or cacophony? *Patient Education and Counseling*, *66*(1), 13–20. doi:10.1016/j.pec.2006.09.008 PMID:17084059

Ayabakan, S., Bardhan, I. R., & Zheng, Z. (2017). A data envelopment analysis approach to estimate it-enabled production capability. *Management Information Systems Quarterly, 41*(1), 189–205. doi:10.25300/MISQ/2017/41.1.09

Aylott, M. (2011). Blurring the boundaries: Technology and the nurse-patient relationship. *British Journal of Nursing (Mark Allen Publishing), 20*(13), 810–812, 814–816. doi:10.12968/bjon.2011.20.13.810

Bah, S., Alharthi, H., El Mahalli, A. A., Jabali, A., Al-Qahtani, M., & Al-kahtani, N. (2011). Annual survey on the level and extent of usage of electronic health records in government-related hospitals in Eastern Province, Saudi Arabia. Perspectives in Health Information Management / AHIMA, American Health Information Management Association.

Baim-Lance, A., Tietz, D., Lever, H., Swart, M., & Agins, B. (2019). Everyday and unavoidable coproduction: Exploring patient participation in the delivery of healthcare services. *Sociology of Health & Illness, 41*(1), 128–142. doi:10.1111/1467-9566.12801 PMID:30084113

Banasiak, N. C., & Meadows-Oliver, M. (2017). Evaluating asthma websites using the Brief DISCERN instrument. *Journal of Asthma and Allergy, 10*, 191–196. doi:10.2147/JAA.S133536 PMID:28670135

Bandon, D., Lovis, C., Geissbühler, A., & Vallée, J. P. (2005). Enterprise-wide PACS: Beyond Radiology, an Architecture to Manage All Medical Images. *Academic Radiology, 12*(8), 1000–1009. doi:10.1016/j.acra.2005.03.075 PubMed

Bansal, G., Zahedi, F. M., & Gefen, D. (2007). The impact of personal dispositions on privacy and trust in disclosing health information online. In *Proceedings of the AMCIS, Keystone, Colorado.*

Bansal, G., Zahedi, F. M., & Gefen, D. (2010). The impact of personal dispositions on information sensitivity, privacy concern and trust in disclosing health information online. *Decision Support Systems, 49*(2), 138–150. doi:10.1016/j.dss.2010.01.010

Bansal, G., Zahedi, F. M., & Gefen, D. (2016). Do context and personality matter? Trust and privacy concerns in disclosing private information online. *Information & Management, 53*(1), 1–21. doi:10.1016/j.im.2015.08.001

Barello, S., Graffigna, G., & Vegni, E. (2012). Patient engagement as an emerging challenge for healthcare services: mapping the literature. *Nursing Research and Practice, 2012*. Retrieved from http://www.ncbi.nlm.nih.gov/pmc/articles/PMC3504449/

Barrows, R. C. Jr, & Clayton, P. D. (1996). Privacy, confidentiality : And electronic medical records. *Journal of the American Medical Informatics Association, 3*(2), 139–148. doi:10.1136/jamia.1996.96236282

Baskerville, R. L., & Stage, J. (1996). Controlling prototype development through risk analysis. *Management Information Systems Quarterly, 20*(4), 482–504. doi:10.2307/249565

Baskerville, R. L., & Wood-Harper, A. T. (1996). A critical perspective on information systems action research. *Journal of Information Technology, 11*, 235–246. doi:10.1177/026839629601100305

Beck, F., Richard, J. B., Nguyen-Thanh, V., Montagni, I., Parizot, I., & Renahy, E. (2014). Use of the internet as a health information resource among French young adults: Results from a nationally representative survey. *Journal of Medical Internet Research, 16*(5), e128. doi:10.2196/jmir.2934 PMID:24824164

Benbasat, I., Gefen, D., & Pavlou, P. A. (2008). Introduction to the JMIS special issue trust in online environments. *Journal of MIS, 25*(1), 5–12.

Benbya, H., & McKelvey, B. (2006). Toward a complexity theory of information systems development. *Information Technology & People, 19*(1), 12–34. doi:10.1108/09593840610649952

Benson, B. (2014). ETL challenges within healthcare business intelligence. Retrieved from https://www.hitechanswers.net/etl-challenges-within-healthcare-business

Ben-Zeev, D., Fathy, C., Jonathan, G., Abuharb, B., Brian, R. M., Kesbeh, L., & Abdelkader, S. (2017). mHealth for mental health in the Middle East: Need, technology use, and readiness among Palestinians in the West Bank. *Asian Journal of Psychiatry, 27*, 1–4. doi:10.1016/j.ajp.2017.02.010 PMID:28558877

Ben-Zeev, D., Scherer, E. A., Gottlieb, J. D., Rotondi, A. J., Brunette, M. F., Achtyes, E. D., & Mohr, D. C. (2016). mHealth for schizophrenia: Patient engagement with a mobile phone intervention following hospital discharge. *JMIR Mental Health, 3*(3), 1–9. doi:10.2196/mental.6348 PMID:27465803

Berg, M. (2003). *Health information management: Integrating information and communication technology in health care work*. Abingdon, UK: Routledge. doi:10.4324/9780203563298

Bexelius, C., Löf, M., Sandin, S., Trolle Lagerros, Y., Forsum, E., & Litton, J. E. (2010). Measures of physical activity using cell phones: Validation using criterion methods. *Journal of Medical Internet Research, 12*(1), e2. doi:10.2196/jmir.1298 PMID:20118036

Bhardwaj, R., Nambiar, A., & Dutta, D. (2017). A study of machine learning in healthcare. *Proceedings of 2017 IEEE 41st Annual Computer Software and Applications Conference*, Torino, Italy: IEEE Computer Society, 236-241. 10.1109/COMPSAC.2017.164

Bhavnani, S. K. (2002, April). Domain-specific search strategies for the effective retrieval of healthcare and shopping information. In CHI'02 Extended Abstracts on Human Factors in Computing Systems (pp. 610-611). ACM. doi:10.1145/506443.506508

Biernatzki, L., Kuske, S., Genz, J., Ritschel, M., Stephan, A., Bächle, C., ... Icks, A. (2018). Information needs in people with diabetes mellitus: A systematic review. *Systematic Reviews, 7*(1), 1–21. doi:10.118613643-018-0690-0 PMID:29444711

Biostrap. (2019). Hack your health: Biostrap helps you measurably improve your sleep, recovery, and performance. Retrieved from https://biostrap.com/

Birkhead, G. S., Klompas, M., & Shah, N. R. (2015). Uses of electronic health records for public health surveillance to advance public health. *Annual Review of Public Health, 36*(1), 345–359. doi:10.1146/annurev-publhealth-031914-122747 PMID:25581157

Bisson, J., Cosgrove, S., Lewis, C., & Roberts, N. P. (2015). Post-traumatic stress disorder. *Clinical Review, 351*, 1–7. PMID:26611143

Blankenburg, R., Hilton, J. F., Yuan, P., Rennke, S., Monash, B., & Harman, S. M., ... Huynh, E. (2018). Shared Decision-Making During Inpatient Rounds: Opportunities for Improvement in Patient Engagement and Communication. *Journal of Hospital Medicine, 13*(7), 453–461. PMID:29401211

Blau, M. (2017). Health wearables raise new privacy concerns. *The Boston Globe*. Retrieved from https://www.bostonglobe.com/business/2017/08/09/health-wearables-raise-new-privacy-concerns/0W2X9iNuLttoa7dUTFTzLJ/story.html

Bodemer, N., & Gaissmaier, W. (2012). Risk communication in health (pp. 621–660). New York, NY: Springer Netherlands.

Bodenheimer, T. (2008). Coordinating care—A perilous journey through the health care system. *The New England Journal of Medicine, 358*(10), 1064–1071. doi:10.1056/NEJMhpr0706165 PubMed

Bodenheimer, T., Wagner, E. H., & Grumbach, K. (2002). Improving primary care for patients with chronic illness. *Journal of the American Medical Association, 288*(14), 1775–1779. doi:10.1001/jama.288.14.1775 PMID:12365965

Boonstra, A., & Broekhuis, M. (2010). Barriers to the acceptance of electronic medical records by physicians from systematic review to taxonomy and interventions. *BMC Health Services Research, 10*(1), 231. doi:10.1186/1472-6963-10-231 PMID:20691097

Bosslet, G. T. (2011). Commentary: The good, the bad, and the ugly of social media. *Academic Emergency Medicine, 18*(11), 1221–1222. doi:10.1111/j.1553-2712.2011.01197.x

Boulton, C. (2018). Virtual healthcare gets real, as telehealth turns to AI. *CIO*. Retrieved from https://www.cio.com/article/3321736/health-care-industry/virtual-healthcare-gets-real-as-telehealth-turns-to-ai.html

Boyer, C., Selby, M., & Appel, R. D. (1998). The Health On the Net Code of Conduct for medical and health web sites. *Studies in Health Technology and Informatics, 52*(Pt 2), 1163–1166. PMID:10384641

Brabin, L., Roberts, S. A., Stretch, R., Baxter, D., Chambers, G., Kitchener, H., & McCann, R. (2008). Uptake of first two doses of human papillomavirus vaccine by adolescent schoolgirls in Manchester: Prospective cohort study. *BMJ (Clinical Research Ed.), 336*(7652), 1056–1058. doi:10.1136/bmj.39541.534109.BE PMID:18436917

Bragge, P., Gruen, R. L., Chau, M., Forbes, A., & Taylor, H. R. (2011). Screening for presence or absence of diabetic retinopathy: A meta-analysis. *Archives of Ophthalmology, 129*(4), 435–444. doi:10.1001/archophthalmol.2010.319 PMID:21149748

Brannigan, V. M. (1992). Protecting the privacy of patient information in clinical networks: Regulatory effectiveness analysis. *Annals of the New York Academy of Sciences, 670*(1 Extended Clin), 190–201. doi:10.1111/j.1749-6632.1992.tb26090.x

Braverman, A. M., Kunkel, E. J., Katz, L., Katona, A., Heavens, T., Miller, A., & Arfaa, J. J. (2015). Do I buy it? How AIDET™ training changes residents' values about patient care. *Journal of Patient Experience, 2*(1), 13–20. doi:10.1177/237437431500200104 PMID:28725811

Bravo, P., Edwards, A., Barr, P. J., Scholl, I., Elwyn, G., & Mcallister, M. (2015). Conceptualising patient empowerment: A mixed methods study. *BMC Health Services Research, 15*(1), 525. doi:10.118612913-015-0907-z PMID:26126998

Breckons, M., Jones, R., Morris, J., & Richardson, J. (2008). What do evaluation instruments tell us about the quality of complementary medicine information on the internet? *Journal of Medical Internet Research, 10*(1), e3. doi:10.2196/jmir.961 PMID:18244894

Brewer, N. T., & Fazekas, K. I. (2007). Predictors of HPV vaccine acceptability: A theory-informed, systematic review. *Preventive Medicine, 45*(2–3), 107–114. doi:10.1016/j.ypmed.2007.05.013 PMID:17628649

Brian, R. M., & Ben-Zeev, D. (2014). Mobile health (mHealth) for mental health in Asia: Objectives, strategies, and limitations. *Asian Journal of Psychiatry, 10*, 96–100. doi:10.1016/j.ajp.2014.04.006 PMID:25042960

Bromwich, M., & Bromwich, R. (2016). Privacy risks when using mobile devices in health care. CMAJ : Canadian Medical Association Journal = Journal de l'Association Medicale Canadienne, 188(12), 855–856. doi:10.1503/cmaj.160026

Brotherton, J. M., Pitcher, H., Passaris, I., Deeks, S. L., Webby, R., & Campbell-Lloyd, S., … Watson, M. (2008). Interim estimates of human papillomavirus vaccination coverage in the school-based program in Australia. *Communicable Diseases Intelligence Quarterly Report, 32*(4), 457–461. PMID:19374275

Bruckner, T. A., Scheffler, R. M., Shen, G., Yoon, J., Chisholm, D., Morris, J., & Saxena, S. (2011). The mental health workforce gap in low-and middle-income countries: A needs-based approach. *Bulletin of the World Health Organization, 89*(3), 184–194. doi:10.2471/BLT.10.082784 PMID:21379414

Bulsara, C., Styles, I., Ward, A. M., & Bulsara, M. (2006). The Psychometrics of Developing the Patient Empowerment Scale. *Journal of Psychosocial Oncology*, *24*(2), 1–16. doi:10.1300/J077v24n02_01 PMID:17046803

Bunderson, J. S., & Reagans, R. E. (2011). Power, status, and learning in organizations. *Organization Science*, *22*(5), 1182–1194. doi:10.1287/orsc.1100.0590

Buntin, M. B., Burke, M. F., Hoaglin, M. C., & Blumenthal, D. (2011). The benefits of health information technology: A review of the recent literature shows predominantly positive results. *Profiles of Innovation in Healthcare Delivery*, *30*(3). doi:10.1377/hlthaff.2011.0178

Bureau of Labor Statistics, U.S. Department of Labor. (2018). Occupational Outlook Handbook: Diagnostic Medical Sonographers and Cardiovascular Technologists and Technicians, Including Vascular Technologists. Retrieved from https://www.bls.gov/ooh/Healthcare/Diagnostic-medical-sonographers.htm

Burke, C. S., Stagl, K. C., Salas, E., Pierce, L., & Kendall, D. (2006). Understanding team adaptation: A conceptual analysis and model. *The Journal of Applied Psychology*, *91*(6), 1189–1207. doi:10.1037/0021-9010.91.6.1189 PMID:17100478

Burn-Murdoch, J. (2013, April 12). Data protection law is in danger of lagging behind technological change. *The Guardian*.

Burns, M. N., Begale, M., Duffecy, J., Gergle, D., Karr, C. J., Giangrande, E., & Mohr, D. C. (2011). Harnessing context sensing to develop a mobile intervention for depression. *Journal of Medical Internet Research*, *13*(3), e55. doi:10.2196/jmir.1838 PMID:21840837

Bylund, C. L., Gueguen, J. A., Sabee, C. M., Imes, R. S., Li, Y., & Sanford, A. A. (2007). Provider–patient dialogue about Internet health information: An exploration of strategies to improve the provider–patient relationship. *Patient Education and Counseling*, *66*(3), 346–352. doi:10.1016/j.pec.2007.01.009 PMID:17329062

Cabey, W. V., Shea, J. A., Kangovi, S., Kennedy, D., Onwuzulike, C., & Fein, J. (2018). Understanding Pediatric Caretakers' Views on Obtaining Medical Care for Low-acuity Illness. *Academic Emergency Medicine*, *25*(9), 1004–1013. doi:10.1111/acem.13436 PMID:29741232

Caldicott, F. (2013). Information: To share or not to share. Information Governance Review. Information: To Share or Not to Share.

Callen, J., Paoloni, R., Li, J., Stewart, M., Gibson, K., Georgiou, A., ... Westbrook, J. (2013). Perceptions of the effect of information and communication technology on the quality of care delivered in emergency departments: A cross-site qualitative study. *Annals of Emergency Medicine*, *61*(2), 131–144. doi:10.1016/j.annemergmed.2012.08.032 PubMed

Campaign, G. I. L. (2001). *Privacy and Human Rights: An International Survey of Privacy Laws and Practice*. Global Internet Liberty Campaign.

Campbell, B., Caine, K., Connelly, K., Doub, T., & Bragg, A. (2015). Cell phone ownership and use among mental health outpatients in the USA. *Personal and Ubiquitous Computing*, *19*(2), 367–378. doi:10.100700779-014-0822-z

Cancela, J., Mascato, S. V., Gatsios, D., Rigas, G., Marcante, A., Gentile, G., & Konitsiotis, S. (2016). Monitoring of motor and non-motor symptoms of Parkinson's disease through a mHealth platform. Paper presented at the *38th Annual International Conference of the IEEE Engineering in Medicine and Biology Society*, Orlando, FL. 10.1109/EMBC.2016.7590789

Cannataci, J. A. (2017). Report of the Special Rapporteur on the right to privacy A/HRC/34/60.

Carman, K. L., Dardess, P., Maurer, M., Sofaer, S., Adams, K., Bechtel, C., & Sweeney, J. (2013). Patient and family engagement: A framework for understanding the elements and developing interventions and policies. *Health Affairs*, *32*(2), 223–231. doi:10.1377/hlthaff.2012.1133 PMID:23381514

Carrasco, M. P., Salvador, C. H., Sagredo, P. G., Márquez-Montes, J., González de Mingo, M. A., Fragua, J. A., ... Monteagudo, J. L. (2008). Impact of patient-general practitioner short-messages-based interaction on the control of hypertension in a follow-up service for low-to-medium risk hypertensive patients: A randomized controlled trial. *IEEE Transactions on Information Technology in Biomedicine*, *12*(6), 780–791. doi:10.1109/TITB.2008.926429 PMID:19000959

Carrasqueiro, S., Esteves, A., Marques, L., Martins, D., Pereira, C., & Ramalho, A. (2017). EU state of play on telemedicine services and uptake recommendations (Report No. D7.1.2). Retrieved from https://ec.europa.eu/health/sites/health/files/ehealth/docs/ev_20171128_co09_en.pdf

Carswell, K., Harper-Shehadeh, M., Watts, S., van't Hof, E., Ramia, J. A., Heim, E., ... van Ommeren, M. (2018). Step-by-Step: A new WHO digital mental health intervention for depression. *mHealth*, *4*, 1–7. doi:10.21037/mhealth.2018.08.01 PMID:30225240

Casella, E., Mills, J., & Usher, K. (2014). Social media and nursing practice: Changing the balance between the social and technical aspects of work. *Collegian (Royal College of Nursing, Australia)*, *21*(2), 121–126. doi:10.1016/j.colegn.2014.03.005

Castro, E. M., Van Regenmortel, T., Vanhaecht, K., Sermeus, W., & Van Hecke, A. (2016). Patient empowerment, patient participation and patient-centeredness in hospital care: A concept analysis based on a literature review. *Patient Education and Counseling*, *99*(12), 1923–1939. doi:10.1016/j.pec.2016.07.026 PMID:27450481

Cerezo, P. G., Juvé-Udina, M.-E., & Delgado-Hito, P. (2016). Concepts and measures of patient empowerment: A comprehensive review. *Revista da Escola de Enfermagem da U S P.*, *50*(4), 667–674. doi:10.1590/S0080-623420160000500018 PMID:27680054

Chakravarthy, B. S. (1982). Adaptation: A promising metaphor for strategic management. *Academy of Management Review*, *7*(1), 35–44. doi:10.5465/amr.1982.4285438

Chandrashekar, P. (2018). Do mental health mobile apps work: Evidence and recommendations for designing high-efficacy mental health mobile apps. *mHealth*, *4*, 1–4. doi:10.21037/mhealth.2018.03.02 PMID:29682510

Chang, J., Savage, S. J., & Waldman, D. M. (2017). Estimating willingness to pay for online health services with discrete-choice experiments. *Applied Health Economics and Health Policy*, *15*(4), 491–500. doi:10.100740258-017-0316-z PMID:28290107

Chan, V. (2017). Schizophrenia and psychosis: Diagnosis, current research trends, and model treatment approaches with implications for transitional age youth. *Child and Adolescent Psychiatric Clinics*, *26*(2), 341–366. doi:10.1016/j.chc.2016.12.014 PMID:28314460

Charnock, D., Shepperd, S., Needham, G., & Gann, R. (1999). DISCERN: An instrument for judging the quality of written consumer health information on treatment choices. *Journal of Epidemiology and Community Health*, *53*(2), 105–111. doi:10.1136/jech.53.2.105 PMID:10396471

Chatterjee, S., Byun, J., Dutta, K., Pedersen, R. U., Pottathil, A., & Xie, H. (2018). Designing an Internet-of-Things (IoT) and sensor-based in-home monitoring system for assisting diabetes patients: Iterative learning from two case studies. *European Journal of Information Systems*, *27*(6), 670–685. doi:10.1080/0960085X.2018.1485619

Chaudhry, B., Wang, J., Wu, S., Maglione, M., Mojica, W., Roth, E., ... Shekelle, P. G. (2006). Systematic review: Impact of health information technology on quality, efficiency, and costs of medical care. *Annals of Internal Medicine*, *144*(10), 742–752. doi:10.7326/0003-4819-144-10-200605160-00125 PMID:16702590

Chen, B., & Butte, A. J. (2016). Leveraging big data to transform target selection and drug discovery. *Clinical Pharmacology and Therapeutics*, *99*(3), 285–297. doi:10.1002/cpt.318 PMID:26659699

Chen, J. (2017). Playing to our human strengths to prepare medical students for the future. *Korean Journal of Medical Education*, *29*(3), 193–197. doi:10.3946/kjme.2017.65 PMID:28870022

Chen, Y., Argentinis, J. D. E., & Weber, G. (2016). IBM Watson: How cognitive computing can be applied to big data challenges in life sciences research. *Clinical Therapeutics*, *38*(4), 688–701. doi:10.1016/j.clinthera.2015.12.001 PMID:27130797

Chikhaoui, E., Sarabdeen, J., & Parveen, R. (2016). Privacy and security issues in the use of clouds in E-Health in the Kingdom Of Saudi Arabia. In Communications of the IBIMA (pp. 1–18). doi:10.5171/2017.369309

Chow, P. I., Showalter, S. L., Gerber, M. S., Kennedy, E., Brenin, D. R., Schroen, A. T., ... Cohn, W. F. (2019). Use of Mental Health Apps by Breast Cancer Patients and Their Caregivers in the United States: Protocol for a Pilot Pre-Post Study. *JMIR Research Protocols*, *8*(1). doi:10.2196/11452

Chua, S. L., & Chow, W. L. (2019). Development of predictive scoring model for risk stratification of no-show at a public hospital specialist outpatient clinic. *Proceedings of Singapore Healthcare*, *28*(2), 96–104. doi:10.1177/2010105818793155

Chu, J. T. W., Whittaker, R., Jiang, Y., Wadham, A., Stasiak, K., Shepherd, M., & Bullen, C. (2018). Evaluation of MyTeen–a SMS-based mobile intervention for parents of adolescents: A randomised controlled trial protocol. *BMC Public Health*, *18*(1), 1–8. doi:10.118612889-018-6132-z PMID:30367613

Cilliers, L. (2014). Using the cloud to provide telemedicine services in a developing country. *South African Journal of Information Management*, *16*(1), 1–7. doi:10.4102ajim.v16i1.611

Clark, K. (2005). Serving underserved communities with instructional technologies: Giving them what they need, not what you want. *Urban Education*, *40*(4), 430–445. doi:10.1177/0042085905276388

Close, S., Smaldone, A., Fennoy, I., Reame, N., & Grey, M. (2013). Using information technology and social networking for recruitment of research participants: Experience from an exploratory study of pediatric Klinefelter syndrome. *Journal of Medical Internet Research*, *15*(3), e48. doi:10.2196/jmir.2286 PubMed

Cobb, N. K., & Graham, A. L. (2012). Health behavior interventions in the age of facebook. *American Journal of Preventive Medicine*, *43*(5), 571–572. doi:10.1016/j.amepre.2012.08.001

Codari, M., Pesapane, F., & Sardanelli, F. (2018). Artificial intelligence in medical imaging: Threat or opportunity? Radiologists again at the forefront of innovation in medicine. *European Radiology Experimental*, *2*(1), 35.

Cohen, J. K. (2019). CEO power panel: Patient access is next frontier for health systems. *Modern Healthcare*, *49*(20), 32. Retrieved from https://www.modernhealthcare.com/providers/ceo-power-panel-patient-access-next-frontier-health-systems

Colineau, N., & Paris, C. (2010). Talking about your health to strangers: Understanding the use of online social networks by patients. *New Review of Hypermedia and Multimedia*, *16*(1-2), 141–160. doi:10.1080/13614568.2010.496131

Collingwood, L. H. (2013). Privacy protection under the English legal system: is it adequate given the challenges raised by online communicating between individuals? (Doctoral dissertation, Kingston University).

Colombo, C., Mosconi, P., Confalonieri, P., Baroni, I., Traversa, S., Hill, S. J., ... Filippini, G. (2014). Web search behavior and information needs of people with multiple sclerosis: Focus group study and analysis of online postings. *Interactive Journal of Medical Research*, *3*(3), e12. doi:10.2196/ijmr.3034 PMID:25093374

Conboy, K. (2009). Agility from first principles: Reconstructing the concept of agility in information systems development. *Information Systems Research*, *20*(3), 329–354. doi:10.1287/isre.1090.0236

Conger, J. A., & Kanungo, R. N. (1988). The empowerment process: Integrating theory and practice. *Academy of Management Review*, *13*(3), 471–482. doi:10.5465/amr.1988.4306983

Cooper-Patrick, L., Gallo, J. J., Gonzales, J. J., Vu, H. T., Powe, N. R., Nelson, C., & Ford, D. E. (1999). Race, gender, and partnership in the patient-physician relationship. *Journal of the American Medical Association*, *282*(6), 583–589. doi:10.1001/jama.282.6.583 PMID:10450723

Copelton, D. A., & Valle, G. (2009). "You don't need a prescription to go gluten-free": The scientific self-diagnosis of celiac disease. *Social Science & Medicine*, *69*(4), 623–631. doi:10.1016/j.socscimed.2009.05.012 PMID:19559513

Corbett, E. (2017). The real-world benefits of machine learning in healthcare. Retrieved from https://www.healthcatalyst.com/clinical-applications-of-machine-learning-in-healthcare

Corfield, J. M., Abouassaly, R., & Lawrentschuk, N. (2018). Health information quality on the internet for bladder cancer and urinary diversion: A multi-lingual analysis. *Minerva Urologica e Nefrologica = The Italian. Journal d'Urologie et de Nephrologie*, *70*(2), 137–143. doi:10.23736/S0393-2249.17.02952-6 PMID:28707843

Coughlin, S.S., Whitehead, M., Sheats, J.Q., Mastromonico, J., & Smith, S. (2016). A Review of Smartphone Applications for Promoting Physical Activity. Jacobs J. Community Med, 2, 021.

Coulter, A. (2012). Patient engagement-What works? *The Journal of Ambulatory Care Management*, *35*(2), 80–89. doi:10.1097/JAC.0b013e318249e0fd PMID:22415281

Coulter, A., & Ellins, J. (2007). Effectiveness of strategies for informing, educating, and involving patients. *BMJ (Clinical Research Ed.)*, *335*(7609), 24–27. doi:10.1136/bmj.39246.581169.80 PMID:17615222

Creswell, J. W., & Poth, C. N. (2017). Qualitative inquiry and research design: Choosing among five approaches. Thousand Oaks, CA: Sage.

Cullen, M. W., Ijioma, N. N., Jayaram, N., Kithcart, A. P., Narang, A., Rajagopalan, B., ... Sinha, S. S. (2016). The supply and demand of the cardiovascular workforce: Striking the right balance. *Journal of the American College of Cardiology*, *68*(15), 1680–1689.

D'Abate, F., & La Leggia, A. (2017, June 16). The role of sonographers: future professionals across Europe? Retrieved from https://healthcare-in-europe.com/en/news/the-role-of-sonographers-future-professionals-across-europe.html

Dadgar, M., & Joshi, K. D. (2018). The role of Information and Communication Technology in self-management of chronic diseases: An Empirical Investigation through Value Sensitive Design. *Journal of the Association for Information Systems*, *19*(2), 86–112. doi:10.17705/jais1.00485

Daggy, J., Lawley, M., Willis, D., Thayer, D., Suelzer, C., DeLaurentis, P.-C., ... Sands, L. (2010). Using no-show modeling to improve clinic performance. *Health Informatics Journal*, *16*(4), 246–259. doi:10.1177/1460458210380521 PMID:21216805

Dalal, S., & Bruera, E. (2012). Assessing cancer pain. *Current Pain and Headache Reports*, *16*(4), 314–324. doi:10.100711916-012-0274-y PMID:22585314

Dambacher, M., Haffke, P., Groß, D., & Hübner, R. (2016). Graphs versus numbers: How information format affects risk aversion in gambling. *Judgment and Decision Making*, *11*(3), 223–242.

Dantas, L. F., Fleck, J. L., Oliveira, F. L. C., & Hamacher, S. (2018). No-shows in appointment scheduling--a systematic literature review. *Health Policy (Amsterdam)*, *122*(4), 412–421. doi:10.1016/j.healthpol.2018.02.002 PMID:29482948

Data Bridge Market Research. (2016). Europe Departmental PACS Market – Industry Trends and Forecast to 2024 (Report No. DBMR-1215). Retrieved from https://databridgemarketresearch.com/reports/europe-departmental-pacs-market/

Daugherty Douglas, M., Xu, J., Heggs, A., Wrenn, G., Mack, D., & Rust, G. (2016). Assessing telemedicine utilization by using Medicaid claims data. *Psychiatric Services (Washington, D.C.)*, *68*(2), 173–178. doi:10.1176/appi.ps.201500518 PMID:27691381

Davey, S., & Davey, A. (2014). Mobile-health technology: Can it Strengthen and improve public health systems of other developing countries as per Indian strategies? A systematic review of the literature. *International Journal of Medicine and Public Health*, *4*(1), 40–45. doi:10.4103/2230-8598.127121

Davidson, T. M., Bunnell, B. E., Saunders, B. E., Hanson, R. F., Danielson, C. K., Cook, D., ... Walker, J. H. (2019). Pilot Evaluation of a Tablet-Based Application to Improve Quality of Care in Child Mental Health Treatment. *Behavior Therapy*, *50*(2), 367–379. doi:10.1016/j.beth.2018.07.005 PMID:30824252

Davis, F. D. (1989). Perceived Usefulness, Perceived ease of use and user acceptance of information technology. *Management Information Systems Quarterly*, *13*(3), 319–340. doi:10.2307/249008

Davis, N. O., Bower, J., & Kollins, S. H. (2018). Proof-of-concept study of an at-home, engaging, digital intervention for pediatric ADHD. *PLoS One*, *13*(1). doi:10.1371/journal.pone.0189749 PMID:29324745

Davison, C., Smith, G. D., & Frankel, S. (1991). Lay epidemiology and the prevention paradox: The implications of coronary candidacy for health education. *Sociology of Health & Illness*, *13*(1), 1–19. doi:10.1111/1467-9566.ep11340301

De Cnudde, S., Martens, D., & Provost, F. (2018). An exploratory study towards applying and demystifying deep learning classification on behavioral big data. *University of Antwerp Working Paper*, 1-32.

De Rosis, S., & Barsanti, S. (2016). Patient satisfaction, e-health and the evolution of the patient – general practitioner relationship : Evidence from an Italian survey. *Health Policy (Amsterdam)*, *120*(11), 1279–1292. doi:10.1016/j.healthpol.2016.09.012 PMID:27836231

Deandrea, S., Montanari, M., Moja, L., & Apolone, G. (2008). Prevalence of undertreatment in cancer pain. A review of published literature. *Annals of Oncology: Official Journal of the European Society for Medical Oncology*, *19*(12), 1985–1991. doi:10.1093/annonc/mdn419 PMID:18632721

Della Mea, V. (2001). What is e-health?: The death of telemedicine? *Journal of Medical Internet Research*, *3*(2), E22. doi:10.2196/jmir.3.2.e22

Dempsey, A. F., Zimet, G. D., Davis, R. L., & Koutsky, L. (2006). Factors that are associated with parental acceptance of human papillomavirus vaccines: A randomized intervention study of written information about HPV. *Pediatrics*, *117*(5), 1486–1493. doi:10.1542/peds.2005-1381 PMID:16651301

Denecke, K., Bamidis, P., Bond, C., Gabarron, E., Househ, M., Lau, A. Y., ... Hansen, M. (2015a). Ethical issues of social media usage in healthcare. *Yearbook of Medical Informatics*, *10*(1), 137–147. doi:10.15265/IY-2015-001

Deng, X., Joshi, K. D., & Galliers, R. D. (2016). The Duality of Empowerment and Marginalization in Microtask Crowdsourcing: Giving Voice to the Less Powerful Through Value Sensitive Design. *Management Information Systems Quarterly*, *40*(2), 279–302. doi:10.25300/MISQ/2016/40.2.01

Deng, X., Khuntia, J., & Ghosh, K. (2013). Psychological Empowerment of Patients with Chronic Diseases: The Role of Digital Integration. *Thirty Fourth International Conference on Information Systems* (pp. 1–20).

Denney, M. J., Long, D. M., Armistead, M. G., Anderson, J. L., & Conway, B. N. (2016). Validating the extract, transform, load process used to populate a large clinical research database. *International Journal of Medical Informatics, 94*, 271–274. doi:10.1016/j.ijmedinf.2016.07.009 PMID:27506144

Dennison, L., Smith, E. M., Bradbury, K., & Galea, I. (2016). How do people with multiple sclerosis experience prognostic uncertainty and prognosis communication? A qualitative study. *PLoS One, 11*(7). doi:10.1371/journal.pone.0158982 PMID:27434641

Dennis, T. A., & O'Toole, L. J. (2014). Mental health on the go: Effects of a gamified attention-bias modification mobile application in trait-anxious adults. *Clinical Psychological Science, 2*(5), 576–590. doi:10.1177/2167702614522228 PMID:26029490

Denny-Smith, T., Bairan, A., & Page, M. C. (2006). A survey of female nursing students' knowledge, health beliefs, perceptions of risk, and risk behaviors regarding human papillomavirus and cervical cancer. *Journal of the American Academy of Nurse Practitioners, 18*(2), 62–69. doi:10.1111/j.1745-7599.2006.00100.x PMID:16460412

Department of Health and Human Services USA. (2019). Merit-based Incentive Payment System (MIPS) overview. Retrieved from https://qpp.cms.gov/mips/overview

Department of Statistics Singapore. (2013). Waiting Time Policies in the Health Sector. Retrieved from https://www.singstat.gov.sg/find-data/search-by-theme/population/population-and-population-structure/latest-data

DeSouza, S. I., Rashmi, M. R., Vasanthi, A. P., Joseph, S. M., & Rodrigues, R. (2014). Mobile phones: The next step towards healthcare delivery in rural India? *PLoS One, 9*(8). doi:10.1371/journal.pone.0104895 PMID:25133610

Deterding, S., Dixon, D., Khaled, R., & Nacke, L. (2011). From game design elements to gamefulness. *Proceedings of the 16th International Academic MindTrek Conference on Envisioning Future Media Environments – MindTrek 11*. 10.1145/2181037.2181040

Devi, S. (2011). Facebook friend request from a patient? *Lancet, 377*(9772), 1141–1142. doi:10.1016/S0140-6736(11)60449-2

Dhanireddy, S., Walker, J., Reisch, L., Oster, N., Delbanco, T., & Elmore, J. G. (2014). The urban underserved: Attitudes towards gaining full access to electronic medical records. *Health Expectations, 17*(5), 724–732. doi:10.1111/j.1369-7625.2012.00799.x PMID:22738155

Dibbern, J., Goles, T., Hirschheim, R., & Jayatilaka, B. (2004). Information systems outsourcing: A survey and analysis of the literature. *SIGMIS Database, 35*(4), 6–102. doi:10.1145/1035233.1035236

Dimatteo, M. R., Giordani, P. J., Lepper, H. S., & Croghan, T. W. (2002). Patient Adherence and Medical Treatment Outcomes. *Medical Care, 40*(9), 794–811. doi:10.1097/00005650-200209000-00009 PMID:12218770

Dimoka, A. (2010). What does the brain tell us about trust and distrust? Evidence from a functional neuroimaging study. *Management Information Systems Quarterly, 34*(2), 373–396. doi:10.2307/20721433

Dinesen, B., Nonnecke, B., Lindeman, D., Toft, E., Kidholm, K., Jethwani, K., . . . Albert, N. M. (2018). Fair Health. FH Healthcare Indicators™ and FH Medical Price Index™: a new view of place of service trends and medical pricing. Retrieved from https://s3.amazonaws.com/media2.fairhealth.org/whitepaper/asset/FH%20Medical%20Price%20Index%20and%20FH%20Healthcare%20Indicators--white%20paper.pdf

Dobkin, B. H. (2013). Wearable motion sensors to continuously measure real-world physical activities. *Current Opinion in Neurology, 26*(6), 602–608. doi:10.1097/WCO.0000000000000026 PMID:24136126

Doescher, M. P., Saver, B. G., Franks, P., & Fiscella, K. 2000. Racial and ethnic disparities in perceptions of physician style and trust. *Meyers Primary Care Institute Publications and Presentations, 553.*

Doll, W., & Deng, X. (2010). A technology empowerment model for engineering work. *ACM SIGMIS Database: the DATABASE for Advances in Information Systems, 41*(4), 52–74. doi:10.1145/1899639.1899643

Domecq, J. P., Prutsky, G., Elraiyah, T., Wang, Z., Nabhan, M., & Shippee, N. … Erwin, P. (2014). Patient engagement in research: a systematic review. *BMC Health Services Research, 14*(1), 89. Retrieved from https://bmchealthservres.biomedcentral.com/articles/10.1186/1472-6963-14-89

Domingos, P. M. (2012). A few useful things to know about machine learning. *Communications of the ACM, 55*(10), 78–87. doi:10.1145/2347736.2347755

Dou, K., Yu, P., Deng, N., Liu, F., Guan, Y., Li, Z., ... Duan, H. (2017). Patients' acceptance of smartphone health technology for chronic disease management: A theoretical model and empirical test. *JMIR mHealth and uHealth, 5*(12), e177. doi:10.2196/mhealth.7886 PMID:29212629

Dror, Y. (1958). Law and Social Change. *Tulane Law Review*, 33.

Dubey, V., Mathew, R., Iglar, K., Moineddin, R., & Glazier, R. (2006). Improving preventive service delivery at adult complete health check-ups: The Preventive health Evidence-based Recommendation Form (PERFORM) cluster randomized controlled trial. *BMC Family Practice, 7*(1), 44. doi:10.1186/1471-2296-7-44 PMID:16836761

Dufour, S., Lessard, D., & Chamberland, C. (2014). Facilitators and barriers to implementation of the AIDES initiative, a social innovation for participative assessment of children in need and for coordination of services. *Evaluation and Program Planning, 47*, 64–70. doi:10.1016/j.evalprogplan.2014.07.006 PMID:25150926

Dullet, N. W., Geraghty, E. M., Kaufman, T., Kissee, J. L., King, J., Dharmar, M., ... Marcin, J. P. (2017). Impact of a university-based outpatient telemedicine program on time savings, travel costs, and environmental pollutants. *Value in Health, 20*(4), 542–546. doi:10.1016/j.jval.2017.01.014 PMID:28407995

Durand, A. C., Palazzolo, S., Tanti-Hardouin, N., Gerbeaux, P., Sambuc, R., & Gentile, S. (2012). Nonurgent patients in emergency departments: Rational or irresponsible consumers? Perceptions of professionals and patients. *BMC Research Notes, 5*(1), 525. doi:10.1186/1756-0500-5-525 PMID:23006316

Durkan, P., Durkin, M., & Gillen, J. (2003). Exploring efforts to engender on-line trust. *International Journal of Entrepreneurial Behaviour & Research, 9*(3), 93–110. doi:10.1108/13552550310476184

EANM Technologists Committee. (2018). *Competencies for the European Nuclear Medicine technologists.* Staffordshire, U.K: BNMS Technology Group.

Eastwood, B. (2012). 10 ways telemedicine is changing healthcare IT. *CIO.* Retrieved from https://www.cio.com/article/2390576/healthcare/10-ways-telemedicine-is-changing-healthcare-it.html

Ebad, S. A., Jaha, E. S., & Al-Qadhi, M. A. (2014). Analyzing privacy requirements: A case study of healthcare in Saudi Arabia. *Informatics for Health & Social Care, 41*(1), 47–63. doi:10.3109/17538157.2014.965301

Edwards, B. K., Noone, A. M., Mariotto, A. B., Simard, E. P., Boscoe, F. P., Henley, S. J., ... Ward, E. M. (2014). Annual report to the nation on the status of cancer, 1975-2010, featuring prevalence of comorbidity and impact on survival among persons with lung, colorectal, breast, or prostate cancer. *Cancer, 120*(9), 1290–1314. doi:10.1002/cncr.28509 PMID:24343171

Edwards, L. (2016). Privacy, Security and data protection in smart cities: A critical EU law perspective. *European Data Protection Law Review, 2*(1), 28–58. doi:10.21552/EDPL/2016/1/6

Eisenhardt, K. M. (1985). Control: Organizational and Economic approaches. *Management Science. Linthicum, 31*(2), 134.

Eisenhart, S. (2019). Final guidance from US FDA on clinical evaluation of software as a medical device (SaMD). *Emergo*. Retrieved from https://www.emergobyul.com/blog/2017/12/final-guidance-us-fda-clinical-evaluation-software-medical-device-samd

Electronic Frontier Foundation. (2014). *NECESSARY & PROPORTIONATE: International Principles on the Application of Human Rights Law to Communications Surveillance*. Retrieved from http://www.ohchr.org/Documents/Issues/Privacy/ElectronicFrontierFoundation.pdf

Elhauge, E. (2010). *The fragmentation of U.S. health care: Causes and solutions*. New York, NY: Oxford University Press; doi:10.1093/acprof:oso/9780195390131.001.0001.

Elvira, C., Ochoa, A., Gonzalvez, J. C., & Mochón, F. (2018). Machine-Learning-Based No Show Prediction in Outpatient Visits. *International Journal of Interactive Multimedia & Artificial Intelligence, 4*(7), 29–34. doi:10.9781/ijimai.2017.03.004

Eng, D., Lee, J. M., Eng, D. S., & Lee, J. M. (2013). The promise and peril of mobile health applications for diabetes and endocrinology. *Pediatric Diabetes, 14*(4), 231–238. doi:10.1111/pedi.12034 PMID:23627878

Eng, T. R. (2002). eHealth research and evaluation: Challenges and opportunities. *Journal of Health Communication, 7*(4), 267–272. doi:10.1080/10810730290001747 PMID:12356287

Epic.org. (2019). Big data and the future of privacy. Retrieved from https://epic.org/privacy/big-data/

Epp, C. D., Horne, J., Scolieri, B. B., Kane, I., & Bowser, A. S. (2018, September). PsychOut! a Mobile App to Support Mental Status Assessment Training. In *European Conference on Technology Enhanced Learning* (pp. 216-230). Cham, Switzerland: Springer.

Eskildsen, N. B., Joergensen, C. R., Thomsen, T. G., Ross, L., Dietz, S. M., Groenvold, M., & Johnsen, A. T. (2017). Patient empowerment: A systematic review of questionnaires measuring empowerment in cancer patients. *Acta Oncologica, 56*(2), 156–165. doi:10.1080/0284186X.2016.1267402 PMID:28077053

EU eHealth Stakeholder Group. (2014). Widespread Deployment of Telemedicine Services in Europe. (Report No. DAE KA 13/2). Retrieved from http://www.vitlab-resater.eu/sites/default/files/TelemedicinedeploymentreportEHSG.pdf

euro.who.int. (2019). Data and statistics. Retrieved from http://www.euro.who.int/en/health-topics/Health-systems/health-workforce/data-and-statistics

Europe, W. H. O. (2016). Strengthening people-centred health systems in the WHO European Region: framework for action on integrated health services delivery. Retrieved from http://www.euro.who.int/__data/assets/pdf_file/0004/315787/66wd15e_FFA_IHSD_160535.pdf?ua=1

European Commission. (2017). Expert Group on Health Systems Performance Assessment, BLOCKS. Tools and methodologies to assess integrated care in Europe. Retrieved from http://ec.europa.eu/health/sites/health/files/systems_performance_assessment/docs/2017_blocks_en_0.pdf

European Commission. eHealth. (2012). Communication from the Commission To the European Parliament, the Council, The European Economic and Social Committee and The Committee of the Regions (Report No. COM 736). Retrieved from https://eur-lex.europa.eu/legal-content/EN/TXT/PDF/?uri=CELEX:52012DC0736&from=EN

European Multiple Sclerosis Platform. (2014). Defeating MS together: The European code of good practice in MS. Retrieved from http://www.emsp.org/wp-content/uploads/2015/06/140824-Revised-Code-of-Good-Practice.pdf

European Union. (2016). Regulation 2016/679 of the European Parliament and the Council of the European Union. *Official Journal of the European Communities, 2014*(April), 1–88.

Everstine, L., Everstine, D. S., Heymann, G. M., True, R. H., Frey, D. H., Johnson, H. G., & Seiden, R. H. (1980). Privacy and confidentiality in psychotherapy. *The American Psychologist, 35*(9), 828–840. doi:10.1037/0003-066X.35.9.828

Eysenbach, G. (2001). What is e-health? *Journal of Medical Internet Research, 3*(2), e20. Retrieved from http://www.ncbi.nlm.nih.gov/pmc/articles/PMC1761894/. doi:10.2196/jmir.3.2.e20 PMID:11720962

Farion, K. J., Wright, M., Zemek, R., Neto, G., Karwowska, A., Tse, S., ... Barrowman, N. (2015). Understanding Low-Acuity Visits to the Pediatric Emergency Department. *PLoS One*, 10. PMID:26083338

Farnan, J. M., Sulmasy, L. S., Worster, B. K., Chaudhry, H. J., Rhyne, J. A., & Arora, V. M. (2013). Online medical professionalism: Patient and public relationships: Policy Statement From the American College of Physicians and the Federation of State Medical Boards. *Annals of Internal Medicine, 158*(8), 620. doi:10.7326/0003-4819-158-8-201304160-00100

FDA News Release. (2018). FDA permits marketing of artificial intelligence-based device to detect certain diabetes-related eye problems. Retrieved from https://www.fda.gov/NewsEvents/Newsroom/PressAnnouncements/ucm604357.htm

Fernandez-Luque, L., Elahi, N., Grajales, F. J., & Iii, F. J. G. (2009). An analysis of personal medical information disclosed in youtube videos created by patients with multiple sclerosis. In Studies in Health Technology and Informatics (pp. 292–296). doi:10.3233/978-1-60750-044-5-292

Feste, C., & Anderson, R. M. (1995). Empowerment: From Philosophy to Practice. *Patient Education and Counseling, 26*(1), 139–144. doi:10.1016/0738-3991(95)00730-N PMID:7494713

Fetterman, D. M. (2009). Ethnography: Step-by-step. Thousand Oaks, CA: Sage.

Fetterolf, D. E. (1999). A Framework for Evaluating Underutilization of Health Care Services. *American Journal of Medical Quality, 14*(2), 89–97. doi:10.1177/106286069901400204 PMID:10446670

Fink, J. (2011, Nov. 19). Five nurses fired for Facebook postings. Scrubs.

Finucane, M. L., Slovic, P., Hibbard, J. H., Peters, E., Mertz, C. K., & MacGregor, D. G. (2002). Aging and decision-making competence: An analysis of comprehension and consistency skills in older versus younger adults considering health-plan options. *Journal of Behavioral Decision Making, 15*(2), 141–164. doi:10.1002/bdm.407

Fiscella, K. (2005). Health vulnerability. *Journal of the American Medical Association, 293*(15), 1924–1925. doi:10.1001/jama.293.15.1924

Fiscella, K., & Shin, P. (2005). The inverse care law: Implications for healthcare of vulnerable populations. *The Journal of Ambulatory Care Management, 28*(4), 304–312. doi:10.1097/00004479-200510000-00005 PMID:16172559

Fishbein, M., & Ajzen, I. (1975). *Belief, Attitude, Intention and Behavior: An Introduction to Theory and Research.* Reading, MA: Addison-Wesley Publishing Company.

Fisher, J., & Clayton, M. (2012). Who gives a Tweet: Assessing patients' interest in the use of social media for health care. *Worldviews on Evidence-Based Nursing, 9*(2), 100–108. doi:10.1111/j.1741-6787.2012.00243.x

Flesch, R. (1948). A new readability yardstick. *The Journal of Applied Psychology, 32*(3), 221–233. doi:10.1037/h0057532 PMID:18867058

Flickinger, T. E., Saha, S., Moore, R. D., & Beach, M. C. (2013). Higher quality communication and relationships are associated with improved patient engagement in HIV care. *Journal of Acquired Immune Deficiency Syndromes, 63*(3), 362–366. doi:10.1097/QAI.0b013e318295b86a PMID:23591637

FlyData. (2019). The 6 challenges of big data integration. Retrieved from https://www.flydata.com/the-6-challenges-of-big-data-integration/

Folkman, S. (2000). Privacy and Confidentiality. In B. D. Sales, & S. Folkman (Eds.), *Ethics in research with human participants* (1st ed., p. 215). American Psychological Association.

Fong, D. S., Aiello, L., Gardner, T. W., King, G. L., Blankenship, G., Cavallerano, J. D., ... Klein, R. (2003). Diabetic retinopathy. *Diabetes Care*, *26*(1), 226–229. doi:10.2337/diacare.26.1.226 PMID:12502685

Forbes, K. (2011). Pain in patients with cancer: The World Health Organization analgesic ladder and beyond. *Clinical Oncology (Royal College of Radiologists (Great Britain))*, *23*(6), 379–380. doi:10.1016/j.clon.2011.04.016 PMID:21636259

Forrest, C. B., Glade, G. B., Baker, A. E., Bocian, A., von Schrader, S., & Starfield, B. (2000). Coordination of specialty referrals and physician satisfaction with referral care. *Archives of Pediatrics & Adolescent Medicine*, *154*(5), 499–506. doi:10.1001/archpedi.154.5.499 PubMed

Fox, S., & Duggan, M. (2013). Health Online 2013. *Pew Internet and American Life Project*, 1–55.

Fox, G., & Connolly, R. (2018). Mobile health technology adoption across generations: Narrowing the digital divide. *Information Systems Journal*, *28*(6), 995–1019. doi:10.1111/isj.12179

Free, C., Phillips, G., Galli, L., Watson, L., Felix, L., Edwards, P., ... Haines, A. (2013). The Effectiveness of Mobile-Health Technology-Based Health Behaviour Change or Disease Management Interventions for Health Care Consumers: A Systematic Review. *PLoS Medicine*, *10*(1). doi:10.1371/journal.pmed.1001362 PMID:23349621

Friedman, B., & Kahn, P. H. Jr. (2007). Human values, ethics, and design. In *The human-computer interaction handbook* (pp. 1223–1248). Boca Raton, FL: CRC Press.

Frost & Sullivan. (2011). *Drowning in big data? Reducing information technology complexities and costs for healthcare organizations*. Mountain View, CA. Retrieved from https://www.emc.com/collateral/analyst-reports/frost-sullivan-reducing-information-technology-complexities-ar.pdf

Fu, L. Y., Bonhomme, L.-A., Cooper, S. C., Joseph, J. G., & Zimet, G. D. (2014). Educational interventions to increase HPV vaccination acceptance: A systematic review. *Vaccine*, *32*(17), 1901–1920. doi:10.1016/j.vaccine.2014.01.091 PMID:24530401

Funk, E., Riddell, J., Ankel, F., & Cabrera, D. (2018). Blockchain Technology: A Data Framework to Improve Validity, Trust, and Accountability of Information Exchange in Health Professions Education. *Academic Medicine : Journal of the Association of American Medical Colleges*, *93*(12), 1791–1794. doi:10.1097/ACM.0000000000002326 PMID:29901658

Funnell, M. M., Anderson, R. M., Arnold, M. S., Barr, P. A., Donnelly, M., Johnson, P. D., ... White, N. H. (1991). Empowerment: An idea whose time has come in diabetes education. *The Diabetes Educator*, *17*(1), 37–41. doi:10.1177/014572179101700108 PMID:1986902

Future II Study Group. (2007). Quadrivalent vaccine against human papillomavirus to prevent high-grade cervical lesions. *The New England Journal of Medicine*, *356*(19), 1915–1927. doi:10.1056/NEJMoa061741 PMID:17494925

Gaggioli, A., Pioggia, G., Tartarisco, G., Baldus, G., Corda, D., Cipresso, P., & Riva, G. (2013). A mobile data collection platform for mental health research. *Personal and Ubiquitous Computing*, *17*(2), 241–251. doi:10.100700779-011-0465-2

Galanakis, M., Tsoli, M., & Darviri, S. (2016). The Effects of Patient Empowerment Scale in Chronic Dis-eases. *Psychology (Irvine, Calif.)*, *7*(11), 1369–1390. doi:10.4236/psych.2016.711138

Galea, S., Tracy, M., Hoggatt, K. J., DiMaggio, C., & Karpati, A. (2011). Estimated deaths attributable to social factors in the United States. *American Journal of Public Health, 101*(8), 1456–1465. doi:10.2105/AJPH.2010.300086 PMID:21680937

Galewitz, P. (2018). Number Of U.S. Kids Who Don't Have Health Insurance Is On The Rise. Retrieved from https://www.npr.org/sections/health-shots/2018/11/29/671666280/number-of-u-s-kids-who-dont-have-health-insurance-is-on-the-rise

Gammage, J. (2019). Philly sheriff tells feds: ICE agents must now identify themselves to deputies in city Courtrooms. Retrieved from https://www.philly.com/news/ice-immigrant-immigration-philly-sheriff-jewell-williams-20190402.html

Gandhi, T. K., Sittig, D. F., Franklin, M., Sussman, A. J., Fairchild, D. G., & Bates, D. W. (2000). Communication breakdown in the outpatient referral process. *Journal of General Internal Medicine, 15*(9), 626–631. doi:10.1046/j.1525-1497.2000.91119.x PubMed

Gao, J., & Koronios A. (2010). Mobile Application Development for Senior Citizens. PACIS 2010 Proceedings, 65.

García, I. P., Sánchez, C. M., Espílez, Á. S., García-Magariño, I., Guillén, G. A., & García-Campayo, J. (2017). Development and initial evaluation of a mobile application to help with mindfulness training and practice. *International Journal of Medical Informatics, 105*, 59–67. doi:10.1016/j.ijmedinf.2017.05.018 PMID:28750912

Garets, D., & Davis, M. (2006). Electronic medical records vs. electronic health records: Yes, there is a difference. Retrieved from https://www.google.com/url?sa=t&rct=j&q=&esrc=s&source=web&cd=2&ved=2ahUKEwjHka6xjsjiAhVNnKwKHai7DhsQFjABegQIARAC&url=https%3A%2F%2Fwww.aao.org%2Fasset.axd%3Fid%3D8e9b1f20-0ed6-4d2b-92f8-e28fbaf378ec%26t%3D634962799822530000&usg=AOvVaw2IZUASCFHwbgR_kQ7BLvfo

Garland, S. M., Hernandez-Avila, M., Wheeler, C. M., Perez, G., Harper, D. M., Leodolter, S., ... Koutsky, L. A. (2007). Quadrivalent vaccine against human papillomavirus to prevent anogenital diseases. *The New England Journal of Medicine, 356*(19), 1928–1943. doi:10.1056/NEJMoa061760 PMID:17494926

Garner, S. L., George, C. E., Young, P., Hitchcock, J., Koch, H., & Green, G. … Gift, N. (2019). Effectiveness of an mhealth application to improve hypertension health literacy in India. *WHO-South East Asia Journal of Public Health, Under Review*. Retrieved from https://www.journals.elsevier.com/public-health

Garner, S. L., Sudia, T., & Rachaprolu, S. (2018). Smart phone accessibility and mHealth use in a limited resource setting. *International Journal of Nursing Practice, 24*(1), e12609. doi:10.1111/ijn.12609 PMID:29159919

Gefen, D. (2000). E-commerce: The role of familiarity and trust. Omega. *International Journal of Management Sciences, 28*(6), 725–737.

Gefen, D., & Carmel, E. (2008). Is the world really flat? A look at offshoring in an online programming marketplace. *Management Information Systems Quarterly, 32*(2), 367–384. doi:10.2307/25148844

Gefen, D., Karahanna, E., & Straub, D. W. (2003). Trust and TAM in online shopping: An integrated model. *Management Information Systems Quarterly, 27*(1), 51–90. doi:10.2307/30036519

Gefen, D., & Pavlou, P. A. (2012). The Boundaries of Trust and Risk: The Quadratic Moderating Role of Institutional Structures. *Information Systems Research, 23*(3), 940–959. doi:10.1287/isre.1110.0395

Gefen, D., & Ridings, C. (2003). IT acceptance: Managing user - IT group boundaries. *ACM SIGMIS Database, 34*(3), 25–40. doi:10.1145/937742.937746

Gefen, D., Rose, G. M., Warkentin, M., & Pavlou, P. A. (2005). Cultural diversity and trust in IT adoption: A comparison of potential e-voters in the USA and South Africa. *Journal of Global Information Management, 13*(1), 54–78. doi:10.4018/jgim.2005010103

Gefen, D., & Straub, D. W. (1997). Gender Differences in Perception and Adoption of E-mail: An Extension to the Technology Acceptance Model. *Management Information Systems Quarterly*, *21*(4), 389–400. doi:10.2307/249720

Gefen, D., Wyss, S., & Lichtenstein, Y. (2008). Business familiarity as risk mitigation in software development outsourcing contracts. *Management Information Systems Quarterly*, *32*(3), 531–551. doi:10.2307/25148855

Gemmill, E. L., & Peterson, M. (2006). Technology Use Among College Students: Implications for Student Affairs Professionals. *Journal of Student Affairs Research and Practice*, *43*(2). doi:10.2202/1949-6605.1640

General Medical Council. (2018). Confidentiality - GMC good medical practice. Retrieved from https://www.gmc-uk.org/ethical-guidance/ethical-guidance-for-doctors/confidentiality

George, D. R., Rovniak, L. S., & Kraschnewski, J. L. (2013). Dangers and opportunities for social media in medicine. *Clinical Obstetrics and Gynecology*, *56*(3), 453–462. doi:10.1097/GRF.0b013e318297dc38

Gheorghe, M. (2014). Mobile cloud computing for telemedicine solutions. *Informações Econômicas*, *18*(4), 50–61. doi:10.12948/issn14531305/18.4.2014.05

Ghosh, K., Khuntia, J., Chawla, S., & Deng, X. (2014). Media Reinforcement for Psychological Empowerment in Chronic Disease Management. CAIS, 34, 22.

Gibson, C. H. (1991). A Concept Analysis of Empowerment. *Journal of Advanced Nursing*, *16*(3), 354–361. doi:10.1111/j.1365-2648.1991.tb01660.x PMID:2037742

Gimpe, H., Nißen, M., & Görlitz, R. (2013). Quantifying the quantified self: A study on the motivations of patients to track their own health. In *International Conference on Information Systems ICIS 2013*, Milan, Italy: Association for Information Systems.

Glanz, K., Rimer, B. K., & Viswanath, K. (2008). *Health behavior and health education: theory, research, and practice*. Hoboken, NJ: John Wiley & Sons.

Glowacka, K. J., Henry, R. M., & May, J. H. (2009). A hybrid data mining/simulation approach for modelling outpatient no-shows in clinic scheduling. *The Journal of the Operational Research Society*, *60*(8), 1056–1068. doi:10.1057/jors.2008.177

Goetz, T. (2010). *The decision tree: Taking control of your health in the new era of personalized medicine*. Emmaus, PA: Rodale.

Goffman, R. M., Harris, S. L., May, J. H., Milicevic, A. S., Monte, R. J., Myaskovsky, L., ... Vargas, D. L. (2017). Modeling patient no-show history and predicting future outpatient appointment behavior in the veterans health administration. *Military Medicine*, *182*(5–6), e1708–e1714. doi:10.7205/MILMED-D-16-00345 PMID:29087915

Goldner, E. M., Jeffries, V., Bilsker, D., Jenkins, E., Menear, M., & Petermann, L. (2011). Knowledge translation in mental health: A scoping review. *Healthcare Policy*, *7*(2), 83. PMID:23115572

Good Things Foundation. (2017). The Real Digital Divide? Retrieved from https://www.goodthingsfoundation.org/sites/default/files/research-publications/ofcom_report_v4_links.pdf

Goodman, K. W., Miller, R. A., & Informatics, H. (2006). Ethics and health informatics : Users, standards, and outcomes. In E. H. Shortliffe, & J. J. Cimino (Eds.), *Biomedical Informatics Computer Applications in Health Care and Biomedicine* (3rd ed., pp. 379–402). New York, NY: Springer. doi:10.1007/0-387-36278-9_10

Goss, P. E., Strasser-Weippl, K., Lee-Bychkovsky, B. L., Fan, L., Li, J., Chavarri-Guerra, Y., ... Chan, A. (2014). Challenges to effective cancer control in China, India, and Russia. *The Lancet Oncology*, *15*(5), 489–538. doi:10.1016/S1470-2045(14)70029-4 PMID:24731404

Gouge, C. (2018). "Getting the knowledge right": Patient communication, agency, and knowledge. *The Journal of Medical Humanities*, *39*(4), 535–551. doi:10.100710912-016-9389-1 PMID:27017829

Grace College. (2019). Rapid Growth: The past, present and future of wearable technology. Retrieved from https://online.grace.edu/news/business/the-past-present-future-of-wearable-technology/

Grando, M. A., Rozenblum, R., & Bates, D. W. (2015). Information technology for patient empowerment in healthcare. Berlin, Germany: H. Walter de Gruyter GmbH & K. G. Co. doi:10.1515/9781614514343

Grant, M. J., & Booth, A. (2009). A typology of reviews: An analysis of 14 review types and associated methodologies. *Health Information and Libraries Journal*, *26*(2), 91–108. doi:10.1111/j.1471-1842.2009.00848.x PMID:19490148

Greco, M. T., Roberto, A., Corli, O., Deandrea, S., Bandieri, E., Cavuto, S., & Apolone, G. (2014). Quality of cancer pain management: An update of a systematic review of undertreatment of patients with cancer. *Journal of Clinical Oncology*, *32*(36), 4149–4154. doi:10.1200/JCO.2014.56.0383 PMID:25403222

Green, J. (2019). How much EHR costs and how to set your budget. Retrieved from https://www.ehrinpractice.com/ehr-cost-and-budget-guide.html

Greenspun, H., & Coughlin, S. (2012). mHealth in an mWorld: How mobile technology is transforming health care. Deloitte Center for Health Solutions, 1-21.

Groves, P., Kayyali, B., Knott, D., & Kuiken, V. S. (2013). *The "big data" revolution in healthcare. Accelerating value and innovation.* Retrieved from http://www.pharmatalents.es/assets/files/Big_Data_Revolution.pdf

Gruessner, V. (n.d.). Why mobile security risks are healthcare's biggest liability. Retrieved from https://mhealthintelligence.com/news/why-mobile-security-risks-are-healthcares-biggest-liability

Gruman, J., Rovner, M. H., French, M. E., Jeffress, D., Sofaer, S., Shaller, D., & Prager, D. J. (2010). From patient education to patient engagement: Implications for the field of patient education. *Patient Education and Counseling*, *78*(3), 350–356. doi:10.1016/j.pec.2010.02.002 PMID:20202780

Gulati, R. (1995). Does Familiarity Breed Trust? The implications of repeated ties for contractual choice in alliances. *Academy of Management Journal*, *38*(1), 85–112.

Gunawardena, C. N., Hermans, M. B., Sanchez, D., Richmond, C., Bohley, M., & Tuttle, R. (2009). A theoretical framework for building online communities of practice with social networking tools. *Educational Media International*, *46*(1), 3–16. doi:10.1080/09523980802588626

Guruge, S., & Butt, H. (2015). A scoping review of mental health issues and concerns among immigrant and refugee youth in Canada: Looking back, moving forward. *Canadian Journal of Public Health*, *106*(2), e72–e78. doi:10.17269/CJPH.106.4588 PMID:25955675

Hacker, K., Chu, J., Leung, C., Marra, R., Pirie, A., Brahimi, M., ... Marlin, R. P. (2011). The impact of Immigration and Customs Enforcement on immigrant health: Perceptions of immigrants in Everett, Massachusetts, USA. *Social Science & Medicine*, *73*(4), 586–594. doi:10.1016/j.socscimed.2011.06.007 PMID:21778008

Hajek, A., Bock, J. O., & König, H. H. (2017). Association of general psychological factors with frequent attendance in primary care: A population-based cross-sectional observational study. *BMC Family Practice*, *18*(1), 48. doi:10.118612875-017-0621-5 PMID:28340559

Hall, M. T., Simms, K. T., Lew, J.-B., Smith, M. A., Brotherton, J. M. L., Saville, M., ... Canfell, K. (2019). The projected timeframe until cervical cancer elimination in Australia: A modelling study. *The Lancet Public Health, 4*(1), e19–e27. doi:10.1016/S2468-2667(18)30183-X PMID:30291040

Hall, M., Hanna, L.-A., & Huey, G. (2013). Use and views on social networking sites of pharmacy students in the United Kingdom. *American Journal of Pharmaceutical Education, 77*(1), 9. doi:10.5688/ajpe7719

Hamari, J., Koivisto, J., & Pakkanen, T. (2014). Do Persuasive Technologies Persuade? - A Review of Empirical Studies. Persuasive Technology Lecture Notes in Computer Science, 118-136. doi:10.1007/978-3-319-07127-5_11

Hamm, M. P., Chisholm, A., Shulhan, J., Milne, A., Scott, S. D., Given, L. M., & Hartling, L. (2000). Social media use among patients and caregivers: a scoping review. doi:10.1136/bmjopen-2013

Han, J. J., & Nesbitt, T. (2016). Personalized telehealth in the future: A global research agenda. *Journal of Medical Internet Research, 18*(3), 1–31. PMID:26932229

Han, P. K., Klein, W. M., & Arora, N. K. (2011). Varieties of uncertainty in health care: A conceptual taxonomy. *Medical Decision Making, 31*(6), 828–838. doi:10.1177/0272989X10393976 PMID:22067431

Harris, M. (2001). The rise of anthropological theory: A history of theories of culture. Thousand Oaks, CA: AltaMira Press.

Harrison, V., Proudfoot, J., Wee, P. P., Parker, G., Pavlovic, D. H., & Manicavasagar, V. (2011). Mobile mental health: Review of the emerging field and proof of concept study. *Journal of Mental Health (Abingdon, England), 20*(6), 509–524. doi:10.3109/09638237.2011.608746 PMID:21988230

Hartzler, A. L., Venkatakrishnan, A., Mohan, S., Silva, M., Lozano, P., Ralston, J. D., & Pirolli, P. (2016). Acceptability of a team-based mobile health (mHealth) application for lifestyle self-management in individuals with chronic illnesses. Paper presented at the *38th Annual International Conference of the IEEE Engineering in Medicine and Biology Society (EMBC)*, Orlando, FL. 10.1109/EMBC.2016.7591428

Hasanain, R. A., Vallmuur, K., & Clark, M. (2015). Electronic medical record systems in Saudi Arabia: Knowledge and preferences of healthcare professionals. *Journal of Health Informatics in Developing Countries, 9*(1), 23–31.

Hay, J., Coups, E., & Ford, J. (2006). Predictors of Perceived Risk for Colon Cancer in a National Probability Sample in the United States. *Journal of Health Communication, 11*(S1), 71–92. doi:10.1080/10810730600637376 PMID:16641075

Haynes, B. (2007). Of studies, syntheses, synopses, summaries, and systems: The "5S" evolution of information services for evidence-based healthcare decisions. *Evidence-Based Nursing, 10*(1), 6–7. doi:10.1136/ebn.10.1.6 PMID:17218282

Head, B., & Alford, J. (2013). Wicked problems: Implications for public policy and management. *Administration & Society, 47*(6), 711–739. doi:10.1177/0095399713481601

Health and Economic Costs of Chronic Disease | CDC. (n.d.). Retrieved from https://www.cdc.gov/chronicdisease/about/costs/index.htm#ref1

Health Education England, Skills for Health, and Skills for Care (2017). Person-Centred Approaches: Empowering people in their lives and communities to enable an upgrade in prevention, wellbeing, health, care and support. Retrieved from http://www.skillsforhealth.org.uk/images/pdf/Person-Centred-Approaches-Framework.pdf?s=form

Health Foundation. (2013). Implementing Shared Decision Making. Retrieved from http://www.health.org.uk/sites/health/files/ImplementingSharedDecisionMaking.pdf

Health Literacy, U. K. (2019). Why is Health Literacy Important? Retrieved from http://www.healthliteracy.org.uk/index.php/about-health-literacy

Health On the Net Foundation. (2017). HONcode Toolbar. Retrieved from https://www.hon.ch/HONcode/Patients/Visitor/visitor.html

Health Resources & Services Administration. (2019). Telehealth programs. Retrieved from https://www.hrsa.gov/rural-health/telehealth/index.html

Health, I. T. gov. (2019). What is an electronic health record (EHR)? Retrieved from https://www.healthit.gov/faq/what-electronic-health-record-ehr

Health, M. (2013). Saudi Arabia Ministry of Health Achievements 2013.

Hebert, E., Ferguson, W., McCullough, S., Chan, M., Drobakha, A., Ritter, S., & Mehta, K. (2016). mBody health: Digitizing disabilities in Sierra Leone. Paper presented at the *IEEE Global Humanitarian Technology Conference (GHTC)*, Seattle, WA. 10.1109/GHTC.2016.7857357

Heesen, C., Kaspar, J., Kopke, S., Richter, T., Segal, J., & Mulhauser, I. (2007). Informed shared decision making in multiple-sclerosis – inevitable or impossible? *Journal of the Neurological Sciences*, *259*(1-2), 109–117. doi:10.1016/j.jns.2006.05.074 PMID:17400253

Heinonen, R., Luoto, R., Lindfors, P., & Nygard, C. H. (2012). Usability and feasibility of mobile phone diaries in an experimental physical exercise study. *Telemedicine Journal and e-Health*, *18*(2), 115–119. doi:10.1089/tmj.2011.0087 PMID:22283356

Hellman, M. (2018). Social causes of depression, anxiety and stress. *Nordisk Alkohol- & Narkotikatidskrift*, *35*(3), 149–151. doi:10.1177/1455072518773613

Herselman, M., Botha, A., Toivanen, H., Myllyoja, J., Fogwill, T., & Alberts, R. A digital health innovation ecosystem for South Africa. Paper presented at 2016 IST Africa Conference, Durban, South Africa.

Herz, M. (2009). Law lags behind: FOIA and affirmative disclosure of information. *Cardozo Public Law, Policy, and Ethics Journal*, *7*(3).

Herzog, T. J., Huh, W. K., Downs, L. S., Smith, J. S., & Monk, B. J. (2008). Initial lessons learned in HPV vaccination. *Gynecologic Oncology*, *109*(2), S4–S11. doi:10.1016/j.ygyno.2008.01.018 PMID:18482557

Heyboer, K. (2010, March 26). Medical students' cadaver photos gets scrutiny after images show up online. New Jersey Real-Time News.

Hinchliffe, A., & Mummery, W. K. (2008). Applying usability testing techniques to improve a health promotion website. *Health Promotion Journal of Australia: Official Journal of Australian Association of Health Promotion Professionals*, *19*(1), 29–35. doi:10.1071/HE08029 PMID:18481929

Hodge, J. G. Jr, Gostin, L. O., & Jacobson, P. D. (1999). Legal issues concerning electronic health information: Privacy, quality, and liability. *Journal of the American Medical Association*, *182*(15), 1466–1471. doi:10.1001/jama.282.15.1466

Hofmann, B., & Svenaeus, F. (2018). How medical technologies shape the experience of illness. *Life Sciences, Society and Policy*, *14*(1), 3. doi:10.118640504-018-0069-y PMID:29397458

Holcomb, B., Bailey, J. M., Crawford, K., & Ruffin, M. T. (2004). Adults' knowledge and behaviors related to human papillomavirus infection. *The Journal of the American Board of Family Practice*, *17*(1), 26–31. doi:10.3122/jabfm.17.1.26 PMID:15014049

Holmström, I., & Röing, M. (2010). The relation between patient-centeredness and patient empowerment: A discussion on concepts. *Patient Education and Counseling*, *79*(2), 167–172. doi:10.1016/j.pec.2009.08.008 PMID:19748203

Hoque, R., & Sorwar, G. (2017). Understanding factors influencing the adoption of mHealth by the elderly: An extension of the UTAUT model. *International Journal of Medical Informatics*, *101*, 75–84. doi:10.1016/j.ijmedinf.2017.02.002 PMID:28347450

House of Commons. (2014). Managing the care of people with long term health conditions. Retrieved from https://www.publications.parliament.uk/pa/cm201415/cmselect/cmhealth/401/401.pdf

Hoyt, R., Snider, D., Thompson, C., & Mantravadi, S. (2016). IBM Watson Analytics: Automating visualization, descriptive, and predictive statistics. *JMIR Public Health and Surveillance*, *2*(2), 157–183. doi:10.2196/publichealth.5810 PMID:27729304

Hsiao, C. J., Hing, E., Socey, T. C., & Cai, B. (2010). Electronic medical record/electronic health record systems of office-based physicians: United States, 2009 and preliminary 2010 state estimates. National Center for Health Statistics, 2001-2011. Available from http://www.cdc.gov/nchs/data/hestat/emr_ehr_09/emr_ehr_09.htm

Hsiao, C.-J., & Hing, E. (2012). Use and characteristics of electronic health record systems among office-based physician practices: United States, 2001-2012. *National Center for Health Statistics Data Brief, 111*(December), 1–8. Retrieved from https://www.cdc.gov/nchs/data/databriefs/DB111.pdf

Hsiao, C.-J., & Hing, E. (2015). *Use and characteristics of electronic health record systems among office-based physician practices: United States, 2001--2013. NCHS data brief, no 143. Hyattsville, MD: National Center for Health Statistics. 2014*. Hyattsville, MD: National Center for Health Statistics. Available at Http://Www.Cdc.Gov/Nchs/Data/Databriefs/Db143.Htm

Huang, K.-Y., & Ran, W. (2014). Not Just for Support: Companionship Activities in Healthcare Virtual Support Communities. *Communications of the Association for Information Systems*, *34*(29).

Huang, Y., & Hanauer, D. A. (2014). Patient no-show predictive model development using multiple data sources for an effective overbooking approach. *Applied Clinical Informatics*, *5*(3), 836–860. doi:10.4338/ACI-2014-04-RA-0026 PMID:25298821

Huckman, R. S., & Stern, A. D. (2018). Why Apps for Managing Chronic Disease Haven't Been Widely Used, and How to Fix It. *Harvard business Review*. Retrieved from https://hbr.org/2018/04/why-apps-for-managing-chronic-disease-havent-been-widely-used-and-how-to-fix-it

Hudspeth, J., & Morse, M. (2017). Health Information and Global Health Inequity: Point-of-Care Knowledge Systems as a Foundation for Progress. *Journal of General Internal Medicine*, *32*(5), 572–575. doi:10.100711606-016-3909-6 PMID:27798781

Hunt, D. (2019)Average Cost of an ER visit. Retrieved from https://www.thebalance.com/average-cost-of-an-er-visit-4176166

Hurst, J. (2018). The Best Apps and Tools for Older People. Retrieved from https://www.lifehack.org/278271/the-best-apps-and-tools-for-older-people

Hu, W., & Ding, G. (2015). The application of intelligent pain management system in cancer pain patients. *Chinese Journal of Pain Medicine*, *21*(2), 107–110.

Igoe, K. (2017). Mental health on the line: use of telemedicine for mental health in rural areas on the rise but uneven. Retrieved from https://hms.harvard.edu/news/mental-health-line

Ingledue, K., Cottrell, R., & Bernard, A. (2004). College women's knowledge, perceptions, and preventive behaviors regarding human papillomavirus infection and cervical cancer. *American Journal of Health Studies*, *19*(1), 28.

Irizarry, T., Dabbs, A. D., & Curran, C. R. (2015). Patient portals and patient engagement: A state of the science review. *Journal of Medical Internet Research, 17*(6), e148. doi:10.2196/jmir.4255 PMID:26104044

Isaac, T., Zheng, J., & Jha, A. (2012). Use of UpToDate and outcomes in US hospitals. *Journal of Hospital Medicine, 7*(2), 85–90. doi:10.1002/jhm.944 PMID:22095750

Iyawa, G. E. (2017c). *A Namibian digital health innovation ecosystem framework.* (PhD thesis, University of South Africa).

Iyawa, G. E., & Hamunyela, S. (2019). mHealth apps and services for maternal healthcare in developing countries. Paper presented at *2019 IST Africa Conference*, Nairobi, Kenya.

Iyawa, G. E., Herselman, M., & Botha, A. (2017a). A scoping review of digital health innovation ecosystem. Paper presented at *2017 IST Africa Conference*, Windhoek, Namibia. 10.23919/ISTAFRICA.2017.8102325

Iyawa, G. E., Velusamy, V., & Palinasamy, S. (2019). Wearable technologies for glucose monitoring: A systematic mapping study of publication trends. In: The IoT and the Next Revolution Automating the World.

Iyawa, G. E., Botha, A., & Herselman, E. (2016b). Identifying and defining the terms related to a Digital Health Innovation Ecosystem. In M. Herselman, & A. Botha (Eds.), *Strategies, Approaches and Experiences: Towards Building a South African Digital Health Innovation Ecosystem* (pp. 30–54). Pretoria, South Africa: CSIR.

Iyawa, G. E., Herselman, M., & Botha, A. (2016a). Digital health innovation ecosystems: From systematic literature to conceptual framework. *Procedia Computer Science, 100*, 244–252. doi:10.1016/j.procs.2016.09.149

Iyawa, G. E., Herselman, M., & Botha, A. (2017b). Identifying essential components of a digital health innovation ecosystem for the Namibian context: Findings from a Delphi study. *The Electronic Journal on Information Systems in Developing Countries, 82*(1), 1–40. doi:10.1002/j.1681-4835.2017.tb00601.x

Iyawa, G. E., Herselman, M., & Botha, A. (2017d). Potential stakeholders and perceived benefits of a Digital Health Innovation Ecosystem for the Namibian context. *Procedia Computer Science, 121*, 431–438. doi:10.1016/j.procs.2017.11.058

Iyawa, G. E., Herselman, M., & Botha, A. (2019). Digital Health Innovation Ecosystem: Identifying key participants, benefits, challenges and guidelines for the Namibian context. *International Journal of Reliable and Quality E-Healthcare, 8*(2), 1–14. doi:10.4018/IJRQEH.2019040101

Iyengar, S., & Lepper, M. (2000). When Choice is Demotivating: Can One Desire Too Much of a Good Thing? *Journal of Personality and Social Psychology, 79*(6), 995–1006. doi:10.1037/0022-3514.79.6.995 PMID:11138768

iYogi. (2018). 10 Best Medical Apps for Seniors. Retrieved from www.iyogi.com/editors-pick/10-best-medical-apps-for-seniors.html

Jabali, A. K., & Jarrar, M. (2018). Electronic health records functionalities in Saudi Arabia: Obstacles and major challenges. *Global Journal of Health Science, 10*(4), 50. doi:10.5539/gjhs.v10n4p50

Jacobsen, R., Liubarskiene, Z., Moldrup, C., Christrup, L., Sjogren, P., & Samsanaviciene, J. (2009). Barriers to cancer pain management: A review of empirical research. *Medicina (Kaunas, Lithuania), 45*(6), 427–433. doi:10.3390/medicina45060055 PMID:19605961

Jain, N., Euler, G. L., Shefer, A., Lu, P., Yankey, D., & Markowitz, L. (2009). Human papillomavirus (HPV) awareness and vaccination initiation among women in the United States, National Immunization Survey: Adult 2007. *Preventive Medicine, 48*(5), 426–431. doi:10.1016/j.ypmed.2008.11.010 PMID:19100762

Jain, N., Singh, H., Koolwal, G. D., Kumar, S., & Gupta, A. (2015). Opportunities and barriers in service delivery through mobile phones (mHealth) for Severe Mental Illnesses in Rajasthan, India: A multi-site study. *Asian Journal of Psychiatry*, *14*, 31–35. doi:10.1016/j.ajp.2015.01.008 PMID:25701069

James, J. (2010). Penetration and growth rates of mobile phones in developing countries: An analytical classification. *Social Indicators Research*, *99*(1), 135–145. doi:10.100711205-009-9572-0 PMID:20835391

James, R. (1975). Why privacy is important. *Philosophy & Public Affairs*, *4*(4), 323–333.

Jamoom, E., & Yang, N. (2016). *Table of electronic health record adoption and use State Variation in Electronic Sharing of Information in Physician Offices: United States, 2015*. Atlanta, GA. Retrieved from https://www.cdc.gov/nchs/products/databriefs/db261.htm

Jan, R. L., Wang, J. Y., Huang, M. C., Tseng, S. M., Su, H. J., & Liu, L. F. (2007). An Internet-based interactive telemonitoring system for improving childhood asthma outcomes in Taiwan. *Telemedicine Journal and e-Health*, *13*(3), 257–268. doi:10.1089/tmj.2006.0053 PMID:17603828

Jauho, M. (2017). Contesting lifestyle risk and gendering coronary candidacy: Lay epidemiology of heart disease in Finland in the 1970s. *Sociology of Health & Illness*, *39*(7), 1005–1018. doi:10.1111/1467-9566.12542 PMID:28236330

Jean, B., Koffi, B., Yazdanmehr, A., & Mahapatra, R. (2018). Mobile Health Mobile Health Privacy Concerns-A Systematic Review. *Twenty-fourth Americas Conference on Information Systems.*

Jefferies, J. (2014). Fear of Deportation in High School: Implications for Breaking the Circle of Silence Surrounding Migration Status AU - Jefferies, Julián. *Journal of Latinos and Education*, *13*(4), 278–295. doi:10.1080/15348431.2014.887469

Jemmott, J. B., Croyle, R. T., & Ditto, P. H. (1988). Commonsense epidemiology: Self-based judgments from laypersons and physicians. *Health Psychology*, *7*(1), 55–73. doi:10.1037/0278-6133.7.1.55 PMID:3257734

Jibb, L. A., Stevens, B. J., Nathan, P. C., Seto, E., Cafazzo, J. A., & Stinson, J. N. (2014). A smartphone-based pain management app for adolescents with cancer: Establishing system requirements and a pain care algorithm based on literature review, interviews, and consensus. *JMIR Research Protocols*, *3*(1), e15. doi:10.2196/resprot.3041 PMID:24646454

Johnson, M. O., Rose, C. D., Dilworth, S. E., & Neilands, T. B. (2012). Advances in the conceptualization and measurement of Health Care Empowerment: Development and validation of the Health Care Empowerment inventory. *PLoS One*, *7*(9). doi:10.1371/journal.pone.0045692 PMID:23029184

Jorunn, L. H., Beatrix, V., Clemens, B., Chris, T., Taraldsen, K., Pijnappels, M., ... Mellone, S. (2017). Mobile Health Applications to Promote Active and Healthy Ageing. *Sensors (Basel)*, *17*(3), 622. doi:10.339017030622 PMID:28335475

Jo, S. M., & Chung, K. Y. (2015). Design of access control system for telemedicine secure XML documents. *Multimedia Tools and Applications*, *74*(4), 2257–2271. doi:10.100711042-014-1938-x

Jotterand, F., Amodio, A., & Elger, B. S. (2016). Patient education as empowerment and self-rebiasing. *Medicine, Health Care, and Philosophy*, *19*(4), 553–561. doi:10.100711019-016-9702-9 PMID:27179973

Jutel, A., & Lupton, D. (2015). Digitizing diagnosis: A review of mobile applications in the diagnostic process. *Diagnosis*, *2*(2), 89–96. doi:10.1515/dx-2014-0068 PMID:29540025

Kagolianni, A. (2011). Factors affect in patient adherence to medication regimen. *Health Science Journal*, *5*(3), 157–158.

Kahn, J. A., Slap, G. B., Bernstein, D. I., Tissot, A. M., Kollar, L. M., Hillard, P. A., & Rosenthal, S. L. (2007). Personal meaning of human papillomavirus and Pap test results in adolescent and young adult women. *Health Psychology*, *26*(2), 192–200. doi:10.1037/0278-6133.26.2.192 PMID:17385971

Kaltenbach, T. (2016). Digital and disrupted: All change for healthcare. *Roland Berger Publication: Think Act*. Retrieved from https://www.rolandberger.com/de/Publications/Digital-and-disrupted-All-change-for-healthcare.html

Kalyanpur, A., Singh, J., & Bedi, R. (2010). Practical issues in picture archiving and communication system and networking. *The Indian Journal of Radiology & Imaging*, *20*(1), 2. doi:10.4103/0971-3026.59743 PubMed

Kamdar, M. M., Centi, A. J., Fischer, N., & Jethwani, K. (2018). A randomized controlled trial of a novel artificial-intelligence based smartphone application to optimize the management of cancer-related pain. Paper presented at the *2018 Palliative and Supportive Care on Oncology Symposium*, San Diego, CA. 10.1200/JCO.2018.36.34_suppl.76

Kamoun, F., & Nicho, M. (2014). Human and organizational factors of healthcare data breaches: The Swiss cheese model of data breach causation and prevention. [IJHISI]. *International Journal of Healthcare Information Systems and Informatics*, *9*(1), 42–60. doi:10.4018/ijhisi.2014010103

Kampmeijer, R., Pavlova, M., Tambor, M., Golinowska, S., & Groot, W. (2016). The use of e-health and m-health tools in health promotion and primary prevention among older adults: A systematic literature review. *BMC Health Services Research*, *16*(S5), 290. doi:10.118612913-016-1522-3

Kaplan, R. M., & Stone, A. A. (2013). Bringing the laboratory and clinic to the community: Mobile technologies for health promotion and disease prevention. *Annual Review of Psychology*, *64*(1), 471–498. doi:10.1146/annurev-psych-113011-143736 PMID:22994919

Kappelman, L. A., McKeeman, R., & Zhang, L. (2006). Early warning signs of IT project failure: The dominant dozen. *Information Systems Management*, *23*(4), 31–36. doi:10.1201/1078.10580530/46352.23.4.20060901/95110.4

Karasouli, E., & Adams, A. (2014). Assessing the Evidence for e-Resources for Mental Health Self-Management: A Systematic Literature Review. *JMIR Mental Health*, *1*(1), e3. doi:10.2196/mental.3708 PMID:26543903

Kay, M., Santos, J., & Takane, M. (2011). mHealth: New horizons for health through mobile technologies. *World Health Organization, 64*(7), 66-71.

Kenny, G., & Connolly, R. (2017). Towards an Inclusive World : Exploring M-Health Adoption Across Generations. *Twenty-fifth European Conference on Information Systems (ECIS)*, Guimarães, Portugal, (pp. 1129-1144).

Keselman, A., & Smith, C. A. (2012). A classification of errors in lay comprehension of medical documents. *Journal of Biomedical Informatics*, *45*(6), 1151–1163. doi:10.1016/j.jbi.2012.07.012 PMID:22925723

Kester, L. M., Shedd-Steele, R. B., Dotson-Roberts, C. A., Smith, J., & Zimet, G. D. (2014). The effects of a brief educational intervention on human papillomavirus knowledge and intention to initiate HPV vaccination in 18--26 year old young adults. *Gynecologic Oncology*, *132*, S9–S12. doi:10.1016/j.ygyno.2013.12.033 PMID:24384459

Khanna, S., Sattar, A., & Hansen, D. (2013). Artificial intelligence in health – the three big challenges. *The Australasian Medical Journal*, *6*(5), 315–317. doi:10.4066/AMJ.2013.1758 PMID:23745154

Khazaal, Y., Chatton, A., Cochand, S., Coquard, O., Fernandez, S., Khan, R., ... Zullino, D. (2009). Brief DISCERN, six questions for the evaluation of evidence-based content of health-related websites. *Patient Education and Counseling*, *77*(1),.33–37. doi:10.1016/j.pec.2009.02.016 PMID:19372023

Khennou, F., Khamlichi, Y. I., & Chaoui, N. E. H. (2018). Improving the Use of Big Data Analytics within Electronic Health Records: A Case Study based OpenEHR. *Procedia Computer Science*, *127*, 60–68. doi:10.1016/j.procs.2018.01.098

Khuntia, J., Yim, D., Tanniru, M., & Lim, S. (2017). Patient empowerment and engagement with a health infomediary. *Health Policy and Technology*, *6*(1), 40–50. doi:10.1016/j.hlpt.2016.11.003

Kimball, T. G. (2018). How wearable technology changes our approach to healthcare. *MAP Health Management*. Retrieved from https://thisismap.com//insights/map-blog/how-wearable-technology-changes-our-approach-healthcare

Kincaid, J. P., Fishburne, R. P., Rogers, R. L., & Chissom, B. S. (1975). *Derivation of New Readability Formulas (Automated Readability Index, Fog Count and Flesch Reading Ease Formula) for Navy Enlisted Personnel*. Memphis, TN. doi:10.21236/ADA006655

King, T. E., Jr. & Wheeler, M. B. (2007). Medical management of vulnerable and underserved patients: principles, practice, and populations: New York, NY: McGraw-Hill Medical Publishing Division.

King, D., Karthikesalingam, A., Hughes, C., Montgomery, H., Raine, R., Rees, G., & Team, O. (2018). Letter in response to Google DeepMind and healthcare in an age of algorithms. *Health and Technology*, *8*(1–2), 11–13. doi:10.100712553-018-0228-4

Kings Fund. (2016). A Digital NHS? Retrieved from https://www.kingsfund.org.uk/sites/default/files/field/field_publication_file/A_digital_NHS_Kings_Fund_Sep_2016.pdf

Kings Fund. (2019). The NHS long-term plan explained. Retrieved from https://www.kingsfund.org.uk/sites/default/files/field/field_publication_file/A_digital_NHS_Kings_Fund_Sep_2016.pdf

Klasnja, P., & Pratt, W. (2012). Healthcare in the pocket: Mapping the space of mobile-phone health interventions. *Journal of Biomedical Informatics*, *45*(1), 184–198. doi:10.1016/j.jbi.2011.08.017 PMID:21925288

Klecun, E. (2016). Transforming healthcare: Policy discourses of IT and patient-centred care. *European Journal of Information Systems*, *25*(1), 64–76. doi:10.1057/ejis.2014.40

Knight, L. V., & Mattick, K. (2006). "When I first came here, I thought medicine was black and white": Making sense of medical students' ways of knowing. *Social Science & Medicine*, *63*(4), 1084–1096. doi:10.1016/j.socscimed.2006.01.017 PMID:16519978

Kodner, L. D., & Spreeuwenberg, C. (2002). Integrated care: Meaning, logic, applications, and implications – a discussion paper. *International Journal of Integrated Care*, *2*(4), e12. doi:10.5334/ijic.67 PMID:16896389

Koh, H. K., Berwick, D. M., Clancy, C. M., Baur, C., Brach, C., Harris, L. M., & Zerhusen, E. G. (2012). New federal policy initiatives to boost health literacy can help the nation move beyond the cycle of costly "crisis care.". *Health Affairs*, *31*(2), 434–443. doi:10.1377/hlthaff.2011.1169 PMID:22262723

Koh, H. K., Brach, C., Harris, L. M., & Parchman, M. L. (2013). A proposed "health literate care model" would constitute a systems approach to improving patients' engagement in care. *Health Affairs*, *32*(2), 357–367. doi:10.1377/hlthaff.2012.1205 PMID:23381529

Köpke, S., Solari, A., Khan, F., Heesen, C., & Giordano, A. (2014). Information provision for people with multiple sclerosis. *Cochrane Database of Systematic Reviews*, *4*. PMID:24752330

Kripalani, S., LeFevre, F., Phillips, C. O., Williams, M. V., Basaviah, P., & Baker, D. W. (2007). Deficits in communication and information transfer between hospital-based and primary care physicians: Implications for patient safety and continuity of care. *Journal of the American Medical Association*, *297*(8), 831–841. doi:10.1001/jama.297.8.831 PubMed

Kuhn, T. (2011). Health Information Technology and Privacy- American College of Physicians A Position Paper July 2011.

Kurniawan, S. (2008). Older people and mobile phones: A multi-method investigation. *International Journal of Human-Computer Studies*, *66*(12), 889–901. doi:10.1016/j.ijhcs.2008.03.002

Kutner, M., Greenburg, E., Jin, Y., & Paulsen, C. (2006). The Health Literacy of America's Adults: Results from the 2003 National Assessment of Adult Literacy. NCES 2006-483. National Center for Education Statistics. Available from https://files.eric.ed.gov/fulltext/ED493284.pdf

Kuzeyli Yildirim, Y., & Uyar, M. (2006). Barriers to effective cancer pain management. *The Journal of the Turkish Society of Algology*, *18*(3), 12–19. Retrieved from https://www.ncbi.nlm.nih.gov/pubmed/17089225 PMID:17089225

Kvedar, J. C., Colman, C., & Cella, G. (2015). The internet of healthy things. Boston, MA: Partners Connected Health.

Kwag, K. H., González-Lorenzo, M., Banzi, R., Bonovas, S., & Moja, L. (2016). Providing Doctors With High-Quality Information: An Updated Evaluation of Web-Based Point-of-Care Information Summaries. *Journal of Medical Internet Research*, *18*(1), e15. doi:10.2196/jmir.5234 PMID:26786976

Kwon, H. E., Dewan, S., Oh, W., & Kim, T. (2017). Efficacy of a Health App for Obesity and Overweight Management: A Hidden Markov Model. *International Conference on Information Systems*, 1-17.

Kwon, J. H. (2014). Overcoming barriers in cancer pain management. *Journal of Clinical Oncology*, *32*(16), 1727–1733. doi:10.1200/JCO.2013.52.4827 PMID:24799490

Lafolla, T. (2017). *History of Telemedicine Infographic*. Retrieved from http://blog.evisit.com/history-telemedicine-infographic

Laird, E. A., Ryan, A., McCauley, C., Bond, R. B., Mulvenna, M. D., Curran, K. J., & Gibson, A. (2018). Using Mobile Technology to Provide Personalized Reminiscence for People Living with Dementia and Their Carers: Appraisal of Outcomes from a Quasi-Experimental Study. *JMIR Mental Health*, *5*(3), e57. doi:10.2196/mental.9684 PMID:30206053

Laja, S. (2011, Nov. 9). Trusts reveal staff abuse of social media | Healthcare Professionals Network | The Guardian. *The Guardian*.

Lambert, E. C. (2001). College students' knowledge of human papillomavirus and effectiveness of a brief educational intervention. *The Journal of the American Board of Family Practice*, *14*(3), 178–183. PMID:11355049

Lamkin, P. (2016). Wearable tech market to be worth $34 billion by 2020. *Forbes*. Retrieved from https://www.forbes.com/sites/paullamkin/2016/02/17/wearable-tech-market-to-be-worth-34-billion-by-2020/#67333e973cb5

Lamkin, P. (2017). Smartwatch sales to double in next 5 years. *Forbes*. Retrieved from https://www.forbes.com/sites/paullamkin/2017/11/29/smartwatch-sales-to-double-in-next-5-years/#2a7c2b8d35ed

Lanamäki, A., Stendal, K., & Thapa, D. (2011). Mutual informing between IS academia and practice: Insights from KIWISR-5. *Communications of the Association for Information Systems*, 123–132.

Langer, S. (2009). Issues surrounding PACS archiving to external, third-party DICOM archives. *Journal of Digital Imaging*, *22*(1), 48–52. doi:10.1007/s10278-008-9125-0 PubMed

Lapowsky, I. (2017). The VA's new app tries to reach vets wherever they live. *Wired*. Retrieved from https://www.wired.com/story/va-video-telemedicine-app/

Larsen, M. E., Cummins, N., Boonstra, T. W., O'Dea, B., Tighe, J., Nicholas, J., . . . Christensen, H. (2015). The use of technology in suicide prevention. Paper presented at the *37th annual international conference of the IEEE engineering in Medicine and Biology Society (EMBC)*, Milano, Italy. 10.1109/EMBC.2015.7320081

Lebied, M. (2018). 12 examples of big data analytics in healthcare that can save people. Retrieved from https://www.datapine.com/blog/big-data-examples-in-healthcare/

Lebied, M. (2019). Examples of big data in healthcare that can save people.

Lederer, N., Grechenig, T., & Baranyi, R. (2014). unCUT: bridging the gap from paper diary cards towards mobile electronic monitoring solutions in borderline and self-injury. Paper presented at the *IEEE 3nd International Conference on Serious Games and Applications for Health (SeGAH)*, Rio de Janeiro, Brazil. 10.1109/SeGAH.2014.7067092

Lee, G., & Xia, W. (2005). The ability of information systems development project teams to respond to business and technology changes: A study of flexibility measures. *European Journal of Information Systems*, *14*(1), 75–92. doi:10.1057/palgrave.ejis.3000523

Lee, R. A., & Jung, M. E. (2018). Evaluation of an mHealth App (DeStressify) on University Students' Mental Health: Pilot Trial. *JMIR Mental Health*, *5*(1), e2. doi:10.2196/mental.8324 PMID:29362209

Lejbkowicz, I., Caspi, O., & Miller, A. (2012). Participatory medicine and patient empowerment towards personalized healthcare in multiple sclerosis. *Expert Review of Neurotherapeutics*, *12*(3), 343–352. doi:10.1586/ern.11.161 PMID:22364333

Lejbkowicz, I., Paperna, T., Stein, N., Dishon, S., & Miller, A. (2010). Internet Usage by Patients with Multiple Sclerosis: Implications to Participatory Medicine and Personalized Healthcare. *Multiple Sclerosis International*, *2010*, 1–7. doi:10.1155/2010/640749 PMID:22096625

Lesage, P., & Portenoy, R. K. (1999). Trends in cancer pain management. *Cancer Control*, *6*(2), 136–145. doi:10.1177/107327489900600202 PMID:10758542

Lester, R. T., Ritvo, P., Mills, E. J., Kariri, A., Karanja, S., Chung, M. H., ... Plummer, F. A. (2010). Effects of a mobile phone short message service on antiretroviral treatment adherence in Kenya (WelTel Kenya1): A randomised trial. *Lancet*, *376*(9755), 1838–1845. doi:10.1016/S0140-6736(10)61997-6 PMID:21071074

Leung, R., Tang, C., Haddad, S., McGrenere, J., Graf, P., & Ingriany, V. (2012). How older adults learn to use mobile devices: Survey and field investigations. ACM Trans, 3, Article 11.

Levin-Zamir, D., Baron-Epel, O. B., Cohen, V., & Elhayany, A. (2016). The association of health literacy with health behavior, socioeconomic indicators, and self-assessed health from a national adult survey in Israel. Journal of Health Communication, 21(sup2), 61-68.

Levy, A. G., Weinstein, N., Kidney, E., Scheld, S., & Guarnaccia, P. (2008). Lay and expert interpretations of cancer cluster evidence. *Risk Analysis: An International Journal*, *28*(6), 1531–1538. doi:10.1111/j.1539-6924.2008.01110.x PMID:18795998

Lewis, J. E., & Neider, M. B. (2017). Designing wearable technology for an aging population. *Ergonomics in Design*, *25*(3), 4–10. doi:10.1177/1064804616645488

Lewis, T. L., & Wyatt, J. C. (2014). mHealth and mobile medical Apps: A framework to assess risk and promote safer use. *Journal of Medical Internet Research*, *16*(9), e210. doi:10.2196/jmir.3133

Liberati, E. G., Gorli, M., Moja, L., Galuppo, L., Ripamonti, S., & Scaratti, G. (2015). Exploring the practice of patient centered care: The role of ethnography and reflexivity. *Social Science & Medicine*, *133*, 45–52. doi:10.1016/j.socscimed.2015.03.050 PMID:25841094

Li, I., Dey, A., & Forlizzi, J. (2010). A stage-based model of personal informatics systems. *Proceedings of the 28th International Conference on Human Factors in Computing Systems - CHI 10*. 10.1145/1753326.1753409

Lin, C. J., Hsieh, T. L., & Shiang, W. J. (2009). Exploring the Interface Design of Mobile Phone for the Elderly. *Human Centered Design, 5619*, 476–481. doi:10.1007/978-3-642-02806-9_55

Linder, L. A., Ameringer, S., Baggott, C., Erickson, J., Macpherson, C. F., Rodgers, C., & Stegenga, K. (2015). *Measures and Methods for Symptom and Symptom Cluster Assessment in Adolescents and Young Adults with Cancer, 31*(3), 206–215.

Lipschitz, J., Miller, C. J., Hogan, T. P., Burdick, K. E., Lippin-Foster, R., Simon, S. R., & Burgess, J. (2019). Adoption of Mobile Apps for Depression and Anxiety: Cross-Sectional Survey Study on Patient Interest and Barriers to Engagement. *JMIR Mental Health, 6*(1), e11334. doi:10.2196/11334 PMID:30681968

Liu, F., Guo, X., & Ju, X. (2018). Routine Use of Mobile Health Services: Promotion or Prevention. *International Conference on Information Systems* (pp. 1–10).

Lotsch, J., & Ultsch, A. (2018). Machine learning in pain research. *Pain, 159*(4), 623–630. doi:10.1097/j.pain.0000000000001118 PMID:29194126

Loukanova, S., Molnar, R., & Bridges, J. F. P. (2007). Promoting patient empowerment in the healthcare system: Highlighting the need for patient-centered drug policy. *Expert Review of Pharmacoeconomics & Outcomes Research, 7*(3), 281–289. doi:10.1586/14737167.7.3.281 PMID:20528314

Lovatt, M., Eadie, D., Meier, P. S., Li, J., Bauld, L., Hastings, G., & Holmes, J. (2015). Lay epidemiology and the interpretation of low-risk drinking guidelines by adults in the United Kingdom. *Addiction (Abingdon, England), 110*(12), 1912–1919. doi:10.1111/add.13072 PMID:26212155

Lupton, D. (2013). Quantifying the body: Monitoring and measuring health in the age of mHealth technologies. *Critical Public Health, 23*(4), 393–403. doi:10.1080/09581596.2013.794931

Lupton, D., & Maslen, S. (2019). How women use digital technologies for health: Qualitative interview and focus group study. *Journal of Medical Internet Research, 21*(1), e11481. doi:10.2196/11481 PMID:30681963

Mackert, M., Mabry-Flynn, A., Champlin, S., Donovan, E. E., & Pounders, K. (2016). Health literacy and health information technology adoption: The potential for a new digital divide. *Journal of Medical Internet Research, 18*(10), e264. doi:10.2196/jmir.6349 PMID:27702738

Mail, D. (2011, Jan. 3). Four nursing students expelled from university after posting pictures of themselves posing with a human placenta on Facebook. *Daily Mail.*

Mak, W. W. S., Wong, C. C. Y., Chan, A. T. Y., & Lau, J. T. F. (2019). Mobile self-compassion programme for promotion of public mental health: A randomised controlled trial. *Hong Kong Medical Journal, 25*(1 Supplement 2). PMID:30674702

Malhotra, N. K., Jain, A. K., & Lagakos, S. W. (1982). The Information Overload Controversy: An Alternative Viewpoint. *Journal of Marketing, 46*(2), 27–37. doi:10.1177/002224298204600204

Manda, T. D., & Herstad, J. (2015). Enacting technology: Accounting for the interplay between mHealth solutions and existing paper-based data reporting practices. *Information Technology & People, 28*(3), 442–465. doi:10.1108/ITP-02-2014-0045

Mankodiya, K., Sharma, V., Martins, R., Pande, I., Jain, S., Ryan, N., & Gandhi, R. (2013, December). Understanding User's Emotional Engagement to the Contents on a Smartphone Display: Psychiatric Prospective. Paper presented at *2013 IEEE 10th International Conference on Ubiquitous Intelligence and Computing and 2013 IEEE 10th International Conference on Autonomic and Trusted Computing*, Sorrento Pennisula, Italy. 10.1109/UIC-ATC.2013.98

Mantwill, S., & Schulz, P. J. (2017). Low health literacy and healthcare utilization among immigrants and non-immigrants in Switzerland. *Patient Education and Counseling, 100*(11), 2020–2027. doi:10.1016/j.pec.2017.05.023 PMID:28559092

Manyika, J., Chui, M., Brown, B., Bughin, J., Dobbs, R., Roxburgh, C., & Byers, A. H. (2011). *Big data: The next frontier for innovation, competition, and productivity*. Seoul Korea. Retrieved from https://www.mckinsey.com/~/media/McKinsey/Business Functions/McKinsey Digital/Our Insights/Big data The next frontier for innovation/MGI_big_data_full_report.ashx

Marceau, L. D., Link, C., Jamison, R. N., & Carolan, S. (2007). Electronic diaries as a tool to improve pain management: Is there any evidence? *Pain Medicine, 8*(suppl_3), S101-S109. doi:10.1111/j.1526-4637.2007.00374.x

Marcolino, M. S., Oliveira, J. A. Q., D'Agostino, M., Ribeiro, A. L., Alkmim, M. B. M., & Novillo-Ortiz, D. (2018). The impact of mHealth interventions: Systematic review of systematic reviews. *JMIR mHealth and uHealth, 6*(1), e23. doi:10.2196/mhealth.8873 PMID:29343463

Margalit, R. S., Roter, D., Dunevant, M. A., Larson, S., & Reis, S. (2006). Electronic medical record use and physician–patient communication: An observational study of Israeli primary care encounters. *Patient Education and Counseling, 61*(1), 134–141. doi:10.1016/j.pec.2005.03.004 PMID:16533682

Marie Curie. (2017). The Long and Winding Road. Retrieved from https://www.mariecurie.org.uk/globalassets/media/documents/policy/campaigns/the-long-and-winding-road.pdf

MarketWatch. (2018). The global telemedicine market is accounted for $21.56 billion in 2017 and is expected to reach $93.45 billion by 2026 growing at a CAGR of 17.7% during the forecast period. *PRNewswire*. Retrieved from https://www.marketwatch.com/press-release/the-global-telemedicine-market-is-accounted-for-2156-billion-in-2017-and-is-expected-to-reach-9345-billion-by-2026-growing-at-a-cagr-of-177-during-the-forecast-period-2018-08-30

Markman, M. (2019). 16% HPV Vaccination Rate Among US Adolescents "Inadequate." Retrieved from https://www.medscape.com/viewarticle/908885

Marnocha, S., Marnocha, M. R., & Pilliow, T. (2015). Unprofessional content posted online among nursing students. *Nurse Educator*, *40*(3), 119–123. doi:10.1097/NNE.0000000000000123

Marrie, R. A., Salter, A. R., Tyry, T., Fox, R. J., & Cutter, G. R. (2013). Preferred sources of health information in persons with multiple sclerosis: Degree of trust and information sought. *Journal of Medical Internet Research*, *15*(4), e67. doi:10.2196/jmir.2466 PMID:23635393

Marshall, D. A., Burgos-Liz, L., Pasupathy, K. S., Padula, W. V., IJzerman, M. J., Wong, P. K., ... Osgood, N. D. (2016). Transforming healthcare delivery: Integrating dynamic simulation modelling and big data in health economics and outcomes research. *PharmacoEconomics*, *34*(2), 115–126. doi:10.100740273-015-0330-7 PMID:26497003

Martensson, P., & Lee, A. S. (2004). Dialogical action research at Omega Corporation. *Management Information Systems Quarterly*, *28*(3), 507–536. doi:10.2307/25148648

Martína, L., Martinb, S., & Medranoa, C. (2011). Mobile applications in an aging society: Status and trends Inmaculada Plazaa. *Journal of Systems and Software*, *84*(11), 1977–1988. doi:10.1016/j.jss.2011.05.035

Mathur, G., Nain, S., & Sharma, P. K. (2015). Cancer: An overview. *Academic Journal of Cancer Research, 1*(1), 01-09.

Maunsell, E., Lauzier, S., Brunet, J., Pelletier, S., Osborne, R. H., & Campbell, H. S. (2014). Health-related empowerment in cancer: Validity of scales from the Health Education Impact Questionnaire. *Cancer*, *120*(20), 3228–3236. doi:10.1002/cncr.28847 PMID:24988944

Maxmen, A. (2018). *Deep learning sharpens views of cells and genes*. Retrieved from https://www.scientificamerican.com/article/deep-learning-sharpens-views-of-cells-and-genes/

Mayer, R. C., Davis, J. H., & Schoorman, F. D. (1995). An integrative model of organizational trust. *Academy of Management Review*, *20*(3), 709–734. doi:10.5465/amr.1995.9508080335

Maynard, M. T., Gilson, L. L., & Mathieu, J. E. (2012). Empowerment-Fad or Fab? A Multilevel Review of the Past Two Decades of Research. *Journal of Management*, *38*(4), 1231–1281. doi:10.1177/0149206312438773

McAllister, M., Dunn, G., Payne, K., Davies, L., & Todd, C. (2012). Patient empowerment: The need to consider it as a measurable patient-reported outcome for chronic conditions. *BMC Health Services Research*, *12*(1), 157. doi:10.1186/1472-6963-12-157 PMID:22694747

McCaffery, K., & Irwig, L. (2005). Australian women's needs and preferences for information about human papillomavirus in cervical screening. *Journal of Medical Screening*, *12*(3), 134–141. doi:10.1258/0969141054855238 PMID:16156944

McCree, D. H., Sharpe, P. A., Brandt, H. M., & Robertson, R. (2006). Preferences for sources of information about abnormal Pap tests and HPV in women tested for HPV. *Preventive Medicine*, *43*(3), 165–170. doi:10.1016/j.ypmed.2006.04.001 PMID:16701815

McElroy, E., & Shevlin, M. (2014). The development and initial validation of the cyberchondria severity scale (CSS). *Journal of Anxiety Disorders*, *28*(2), 259–265. doi:10.1016/j.janxdis.2013.12.007 PMID:24508033

McGaughey, R., Zeltmann, S. M., & McMurtrey, M. (2013). Motivations and obstacles to smartphone use by the elderly: Developing a research framework. *International. Journal of Electronic Finance*, *7*(3/4), 177–195. doi:10.1504/IJEF.2013.058601

McGinnis, J. M., Russo, P. M., & Knickman, J. R. (2002). The case for more active policy attention to health promotion. *Health Affairs*, *21*(2), 78–93. doi:10.1377/hlthaff.21.2.78 PMID:11900188

McKee, R. (2013). Ethical issues in using social media for health and health care research. *Health Policy (Amsterdam)*, *110*(2–3), 298–301. doi:10.1016/j.healthpol.2013.02.006

Mckenzie, I. S., Morant, S. V., Bloomfield, G. A., MacDonald, T. M., & O'Riordan, J. (2013). Incidence and prevalence of multiple sclerosis in the UK 1990–2010: A descriptive study in the general practice research database. *Journal of Neurology, Neurosurgery, and Psychiatry*, *85*(1), 76–84. doi:10.1136/jnnp-2013-305450 PMID:24052635

McKinsey. (2013). mHealth: A new vision for healthcare. McKinsey & Company, 1-20.

McKnight, D. H., Cummings, L. L., & Chervany, N. L. (1998). Initial trust formation in new organizational relationships. *Academy of Management Review*, *23*(3), 473–490. doi:10.5465/amr.1998.926622

McQuade, D. (2015). Alice Goffman's Book on "Fugitive Life" in Philly Under Attack. Retrieved from https://www.phillymag.com/news/2015/06/11/alice-goffman-book-philadelphia-on-the-run-criticism/

Medford-Davis, L. N., Eswaran, V., Shah, R. M., & Dark, C. (2015). The Patient Protection and Affordable Care Act's effect on emergency medicine: A synthesis of the data. *Annals of Emergency Medicine*, *66*(5), 496–506. doi:10.1016/j.annemergmed.2015.04.007 PMID:25976250

Medpac. (2012, June). Report to the Congress: Medicare and the Health Care Delivery System. Retrieved from http://www.medpac.gov/docs/default-source/reports/jun12_entirereport.pdf

Meeker, M. (2015). 2015 Internet Trends. Retrieved from https://www.kleinerperkins.com/perspectives/2015-Internet-trends

Mehta, N., & Rahimy, E. (2018). Artificial intelligence for automated detection of diabetic retinopathy. Retina Roundup. Retrieved from https://retinaroundup.com/2018/06/08/artificial-intelligence-for-automated-detection-of-diabetic-retinopathy/

Mehta, P., Sharma, M., & Lee, R. C. (2014). Designing and evaluating a health belief model-based intervention to increase intent of HPV vaccination among college males. *International Quarterly of Community Health Education, 34*(1), 101–117. doi:10.2190/IQ.34.1.h PMID:24366025

Meng, F., Zhang, X., Guo, X., Lai, K. H., & Zhao, X. (2019). How Do Patients with Chronic Diseases Make Usage Decisions regarding Mobile Health Monitoring Service? *Journal of Healthcare Engineering*, 2019. PMID:30931088

Menon, V., Selvakumar, N., Kattimani, S., & Andrade, C. (2018). Therapeutic effects of mobile-based text message reminders for medication adherence in bipolar I disorder: Are they maintained after intervention cessation? *Journal of Psychiatric Research, 104*, 163–168. doi:10.1016/j.jpsychires.2018.07.013 PMID:30081390

MHealth: New horizons for health through mobile technologies. (2011). Geneva, Switzerland: World Health Organization.

Michaud, T. L., Zhou, J., McCarthy, M. A., Siahpush, M., & Su, D. (2018). Costs of home-based telemedicine programs: A systematic review. *International Journal of Technology Assessment in Health Care, 34*(4), 410–418. doi:10.1017/S0266462318000454 PMID:30058505

Michelle, T. Q. Y., Jarzabek, S., & Wadhwa, B. (2014, September). CBT Assistant: mHealth App for Psychotherapy. Paper presented at *IEEE Global Humanitarian Technology Conference-South Asia Satellite*, Trivandrum, India.

Michie, S., Lester, K., Pinto, J., & Marteau, T. M. (2005). Communicating risk information in genetic counseling: An observational study. *Health Education & Behavior, 32*(5), 589–598. doi:10.1177/1090198105278562 PMID:16148206

MicroMarket Monitor. (2015). Europe Departmental Picture Archiving and Communication System (PACS) Market by Product (Radiology PACS, Cardiology PACS, Others), by Deployment), by End User (Hospitals, Laboratories, Physicians), by Component - Analysis and Forecast to 2019 (Report No. DE 1001). Retrieved from http://www.micromarketmonitor.com/market/europe-departmental-pacs-5624333279.html

Middleton, C., Scheepers, R., & Tuunainen, V. K. (2014). When mobile is the norm: Researching mobile information systems and mobility as post-adoption phenomena. *European Journal of Information Systems, 23*(5), 503–512. doi:10.1057/ejis.2014.21

Miller, A. D., Pollack, A. H., & Pratt, W. (2016). Bursting the information bubble: Identifying opportunities for pediatric patient-centered technology. *American Medical Informatics Association Annual Symposium Proceedings, 2016*, 894. PMID:28269886

Miller, A. S., Cafazzo, J. A., & Seto, E. (2014). A game plan: Gamification design principles in mHealth applications for chronic disease management. *Health Informatics Journal, 22*(2), 184–193. doi:10.1177/1460458214537511 PMID:24986104

Ministry of Health Singapore. (2012). MOH 2012 Committee of Supply Speech Healthcare 2020: Improving Accessibility, Quality and Affordability for Tomorrow's Challenges (Part 1 of 2). Retrieved from https://www.moh.gov.sg/news-highlights/details/moh-2012-committee-of-supply-speech-healthcare-2020-improving-accessibility-quality-and-affordability-for-tomorrow-s-challenges-(part-1-of-2)

Ministry of Health Singapore. (2017). SOC Waiting Times. Retrieved from https://www.moh.gov.sg/news-highlights/details/moh-2012-committee-of-supply-speech-healthcare-2020-improving-accessibility-quality-and-affordability-for-tomorrow-s-challenges-(part-1-of-2)

Ministry of Health Singapore. (2018). Admission and Outpatient Attendances. Retrieved from https://www.moh.gov.sg/resources-statistics/singapore-health-facts/admissions-and-outpatient-attendances

Miniwatts Marketing Group. (2019). Statistics about the Internet. Retrieved from https://www.internetworldstats.com/stats.htm

Moccia, M., Carotenuto, A., Massarelli, M., Lanzillo, R., & Brescia Morra, V. (2016). Can people with multiple sclerosis actually understand what they read in the Internet age? *Journal of Clinical Neuroscience*, *25*, 167–168. doi:10.1016/j.jocn.2015.10.003 PMID:26526382

Moh, S. (2017). National E- Health Strategy - MOH Initiatives 2030. Retrieved from https://www.moh.gov.sa/en/Ministry/nehs/Pages/vision2030.aspx

Moorhead, S. A., Hazlett, D. E., Harrison, L., Carroll, J. K., Irwin, A., & Hoving, C. (2013). A new dimension of health care: Systematic review of the uses, benefits, and limitations of social media for health communication. *Journal of Medical Internet Research*, *15*(4), e85. doi:10.2196/jmir.1933

Morgan, L. (2018). What is ETL: Extract, transform, load. Retrieved from https://www.datamation.com/big-data/what-is-etl-extract-transform-load.html

Morris, M. E., Kathawala, Q., Leen, T. K., Gorenstein, E. E., Guilak, F., DeLeeuw, W., & Labhard, M. (2010). Mobile therapy: Case study evaluations of a cell phone application for emotional self-awareness. *Journal of Medical Internet Research*, *12*(2), e10. doi:10.2196/jmir.1371 PMID:20439251

Morton, S., Shih, S. C., Winther, C. H., Tinoco, A., Kessler, R. S., & Scholle, S. H. (2015). Health IT–enabled care coordination: A national survey of patient-centered medical home clinicians. *Annals of Family Medicine*, *13*(3), 250–256. doi:10.1370/afm.1797 PubMed

Motiwalla, L., & Li, X.-B. (2013). Developing privacy solutions for sharing and analyzing healthcare data. *International Journal of Business Information Systems*, *13*(2), 199–216. doi:10.1504/IJBIS.2013.054335 PMID:24285983

Mousseau, S., Lapointe, A., & Gravel, J. (2018). Diagnosing acute otitis media using a smartphone otoscope; a randomized controlled trial. *The American Journal of Emergency Medicine*, *36*(10), 1796–1801. doi:10.1016/j.ajem.2018.01.093 PMID:29544905

Multiple Sclerosis International Federation. (2013). Atlas-of-MS. Retrieved from https://www.msif.org/wp-content/uploads/2014/09/Atlas-of-MS.pdf

Mulvaney, S. A., Anders, S., Smith, A. K., Pittel, E. J., & Johnson, K. B. (2012). A pilot test of a tailored mobile and web-based diabetes messaging system for adolescents. *Journal of Telemedicine and Telecare*, *18*(2), 115–118. doi:10.1258/jtt.2011.111006 PMID:22383802

Mumford, E. (2001). Advice for action researchers. *Information Technology & People*, *14*(1), 12–27. doi:10.1108/09593840110384753

Munie, K., & Thakur, S. (2017). Digital affect ability: Therapeutic lens on value. *Accenture Strategy*. Retrieved from https://www.accenture.com/t20170321T020154__w__/ie-en/_acnmedia/PDF-47/Accenture-Strategy-Digital-Affect-ability-PoV.pdf

Musiat, P., Goldstone, P., & Tarrier, N. (2014). Understanding the acceptability of e-mental health-attitudes and expectations towards computerised self-help treatments for mental health problems. *BMC Psychiatry*, *14*(1), 109. doi:10.1186/1471-244X-14-109

Muthuraman, K., & Lawley, M. (2008). A stochastic overbooking model for outpatient clinical scheduling with no-shows. *IIE Transactions*, *40*(9), 820–837. doi:10.1080/07408170802165823

Naiker, U., FitzGerald, G., Dulhunty, J. M., & Rosemann, M. (2018). Time to wait: A systematic review of strategies that affect out-patient waiting times. *Australian Health Review*, *42*(3), 286–293. doi:10.1071/AH16275 PMID:28355525

Nair, S. C., & Ibrahim, H. (2015). Assessing subject privacy and data confidentiality in an emerging region for clinical trials: United Arab Emirates. *Accountability in Research*, *22*(4), 205–220. doi:10.1080/08989621.2014.942452

Nambisan, P. (2017). Factors that impact Patient Web Portal Readiness (PWPR) among the underserved. *International Journal of Medical Informatics*, *102*, 62–70. doi:10.1016/j.ijmedinf.2017.03.004 PMID:28495349

Narayan, D. (2005). Conceptual Framework and Methodological Challenges. In D. Narayan (Ed.), *Measuring Empowerment* (pp. 3–38). Washington, D.C.: The World Bank.

National Cancer Institute. (2018). Cervix Uteri Cancer.

Nelson, R. R. (2007). IT project management: Infamous failures, classic mistakes, and best practices. *MIS Quarterly Executive*, *6*(2).

Nelson, R., & Staggers, N. (2014). *Health Informatics : An Interprofessional Approach*. Elsevier Health Sciences.

Neter, E., & Brainin, E. (2019). Association Between Health Literacy, eHealth Literacy, and Health Outcomes Among Patients With Long-Term Conditions. *European Psychologist*, *24*(1), 68–81. doi:10.1027/1016-9040/a000350

Neurological Alliance. (2017). Falling short: How has neurology patient experience changed since 2014? Retrieved from http://neural.org.uk/store/assets/files/668/original/Neurological_Alliance_-_Falling_Short_-_How_has_neurology_patient_experience_changed_since_2014.pdf

Ng, J. H., Sobel, K., Roth, L., Byron, S., Lindley, M. C., & Stokley, S. (2017). Supporting human papillomavirus vaccination in adolescents: Perspectives from commercial and medicaid health plans. *Journal of Public Health Management and Practice: JPHMP*, *23*(3), 283–290. doi:10.1097/PHH.0000000000000440 PMID:27798527

NHS. (2014). Five year forward view. Retrieved from https://www.england.nhs.uk/wp-content/uploads/2014/10/5yfv-web.pdf

NHS. (2017). Next steps on the NHS five year forward view (2017). Retrieved from https://www.england.nhs.uk/wp-content/uploads/2017/03/NEXT-STEPS-ON-THE-NHS-FIVE-YEAR-FORWARD-VIEW.pdf

NHS. (2019). The long term plan. Retrieved from https://www.longtermplan.nhs.uk/wp-content/uploads/2019/01/nhs-long-term-plan.pdf

Niccolai, L. M., & Hansen, C. E. (2015). Practice-and community-based interventions to increase human papillomavirus vaccine coverage: A systematic review. *JAMA Pediatrics*, *169*(7), 686–692. doi:10.1001/jamapediatrics.2015.0310 PMID:26010507

Niculescu, A. B., Le-Niculescu, H., Levey, D. F., Roseberry, K., Soe, K. C., Rogers, J., ... White, F. A. (2019). Towards precision medicine for pain: Diagnostic biomarkers and repurposed drugs. *Molecular Psychiatry*. doi:10.103841380-018-0345-5

Nielsen, J. (2012). Usability 101: Introduction to Usability. Retrieved from https://www.nngroup.com/articles/usability-101-introduction-to-usability

Niendam, T. A., Tully, L. M., Iosif, A. M., Kumar, D., Nye, K. E., Denton, J. C., & Pierce, K. M. (2018). Enhancing early psychosis treatment using smartphone technology: A longitudinal feasibility and validity study. *Journal of Psychiatric Research*, *96*, 239–246. doi:10.1016/j.jpsychires.2017.10.017 PMID:29126059

Noar, S. M., & Willoughby, J. F. (2012). eHealth interventions for HIV prevention. *AIDS Care*, *24*(8), 945–952. doi:10.1080/09540121.2012.668167 PubMed

Noel, V. A., Acquilano, S. C., Carpenter-Song, E., & Drake, R. E. (2019). Use of mobile and computer devices to support recovery in people with serious mental illness: Survey study. *JMIR Mental Health*, *6*(2), 1–5. doi:10.2196/12255 PMID:30785401

Nordfeldt, S., Ängarne-Lindberg, T., Nordwall, M., Ekberg, J., & Berterö, C. (2013). As Facts and Chats Go Online, What Is Important for Adolescents with Type 1 Diabetes ?, *PLoS ONE 8*(6). doi:10.1371/journal.pone.0067659

Noteboom, C., & Al-Ramahi, M. (2018). What are the Gaps in Mobile Patient Portal? Mining Users Feedback Using Topic Modeling. *Proceedings of the 51st Hawaii International Conference on System Sciences*, 1-16. 10.24251/HICSS.2018.072

Nouri, R., Niakan, R., Kalhori, S., Ghazisaeedi, M., Marchand, G., & Yasini, M. (2018). Criteria for assessing the quality of mHealth apps: A systematic review. *Journal of the American Medical Informatics Association*, *25*(8), 1089–1098. doi:10.1093/jamia/ocy050 PMID:29788283

Nuij, C., van Ballegooijen, W., Ruwaard, J., De Beurs, D., Mokkenstorm, J., van Duijn, E., ... Kerkhof, A. (2018). Smartphone-based safety planning and self-monitoring for suicidal patients: Rationale and study protocol of the CASPAR (Continuous Assessment for Suicide Prevention and Research) study. *Internet Interventions*, *13*, 16–23. doi:10.1016/j.invent.2018.04.005 PMID:30206514

Nutbeam, D. (2000). Health literacy as a public health goal: A challenge for contemporary health education and communication strategies into the 21st century. *Health Promotion International*, *15*(3), 259–267. doi:10.1093/heapro/15.3.259

Nuti, S. V., Wayda, B., Ranasinghe, I., Wang, S., Dreyer, R. P., Chen, S. I., & Murugiah, K. (2014). The use of google trends in health care research: A systematic review. *PLoS One*, *9*(10). doi:10.1371/journal.pone.0109583 PMID:25337815

Nyongesa, H., Munguti, C., Omondi, C., & Mokua, W. (2014). Harnessing the power of social media in optimizing health outcomes. *The Pan African Medical Journal*, *18*, 1–5. doi:10.11604/pamj.2014.18.290.4634

O'Malley, A. S., & Reschovsky, J. D. (2011). Referral and consultation communication between primary care and specialist physicians: Finding common ground. *Archives of Internal Medicine*, *171*(1), 56–65. PubMed

O'Reilly, G. A., & Spruijt-Metz, D. (2013). Current mHealth technologies for physical activity assessment and promotion. *American Journal of Preventive Medicine*, *45*(4), 501–507. doi:10.1016/j.amepre.2013.05.012 PMID:24050427

OECD/EU. (2018). *Health at a Glance: Europe 2018: State of Health in the EU Cycle. Paris/EU*. Brussels, Belgium: OECD Publishing.

Office of Public and Intergovernmental Affairs. (2018). VA expands telehealth by allowing health care providers to treat patients across state lines. Retrieved from https://www.va.gov/opa/pressrel/pressrelease.cfm?id=4054

Oglevee, C., & Pianykh, O. (2015). Losing Images in Digital Radiology: More than You Think. *Journal of Digital Imaging*, *28*(3), 264–271. doi:10.1007/s10278-014-9748-2 PubMed

OneView. (2019). The eight principles of patient-centered care. Retrieved from https://www.oneviewhealthcare.com/the-eight-principles-of-patient-centered-care/

Ong, T., Kahn, M. G., Kwan, B. M., Yamashita, T., Brandt, E., Hosokawa, P., ... Schilling, L. M. (2017). Dynamic-ETL: A hybrid approach for health data extraction, transformation and loading. *BMC Medical Informatics and Decision Making*, *17*(1), 134. doi:10.118612911-017-0532-3 PMID:28903729

Ong, T., Pradhananga, R., Holve, E., & Kahn, M. G. (2017). A framework for classification of electronic health data extraction-transformation-loading challenges in data network participation. *EGEMs: The Journal for Electronic Health Data and Methods*, *5*(1), 10. doi:10.5334/egems.222 PMID:29930958

Ontario, H. Q. (2013). Electronic tools for health information exchange: An evidence-based analysis. *Ontario Health Technology Assessment Series*, *13*(11), 1–76. Available from http://www.hqontario.ca/en/documents/eds/2013/full-report-OCDM-etools.pdf PubMed

Oracle. (2019). What is big data? Retrieved from https://www.oracle.com/big-data/guide/what-is-big-data.html

Oreglia, E., & Srinivasan, J. (2016). ICT, Intermediaries, and the transformation of gendered power structures. *Management Information Systems Quarterly*, *40*(2), 501–510. doi:10.25300/MISQ/2016/40.2.13

Osma, J., Plaza, I., Crespo, E., Medrano, C., & Serrano, R. (2014). Proposal of use of smartphones to evaluate and diagnose depression and anxiety symptoms during pregnancy and after birth. Paper presented at *IEEE-EMBS International Conference on Biomedical and Health Informatics*, Valencia, Spain. 10.1109/BHI.2014.6864423

Paiva, A. L., Lipschitz, J. M., Fernandez, A. C., Redding, C. A., & Prochaska, J. O. (2014). Evaluation of the acceptability and feasibility of a computer-tailored intervention to increase human papillomavirus vaccination among young adult women. *Journal of American College Health*, *62*(1), 32–38. doi:10.1080/07448481.2013.843534 PMID:24313694

Palermo, T. M. (2009). Assessment of chronic pain in children: Current status and emerging topics. *Pain Research & Management*, *14*(1), 21–26. doi:10.1155/2009/236426 PMID:19262912

Panlaqui, O., Broadfield, E., Champion, R., Edington, J., & Kennedy, S. (2017). Outcomes of telemedicine intervention in a regional intensive care unit: A before and after study. *Australian Society of Anaesthetists*, *45*(5), 605–610. PMID:28911290

Pan, Z., Cheok, A. D., Yang, H., Zhu, J., & Shi, J. (2006). Virtual reality and mixed reality for virtual learning environments. *Computers & Graphics*, *30*(1), 20–28. doi:10.1016/j.cag.2005.10.004

Papa, D., Simas, T. A. M., Reynolds, M., & Melnitsky, H. (2009). Assessing the role of education in women's knowledge and acceptance of adjunct high-risk human Papillomavirus testing for cervical cancer screening. *Journal of Lower Genital Tract Disease*, *13*(2), 66–71. doi:10.1097/LGT.0b013e31818a53f0 PMID:19387125

Parent, W. A. (1983). A new definition of privacy for the law. *Law and Philosophy*, *2*(3), 305–338. doi:10.1007/BF00144949

Park, E., & Kwon, M. (2018). Health-related internet use by children and adolescents: Systematic review. *Journal of Medical Internet Research*, *20*(4), 1–30. doi:10.2196/jmir.7731 PMID:29615385

Parke, D. W. II, Rich, W. L. III, Sommer, A., & Lum, F. (2017). The American Academy of Ophthalmology's IRIS®Registry (Intelligent Research in Sight Clinical Data): A look back and a look to the future. *Ophthalmology*, *124*(11), 1572–1574. doi:10.1016/j.ophtha.2017.08.035 PMID:29055362

Parms, J. (2017). More info, more problems: Privacy and security issues in the age of big data. Retrieved from https://www.business.com/articles/privacy-and-security-issues-in-the-age-of-big-data/

Pass, J. H., Patel, A. H., Stuart, S., Barnacle, A. M., & Patel, P. A. (2018). Quality and readability of online patient information regarding sclerotherapy for venous malformations. *Pediatric Radiology*, *48*(5), 708–714. doi:10.100700247-018-4074-3 PMID:29396791

Patient Information Forum. (2017). Perfect patient information journey: Phase 1 summary report. Retrieved from https://www.pifonline.org.uk/wp-content/uploads/2017/05/PIF-PPI-Journey-4May17-final.pdf

Patient Information Forum. (2018). Perfect patient information journey: 7 steps for health services to improve information for people with long term condition. Retrieved from https://www.pifonline.org.uk/wp-content/uploads/2014/11/PIF-PPI-Journey-Final-25Jun18-1-website-version.pdf

Patient Information Forum. (2019). NHS plan promise empowered and informed patients via digital tools. Retrieved from https://www.pifonline.org.uk/blog/nhs-plan-promises-empowered-informed-patients-via-digital-tools/

Patten, K., Whitworth, B., Fjermestad, J., & Mahindra, E. (2005). Leading IT flexibility: anticipation, agility and adaptability. In *Americas Conference on Information Systems Proceedings*, Omaha, NE: Association for Information Systems.

Pattinson, S. D. (2017). Medical Law and Ethics (5th ed.). London, UK: Sweet and Maxwell.

Pavlou, P. A., & Gefen, D. (2005). Psychological contract violation in online marketplaces: Antecedents, consequences, and moderating role. *Information Systems Research*, *16*(4), 372–399. doi:10.1287/isre.1050.0065

Paz-Fuchs, A., Mandelkern, R., & Galnoor, I. (Eds.). (2018). The privatization of Israel: the withdrawal of state responsibility. Berlin, Germany: Springer. doi:10.1057/978-1-137-58261-4

Pegah, N. B., Mahdavi, M., Shahram, E. B., & Arasteh, S. (2018). Security analysis of a key based color image watermarking vs. a non-key based technique in telemedicine applications. *Multimedia Tools and Applications*, *77*(24), 31713–31735. doi:10.100711042-018-6218-8

Peleg, M., Michalowski, W., Wilk, S., Parimbelli, E., Bonaccio, S., O'Sullivan, D., ... Carrier, M. (2018). Ideating Mobile Health Behavioral Support for Compliance to Therapy for Patients with Chronic Disease: A Case Study of Atrial Fibrillation Management. *Journal of Medical Systems*, *42*(11), 234. doi:10.100710916-018-1077-4 PMID:30317403

Peleg, M., Shahar, Y., Quaglini, S., Fux, A., García-Sáez, G., Goldstein, A., ... Parimbelli, E. (2017). MobiGuide: A personalized and patient-centric decision-support system and its evaluation in the atrial fibrillation and gestational diabetes domains. *User Modeling and User-Adapted Interaction*, *27*(2), 159–213. doi:10.100711257-017-9190-5

Pennic, F. (2015). 66% of Americans would use mobile health apps to manage their health. *HIT Consultant*. Retrieved from https://hitconsultant.net/2015/02/24/66-of-americans-would-use-mobile-health-apps/#.XGxlKeRKiUk

Perera, G., Holbrook, A., Thabane, L., Foster, G., & Willison, D. J. (2011). Views on health information sharing and privacy from primary care practices using electronic medical records. *International Journal of Medical Informatics*, *80*(2), 94–101. doi:10.1016/j.ijmedinf.2010.11.005 PMID:21167771

Perkins, R. B., & Clark, J. A. (2012). What affects human papillomavirus vaccination rates? A qualitative analysis of providers' perceptions. *Women's Health Issues*, *22*(4), e379–e386. doi:10.1016/j.whi.2012.04.001 PMID:22609253

Permwonguswa, S., Khuntia, J., Yim, D., & Gregg, D. (2017). Empowerment and knowledge sharing in health infomediary: empirical evidence from reconstructive surgery patients. In *Twenty-third Americas Conference on Information Systems*, Boston, MA.

Petersen, K., Feldt, R., Mujtaba, S., & Mattsson, M. (2008). Systematic mapping studies in software engineering. *EASE*, *8*, 68–77.

Pham, J. A. O. (2018). Nation's Progress on Children's Health Coverage Reverses Course. Retrieved from https://ccf.georgetown.edu/wp-content/uploads/2018/11/UninsuredKids2018_Final_asof1128743pm.pdf

Pham, T., Tran, T., Phung, D., & Venkatesh, S. (2017). Predicting healthcare trajectories from medical records: A deep learning approach. *Journal of Biomedical Informatics*, *69*, 218–229. doi:10.1016/j.jbi.2017.04.001 PMID:28410981

PhiladelphiaC. H. O. (2018). About Us. Retrieved from https://www.chop.edu/about-us/about

Phills, J. A., Deiglmeier, K., & Miller, D. T. (2008, Fall). Rediscovering social innovation. Stanford Social Innovation Review; Stanford, 6(4), 34–43.

Pichler, H., & Hesson, A. (2016). Discourse-pragmatic variation across situations, varieties, ages: I don't know in sociolinguistic and medical interviews. *Language & Communication*, *49*, 1–18. doi:10.1016/j.langcom.2016.04.002

Picture archiving and communication system. (2019, Jan. 22). Retrieved from https://en.wikipedia.org/w/index.php?title=Picture_archiving_and_communication_system&action=info

Pilnick, A., & Zayts, O. (2014). "It's just a likelihood": Uncertainty as topic and resource in conveying "positive" results in an antenatal screening clinic. *Symbolic Interaction*, *37*(2), 187–208. doi:10.1002ymb.99

Pinnock, H., Barwick, M., Carpenter, C. R., Eldridge, S., Grandes, G., Griffiths, C. J., ... Taylor, S. J. C. (2017). Standards for Reporting Implementation Studies (StaRI): Explanation and elaboration document. *BMJ Open*, *7*(4). doi:10.1136/bmjopen-2016-013318 PMID:28373250

Politi, D. (2018). ICE Officers Arrest Man Who Was Driving Pregnant Wife to Hospital for C-Section. Retrieved from https://slate.com/news-and-politics/2018/08/joel-arrona-arrested-ice-detains-man-who-was-driving-wife-to-hospital-for-c-section.html

Portenoy, R. K., & Lesage, P. (1999). Management of cancer pain. *Lancet*, *353*(9165), 1695–1700. doi:10.1016/S0140-6736(99)01310-0 PMID:10335806

Powell, J., Inglis, N., Ronnie, J., & Large, S. (2011). The characteristics and motivations of online health information seekers: Cross-sectional survey and qualitative interview study. *Journal of Medical Internet Research*, *13*(1), e20. doi:10.2196/jmir.1600 PMID:21345783

Powles, J., & Hodson, H. (2017). Google DeepMind and healthcare in an age of algorithms. *Health and Technology*, *7*(4), 351–367. doi:10.100712553-017-0179-1

Practical-patient-care.com. (2019). TeleConsult Europe - Maximise radiology efficiency with expertise on demand - Practical Patient Care. Retrieved from http://www.practical-patient-care.com/contractors/imaging-diagnostics-and-analysis/teleconsult-europe/

Prasanna, P. M., Seagull, F. J., & Nagy, P. (2011). Online social networking: A primer for radiology. *Journal of Digital Imaging*, *24*(5), 908–912. doi:10.1007/s10278-011-9371-4 PubMed

Prgomet, M., Georgiou, A., & Westbrook, J. I. (2009). The impact of mobile handheld technology on hospital physicians' work practices and patient care: A systematic review. *Journal of the American Medical Informatics Association*, *16*(6), 792–801. doi:10.1197/jamia.M3215 PMID:19717793

Prior, L. (2003). Belief, knowledge and expertise: The emergence of the lay expert in medical sociology. *Sociology of Health & Illness*, *25*(3), 41–57. doi:10.1111/1467-9566.00339 PMID:14498929

Prior, L., Evans, M. R., & Prout, H. (2011). Talking about colds and flu: The lay diagnosis of two common illnesses among older British people. *Social Science & Medicine*, *73*(6), 922–928. doi:10.1016/j.socscimed.2010.09.054 PMID:21186076

Prociow, P. A., & Crowe, J. A. (2010). Development of mobile psychiatry for bipolar disorder patients. In *2010 Annual International Conference of the IEEE Engineering in Medicine and Biology* (pp. 5484-5487). IEEE. 10.1109/IEMBS.2010.5626759

Project Management Institute, Inc. (2017). *Guide to the Project Management Body of Knowledge* (6th ed.). Newton Square, PA: Project Management Institute. Retrieved from https://www.pmi.org/pmbok-guide-standards/foundational/pmbok

Public Health Institute. (2018). State telehealth laws and reimbursement program policies. Retrieved from http://www.phi.org/resources/?resource=state-telehealth-laws-and-medicaid-program-policies

Pung, A., Fletcher, S. L., & Gunn, J. M. (2018). Mobile app use by primary care patients to manage their depressive symptoms: Qualitative study. *Journal of Medical Internet Research*, *20*(9). doi:10.2196/10035 PMID:30262449

Pyper, C., Amery, J., Watson, M., & Crook, C. (2004). Patients' experiences when accessing their on-line electronic patient records in primary care. *The British Journal of General Practice*, *54*(498), 38–43. PMID:14965405

Quinn, C. C., Shardell, M. D., Terrin, M. L., Barr, E. A., Ballew, S. H., & Gruber-Baldini, A. L. (2011). Cluster-randomized trial of a mobile phone personalized behavioral intervention for blood glucose control. *Diabetes Care*, *34*(9), 1934–1942. doi:10.2337/dc11-0366 PMID:21788632

Raghupathi, W., & Raghupathi, V. (2014). Big data analytics in healthcare: Promise and potential. *Health Information Science and Systems*, *2*(1), 3. doi:10.1186/2047-2501-2-3 PMID:25825667

Rai, A., Chen, L., Pye, J., & Baird, A. (2013). Understanding determinants of consumer mobile health usage intentions, assimilation, and channel preferences. *Journal of Medical Internet Research*, *15*(8), e149. doi:10.2196/jmir.2635 PMID:23912839

Ranney, M. L., Thorsen, M., Patena, J. V., Cunningham, R. M., Boyer, E. W., Walton, M. A., . . . Morrow, K. (2015). "You Need to Get Them Where They Feel it": Conflicting Perspectives on How to Maximize the Structure of Text-Message Psychological Interventions for Adolescents. Paper presented at *2015 48th Hawaii International Conference on System Sciences*, Kauai, Hawaii.

Rapoza, K. (2017). China's aging population becoming more of a problem. Forbes. Retrieved from https://www.forbes.com/sites/kenrapoza/2017/02/21/chinas-aging-population-becoming-more-of-a-problem/#25c770ac140f

Rasool, S., ZeeshanZafar, M., Ali, Z., & Erum, A. (2018). Schizophrenia: An overview. *Clinical Practice (Therapy)*, *15*(5), 847–851.

Rauv, S. (2017, June 14). The impact of technology in healthcare. Retrieved from https://www.elcomcms.com/resources/blog/the-impact-of-technology-in-healthcare-trends-benefits-examples

Razzak, M., Naz, S., & Zaib, A. (2017). *Deep learning for medical image processing: overview, challenges and future.* Retrieved from https://arxiv.org/ftp/arxiv/papers/1704/1704.06825.pdf

Register, M. S. (2019). Let's make sense of MS. Retrieved from https://ukmsregister.org/

Reid, S. C., Kauer, S. D., Hearps, S. J., Crooke, A. H., Khor, A. S., Sanci, L. A., & Patton, G. C. (2011). A mobile phone application for the assessment and management of youth mental health problems in primary care: A randomised controlled trial. *BMC Family Practice*, *12*(1), 131–145. doi:10.1186/1471-2296-12-131 PMID:22123031

Reiter, P. L., Brewer, N. T., Gottlieb, S. L., McRee, A.-L., & Smith, J. S. (2009). Parents' health beliefs and HPV vaccination of their adolescent daughters. *Social Science & Medicine*, *69*(3), 475–480. doi:10.1016/j.socscimed.2009.05.024 PMID:19540642

Reiter, P. L., Stubbs, B., Panozzo, C. A., Whitesell, D., & Brewer, N. T. (2011). HPV and HPV vaccine education intervention: Effects on parents, healthcare staff, and school staff. *Cancer Epidemiology and Prevention Biomarkers*, *20*(11), 2354–2361. doi:10.1158/1055-9965.EPI-11-0562 PMID:21949110

Research2Guidance. (2018). mHealth Economics 2017/2018 – Connectivity in Digital Health. *Research2Guidance*, 1-17.

Reychav, I., McHaney, R., Zhu, L., & Moshonov, R. (2018). Media Impact on Patient Empowerment in Complicated Medical Situations: A TREO Talk Paper. In *Twenty-fourth Americas Conference on Information System*. New Orleans, LA: AIS. Retrieved from https://aisel.aisnet.org/amcis2018/TREOsPDS/Presentations/8/

Reychav, I., Beeri, R., Balapour, A., Raban, D. R., Sabherwal, R., & Azuri, J. (2019). How reliable are self-assessments using mobile technology in healthcare? The effects of technology identity and self-efficacy. *Computers in Human Behavior, 91*, 52–61. doi:10.1016/j.chb.2018.09.024

Reychav, I., Najami, I., Raban, D., McHaney, R., & Azuri, J. (2018). The impact of media type on shared decision processes in third-age populations. *International Journal of Medical Informatics, 112*, 45–58. doi:10.1016/j.ijmedinf.2018.01.004 PMID:29500021

Reychav, I., Parush, A., McHaney, R., Hazan, M., & Moshonov, R. (2018). The use of mobile technology in waiting rooms to leverage women's empowerment: A conceptual context. *Health Informatics Journal, 24*(3), 277–292. doi:10.1177/1460458216671561 PMID:27738260

Reynoldson, C., Stones, C., Bennett, M. I., Jones, R., Allsop, M., Gardner, P., . . . Knapp, P. (2014). Assessing the quality and usability of smartphone apps for pain self-management. *Pain Medicine, 15*(6), 898-909. doi:10.1111/pme.12327

Richardson, S., Kettinger, W., Banks, M., & Quintana, Y. (2014a). IT and Agility in the social enterprise: A case study of St Jude children's Research Hospital's "Cure4Kids" it-platform for international outreach. *Journal of the Association for Information Systems, 15*(1), 1–32. doi:10.17705/1jais.00351

Rider, E. A., Kurtz, S., Slade, D., Longmaid, H. E. III, Ho, M.-J., Pun, J. K., ... Branch, W. T. Jr. (2014). The International charter for human values in healthcare: An interprofessional global collaboration to enhance values and communication in healthcare. *Patient Education and Counseling, 96*(3), 273–280. doi:10.1016/j.pec.2014.06.017 PMID:25103181

Riegelsberger, J., Sasse, M. A., & McCarthy, J. D. (2005). The mechanics of trust: A framework for research and design. *International Journal of Human-Computer Studies, 62*(3), 381–422. doi:10.1016/j.ijhcs.2005.01.001

Riel, N. V., Auwerx, K., Debbaut, P., Hees, S. V., & Schoenmakers, B. (2017). The effect of Dr Google on doctor–patient encounters in primary care: A quantitative, observational, cross-sectional study. *BJGP Open*, 1(2), 1-10. Retrieved from https://bjgpopen.org/content/1/2/bjgpopen17X100833.abstract.

Rimer, B., Harper, H., & Witte, O. (2014). *Accelerating HPV vaccine uptake: urgency for action to prevent cancer. A report to the President of the United States from the President's Cancer Panel*. Bethesda, MD: National Cancer Institute.

Riva, S., Camerini, A., Allam, A., & Schulz, P. J. (2014). Interactive Sections of an Internet-Based Intervention Increase Empowerment of Chronic Back Pain Patients: Randomized Controlled Trial. *Journal of Medical Internet Research, 16*(8), e180. doi:10.2196/jmir.3474 PMID:25119374

Rizia, R., Johnson, N., Patwary, A. K., Ahsan, G. M. T., Ahamed, S. I., Franco, Z., & Flower, M. (2014). Mobile peer-mentoring: An approach to make veterans seek mental health-care support a normality. Paper presented at *10th IEEE International Conference on Collaborative Computing: Networking, Applications and Worksharing*, Miami, Florida.

Roberts, K. J. (1999). Patient Empowerment in the United States: A Critical Commentary. *Health Expectations, 2*(2), 82–92. doi:10.1046/j.1369-6513.1999.00048.x PMID:11281882

Rogers, S., Chamberlin, J., Ellison, M. L., & Crean, T. (1997). A consumer-constructed scale to measure empowerment among users of mental health services. *Psychiatric Services (Washington, D.C.), 48*(8), 1042–1047. doi:10.1176/ps.48.8.1042 PMID:9255837

Rojnic, K. M., Andlauer, O., Burmeister, K., Dvoracek, B., Lencer, R., Koelkebeck, K., & Aukst, M. B. (2018). Effective assessment of psychotropic medication side effects using PsyLOG mobile application. *Schizophrenia Research, 192*, 211–212. doi:10.1016/j.schres.2017.04.038 PMID:28457773

Ronis, S. D., McConnochie, K. M., Wang, H., & Wood, N. E. (2017). Urban Telemedicine Enables Equity in Access to Acute Illness Care. *Telemedicine Journal and e-Health, 23*(2), 105–112. doi:10.1089/tmj.2016.0098 PMID:27383822

Rosenfeld, D., & Weinberg, D. (2012). Domestic practice, situated contingency and adherence to medical directives: A call for research. *Social Theory & Health, 10*(1), 42–60. doi:10.1057th.2011.9

Rosenthal, S. L., Weiss, T. W., Zimet, G. D., Ma, L., Good, M. B., & Vichnin, M. D. (2011). Predictors of HPV vaccine uptake among women aged 19--26: Importance of a physician's recommendation. *Vaccine, 29*(5), 890–895. doi:10.1016/j.vaccine.2009.12.063 PMID:20056186

Rosser, B. A., & Eccleston, C. (2011). Smartphone applications for pain management. *Journal of Telemedicine and Telecare, 17*(6), 308–312. doi:10.1258/jtt.2011.101102 PMID:21844177

Roth, C. J., Lannum, L. M., Dennison, D. K., & Towbin, A. J. (2016). The current state and path forward for enterprise image viewing: HIMSS-SIIM collaborative white paper. *Journal of Digital Imaging, 29*(5), 567–573. doi:10.1007/s10278-016-9887-8 PubMed

Roughead, T., Sewell, D., Ryerson, C. J., Fisher, J. H., & Flexman, A. M. (2016). Internet-based resources frequently provide inaccurate and out-of-date recommendations on preoperative fasting: A systematic review. *Anesthesia and Analgesia, 123*(6), 1463–1468. doi:10.1213/ANE.0000000000001590 PMID:27644057

Rouppret, M., Morgan, T. M., Bostrom, P. J., Cooperberg, M. R., Kutikov, A., Linton, K. D., ... Catto, J. W. F. F. (2014). European Association of Urology (@Uroweb) recommendations on the appropriate use of social media. *European Urology, 66*(4), 628–632. doi:10.1016/j.eururo.2014.06.046

Rudell, E., Peterson, P., Pulim, S., Griffin, A. L., & Bowen, J. D. (2016). Connecting healthcare providers with patients through mobile technology: Formula for shared decision making and improved patient outcomes. *Iproceedings, 2*(1), e3. doi:10.2196/iproc.6224

Rupp, S. (2017). A quick look at the history of telemedicine. Retrieved from https://www.nuemd.com/news/2017/01/04/quick-look-history-telemedicine

Russell, E., & Patrick, K. (2018). Mental health needs our attention. *CMAJ: Canadian Medical Association Journal, 190*(2), E34. doi:10.1503/cmaj.171469 PMID:29335259

Ryan, R. M., Rigby, C. S., & Przybylski, A. (2006). The Motivational Pull of Video Games: A Self-Determination Theory Approach. *Motivation and Emotion, 30*(4), 344–360. doi:10.100711031-006-9051-8

Sade, R. M. (2010). Breaches of health information: Are electronic records different from paper records? *The Journal of Clinical Ethics, 21*(1), 39–41.

Saigi-Rubió, F., Jiménez-Zarco, A., & Torrent-Sellens, J. (2016). Determinants of the intention to use telemedicine: Evidence from primary physicians. *International Journal of Technology Assessment in Health Care, 32*(2), 29–36. doi:10.1017/S0266462316000015 PMID:27472158

Salas, E., Sims, D. E., & Burke, C. S. (2005). Is there a "big five" in teamwork? *Small Group Research, 36*(5), 555–599. doi:10.1177/1046496405277134

Salem, J., Paffenholz, P., Bolenz, C., von Brandenstein, M., Cebulla, A., Haferkamp, A., … Heidenreich, A. (2018). Websites on Bladder Cancer: An Appropriate Source of Patient Information? *Journal of Cancer Education: The Official Journal of the American Association for Cancer Education*. doi:10.100713187-017-1316-2

Samorani, M., & LaGanga, L. (2011). A stochastic programming approach to improve overbooking in clinic appointment scheduling. In *POMS annual meeting proceedings*.

Samorani, M., & LaGanga, L. (2015). Outpatient appointment scheduling given individual day-dependent no-show predictions. *European Journal of Operational Research*, *240*(1), 245–257. doi:10.1016/j.ejor.2014.06.034

Samuel, L. (2017). At a growing number of schools, sick kids can take a virtual trip to the doctor. [July 19]. *Stat*.

Sánchez, A., Plaza, I., Medrano, C. T., & Garcia-Campayo, J. (2015). Proposal of a mobile application for mindfulness practice in elder people. Paper presented at the *IET International Conference on Technologies for Active and Assisted Living*, London, UK. 10.1049/ic.2015.0143

Sandlund, M., Lindgren, H., Pohl, P., Melander-Wikman, A., Bergvall Kåreborn, B., & Lundin Olsson, L. (2016). Towards a mobile exercise application to prevent falls: A participatory design process. *International Journal of Child Health and Human Development*, *9*(3), 389–398.

Sanyal, S. (2018). 5 surprising ways in which telemedicine is revolutionizing healthcare. *Forbes*. Retrieved from https://www.forbes.com/sites/shourjyasanyal/2018/10/31/5-surprising-ways-in-which-telemedicine-is-revolutionizing-healthcare/#68a924e156be

SAS. (2019a). Data warehouse: What it is and why it matters. Retrieved from https://www.sas.com/en_us/insights/data-management/data-warehouse.html

SAS. (2019b). ETL: What it is and why it matters. Retrieved from https://www.sas.com/en_us/insights/data-management/what-is-etl.html

Sawyer, A. C., Kaim, A. L., Reece, C. E., McDonald, D., Le, H. N., Clark, J., ... Sawyer, M. G. (2019). Evaluating the Effectiveness of an App-Based Nurse-Moderated Program for New Mothers with Depression and Parenting Problems (eMums Plus): Protocol for a Pragmatic Randomized Controlled Trial. *JMIR Research Protocols*, *8*(1). doi:10.2196/11549 PMID:30664487

Sayakhot, P., & Carolan-Olah, M. (2016). Internet use by pregnant women seeking pregnancy-related information: A systematic review. *BMC Pregnancy and Childbirth*, *16*(1), 65. doi:10.118612884-016-0856-5 PMID:27021727

Sbaffi, L., & Rowley, J. (2017). Trust and credibility in web-based health information: A review and agenda for future research. *Journal of Medical Internet Research*, *19*(6), e218. doi:10.2196/jmir.7579 PMID:28630033

Schag, C. C., Heinrich, R. L., & Ganz, P. A. (1984). Karnofsky performance status revisited: Reliability, validity, and guidelines. *Journal of Clinical Oncology*, *2*(3), 187–193. doi:10.1200/JCO.1984.2.3.187 PMID:6699671

Scherer, L. D., Ubel, P. A., McClure, J., Greene, S. M., Alford, S. H., Holtzman, L., ... Fagerlin, A. (2013). Belief in numbers: When and why women disbelieve tailored breast cancer risk statistics. *Patient Education and Counseling*, *92*(2), 253–259. doi:10.1016/j.pec.2013.03.016 PMID:23623330

Schmidt, C., Kude, T., Tripp, J., Heinzl, A., & Spohrer, K. (2013). *Team adaptability in agile information systems development*. In *Proceedings of the 34th International Conference on Information Systems*, Milan, Italy: Association of Information Systems.

Schoen, C., Osborn, R., Huynh, P. T., Doty, M., Zapert, K., Peugh, J., & Davis, K. (2005). Taking The Pulse Of Health Care Systems: Experiences Of Patients With Health Problems In Six Countries: Patients' voices can provide policy leaders with a window onto what is happening at the front lines of care. *Health Affairs*, *24*(Suppl1), W5-509–W5-525. doi:10.1377/hlthaff.W5.509

Schroeder, S. A. (2007). We can do better - Improving the health of the American people. *The New England Journal of Medicine*, *357*(12), 1221–1228. doi:10.1056/NEJMsa073350 PMID:17881753

Schwebel, F. J., & Larimer, M. E. (2018). Using text message reminders in health care services: A narrative literature review. *Internet Interventions*, *13*, 82–104. doi:10.1016/j.invent.2018.06.002 PMID:30206523

Sedrati, H., Nejjari, C., Chaqsare, S., & Ghazal, H. (2016). Mental and physical mobile health apps. *Procedia Computer Science*, *100*, 900–906. doi:10.1016/j.procs.2016.09.241

Seldeslachts, U. (2019). PACS Market and Spending Trends Overview. Retrieved from https://ipacso.eu/11-uncategorized/157-pacs-market-and-spending-trends-overview.html

Sennaar, K. (2019a). Machine learning for medical diagnostics – 4 current applications. *Emerj - Artificial Intelligence Research and Insight*. Retrieved from https://emerj.com/ai-sector-overviews/machine-learning-medical-diagnostics-4-current-applications/

Sennaar, K. (2019b). Artificial intelligence in telemedicine and telehealth – 4 current applications. *Emerj - Artificial Intelligence Research and Insight*. Retrieved from https://emerj.com/ai-sector-overviews/artificial-intelligence-in-telemedicine-and-telehealth/

Seppala, J., De Vita, I., Jamsa, T., Miettunen, J., Isohanni, M., Rubinstein, K., … Bulgheroni, M. (2019). Mobile Phone and Wearable Sensor-Based mHealth Approaches for Psychiatric Disorders and Symptoms: Systematic Review. *JMIR Mental Health, 6*(2), 1-14.

Shane, L., III. (2018). VA: Suicide rate for younger veterans increased by more than 10 percent. *Military Times*. Retrieved from https://www.militarytimes.com/news/pentagon-congress/2018/09/26/suicide-rate-spikes-among-younger-veterans/

Shaw, E. K., Howard, J., Clark, E. C., Etz, R. S., Arya, R., & Tallia, A. F. (2013). Decision-making processes of patients who use the emergency department for primary care needs. *Journal of Health Care for the Poor and Underserved*, *24*(3), 1288–1305. doi:10.1353/hpu.2013.0140 PMID:23974399

Shcherbina, A., Mattsson, M. C., Waggott, D., Salisbury, H., Christle, J. W., Hastie, T., ... Ashley, E. A. (2017). Accuracy in wrist-worn, sensor-based measurements of heart rate and energy expenditure in a diverse cohort. *Journal of Personalized Medicine*, *7*(2), 1–12. doi:10.3390/jpm7020003 PMID:28538708

Shead, S. (2017). Google DeepMind is funding NHS research at Moorfields Eye Hospital. *Business Insider*. Retrieved from https://www.businessinsider.com/deepmind-is-funding-nhs-research-2017-7?r=UK

Shickel, B., Tighe, P. J., Bihorac, A., & Rashidi, P. (2017). Deep EHR: A survey of recent advances in deep learning techniques for electronic health record (EHR) analysis. *IEEE Journal of Biomedical and Health Informatics*, *22*(5), 1589–1604. doi:10.1109/JBHI.2017.2767063 PMID:29989977

Silberg, W. M., Lundberg, G. D., & Musacchio, R. A. (1997, April). Assessing, controlling, and assuring the quality of medical information on the Internet: Caveant lector et viewor--Let the reader and viewer beware. *JAMA*. USA.

Sim, D. A., Keane, P. A., Tufail, A., Egan, C. A., Aiello, L. P., & Silva, P. (2015). Automated retinal image analysis for diabetic retinopathy in telemedicine. *Current Diabetes Reports*, *15*(14), 577–590. doi:10.100711892-015-0577-6 PMID:25697773

Similä, H., Immonen, M., Toska-Tervola, J., Enwald, H., Keränen, N., Kangas, M., & Korpelainen, R. (2018). Feasibility of mobile mental wellness training for older adults. *Geriatric Nursing, 39*(5), 499–505. doi:10.1016/j.gerinurse.2018.02.001 PMID:29530292

Simmons, L. A., Wolever, R. Q., Bechard, E. M., & Snyderman, R. (2014). Patient engagement as a risk factor in personalized health care: A systematic review of the literature on chronic disease. *Genome Medicine, 6*(2), 16. doi:10.1186/gm533 PMID:24571651

Singh, R., Mathiassen, L., Stachura, M. E., & Astapova, E. V. (2011). Capabilities in Home Health : IT-Enabled Transformation of Post-Acute Care. *Journal of the Association for Information Dynamic, 12*(2), 163–188. doi:10.17705/1jais.00257

Sixsmith, A. (2013). Chapter 2 Technology and the Challenge of Aging. In A. Sixsmith, & G. Gutman (Eds.), Technologies for Active Aging, 7 International Perspectives on Aging, Springer Science+Business Media, New York, NY. p. 10-11.

Skolbekken, J. A. (2019). Online risk numbers–helpful, meaningless or simply wrong? Reflections on online risk calculators. *Health.* PMID:30678517

Skymind. (2019). Artificial intelligence (AI) vs. machine learning vs. deep learning. Retrieved from https://skymind.ai/wiki/ai-vs-machine-learning-vs-deep-learning

Small, N., Bower, P., Chew-Graham, C. A., Whalley, D., & Protheroe, J. (2013). Patient empowerment in long-term conditions: Development and preliminary testing of a new measure. *BMC Health Services Research, 13*(1), 263. doi:10.1186/1472-6963-13-263 PMID:23835131

Social networking service. (2019, Feb. 18). Retrieved from https://en.wikipedia.org/w/index.php?title=Social_networking_service&oldid=884010054

Solari, A. (2014). Effective communication at the point of multiple sclerosis diagnosis. *Multiple Sclerosis Journal, 20*(4), 397–402. doi:10.1177/1352458514523061 PMID:24503056

Sondaal, S. F. V., Browne, J. L., Amoakoh-Coleman, M., Borgstein, A., Miltenburg, A. S., Verwijs, M., & Klipstein-Grobusch, K. (2016). Assessing the Effect of mhealth interventions in improving maternal and neonatal care in low- and middle-income countries: A systematic review. *PLoS One, 11*(5). doi:10.1371/journal.pone.0154664 PMID:27144393

Spreitzer, G. M. (1995). Psychological Empowerment in the Workplace: Dimensions, Measurement, and Validation. *Academy of Management Journal, 38*(5), 1442–1465.

Srivastava, S., Soman, S., & Rai, A., & Srivastava, P. K. (2017). Deep learning for health informatics: recent trends and future directions. *Proceedings of 2017 International Conference on Advances in Computing, Communications and Informatics (ICACCI)*, Udupi, India. 10.1109/ICACCI.2017.8126082

Srivastava, S. C., Shainesh, G., Barrett, M., Davidson, E., Prabhu, J., & Vargo, S. L. (2015). Bridging the Service Divide Through Digitally Enabled Service Innovations: Evidence from Indian Healthcare Service Providers. *Management Information Systems Quarterly, 39*(1), 245–267. doi:10.25300/MISQ/2015/39.1.11

Stallard, P., Porter, J., & Grist, R. (2018). A smartphone app (BlueIce) for young people who self-harm: Open phase 1 pre-post trial. *JMIR mHealth and uHealth, 6*(1), e32. doi:10.2196/mhealth.8917 PMID:29382632

Stamate, D., Katrinecz, A., Alghamdi, W., Stahl, D., Delespaul, P., van Os, J., & Guloksuz, S. (2017). Predicting Psychosis Using the Experience Sampling Method with Mobile Apps. Paper presented at the *IEEE International Conference on Machine Learning and Applications*, Cancun, Mexico. 10.1109/ICMLA.2017.00-84

Starcevic, V. (2017). Cyberchondria: Challenges of Problematic Online Searches for Health-Related Information. *Psychotherapy and Psychosomatics, 86*(3), 129–133. doi:10.1159/000465525 PMID:28490037

Starcevic, V., & Berle, D. (2013). Cyberchondria: Towards a better understanding of excessive health-related Internet use. *Expert Review of Neurotherapeutics*, *13*(2), 205–213. doi:10.1586/ern.12.162 PMID:23368807

Statista. (2019). Number of social media users worldwide. Retrieved from https://www.statista.com/statistics/278414/number-of-worldwide-social-network-users/

Stevens, G., Mascarenhas, M., & Mathers, C. (2009). Global health risks: Progress and challenges. *Bulletin of the World Health Organization*, *87*(9), 646–646. doi:10.2471/BLT.09.070565 PMID:19784438

Stinson, J. N., Jibb, L. A., Nguyen, C., Nathan, P. C., Maloney, A. M., Dupuis, L. L., ... Orr, M. (2013). Development and testing of a multidimensional iPhone pain assessment application for adolescents with cancer. *Journal of Medical Internet Research*, *15*(3), e51. doi:10.2196/jmir.2350 PMID:23475457

Stoll, R. D., Pina, A. A., Gary, K., & Amresh, A. (2017). Usability of a smartphone application to support the prevention and early intervention of anxiety in youth. *Cognitive and Behavioral Practice*, *24*(4), 393–404. doi:10.1016/j.cbpra.2016.11.002 PMID:29056845

Stone, A. A., & Broderick, J. E. (2007). Real-time data collection for pain: Appraisal and current status. *Pain Medicine*, *8*(Suppl 3), S85–S93. doi:10.1111/j.1526-4637.2007.00372.x PMID:17877531

Storni, C. (2014). Diabetes self-care in-the-wild: Design challenges for personal health record systems and self-monitoring technologies. *Information Technology & People*, *27*(4), 397–420. doi:10.1108/ITP-02-2013-0032

Straus, S., & Haynes, R. B. (2009). Managing evidence-based knowledge: The need for reliable, relevant and readable resources. *Canadian Medical Association Journal*, *180*(9), 942–945. doi:10.1503/cmaj.081697 PMID:19398741

Street, R. L., O'Malley, K. J., Cooper, L. A., & Haidet, P. (2008). Understanding concordance in patient-physician relationships: Personal and ethnic dimensions of shared identity. *Annals of Family Medicine*, *6*(3), 198–205. doi:10.1370/afm.821 PMID:18474881

Studer, Q., Robinson, B. C., & Cook, K. (2010). *The HCAHPS handbook: Hardwire your hospital for pay-for-performance success*. Dover, AR: Fire Starter Pub.

Suarez-Almazor, M. E., Kendall, C. J., & Dorgan, M. (2001). Surfing the Net--information on the World Wide Web for persons with arthritis: Patient empowerment or patient deceit? *The Journal of Rheumatology*, *28*(1), 185–191. PMID:11196523

Sullivan, T. J., Karaki, H. S., Kimoto, R. C., Koch, R. H., Harrison-Noonan, T. J., & Montgomery, R. K. (2018). Cuff designs and methods. *United States Patent application publication.* Retrieved from http://pdfaiw.uspto.gov/.aiw?docid=20180153418

Sun, Y., Jiang, F., Gu, J. J., Wang, Y. K., Hua, H., Li, J., ... Hu, W. (2017). Development and testing of an Intelligent Pain Management System (IPMS) on mobile phones through a randomized trial among Chinese cancer patients: A new approach in cancer pain management. *JMIR mHealth and uHealth*, *5*(7), e108. doi:10.2196/mhealth.7178 PMID:28743681

Susman, G. I., & Dean, J. W., Jr. (1992). Development of a model for predicting design for manufacturability effectiveness. Integrating Design and Manufacturing for Competitive Advantage, 207–227.

Su, Y., Yuan, C., Zhou, Z., Heitner, J., & Campbell, B. (2016). Impact of an SMS advice programme on maternal and newborn health in rural China: Study protocol for a quasi-randomised controlled trial. *BMJ Open*, *6*(8). doi:10.1136/bmjopen-2015-011016 PMID:27515750

Sylvester, G. (2016). *Use of mobile phones by the rural poor: gender perspectives from selected Asian countries*. Ottawa, Canada: IDRC.

Synnot, A. J., Hill, S. J., Garner, K. A., Summers, M. P., Filippini, G., Osborne, R. H., ... Mosconi, P. (2016). Online health information seeking: How people with multiple sclerosis find, assess and integrate treatment information to manage their health. *Health Expectations, 19*(3), 727–737. doi:10.1111/hex.12253 PMID:25165024

Tallon, P. P., & Pinsonneault, A. (2011). Competing perspectives on the link between strategic information technology alignment and organizational agility: Insights from a mediation model. *Management Information Systems Quarterly, 35*(2), 463.

Tangri, V., & Chande, N. (2011). Quality of Internet-based information on gastrointestinal diseases. *Canadian Journal of Gastroenterology, 25*(2), 93–96. doi:10.1155/2011/345076 PMID:21321681

Tan, S. S. L., & Goonawardene, N. (2017). Internet health information seeking and the patient-physician relationship: A systematic review. *Journal of Medical Internet Research, 19*(1), e9. doi:10.2196/jmir.5729 PMID:28104579

Tatikonda, M. V., & Montoya-Weiss, M. M. (2001). Integrating operations and marketing perspectives of product innovation: The influence of organizational process factors and capabilities on development performance. *Management Science, 47*(1), 151–172. doi:10.1287/mnsc.47.1.151.10669

Taylor, S., & Todd, P. (1995). Understanding Information Technology Usage: A Test of Competing Models. *Information Systems Research, 6*(2), 144–176. doi:10.1287/isre.6.2.144

Teng, M. H., Hou, Y. M., Chang, S. H., & Cheng, H. J. (2019). Home-delivered attention bias modification training via smartphone to improve attention control in sub-clinical generalized anxiety disorder: A randomized, controlled multi-session experiment. *Journal of Affective Disorders, 246*, 444–451. doi:10.1016/j.jad.2018.12.118 PMID:30599367

The Centers for Disease Control and Prevention. (2011). *National diabetes fact sheet, 2011*. Retrieved from https://www.cdc.gov/diabetes/pubs/pdf/ndfs_2011.pdf

The Centers for Disease Control and Prevention. (2017). *Diabetes Report Card 2017*. U.S. Department of Health and Human Services. Retrieved from https://www.cdc.gov/diabetes/pdfs/library/diabetesreportcard2017-508.pdf

The Military Time. (2019). Commandos to counselors: A response to the special operations forces mental health crisis. Retrieved from https://www.militarytimes.com/opinion/commentary/2019/02/14/commandos-to-counselors-a-response-to-the-special-operations-forces-mental-health-crisis/

The Saudi Commission for Health Specialties. (2014). *Code of Ethics for Healthcare Practitioners*. Saudi Commission for Health Specialties.

The top 10 causes of death. (n.d.). Retrieved from https://www.who.int/news-room/fact-sheets/detail/the-top-10-causes-of-death

Thomas, K. W., & Velthouse, B. A. (1990). Cognitive elements of empowerment: An "interpretive" model of intrinsic task motivation. *Academy of Management Review, 15*(4), 666–681.

Thompson, L. A., Dawson, K., Ferdig, R., Black, E. W., Boyer, J., Coutts, J., & Paradise Black, N. (2008). The intersection of online social networking with medical professionalism. *Journal of General Internal Medicine, 23*(7), 954–961. doi:10.100711606-008-0538-8

Thorne, S. E. (2009). Is the Story Enough? *Qualitative Health Research, 19*(9), 1183–1185. doi:10.1177/1049732309343951 PMID:19690200

Thorne, S., Con, A., McGuinness, L., McPherson, G., & Harris, S. R. (2004). Health care communication issues in multiple sclerosis: An interpretive description. *Qualitative Health Research, 14*(1), 5–22. doi:10.1177/1049732303259618 PMID:14725173

Thurnheer, S. E., Gravestock, I., Pichierri, G., Steurer, J., & Burgstaller, J. M. (2018). Benefits of mobile apps in pain management: Systematic review. *JMIR mHealth and uHealth*, *6*(10), e11231. doi:10.2196/11231 PMID:30348633

Tiwana, A., & Keil, M. (2009). Control in internal and outsourced software projects. *Journal of Management Information Systems*, *26*(3), 9–44. doi:10.2753/MIS0742-1222260301

Tkachenko, N., Gupta, N., Chotvijit, S., Gilks, C., Jarvis, S., Crosby, H., ... Guo, W. (2017). Google Trends can improve surveillance of Type 2 diabetes. *Scientific Reports*, *7*(1), 1–10. doi:10.103841598-017-05091-9 PMID:28694479

Tomlinson, M., & Lund, C. (2012). Why does mental health not get the attention it deserves? An application of the Shiffman and Smith framework. *PLoS Medicine*, *9*(2). doi:10.1371/journal.pmed.1001178 PMID:22389632

Torous, J., Wisniewski, H., Liu, G., & Keshavan, M. (2018). Mental Health Mobile Phone App Usage, Concerns, and Benefits Among Psychiatric Outpatients: Comparative Survey Study. *JMIR Mental Health*, *5*(4), 1–11. doi:10.2196/11715 PMID:30446484

Torri, E., Mayora, O., Cobo, J., & Palao, D. (2015). Requirements identification for the development of a design involving adaptive ICTs for supporting bipolar disorder treatment in different healthcare contexts. Paper presented at the *Proceedings of the 9th International Conference on Pervasive Computing Technologies for Healthcare*, Istanbul, Turkey. 10.4108/icst.pervasivehealth.2015.259238

Trauth, E., Joshi, K. D., & Yarger, L. K. (2018). ISJ Editorial. *Information Systems Journal*, *28*(6), 989–994. doi:10.1111/isj.12201

Trocin, C., Arkhipova, D., Lee, G., Vaia, G., & Saccavini, C. (2018). The Effect of Network Centrality of Medical Specialists on Their Performance: Evidence from an Italian Health Information Exchange Platform. *International Conference on Information Systems Proceedings*, San Francisco, CA.

Trust, M. S. (2016a). MS forward view: A consensus for the future of MS services. Retrieved from https://www.mstrust.org.uk/sites/default/files/Future%20of%20MS%20Services%20WEB%20FINAL.pdf

Trust, M. S. (2016b) Is MS care fair? Retrieved from https://www.mstrust.org.uk/file/ms-care-media-reportpdf/download?token=R8dXTbMB

Trust, M. S. (2019). Prevalence and incidence of multiple sclerosis. Retrieved from https://www.mstrust.org.uk/a-z/prevalence-and-incidence-multiple-sclerosis

Tuli, A., Singh, P., Sood, M., Deb, K. S., Jain, S., Jain, A., & Verma, R. (2016). Harmony: close knitted mhealth assistance for patients, caregivers and doctors for managing SMIs. Paper presented at the *ACM International Joint Conference on Pervasive and Ubiquitous Computing: Adjunct*, Heidelberg, Germany. 10.1145/2968219.2968301

Tuominen, M., Rajala, A., & Möller, K. (2004). How does adaptability drive firm innovativeness? *Journal of Business Research*, *57*(5), 495–506. doi:10.1016/S0148-2963(02)00316-8

U. S. Department of Commerce. (2017). Health Information Technology Industry Snapshot. Retrieved from https://build.export.gov/build/groups/public/@eg_main/@byind/@healthtech/documents/webcontent/eg_main_114799.pdf

U.S. Census Bureau. (2019). *Census Bureau projects U.S. and world populations on New Year's Day*. Retrieved from https://www.census.gov/newsroom/press-releases/2019/new-years-population.html

U.S. Department of Health and Services. (2018). *Health, United States, 2017 with special feature on mortality*. Hyattsville, MD. Retrieved from https://www.cdc.gov/nchs/data/hus/hus17.pdf

U.S. Food and Drug Administration. (2017). Digital health innovation action plan. Retrieved from https://www.fda.gov/downloads/medicaldevices/digitalhealth/ucm568735.pdf

United Nations Development Programme. (2014). Good health and well-being. Available at https://www.undp.org/content/undp/en/home/sustainable-development-goals/goal-3-good-health-and-well-being.html

US Department of Health and Human Services. (2001, Sept. 5). Protecting the privacy of patients health information. Retrieved from https://aspe.hhs.gov/basic-report/protecting-privacy-patients-health-information

Vahdat, S., Hamzehgardeshi, L., Hessam, S., & Hamzehgardeshi, Z. (2014). Patient involvement in health care decision making: A review. *Iranian Red Crescent Medical Journal*, *16*(1). doi:10.5812/ircmj.12454 PMID:24719703

Välimäki, M., Hätönen, H., & Adams, C. E. (2012). Mobile. net: mobile telephone text messages to encourage adherence to medication and to follow up with people with psychosis: methods and protocol for a multicenter randomized controlled two-armed trial. *JMIR Research Protocols*, *1*(2), e8. doi:10.2196/resprot.2136 PMID:23611874

van den Broek, E., & Sergeeva, A. (2018). Empowering Patients Through Data: Promise versus Practice. Academy of Management Global Proceedings, 97.

van Dijk, L., Groenewegen, P. P., Rademakers, J. J., de Jong, J. D., & Brabers, A. E. M. (2017). What role does health literacy play in patients' involvement in medical decision-making? *PLoS One*, *12*(3). doi:10.1371/journal.pone.0173316 PMID:28257472

Van Uden-Kraan, C. F., Drossaert, C. H. C., Taal, E., Seydel, E. R., & van de Laar, M. A. F. J. (2009). Participation in online patient support groups endorses patients' empowerment. *Patient Education and Counseling*, *74*(1), 61–69. doi:10.1016/j.pec.2008.07.044 PMID:18778909

van Uden-Kraan, C. F., Drossaert, C. H., Taal, E., Shaw, B. R., Seydel, E. R., & van de Laar, M. A. (2008). Empowering Processes and Outcomes of Participation in Online Support Groups for Patients with Breast Cancer, Arthritis, Or Fibromyalgia. *Qualitative Health Research*, *18*(3), 405–417. doi:10.1177/1049732307313429 PMID:18235163

VanEpps, E. M., Volpp, K. G., & Halpern, S. D. (2016). A nudge toward participation: Improving clinical trial enrollment with behavioral economics. *Science Translational Medicine*, *8*(348), 348fs313. doi:10.1126citranslmed.aaf0946 PMID:27440726

Varshney, U. (2014). Mobile health: Four emerging themes of research. *Decision Support Systems*, *66*, 20–35. doi:10.1016/j.dss.2014.06.001

Ventola, C. L. (2014). Social media and health care professionals: Benefits, risks, and best practices. *P&T*, *39*(7), 491.

Viceconti, M., Hunter, P., & Hose, R. (2015). Big data, big knowledge: Big data for personalized healthcare. *IEEE Journal of Biomedical and Health Informatics*, *19*(4), 1209–1215. doi:10.1109/JBHI.2015.2406883 PMID:26218867

Visser, L. M., Bleijenbergh, I. L., Benschop, Y. W. M., Van Riel, A. C., & Bloem, B. R. (2016). Do online communities change power processes in healthcare? Using case studies to examine the use of online health communities by patients with Parkinson's disease. doi:10.1136/bmjopen-2016-012110

Viswanathan, V., Hollebeek, L. D., Malthouse, E. C., Maslowska, E., Jung Kim, S., & Xie, W. (2017). The dynamics of consumer engagement with mobile technologies. *Service Science*, *9*(1), 36–49. doi:10.1287erv.2016.0161

von Muhlen, M., & Ohno-Machado, L. (2012). Reviewing social media use by clinicians. *Journal of the American Medical Informatics Association*, *19*(5), 777–781. doi:10.1136/amiajnl-2012-000990

Vorhies, D. W., Harker, M., & Rao, C. (1999). The capabilities and performance advantages of market-driven firms. *European Journal of Marketing, 33*(11/12), 1171–1202. doi:10.1108/03090569910292339

Vreeland, A., Persons, K. R., Primo, H. R., Bishop, M., Garriott, K. M., Doyle, M. K., ... Bashall, C. (2016). Considerations for exchanging and sharing medical images for improved collaboration and patient care: HIMSS-SIIM collaborative white paper. *Journal of Digital Imaging, 29*(5), 547–558. doi:10.1007/s10278-016-9885-x PubMed

Wadhwa, V. (2014). Laws and ethics can't keep pace with technology. Retrieved from https://www.technologyreview.com/s/526401/laws-and-ethics-cant-keep-pace-with-technology/

Walker, R., Hickey, A., & Freedson, P. (2016). Advantages and Limitations of Wearable Activity Trackers: Considerations for Patients and Clinicians. *Clinical Journal of Oncology Nursing, 20*(6), 606–610. doi:10.1188/16.CJON.606-610 PMID:27857250

Wallace, L. S., Angier, H., Huguet, N., Gaudino, J. A., Krist, A., Dearing, M., . . . DeVoe, J. E. (2017). Patterns of electronic portal use among vulnerable patients in a nationwide practice-based research network: From the OCHIN Practice-based Research Network (PBRN). *HHS Author Manuscripts.* Retrieved from https://www.ncbi.nlm.nih.gov/pmc/articles/PMC5341130/

Wallace, L. S., Angier, H., Huguet, N., Gaudino, J. A., Krist, A., Dearing, M., ... DeVoe, J. E. (2016). Patterns of electronic portal use among vulnerable patients in a nationwide practice-based research network: From the OCHIN Practice-based Research Network (PBRN). *Journal of the American Board of Family Medicine: JABFM, 29*(5), 592–603. doi:10.3122/jabfm.2016.05.160046 PMID:27613792

Wallace, L. S., & Dhingra, L. K. (2014). A systematic review of smartphone applications for chronic pain available for download in the United States. *Journal of Opioid Management, 10*(1). doi:10.5055/jom.2014.0193 PMID:24604571

Waller, J., McCaffery, K., Forrest, S., Szarewski, A., Cadman, L., & Wardle, J. (2003). Awareness of human papillomavirus among women attending a well woman clinic. *Sexually Transmitted Infections, 79*(4), 320–322. doi:10.1136ti.79.4.320 PMID:12902585

Wallerstein, N. (2006). *What is the evidence on effectiveness of empowerment to improve health?* Copenhagen Denmark World Health Organization [WHO] Regional Office for Europe Health Evidence Network. Retrieved from https://www.popline.org/node/175634

Walls, J. G., Widmeyer, G. R., & El Sawy, O. A. (1992). Building an information system design theory for vigilant EIS. *Information Systems Research, 3*(1), 36–59. doi:10.1287/isre.3.1.36

Wallwiener, M., Wallwiener, C. W., Kansy, J. K., Seeger, H., & Rajab, T. K. (2009). Impact of electronic messaging on the patient-physician interaction. *Journal of Telemedicine and Telecare, 15*(5), 243–250. doi:10.1258/jtt.2009.090111

Walsh, B. (2014, March). Google flu trends failure shows drawbacks of big data. *Time.Com.* Retrieved from http://time.com/23782/google-flu-trends-big-data-problems/

Walsham, G. (2017). ICT4D research: Reflections on history and future agenda. *Information Technology for Development, 23*(1), 18–41. doi:10.1080/02681102.2016.1246406

Wang, R., Aung, M. S., Abdullah, S., Brian, R., Campbell, A. T., Choudhury, T., & Tseng, V. W. (2016). CrossCheck: toward passive sensing and detection of mental health changes in people with schizophrenia. Paper presented at the *ACM International Joint Conference on Pervasive and Ubiquitous Computing*, Heidelberg, Germany.

Ward, S. E., Goldberg, N., Miller-McCauley, V., Mueller, C., Nolan, A., Pawlik-Plank, D., ... Weissman, D. E. (1993). Patient-related barriers to management of cancer pain. *Pain, 52*(3), 319–324. doi:10.1016/0304-3959(93)90165-L PMID:7681557

Warkentin, M., Sharma, S., Gefen, D., Rose, G. M., & Pavlou, P. A. (2018). Social identity and trust in internet-based voting adoption. *Government Information Quarterly, 35*(2), 195–209. doi:10.1016/j.giq.2018.03.007

Warren, T., & Ebel, C. (2005). Counseling the patient who has genital herpes or genital human papillomavirus infection. *Infectious Disease Clinics, 19*(2), 459–476. PMID:15963883

Washington, P., Kumar, M., Tibrewal, A., & Sabharwal, A. (2015). ScaleMed: A methodology for iterative mHealth clinical trials. Paper presented at the *17th International Conference on E-health Networking, Application and Services*, Boston, MA. doi:10.1145/2971648.2971740

Waterman, L., Szatala, S., Motta, B. D., Son, C. H., & To, J. (2018). Mellow: A mobile application to help youth in crisis. Extended Abstracts presented at the *2018 CHI Conference on Human Factors in Computing Systems,* Quebec, Canada.

Waters, M. C. (2018). An undocumented immigrant's life of fear and activism. Retrieved from https://www.washingtonpost.com/outlook/an-undocumented-immigrants-life-of-fear-and-activism/2018/10/18/2ab5fb86-a572-11e8-97ce-cc9042272f07_story.html?utm_term=.5cc14827604e

Wavelet Health. (2019). Technology: A fundamentally different approach. Retrieved from https://wavelethealth.com/technology/#data

Webb, D. G., Horne, R., & Pinching, A. J. (2001). Treatment-related empowerment: Preliminary evaluation of a new measure in patients with advanced HIV disease. *International Journal of STD & AIDS, 12*(2), 103–107. doi:10.1258/0956462011916875 PMID:11236098

Weber, B., Reichert, M., & Rinderle-Ma, S. (2008). Change patterns and change support features–enhancing flexibility in process-aware information systems. *Data & Knowledge Engineering, 66*(3), 438–466. doi:10.1016/j.datak.2008.05.001

Webster, J., & Watson, R. (2002). Analyzing the Past to Prepare for the Future: Writing a Literature Review. *MIS Quarterly, 26*(2), 13-23.

Wee, S., & Choong, W. (2019). Gamification: Predicting the effectiveness of variety game design elements to intrinsically motivate users energy conservation behaviour. *Journal of Environmental Management, 233*, 97–106. doi:10.1016/j.jenvman.2018.11.127 PMID:30572268

Welkenhuysen, M., Evers-Kiebooms, G., & d'Ydewalle, G. (2001). The language of uncertainty in genetic risk communication: Framing and verbal versus numerical information. *Patient Education and Counseling, 43*(2), 179–187. doi:10.1016/S0738-3991(00)00161-0 PMID:11369151

Wentzer, H. S., & Bygholm, A. (2013). Narratives of empowerment and compliance: Studies of communication in online patient support groups. *International Journal of Medical Informatics, 82*(12), e386–e394. doi:10.1016/j.ijmedinf.2013.01.008 PMID:23523082

West, J. H., Belvedere, L. M., Andreasen, R., Frandsen, C., Hall, P. C., & Crookston, B. T. (2017). Controlling Your "App"etite: How Diet and Nutrition-Related Mobile Apps Lead to Behavior Change. *JMIR mHealth and uHealth, 5*(7), e95. doi:10.2196/mhealth.7410 PMID:28694241

White, P., & Selwyn, N. (2013). Moving on-line? An analysis of patterns of adult Internet use in the UK. *Information Communication and Society, 16*(1), 1–27. doi:10.1080/1369118X.2011.611816

Whittaker, R. (2012). Issues in mHealth: Findings From Key Informant Interviews. *Journal of Medical Internet Research, 14*(5), e129. doi:10.2196/jmir.1989 PMID:23032424

WHO Global Observatory for eHealth. (2011). *mHealth: New horizons for health through mobile technologies.* (No. 3). Retrieved from http://www.who.int/goe/publications/goe_mhealth_web.pdf

WHO. (2008). Commission on Social Determinants of Health - Final Report. Retrieved from https://www.who.int/social_determinants/thecommission/finalreport/en/

Wicklund, E. (2016). Factors Behind the Adoption of School-based Telehealth. Retrieved from https://mhealthintelligence.com/features/factors-behind-the-adoption-of-school-based-telehealth

Wiener, M., Mahring, M., Saunders, C., & Remus, U. (2016). Control configuration and control enactment in information systems projects: Review and expanded theoretical framework. *Management Information Systems Quarterly, 40*(3), 741–774. doi:10.25300/MISQ/2016/40.3.11

Wikipedia. (2019). Web 2.0. Retrieved from https://en.wikipedia.org/wiki/Web_2.0

Wiljer, D., Urowitz, S., Apatu, E., DeLenardo, C., Eysenbach, G., Harth, T., ... Leonard, K. (2008). Patient accessible electronic health records: Exploring recommendations for successful implementation strategies. *Journal of Medical Internet Research, 10*(4), e34. doi:10.2196/jmir.1061 PMID:18974036

Wilson, J. L., Ferguson, G. M., & Thorn, J. M. (2011). Genetic testing likelihood: The impact of abortion views and quality of life information on women's decisions. *Journal of Genetic Counseling, 20*(2), 143–156. doi:10.100710897-010-9335-8 PMID:21057975

Wilson, T. E., Kay, E. S., Turan, B., Johnson, M. O., Kempf, M. C., Turan, J. M., ... Goparaju, L. (2018). Healthcare empowerment and HIV viral control: Mediating roles of adherence and retention in care. *American Journal of Preventive Medicine, 54*(6), 756–764. doi:10.1016/j.amepre.2018.02.012 PMID:29656911

Winkelstein, P. (2013). Medicine 2.0: Ethical challenges of social media for the health profession. In C. George, D. Whitehouse, & P. Duquenoy (Eds.), *eHealth: Legal, Ethical and Governance Challenges* (pp. 227–243). Berlin, Germany: Springer Berlin Heidelberg; doi:10.1007/978-3-642-22474-4_10

Wolf, M., Kraft, S., Tschauner, K., Bauer, S., Becker, T., & Puschner, B. (2016). User activity in a mobile phone intervention to assist mindfulness exercises in people with depressive symptoms. *Mental Health & Prevention, 4*(2), 57–62. doi:10.1016/j.mhp.2016.02.003

Wong, D. F. K., Zhuang, X. Y., Pan, J. Y., & He, X. S. (2014). A critical review of mental health and mental health-related policies in China: More actions required. *International Journal of Social Welfare, 23*(2), 195–204. doi:10.1111/ijsw.12052

Woolf, S. H. (2008). The Power of Prevention and What It Requires. *Journal of the American Medical Association, 299*(20), 2437. doi:10.1001/jama.299.20.2437 PMID:18505953

World Health Organisation. (2014). Mental health: A state of well-being. Available at https://www.who.int/features/factfiles/mental_health/en/

World Health Organization. (2009). *WHO guidelines on hand hygiene in health care: A summary. First global patient safety challenge. Clean care is safer care.* Geneva, Switzerland: World Health Organization. Retrieved from http://www.who.int/gpsc/5may/tools/who_guidelines-handhygiene_summary.pdf

World Health Organization. (2016). Global diffusion of eHealth: making universal health coverage achievable: report of the third global survey on eHealth (No. 9789241511780). World Health Organization.

World Health Organization. (2016). Health Services Delivery Programme Division of Health Systems and Public Health. Integrated care models: An overview. Retrieved from http://www.euro.who.int/__data/assets/pdf_file/0005/322475/Integrated-care-models-overview.pdf

World Health Organization. (2016). *Human Papillomavirus (HPV) and Cervical Cancer Fact Sheet.* Retrieved from http://www.who.int/mediacentre/factsheets/fs380/en/

World Health Organization. (2016). *WHO | World Health Statistics 2016: Monitoring health for the SDGs.* Retrieved from http://www.who.int/gho/publications/world_health_statistics/2016/en/

World Health Organization. (2017). Cancer Fact Sheet. Retrieved from http://www.who.int/mediacentre/factsheets/fs297/en/

Wozney, L., Radomski, A. D., & Newton, A. S. (2018). The Gobbledygook in Online Parent-Focused Information about Child and Adolescent Mental Health. *Health Communication, 33*(6), 710–715. doi:10.1080/10410236.2017.1306475 PMID:28402141

Wu, J.-H., Wang, S.-C., & Lin, L.-M. (2007). Mobile computing acceptance factors in the healthcare industry: A structural equation model. *International Journal of Medical Informatics, 76*(1), 66–77. doi:10.1016/j.ijmedinf.2006.06.006 PMID:16901749

Wu, J., Hou, S., & Jin, M. (2017). Social Support and User Roles in a Chinese Online Health Community: A LDA Based Text Mining Study. In *International Conference on Smart Health* (pp. 169–176). Retrieved from 10.1007/978-3-319-67964-8_16

Wu, P.-Y., Cheng, C.-W., Kaddi, C. D., Venugopalan, J., Hoffman, R., & Wang, M. D. (2016). --Omic and electronic health record big data analytics for precision medicine. *IEEE Transactions on Biomedical Engineering, 64*(2), 263–273. PMID:27740470

Yakasai, A. B. M., & Jusoh, W. J. W. (2015). Testing the Theory of Planned Behavior in Determining Intention to use Digital Coupon among University Students. *Procedia Economics and Finance, 31*, 186–193. doi:10.1016/S2212-5671(15)01145-4

Yang, J., Weng, L., Chen, Z., Cai, H., Lin, X., Hu, Z., ... Liu, M. (2019). Development and testing of a mobile app for pain management among cancer patients discharged from hospital treatment: Randomized controlled trial. *JMIR mHealth and uHealth, 7*(5), e12542. doi:10.2196/12542 PMID:31144672

Yaraghi, N., Du, A. Y., Sharman, R., Gopal, R. D., & Ramesh, R. (2014). Health information exchange as a multisided platform: Adoption, usage, and practice involvement in service co-production. *Information Systems Research, 26*(1), 1–18. doi:10.1287/isre.2014.0547

Yen, C. C., Chang, L., Tai, B. C., Chan, H. C., Choolani, M., Lim, S., ... Xue, L. (2011). A study on Singaporean women's acceptance of using mobile phones to seek health information. *International Journal of Medical Informatics, 80*(12), e189–e202. doi:10.1016/j.ijmedinf.2011.08.007 PMID:21956003

Young, S. L. (2007). Older adults' user experiences with mobile phones: identification of user clusters and user requirements. (*Dissertation submitted to the Faculty of the Virginia Polytechnic Institute and State University in partial fulfillment of the requirements for the degree of Doctor of Philosophy in Industrial and Systems Engineering).*

Young, R., Burge, S., Kumar, K., Wilson, J., & Ortiz, D. (2018). A time-motion study of primary care physicians' work in the electronic health record era. *Family Medicine, 50*(2), 91–99. doi:10.22454/FamMed.2018.184803 PMID:29432623

Zarcadoolas, C., Vaughon, W. L., Czaja, S. J., Levy, J., & Rockoff, M. L. (2013). Consumers' perceptons of patient accessible electronic medical records. *Journal of Medical Internet Research, 15*(8), e168. doi:10.2196/jmir.2507 PMID:23978618

Zeng, B., Turkcan, A., Lin, J., & Lawley, M. (2010). Clinic scheduling models with overbooking for patients with heterogeneous no-show probabilities. *Annals of Operations Research, 178*(1), 121–144. doi:10.100710479-009-0569-5

Zhang, L., Wang, H., Li, Q., Zhao, M.-H., & Zhan, Q.-M. (2018). Big data and medical research in China. *BMJ (Clinical Research Ed.), 360*, j5910. doi:10.1136/bmj.j5910 PMID:29437562

Zhao, Y., Ni, Q., & Zhou, R. (2018). What factors influence the mobile health service adoption? A meta-analysis and the moderating role of age. *International Journal of Information Management, 43*, 342–350. doi:10.1016/j.ijinfomgt.2017.08.006

Zhao, Y., & Zhang, J. (2017). Consumer health information seeking in social media: A literature review. *Health Information and Libraries Journal, 34*(4), 268–283. doi:10.1111/hir.12192 PMID:29045011

Zheng, Y., & Walsham, G. (2008). Inequality of what? Social exclusion in the e-society as capability deprivation. *Information Technology & People, 21*(3), 222–243. doi:10.1108/09593840810896000

Zhou, B., Bentham, J., Cesare, M. D., Bixby, H., Danaei, G., Cowan, M. J., & Cisneros, J. Z. (2017). Worldwide trends in blood pressure from 1975 to 2015: A pooled analysis of 1479 population-based measurement studies with 19·1 million participants. *Lancet, 389*(10064), 37–55. doi:10.1016/S0140-6736(16)31919-5 PMID:27863813

Ziebland, S., Powell, J., Briggs, P., Jenkinson, C., Wyke, S., Sillence, E., . . . Farmer, A. (2016). Examining the role of patients' experiences as a resource for choice and decision-making in health care: A creative, interdisciplinary mixed-method study in digital health. Retrieved from http://www.ncbi.nlm.nih.gov/books/NBK401199/

Zimic, M., Coronel, J., Gilman, R. H., Luna, C. G., Curioso, W. H., & Moore, D. A. (2009). Can the power of mobile phones be used to improve tuberculosis diagnosis in developing countries? *Transactions of the Royal Society of Tropical Medicine and Hygiene, 103*(6), 638–640. doi:10.1016/j.trstmh.2008.10.015 PMID:19036392

Zimmerman, M. A. (1990). Taking Aim on Empowerment Research: On the Distinction between Individual and Psychological Conceptions. *American Journal of Community Psychology, 18*(1), 169–177. doi:10.1007/BF00922695

Zimmerman, M. A. (1995). Psychological empowerment: Issues and illustrations. *American Journal of Community Psychology, 23*(5), 581–599. doi:10.1007/BF02506983 PMID:8851341

Zucker, L. G. (1986). Production of trust: Institutional sources of economic structure, 1840-1920. In B. M. Staw, & L. L. Cummings (Eds.), *Research in Organizational Behavior* (Vol. 8, pp. 53–111). Greenwich, CT: JAI Press.

About the Contributors

Roger McHaney is Professor and University Distinguished Teaching Scholar at Kansas State University. He currently holds the Daniel D. Burke Chair for Exceptional Faculty and teaches courses in Management Information Systems and Data Analytics. McHaney earned his B.S. and M.B.A. degrees from Lake Superior State University, and his Ph.D. in Computer Information Systems and Quantitative Analysis from the Sam M. Walton College of Business at the University of Arkansas. Prior to obtaining a Ph.D., he worked in various software development and simulation analyst roles at a major industrial automation firm. He joined the Department of Management faculty at Kansas State in Fall, 1995. His main research interests include computer simulation and its intersection with industrial systems, healthcare, big data, and other areas. He has authored and coauthored numerous journal articles, scholarly books, and textbooks.

Iris Reychav Ph.D. is a professor of Industrial Engineering and Management and Head of the Collaborative Learning Technology Lab at Ariel University. Prof. Iris Reychav holds an B.Sc and M.Sc in Industrial Engineering and Management from Ben Gurion University of the Negev, and has 10 years' experience at Motorola in the field of information systems. She earned her Ph.D. from Bar-Ilan University's Graduate School of Business Administration, and did her post- doctoral work at Tel Aviv University in cooperation with INSEAD. Her current research interests include knowledge management technologies, mobile learning and technologies in health and education.

Joseph Azuri is a specialist in family medicine, and teaches in the Family Department of the Sackler Faculty of Medicine in Tel Aviv University. He also works for the Department of Community Medicine for Maccabi Healthcare Services. Dr. Azuri is an expert in patient management issues and community healthcare.

Mark McHaney received his M.D. from the University of Kansas after completing a B.S. in Biology from Kansas State University. He completed a Belleville Family Medicine Residency at Scott AFB. He served as Medical Services Director and Ambulance Services director at Kunsan AFB in the Republic of Korea. He currently is a Family Physician at Wright-Patterson AFB in Dayton, OH. He is BLS, ACLS, and ATLS Certified. Dr. McHaney has a keen interest in technology and its intersection with patient care.

Rami Moshonov has been a senior gynecologist since 1987. He currently practices at Assuta Ramat Hahaial Medical Center with a sub specialty in lower genital tract pathology. He holds several other positions including the head of the Cervical Pathology Clinic since 1989 and the head of ob-gyn department since 1991 at the Assuta Tel Aviv Hospital. He also has served as head of gynecology at Assuta medical centers since 1993. Dr. Moshonov has published prior medical studies in the area of patient empowerment.

* * *

Bella Azaria (MD) is the Chief Medical director of the Assuta Medical Centres network, and a family practice physician at Maccabi health services. Dr. Azaria obtained her medical degrees from the Technion Medical School in Israel and an M.Sc in Health management from Ben Gurion University. She was Commander of the Aviation Medical unit in the Israeli Air Force and served in the Homefront Command as Head of the Medical Preparedness & Response Branch for Hospitals and Community.

Erik Baltaxe is a medical doctor specialized in Internal Medicine and Pulmonary diseases. Currently, he is a Fellow at the Sleep lab and non-invasive ventilation unit at Hospital Clinic (Barcelona) and a pre-doctoral student at the University of Barcelona (SELFIE, NEXCARE, and CONNECARE H2020 projects). Previously, he held the position of senior physician in the Internal Medicine department and the Pulmonary Diseases Institute both at the Chaim Sheba Medical Center at Tel Hashomer (Israel). His main areas of interest are COPD and non-invasive ventilation in chronic complex patients.

Shirly Bar-Lev is a senior lecturer at the department of Industrial Engineering and Management in Ruppin Academic Center. She is also the head of Interdisciplinary Center for Health Informatics, in Ruppin Academic Center. Dr. Bar-Lev conducts research in Health Informatics and specializes in the behavioral consequences of Information Technologies.

Dizza Beimel has a Ph.D. She is a senior lecturer in the Faculty of Engineering. She is also the Head of the Department of Computer and Information Sciences in the Faculty of Engineering, Ruppin Academic Center.

Isaac Cano earned a BSc 2009 in Computer Science, an MSc 2010 in Computer Vision and Artificial Intelligence, and a PhD in 2014 in Digital Health by University of Barcelona – Faculty of Medicine.

Edward T. Chen is a professor of Management Information Systems of Operations and Information Systems Department in the Manning School of Business at University of Massachusetts Lowell. Dr. Chen has published numerous refereed research articles in scholarly journals and refereed chapters in reference books. Dr. Chen has served as vice-president, board director, track chair, and session chair of many IS/IT professional associations and conferences. Professor Chen has also served as journal editor and editorial reviewer for many academic journals. Dr. Chen has received the Irwin Distinguished Paper Award at the Southwestern Federation of Administrative Disciplines conference and the Best Paper Award at the International Conference on Accounting and Information Technology. His main research interests are in the areas of Telemedicine, Project Management, and Software Development.

Ofer Chen is the Deputy Director, Samson Assuta Ashdod University Hospital.

Zhijun Cheng (MD, PhD) is the associate chief physician of the department of anesthesiology at Xinhua Hospital Affiliated to Shanghai Jiao Tong University School of Medicine, Chongming Branch in Shanghai, China.

Wai Leng Chow obtained her bachelors in medicine and surgery (MBBS) from the National University of Singapore. She is a family physician by training and is an experienced researcher in health services research (HSR). Dr. Chow led the team of HSR Analysts in conducting research to support management decision making in Changi General Hospital between 2012-2018. Her research areas include design and implementation research of care models to improve the care of patients, programme evaluation, applied analytics, and health technology assessment for resource allocation. Dr. Chow now serves in the Ministry of Health and oversees the care models in the community.

Siang Li Chua had more than 20 years of experience in Operations Research and Information Technology. She had vast experiences in both private and public services industry such as defense, transport, healthcare, petrochemical, education and insurance. Her technical experiences include applying statistical methods, operations research and artificial intelligence techniques to improve and optimize operations by designing and developing IT solutions. She obtained her Master of Technology (Knowledge Engineering) and Bachelor Degree in Science from the National University of Singapore.

Enrica Croda is Assistant Professor of Economics at Ca' Foscari University of Venice, Italy. She holds a Laurea degree in Economics from Ca' Foscari, and a M.A. and a Ph.D. in Economics from UCLA - University of California at Los Angeles. Dr. Croda's research interests encompass applied microeconomics and econometrics, with an emphasis on health economics and economics of aging.

Jordi de Batlle holds a PhD in Health and Life Sciences (Epidemiology) by the Pompeu Fabra University, Barcelona (Spain). He is a senior research fellow in the Group of Translational Research in Respiratory Medicine (TRRM), at the Biomedical Research Institute of Lleida (IRBLleida). In 2016, he assumed the co-leadership of the WP2 of the EU project CONNECARE (H2020). He is participating in several projects of the TRRM (ISAACC, BIG DATA, and ESCA, among others). Since 2016, he is benefiting from a research contract from the Catalan government: Pla estratègic de recerca i innovació en salut 2016-2020 (PERIS-2016). During his career, he has been granted two European Commission FP7 Marie Curie – COFUND grants. The first was to conduct a two-year post-doc in the Nutritional Epidemiology section of the International Agency for Research on Cancer (IARC-WHO), Lyon, France (2012-2014), focusing on the relationship between vegetal nutrients and breast cancer, as well as the effects of meat products on colorectal cancer. The second was to conduct a 2-year post-doc in the TRRM group, focusing on the management of patients with suspected obstructive sleep apnea in primary care units compared to sleep units. During his Ph.D. in the Centre for Environmental Epidemiology (CREAL) 2004-2011, he studied the measure and effect of diet in chronic obstructive pulmonary disease. His current research interests are on chronic respiratory diseases, sleep apnea, nutritional epidemiology, community-based management of chronic diseases, and big data. In this sense, he has authored more than 50 peer-reviewed research articles in international journals, including first authorship of articles in the most prestigious journals on the fields he has worked (Am J Respir Crit Care Med, J Natl Cancer Inst, Eur J Nutr and Allergy).

Gang Ding (MD, PhD) is a professor and the vice president of Shanghai International Medical Center in China.

Eghosa Edogun works at East Bay Ophthalmology and is a recent graduate of the University of California, Santa Cruz, with a degree in Molecular Cellular and Developmental Biology.

Abba Amsami Elgujja obtained his LLB from University of Maiduguri (2004), bar practice certificate from the Nigeria Law School (2005), and LLM in healthcare laws from University of Salford, Manchester, in 2015. He is presently pursuing a PhD research at the University of Salford, Greater Manchester, in the area of data protection in the healthcare settings in the digital era. His research interest areas include medical negligence and the patient's right to confidentiality in the social media era. He is also a Solicitor and Advocate to the supreme court of Nigeria.

Christopher Gantz is a DBA Candidate at the LeBow College of Business.

David Gefen is a Professor, Provost Distinguished Research Professor, and the Academic Director of the Doctorate in Business Administration (DBA) Program at the LeBow College of Business.

Carolin George is an Assistant Division Head, Community Health.

Gina Green is an Associate Professor of Information Systems, and MSIS Graduate Program Director.

Juan Gu (MD, PhD) is a transnational research scientist at Roswell Park Cancer Institute in Buffalo, NY.

Carolina Gutierrez works at East Bay Ophthalmology and recently graduated from the University of California, Los Angeles, with a Bachelor of Arts in Spanish Language. She is working towards becoming a Pediatrician and working with Doctors without Borders.

Weiwei Hu, a Master of Oncology and Doctor of Hematology, is an experienced physician in the diagnosis and treatment of tumors and cancer pain, and has a deep understanding of tumor immunotherapy.

Hongwei Hua is a physician at Xinhua Hospital Affiliated to Shanghai Jiao Tong University School of Medicine, Chongming Branch in Shanghai, China.

Qian Huang is a physician at Xinhua Hospital Affiliated to Shanghai Jiao Tong University School of Medicine, Chongming Branch in Shanghai, China.

Gloria Ejehiohen Iyawa holds a PhD in Information Systems. She is a Senior Lecturer in the Department of Informatics at the Namibia University of Science and Technology. She serves on four Editorial Committees and acts as reviewer for both National and International journals. Her work is well published in peer-reviewed forums. Her research interests include: Digital Health, Big Data, Software Engineering, and E-Government.

Feng Jiang has an MD and PhD and is an associate professor at Xinhua Hospital Affiliated to Shanghai Jiao Tong University School of Medicine, Chongming Branch in Shanghai, China.

Jeremy Kagan, MSc, is an experienced hi-tech entrepreneur. Jeremy started his career as a Member of Technical Staff at Bell Communications Research in the USA. Jeremy created an award-winning, real-time secure clearing technology for mobile payments and web commerce and brought it to initial soft launch in 63 countries. Since 2016, Jeremy has been developing the Diagnostic Modality Interface Portal for CardioLync, with which they aspire to establish the leading social network for medicine.

Rachelle Kaye is the International Projects Coordinator for Assuta Medical Centers, as well as a member of the core team for implementing digitally-enabled integrated care in Assuta Ashdod Hospital. She is the Assuta manager of CONNECARE, an H2020 project on digitally-enabled integrated care, in which Assuta is a consortium member. Prior to Assuta, she was a senior manager in Maccabi Healthcare Services, Israel's second largest HMO, covering over 2 million people, including holding the positions of Deputy Director of the Medical Department and Director of Strategic Planning. Dr. Kaye established and directed the Maccabi Institute for Health Services Research until 2013. Dr. Kaye is a member of the Board of Directors of EHTEL (the European Health Telematics Association) and acts as a consultant to a number of Israeli and European Organizations, particularly in the area of integrated care and eHealth.

Helen King is a Technical Writer based in York, UK. She gained an M.A. in Technical Communication and E-learning from the University of Limerick in 2018. She has 20 years' experience of vocational education development; writing curriculum and assessment materials for industry and college based qualifications and apprenticeship programmes. She is particularly interested in usability of technology and patient information in healthcare. She is a patient/public representative for the National Institute of Healthcare's Be Part of Research project and information reviewer for the MS Trust. Helen is a Member of the Institute of Scientific and Technical Communicators.

Hope Koch received her Ph.D. in Information and Operations Management from Texas A&M University in 2003. Previously, she worked as a Certified Public Accountant for Wal-Mart Stores, Inc. In 2003, she began her academic career at Baylor University, working as a faculty member in its School of Business Information Systems Program. Today, Dr. Koch holds the Godfrey Sullivan Chair in Information Systems at Baylor University. She has won academic awards from Baylor University, ConocoPhillips, The Southwestern Business Dean's Association, the European Journal of Information Systems, and the Communication of the Association for Information Systems. She is currently part of a team building, implementing, and researching information and communication technologies for development (i.e., ICT4D).

Maarten M. H. Lahr graduated from University of Groningen in 2009 as human movement scientist and behavioral and cognitive neuroscientist. He completed a PhD programme at University Medical Center Groningen, department of Neurology, in 2013. Within his PhD, he performed multi- and interdisciplinary research in the field of organisational models for acute stroke care, together with the faculty of Economics and Business of the University of Groningen and the department of Epidemiology and Medical Technology Assessment of the University of Groningen. In 2013, he was appointed postdoc researcher with Healthy Ageing Team UMCG on an European project aimed at setting up and implementing eHealth and integrated care models for chronic diseases. In this period, he combined his postdoc position with a position as Managing Director of SPRINT center for research excellence, IMDI programme, ZonMw. Starting July 2016, he works as a postdoctoral researcher at the department of Epidemiology, Groningen. His research focuses on modelling and (early) evaluation of innovations and new treatments in healthcare. Lahr (co)supervised many (international) master students, co-authored over 20 papers, and is a commission member of the Dutch Heart Foundation. Recently, he has been awarded two European grants in the field of eHealth and integrated care for chronic diseases.

Danny Lee received his BA in Public Health and BS in Microbial Biology from the University of California, Berkeley, in 2018. He is interested in a wide range of healthcare and public health causes. He is a medical assistant and intends to attend medical school.

Diane Lee is a DBA Candidate at the LeBow College of Business.

Scott Lee, MD, MPH, FACS, is on the Faculty of the UC Berkeley School of Public Health.

Izabella Lejbkowicz is a Clinical Researcher experienced in Digital Health and in the management of clinical trials. She was born in Rio de Janeiro, Brazil, and moved to Israel for her academic studies. She received her BSc. In Microbiology from Bar-Ilan University and her MSc. Degree in Human Genetics from Tel Aviv University. Her research focused on the prenatal diagnosis of Tay-Sachs disease. Dr. Lejbkowicz and her family lived for three years in Montreal, Canada, where she worked as a Research Assistant at the McGill Cancer Center, McGill University, while her husband did his post PhD at the Biochemistry Department, McGill University. Back in Israel, Dr. Izabella Lejbkowicz did her PhD studies in Computers Applications in Medicine at the Technion- Israel Institute of Technology. Her research involved the implementation and evaluation of Expert-systems for radiologic diagnosis, and led to the development of "Bone Browser", an Expert-system to assist in the radiologic diagnosis of bone diseases. Afterwards, Dr. Izabella Lejbkowicz received the Technion's Lady Davis Fellowship for post-doctoral research on web-based applications in medical education. For the past 15 years, Dr. Lejbkowicz has been acting as a Senior Research Assistant at the Technion-Israel Institute of Technology and at Tel Aviv University, and has participated in studies in the fields of Digital Health, Personalized Healthcare, and Multiple Sclerosis. She has also coordinated numerous clinical trials. She has presented her work in congresses and published several papers, among them one article analyzing the use of Electronic Health Records (EHR) in Israeli hospitals, and another bringing an insight on personalized medicine beyond personalized drug treatment. She lives with her husband in Haifa, Israel.

Jing Li is a physician at Xinhua Hospital Affiliated to Shanghai Jiao Tong University School of Medicine, Chongming Branch in Shanghai, China.

Zhijun Liao is a physician at Xinhua Hospital Affiliated to Shanghai Jiao Tong University School of Medicine, Chongming Branch in Shanghai, China.

Julie Langan Martin is a Senior Clinical Lecturer in Psychiatry and Director of the Global Mental Health MSc at the University of Glasgow. Dr Langan Martin's primary interests are in Global Mental Health and the interface between major mental illness (schizophrenia and bipolar disorder) and physical health comorbidity. She is also interested in perinatal mental illness.

Wanano Masikara holds a Bachelor of Science degree in Computer Science. He is the owner and lead software developer of a private software development company called Nanosoft Designs. His research interests include mobile applications, mobile games, and artificial intelligence.

Taiki Nishihara is a recent graduate from the University of California Berkeley, where he studied Molecular Cell Biology with an emphasis in Medical Biology and Physiology. He currently works at East Bay Ophthalmology as a clinical fellow and research coordinator. His current research focuses on the development of a novel smartphone application to increase medication adherence in glaucoma patients.

Caroline Park received her BS in Global Disease Biology from the University of California, Davis. She currently works as a medical assistant at an ophthalmology clinic and is interested in pediatric and emergency medicine.

Gia Park studied Molecular and Cell Biology with a focus on Physiology at University of California, Berkeley. She works at an ophthalmology office in the Bay Area, and is a teaching assistant for a public health course at University of California, Berkeley, titled, "A Global Perspective on Vision." In her free time, Gia enjoys spending time with friends and family, hiking, reading, and serving at her church.

Yagana Parwak graduated from the University of California, Berkeley, where she majored in Public Health and minored in Global Poverty and Practice. She completed her Masters of Science in Global Health at the University of California, San Fransisco.

Josep Roca is Professor of Medicine at the University of Barcelona, senior consultant at Hospital Clínic de Barcelona, and senior researcher at IDIBAPS. He authored more than 300 original articles in peer-reviewed journals and several book chapters, review articles, and books. His two main fields of interest are Chronic diseases: integrated care, systems medicine, predictive medicine, information and communication technologies (ICT).

Reut Ron is a researcher in the Assuta Health Services Research Institute and a research assistant in CONNECARE, an H2020 project to develop and implement a digitally-supported integrated care model. She has experience in promoting, designing, and conducting research. Prior to her position in Assuta, Reut was a research coordinator in the Department of Child and Women's Health at the Gertner Institute for Epidemiology and Health policy research. Reut holds an MSc. in Epidemiology from Tel Aviv University, and is currently doing her doctorate in Health Care Systems at Ben Gurion University.

Stephen Sevalie is at the University of Sierra. His primary interest is in Health Systems and Equity in Mental Health Services and Research.

Darina M. Slattery is Head of Technical Communication and Instructional Design at the University of Limerick, where she has also directed graduate programs. Darina is Vice President of the IEEE Professional Communication Society, and holds a PhD in Computer Science, an MSc in Software Localisation, and a Bachelor of Business Studies with French. She teaches courses on e-learning, instructional design, and technical communication, and has published her research in international refereed journals and conference proceedings. Her current research projects are concerned with learning analytics, online learning/e-learning, virtual teams, content analysis, and flipped classrooms. In addition to teaching at undergraduate and postgraduate level (online and on-campus), Darina facilitates professional development workshops for faculty who wish to move modules and programmes online. She also provides technology-enhanced learning (TEL) consultancy to further education and higher education institutions. Further information is at http://staff.ul.ie/slatteryd.

Yunheng Sun is a physician at Xinhua Hospital Affiliated to Shanghai Jiao Tong University School of Medicine, Chongming Branch in Shanghai, China.

Cristina Trocin is a PhD student in Management at Ca' Foscari University of Venice. She holds a Master's Degree in International Management. She participated in international exchange programs in Management Center of Innsbruck (MCI), Plekhanov Russian University of Economics and American University - Kogod Business School. Her research interests are Digital Platforms, Mobile Health Technology, Organizational Change, and Grounded Theory.

Y. Ken Wang is an associate professor of information systems and director of the computer information systems and technology program at the University of Pittsburgh, Bradford Campus.

Shannon Yee works at East bay Ophthalmology and is a recent graduate of the University of California, Davis, with a degree in Biochemistry and Molecular Biology.

Lin Zhu is a postdoc for industrial management in Ariel University. He graduated from the Southwest Petroleum University with a doctoral degree in project management in 2016. His research interests focus on the knowledge flow network in the energy industry and the knowledge discovery based on data mining.

Index

G

H

I

K

L

M

N

O

P

R

S

T

U

V

W

Ensure Quality Research is Introduced to the Academic Community

Become an IGI Global Reviewer for Authored Book Projects

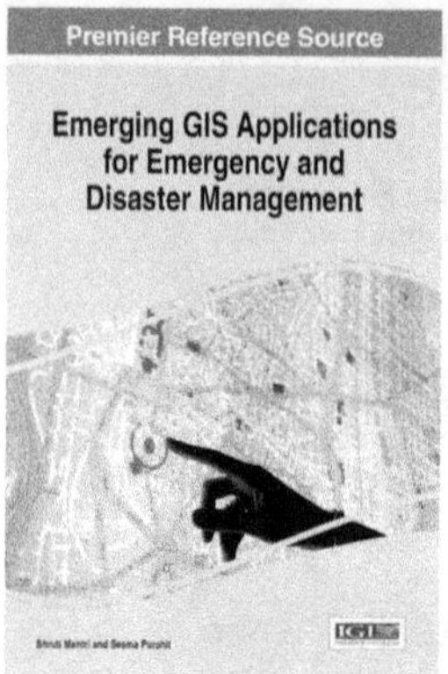

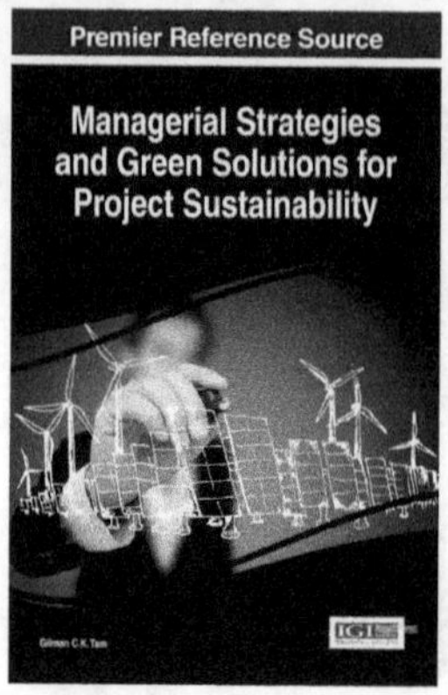

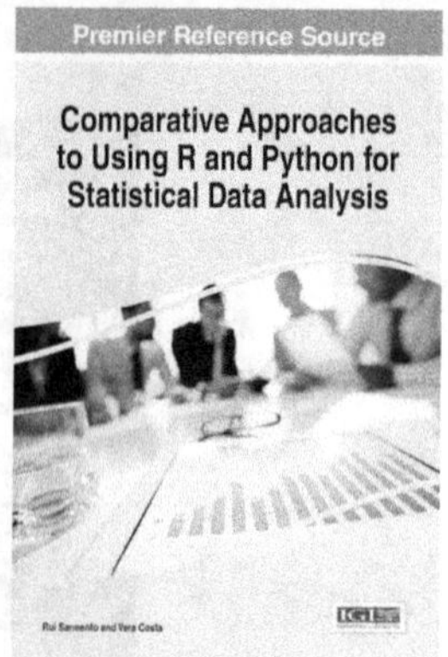

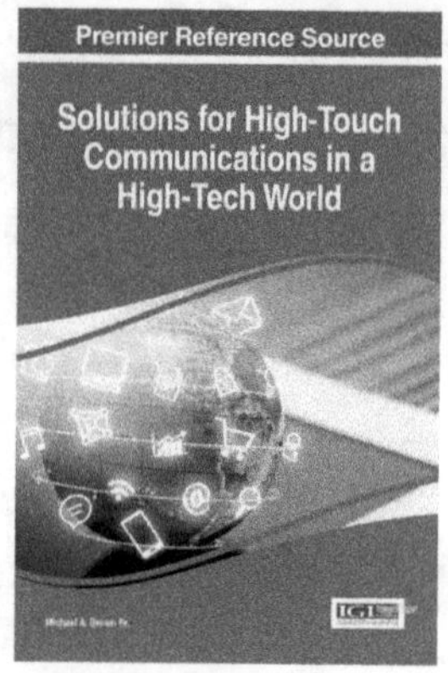

The overall success of an authored book project is dependent on quality and timely reviews.

In this competitive age of scholarly publishing, constructive and timely feedback significantly expedites the turnaround time of manuscripts from submission to acceptance, allowing the publication and discovery of forward-thinking research at a much more expeditious rate. Several IGI Global authored book projects are currently seeking highly-qualified experts in the field to fill vacancies on their respective editorial review boards:

Applications and Inquiries may be sent to:
development@igi-global.com

Applicants must have a doctorate (or an equivalent degree) as well as publishing and reviewing experience. Reviewers are asked to complete the open-ended evaluation questions with as much detail as possible in a timely, collegial, and constructive manner. All reviewers' tenures run for one-year terms on the editorial review boards and are expected to complete at least three reviews per term. Upon successful completion of this term, reviewers can be considered for an additional term.

If you have a colleague that may be interested in this opportunity, we encourage you to share this information with them.

www.ingramcontent.com/pod-product-compliance
Lightning Source LLC
LaVergne TN
LVHW062107300926
849161LV00010B/2390

* 9 7 8 1 7 9 9 8 0 0 4 7 7 *